AF779001

JACC's
Imaging Cases in
Cardiovascular Intervention

JACC's Imaging Cases in Cardiovascular Intervention

Spencer B King III, MD, MACC
Editor in Chief JACC: Cardiovascular Interventions, Emeritus
Professor of Medicine, Emeritus
Emory University School of Medicine
Atlanta, Georgia, USA

Michael McDaniel, MD, FACC, FSCAI
Associate Professor of Medicine
Department of Medicine, Division of Cardiology
Emory University
Atlanta, Georgia, USA

ELSEVIER

Elsevier
1600 John F. Kennedy Blvd.
Ste 1800
Philadelphia, PA 19103-2899

JACC'S IMAGING CASES IN CARDIOVASCULAR INTERVENTION ISBN: 978-0-323-673716

Copyright © 2021 by Elsevier, Inc. All rights reserved.

No part of this publication may be reproduced or transmitted in any form or by any means, electronic or mechanical, including photocopying, recording, or any information storage and retrieval system, without permission in writing from the publisher. Details on how to seek permission, further information about the Publisher's permissions policies and our arrangements with organizations such as the Copyright Clearance Center and the Copyright Licensing Agency, can be found at our website: www.elsevier.com/permissions.

This book and the individual contributions contained in it are protected under copyright by the Publisher (other than as may be noted herein).

Notice

Practitioners and researchers must always rely on their own experience and knowledge in evaluating and using any information, methods, compounds, or experiments described herein. Because of rapid advances in the medical sciences, in particular, independent verification of diagnoses and drug dosages should be made. To the fullest extent of the law, no responsibility is assumed by Elsevier, authors, editors, or contributors for any injury and/or damage to persons or property as a matter of products liability, negligence or otherwise, or from any use or operation of any methods, products, instructions, or ideas contained in the material herein.

Library of Congress Control Number: 2019949248

Content Strategist: Robin Carter
Content Development Specialist: Caroline Dorey-Stein/Kevin Travers
Publishing Services Manager: Deepthi Unni
Project Manager: Beula Christopher
Design Direction: Margaret Reid

Printed in Canada

Last digit is the print number: 9 8 7 6 5 4 3 2 1

ELSEVIER Book Aid International Working together to grow libraries in developing countries
www.elsevier.com • www.bookaid.org

Foreword

Courage that grows from constitution often forsakes a man when he has occasion for it; courage which arises from a sense of duty acts in a uniform manner.

Joseph Addison

On October 27, 1985, the cardiovascular community took a collective gasp as it learned that the founder of coronary angioplasty, Dr. Andreas Grüentzig, and his wife, Margaret Thornton, were tragically killed in a plane crash in Monroe County, Georgia. In October of 1980, Dr. J. Willis Hurst, Dr. Spencer King, Dr. John Douglas, and others recruited Dr. Grüentzig to Emory University School of Medicine in hopes of expanding angioplasty techniques, assuring quality, and educating potential practitioners of the science. Many feared that the burgeoning and exciting field of coronary angioplasty would also be lost with the tragic demise of its most knowledgeable and charismatic proponent. It had only been a short time since Dr. Grüentzig performed the very first successful coronary angioplasty, September 16, 1977, in Zurich, Switzerland. With this bold step, Dr. Grüentzig inspired a new generation of clinicians, forever creating an innovative, nonsurgical approach for the treatment of the world's number-one killer. However, with his untimely death, many feared that the future of coronary angioplasty would possibly die with him. What was once a field of limitless possibility now seemed fraught with obstacles and uncertainty. At the time, one wondered if this young science would have much of a future, having lost its most vocal and knowledgeable advocate.

Dr. Spencer King accepted the tremendous challenge and not only maintained the trajectory of growth and development of coronary angioplasty at Emory, but also enhanced its applicability, safety, and the pathophysiologic understanding of the development and consequences of coronary artery disease. He added significantly to the scientific literature with critical practice-altering research that advanced the science of coronary artery disease treatment and ensured patient safety. Dr. King was instrumental in continuing the growth of coronary intervention and the maturation of the once-promising procedure into a well-researched, scientifically sound, and reproducible technique. He was deliberate in his approach to establishing the field of interventional cardiology. His research provided the scientific basis for the development and success of the technique. He continued the novel teaching approach exampled by Dr. Grüentzig, inviting cardiologists worldwide to come to Emory University School of Medicine to witness the procedure televised live and to learn firsthand about the technique and its benefits, potential complications, and management. This innovative teaching application is now replicated in many disciplines. He championed the establishment of a core curriculum to better teach cardiology fellows, residents, students, and practicing cardiovascular specialists about the knowledge base, technical skills, and appropriate selection of patients with coronary artery disease for the procedure. His adherence to these standards and advocacy aided in the establishment of the American Board of Internal Medicine Interventional Cardiovascular Board of which he was the first chair. Again, ensuring that practitioners of the procedure could obtain the best possible outcomes, Dr. King, along with others, promoted the growth and development of the subspecialty now known as interventional cardiology. There were many who contributed significantly to the development of this field of science. There are too many to mention in this brief Foreword, but few played a more seminal role in interventional cardiology than Dr. King. The manifestation of his contributions is best illustrated by his 10-year tenure—from 2007 to 2017—as the first Editor-in-Chief of the *Journal of the American College of Cardiology: Cardiovascular Interventions*. What follows is a sample of the most enduring images of that era as edited by Dr. Spencer B. King and Dr. Michael McDaniel, associate editor of the journal. This issue represents a profound tribute to a pioneering leader in cardiovascular medicine.

Andreas Grüentzig will forever be remembered as the father of coronary angioplasty, but it was Spencer King who nurtured his invention and brought it to full maturity and created the new subspecialty of interventional cardiology. The pictorial journey that follows represents one of the most storied and productive periods in the history of cardiovascular medicine.

Paul L. Douglass, MD, MACC
Metropolitan Atlanta Cardiology Consultants
Emory University Hospital
Atlanta, Georgia

References

1. Gruentzig AR, Turina M, Schneider J. Experimental percutaneous dilatation of coronary artery stenosis [abstract]. *Circulation.* 1976;(54)(suppl):81.
2. King SB III. The development of interventional cardiology. *J Am Coll Cardiol.* 1998;31(4 suppl B):64B-88B.
3. Hurst JW, King SB III, Greene L. In memory of Andreas Roland Gruentzig and Margaret Anne Thornton Gruentzig. *Am J Cardiol.* 1986; 57;333-336.
4. King SB III, Schlumpf M. Ten-year completed follow-up of percutaneous transluminal coronary angioplasty: the early Zurich experience. *J Am Coll Cardiol.* 1993;22:353-360.

Acknowledgments

We would like to thank the editorial team from Elsevier for their commitment to this project and to Jill Franklin who make our work much more productive and enjoyable.

Most importantly, we thank not only the authors of the more than 250 imaging cases that we selected but also the authors of the 600 cases that were published in the journal and those of the greater than 2000 that were submitted. Almost all of these deserved to be published and they emphasize the value of learning from every patient.

Spencer B. King III
Michael McDaniel

Contents

Chapter 5 Vascular, Congenital, and Other Anatomy and Pathophysiology, 274

Chapter 6 Vascular, Congenital, and Other Interventional Complications, 293

Chapter 7 Vascular, Congenital, and Other Interventional Techniques, 316

VIDEO CONTENTS

Chapter 1
Coronary Anatomy and Pathophysiology

Coronary Anomalies

A Rare Case of Anomalous Original Left Circumflex Artery Stenosis After Artificial Mitral Valve Replacement

Qing Dai, MD, Jie Song, MD, Jian He, MD, Biao Xu, MD

A 72-year-old woman was admitted because of progressive 9-year chest tightness. Nine years ago, she underwent mitral valve replacement using a Hancock II porcine mitral valve bioprosthesis (size 27) (Medtronic, Minneapolis, Minnesota) for posterior mitral valve prolapse. Preoperative coronary angiogram showed anomalous origin of left circumflex artery (LCx) without stenosis (Fig. 1.1A, Online Video 1.1). Postoperative echocardiography showed a left ventricular ejection fraction of 51%.

However, recent echocardiography showed a decreased left ventricular ejection fraction of 36% and segmentally weakened motion of the inferior and lateral wall. Single-photon emission computed tomography showed myocardial ischemia of the inferior and lateral wall. Diagnostic coronary angiogram identified a severe proximal LCx stenosis with distal slow flow (Fig. 1.1B, Online Video 1.2). Both the left anterior descending and right coronary arteries appeared normal. Then percutaneous coronary intervention was performed with a 6F catheter Amplatz L 1.0 guide catheter. After predilation of stenosis with a 2.5-15-mm balloon, intravascular ultrasound catheter detected a marked reduction of vessel lumen without significant atherosclerotic plaques (Fig. 1.2A–B, Online Video 1.3). We then delivered a 3.5–36-mm drug-eluting stent to the proximal LCx. The final angiogram (Fig. 1.1C, Online Video 1.4) and intravascular ultrasound (Fig. 1.2C, Online Video 1.5) showed a good result. Six days later, computed tomography coronary angiography showed that the LCx ectopically originated from the right sinus of Valsalva, coursed posteriorly to the aorta, then traveled tightly around the mitral annulus (Fig. 1.3). The patient has been well after discharge until now.

This is a rare case of anomalous original LCx stenosis after mitral valve replacement. We speculate that compression of the mitral valve bioprosthesis suture ring against the surrounding tissues of the mitral annulus might cause the LCx stenosis. The long-term outcome of artificial mitral valve replacement in such patients should be followed up.

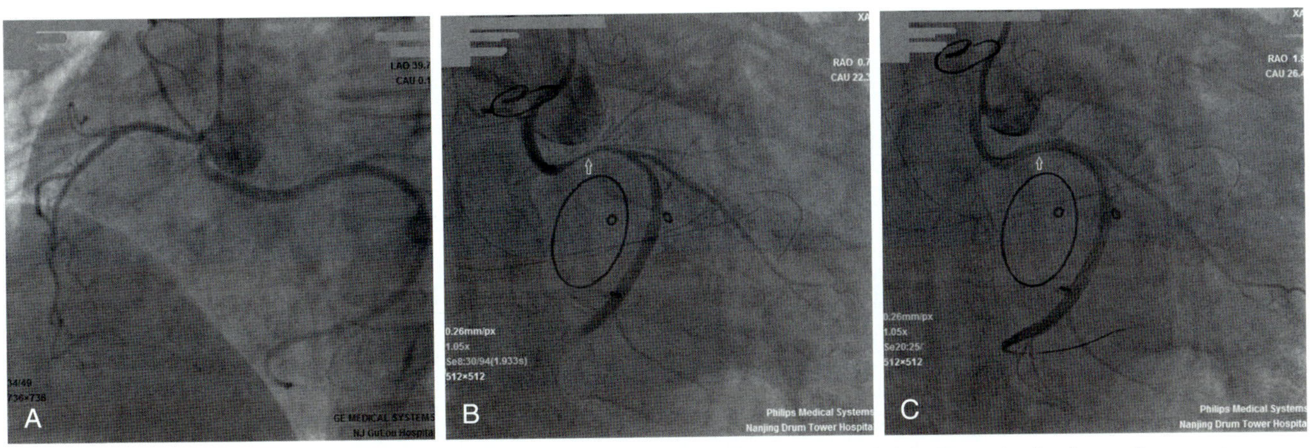

FIG. 1.1 Coronary angiograms showing anomalous origin of the left circumflex artery (LCx) before mitral valve replacement surgery, before and after percutaneous coronary intervention to the LCx stenosis. (A) Before mitral valve replacement surgery, coronary angiogram (left anterior oblique) shows an anomalous origin of the dominant LCx from the right sinus of Valsalva. There is no stenosis in the proximal LCx (Online Video 1.1). (B) Recent angiogram (posteroanterior caudal) shows a severe proximal LCx stenosis (*arrow*) (Online Video 1.2). (C) A similar angiographic view after percutaneous coronary stenting to the LCx shows a good result (*arrow*) (Online Video 1.4).

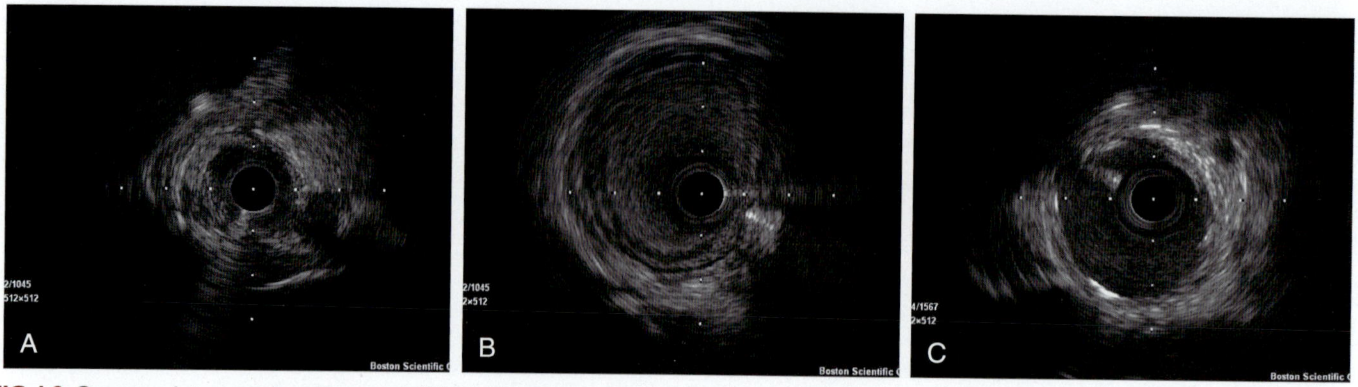

FIG. 1.2 Coronary intravascular ultrasound (IVUS) before and after percutaneous coronary intervention to the LCx stenosis. (A) IVUS reveals a marked reduction of the vessel lumen in the proximal left circumflex artery (LCx) lesion. There is no significant atherosclerotic plaque (Online Video 1.3). (B) IVUS shows a normal reference segment of the LCx. (C) IVUS after percutaneous coronary stenting to the LCx shows a good result (Online Video 1.5).

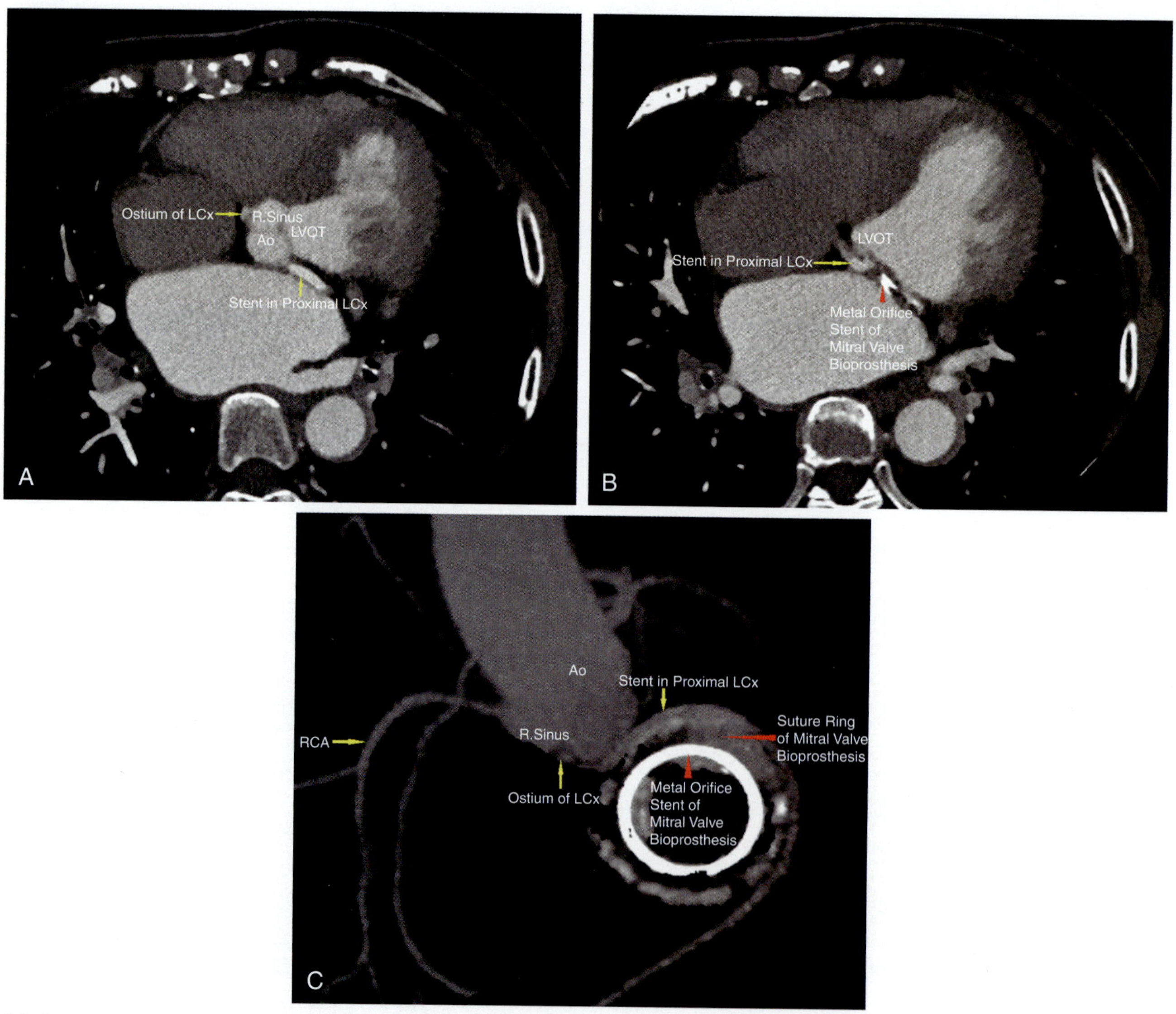

FIG. 1.3 Computed tomography (CT) coronary angiography post-percutaneous coronary intervention showing the course of the anomalous left circumflex artery (*LCx*). (A) CT coronary angiographic image shows the anomalous origin of LCx from the right sinus of Valsalva and the patent stent in proximal LCx. (B) Another CT angiographic image shows proximal LCx coursing posteriorly to aorta, then traveling between LVOT and mitral annulus. (C) CT angiography (three-dimensional reconstruction view) shows the LCx coursing tightly around the suture ring of mitral valve bioprosthesis. *Ao,* aorta; *LVOT,* left ventricular outflow tract; *RCA,* right coronary artery; *R. Sinus,* right sinus of Valsalva.

Anomalous Origin of the Common Left Coronary Artery From the Right Coronary Sinus: An Unusual Anatomic Variation

Pankaj Jariwala, MD, DNB, DNB, MNAMS, Sunitha Lingareddy, MD, Sarat Koduganti, MD, DM

A 56-year-old male patient who was hypertensive and without diabetes had chest discomfort on exertion for the past 3 months. The electrocardiogram result was normal, and two-dimensional echocardiography revealed normal left ventricular function and no left ventricular regional wall motion abnormalities. Hence, he underwent a stress test, results of which were positive for inducible ischemia at low workload.

Coronary angiography showed a small rudimentary left coronary artery. To our surprise, while searching for the left coronary artery its origin was found to be from the right coronary sinus. It had a main stem artery giving separate origins to the left anterior descending, diagonal, and obtuse marginal (first to fifth) coronary arteries. There was an eccentric 80% stenosis of the main stem of the left coronary artery before the origin of the first obtuse marginal artery. The right coronary artery had a normal course, and the posterior descending artery showed 99% stenosis of the proximal segment (Fig. 1.4A–D).

Before planning the patient's revascularization strategy, we performed computed tomography coronary angiography for better delineation of the anatomy of the coronary arteries. Computed tomography coronary angiography determined the coursing of the anomalous left coronary artery and showed no interarterial or intramyocardial course of the coronary arteries (Fig. 1.5A–D).

Percutaneous transluminal coronary angioplasty was performed using two drug-eluting stents to the main stem left coronary artery and posterior descending artery stenoses.

The origin of the left main coronary artery in the right coronary sinus has been described in 0.02% of autopsy series[1] and from 0.05% to 0.19% in angiographic series.[2] A main stem of the left coronary artery arising from the right sinus of Valsalva has four anatomic courses[3]:

1. Anterior course: turns anterior in front of right ventricular outflow tract, as in our case.
2. Interarterial course: between the great vessels, aorta, and pulmonary artery.
3. Septal course: intramyocardial septal continuation.
4. Posterior course: turns posterior behind the aorta.

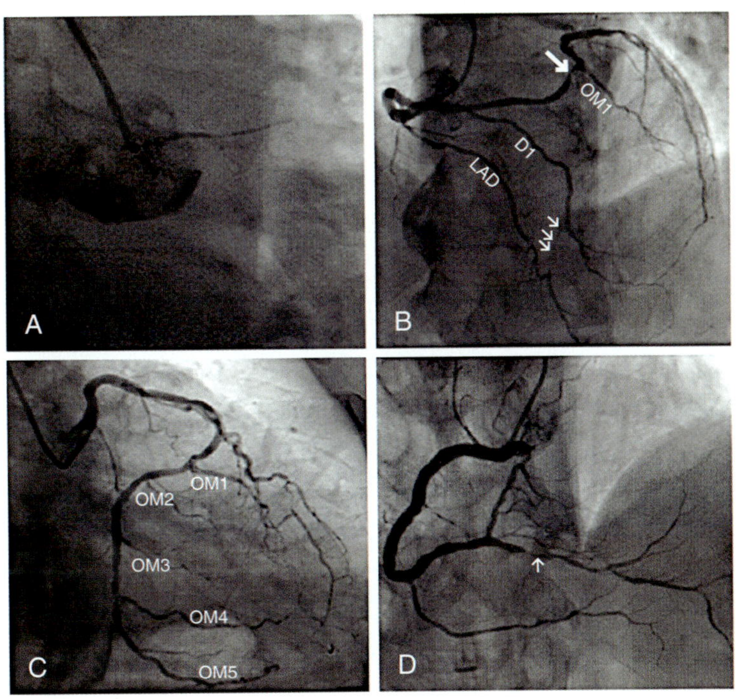

FIG. 1.4 Stepwise figures of transradial coronary angiography. (A) Injection of contrast into the left coronary sinus revealed a small, rudimentary left coronary artery. (B) Origin of the left coronary artery as a main stem from the right coronary sinus giving rise to the left anterior descending coronary artery (*LAD*), diagonal (*D1*) in a left anterior oblique cranial view. There was collateral between the LAD and the diagonal artery (*multiple arrows*). The left coronary main stem had 80% eccentric stenosis before the origin of the first obtuse marginal (*OM1*) (*thick arrow*). (C) Right anterior oblique caudal view showing origins of the first to the fifth obtuse marginal arteries. (D) The right coronary artery had a normal course, and the posterior descending artery had 99% stenosis (*thin arrow*) of its proximal segment. *OM*, obtuse marginal.

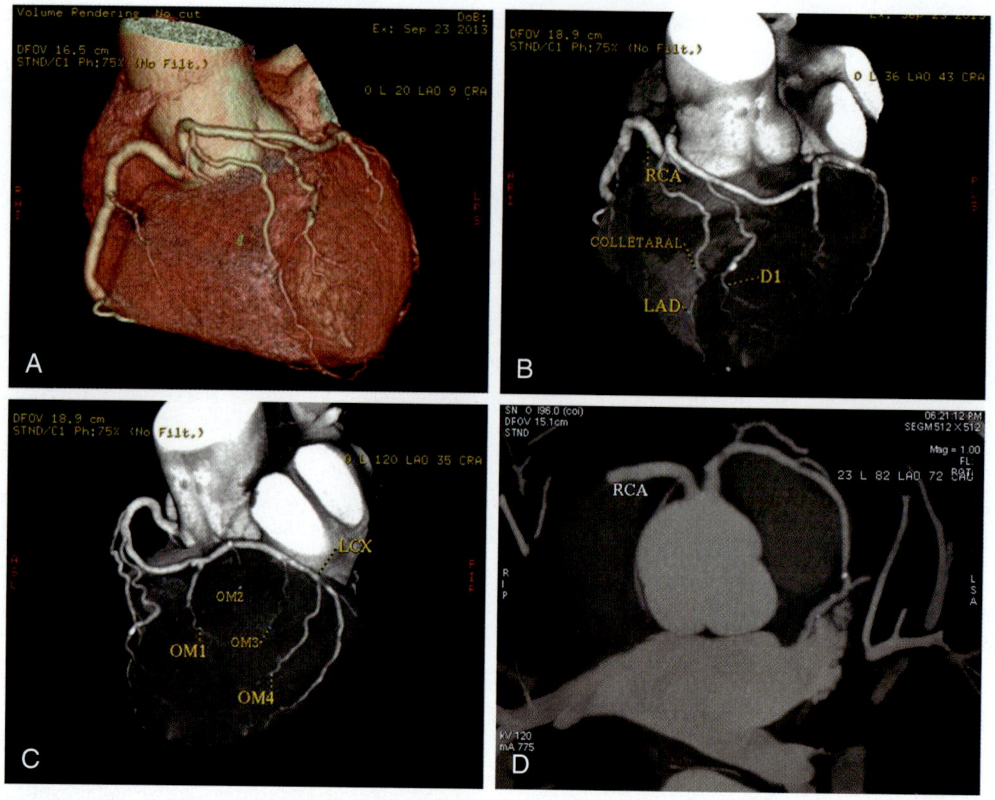

FIG. 1.5 Computed tomography coronary angiography with volume-rendered images to delineate coronary anatomy in three dimensions. (A) The origin of the left coronary artery main stem is from the right coronary sinus adjacent to the origin of the right coronary artery (*RCA*). (B) The anomalous origin of the left coronary artery turns anterior in front of the right ventricular outflow tract to reach the left atrioventricular (*AV*) groove. (C) Before that is the origin to the left anterior descending coronary artery (LAD), which runs normally into the interventricular groove and the diagonal artery. (D) After the left AV groove, there are the origins of obtuse marginal arteries. The right coronary has a normal origin and course. *D1*, diagonal; *LAD*, left anterior descending coronary artery; *LCX*, left circumflex coronary artery; *OM*, obtuse marginal.

Percutaneous angioplasty was performed in view of no interarterial course of the coronary arteries.

References

1. Alexander RW, Griffith GC. Anomalies of the coronary arteries and their clinical significance. *Circulation.* 1956;4:800-805.
2. Kimbiris D. Anomalous origin of the left main coronary artery from the right sinus of Valsalva. *Am J Cardiol.* 1985;55:765-769.
3. Madea B, Dettmeyer R. Sudden death in cases with anomalous origin of the left coronary artery. *Forensic Sci Int.* 1998;96:91-100.

Anomalous Acute Left Main Myocardial Infarction Owing to Compression Between the Pulmonary Artery and the Aorta by Acute Pulmonary Thromboembolism

Koki Shishido, MD, Noriaki Moriyama, MD, Toshimitsu Shimizu, RT, Shigeru Saito, MD

A 62-year-old female tourist without significant cardiovascular risk factors was first seen with acute chest pain. She had arrived from the United States to Japan 5 days earlier by plane. When she had been transferred to our emergency department by ambulance, she was in cardiogenic shock and her initial blood pressure was 63/48 mm Hg. The electrocardiogram demonstrated widespread ST-segment depression plus ST-segment elevation in lead aVR (Fig. 1.6A). The echocardiogram showed severe hypokinesis of left ventricular wall motion with a paradoxical interventricular septum (Online Video 1.6). The emergent coronary angiogram showed very tight narrowing in an anomalous left main coronary artery (LMCA) arising from the right coronary cusp (Fig. 1.6B). A drug-eluting stent (Ultimaster 3.5/18 mm, Terumo Corporation, Tokyo, Japan) was successfully implanted in the LMCA lesion with intraaortic balloon counterpulsation (Fig. 1.6C). Blood pressure, hypotension, and electrocardiogram changes were recovered after primary percutaneous coronary intervention. Two weeks later we could see the patent LMCA stent, which was sandwiched between the pulmonary artery (PA) and aorta by computed tomography imaging (Fig. 1.6D–E). In addition, we could find a lot of thrombus in both pulmonary arteries (Fig. 1.6F–G). We hypothesized that her LMCA was compressed between the ascending aorta and PA because the PA pressure had risen suddenly as the result of a massive acute pulmonary thromboembolism. The pulmonary thrombus improved by use of an anticoagulation drug after a few weeks. The echocardiogram demonstrated good LV function with complete resolution of the right ventricular dysfunction (Online Video 1.7). This case illustrates an unusual etiology of myocardial infarction in LMCA.

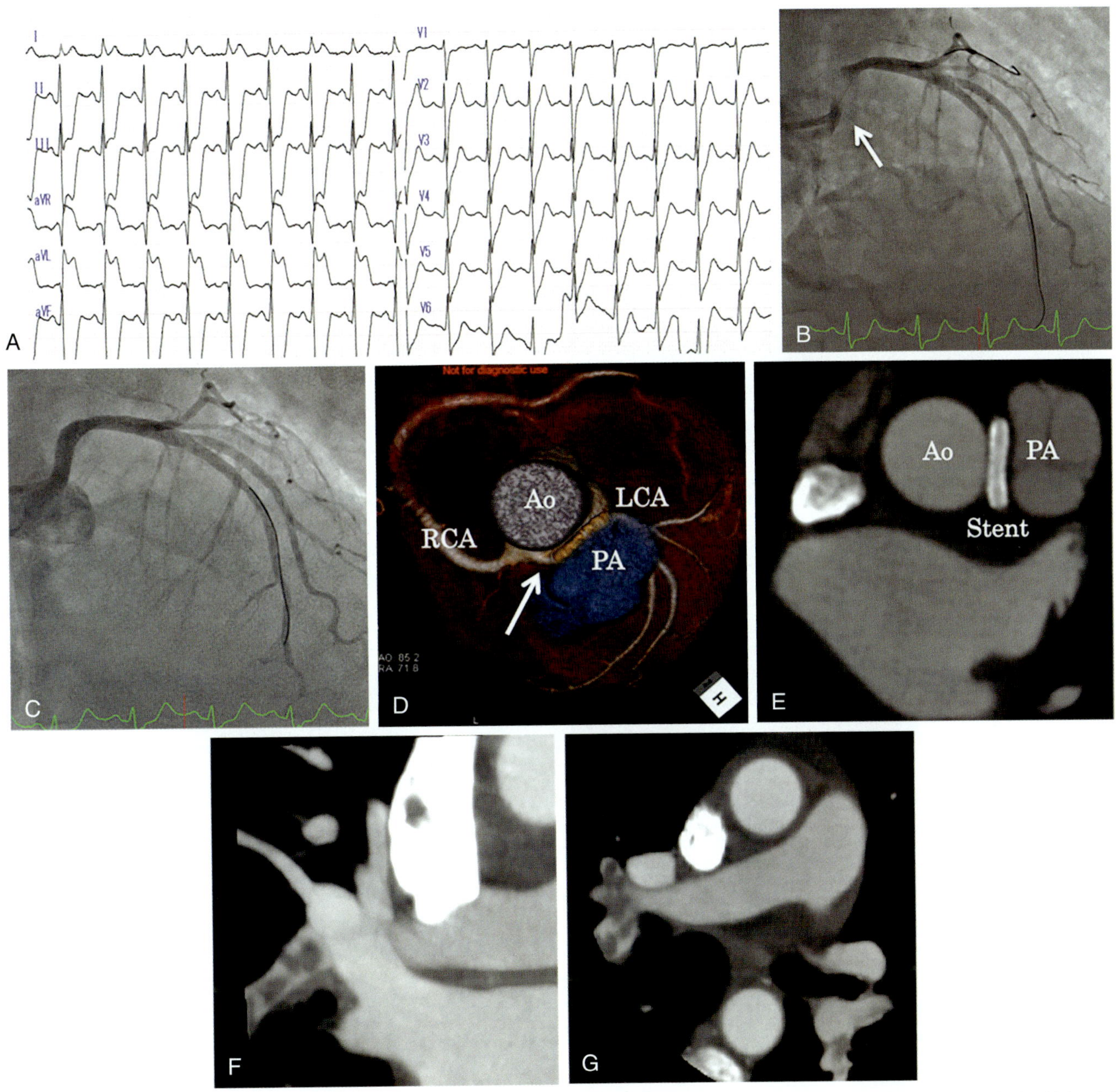

FIG. 1.6 Electrocardiogram, coronary angiograms, and computed tomography scans. (A) Electrocardiogram on admission (Online Video 1.6). (B) Emergent initial coronary angiography. Coronary angiography demonstrated a tight narrowing in the left main coronary artery (LMCA). The left coronary artery (LCA) originated from the right coronary cusp (*arrow*). (C) Final coronary angiography showed a good result after stent implantation. (D and E) Anomalous LCA shown by computed tomography (Online Video 1.7). The LCA originated from the right coronary cusp (*arrow*). The origin of the LCA was close to the origin of the right coronary artery (*RCA*). The implanted stent in the LMCA was compressed between the pulmonary artery (*PA*) and the aorta (*Ao*). (F and G) Pulmonary embolism shown by computed tomography. Computed tomography showed a large thrombus in both pulmonary arteries.

Anomalous Origin of Left Main Coronary Artery From Innominate Artery

Chuan-fen Liu, MD, Cheng-fu Cao, MD, Wei-min Wang, MD, Jian Liu, MD, Ming-yu Lu, MD, Hong Zhao, MD, Yu-liang Ma, MD, Qi Li, MD

A 73-year-old woman was admitted with progressive chest pain for 2 years. She had a history of hypertension for 9 years. Findings on physical examination were normal. Her low-density lipoprotein cholesterol level was 3.04 mmol/L. Electrocardiography and echocardiography results were normal. Cardiac computed tomographic coronary angiography showed an anomalous origin of the left main coronary artery (LMCA) from the innominate artery with ostial severe calcification (Fig. 1.7A).

The patient underwent coronary artery angiography, which confirmed the abnormal origin of the LMCA from the innominate artery and ostial severe stenosis of the LMCA (Fig. 1.7B, Online Video 1.8). The LMCA bifurcated into the normal left anterior descending and left circumflex coronary arteries. The right coronary artery had a 50% stenosis (Online Video 1.9). Intravascular ultrasound was performed to evaluate the LMCA lesion. The intravascular ultrasound image showed that the LMCA ostium had severe stenosis and calcification. The minimal luminal cross-sectional area was 2.87 mm^2 (Fig. 1.7C). A Resolute Integrity 4.0 × 30 mm stent (Medtronic, Minneapolis, Minnesota) was implanted (Fig. 1.7D, Online Video 1.10). Repeat intravascular

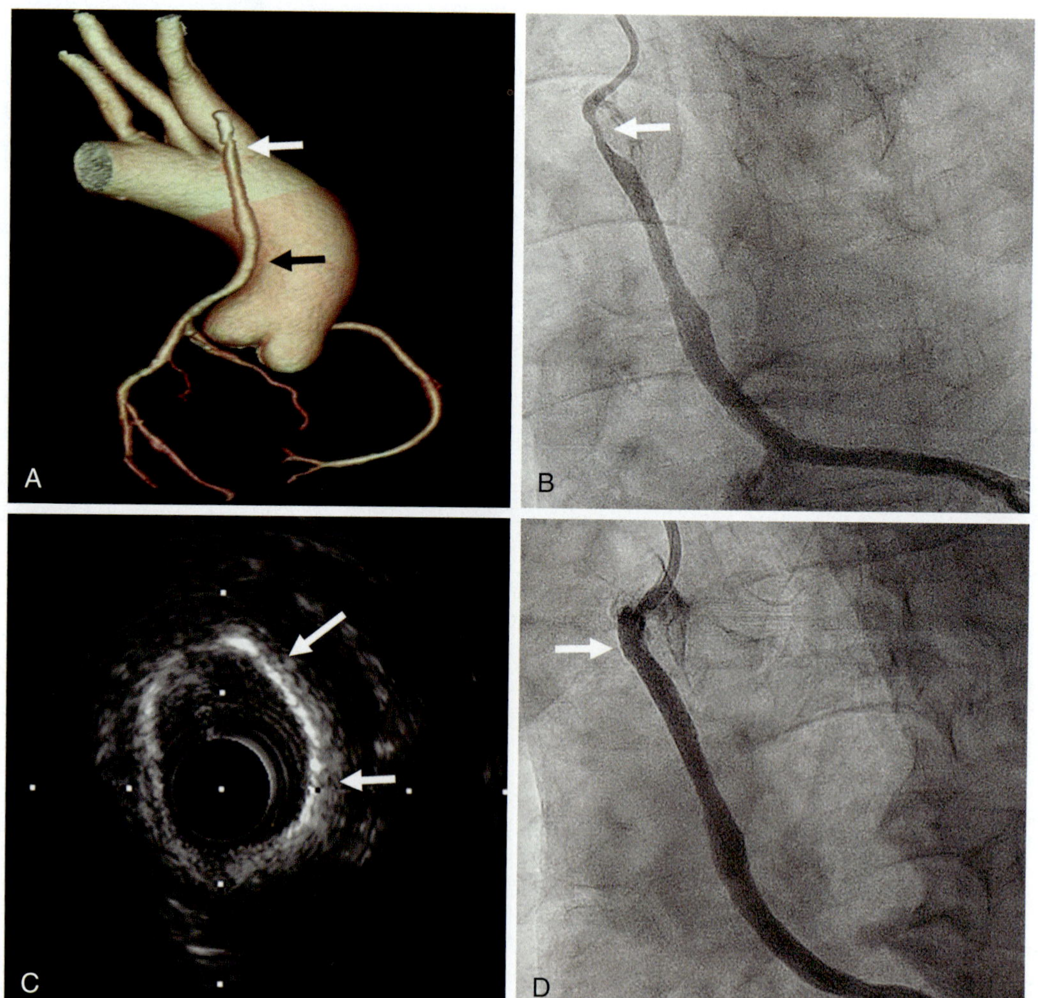

FIG. 1.7 Anomalous origin of left main coronary artery (LMCA) from innominate artery before and after percutaneous coronary intervention. (A) Cardiac computed tomographic coronary angiography shows the anomalous origin of the LMCA from the innominate artery with ostial severe calcification (*arrows*). (B) Coronary angiography indicating the abnormal origin of the LMCA from the innominate artery and ostial severe stenosis of LMCA (*arrow*). See Online Videos 1.8 and 1.9. (C) Intravascular ultrasound image shows severe stenosis and calcification of the LMCA ostium (*arrows*). (D) Final angiographic result of percutaneous coronary intervention showing good stent expansion and apposition (*arrow*). See Online Video 1.10.

ultrasound showed complete stent apposition and full stent expansion.

An anomalous origin of the LMCA from the innominate artery is rare. This patient represented the third published case but the patient was the first to undergo percutaneous coronary intervention.[1,2] Combined computed tomography and coronary angiography are reliable for the diagnosis of LMCA origin from the innominate artery.

References

1. Santucci PA, Bredikis AJ, Kavinsky CJ, Klein LW. Congenital origin of the left main coronary artery from the innominate artery in a 37-year-old man with syncope and right ventricular dysplasia. *Catheter Cardiovasc Interv.* 2001;52:378-381.
2. Duran NE, Duran I, Aykan AC. Congenital anomalous origin of the left main coronary artery from the innominate artery in a 73-year-old woman. *Can J Cardiol.* 2008;24:e108.

Anomalous Origin of the Left Internal Mammary Artery From the Aortic Arch

Alexander Incani, Joseph C. Lee, Karl K. Poon, James A. Crowhurst, BSC, Matthew Pincus, Darren L. Walters, MPhil

A 67-year-old man with diabetes who had a pacemaker for symptomatic bradycardia underwent cardiac catheterization for unstable angina 19 years after coronary artery bypass graft surgery. There were bilateral pedicled internal mammary grafts—from the left internal mammary artery (LIMA) to the left anterior descending coronary artery (LAD) and from the right internal mammary artery to the posterior descending coronary artery—as well as a saphenous venous graft to an obtuse marginal circumflex branch. Angiography revealed a patent right internal mammary artery and posterior descending coronary artery, and a culprit diseased saphenous venous graft (obtuse marginal). The LIMA–LAD could not be engaged at its expected origin from the left subclavian artery (Fig. 1.8A, Online Video 1.11). The LAD was not collateralized, and there was no resting anterior wall motion defect. This prompted examination with cardiac computed tomographic angiography (CCTA) to clarify the origin of an anomalous LIMA.

CCTA revealed a patent pedicled LIMA graft with an unusual origin and course. It arose distal to the left subclavian artery and tracked anteriorly and vertically before looping down the anterior chest wall to supply the LAD (Fig. 1.8B). This was not mentioned in the surgical report. Angiography was resumed; the LIMA graft was selectively engaged uneventfully (Fig. 1.8C, Online Video 1.12).

The LIMA arises from the intrascalenic course of the subclavian in 92% of patients, is interscalenic in 7%, and extrascalenic in 1%.[1] To our knowledge, this is the first described case of an entirely separate origin of the LIMA from the distal aortic arch.

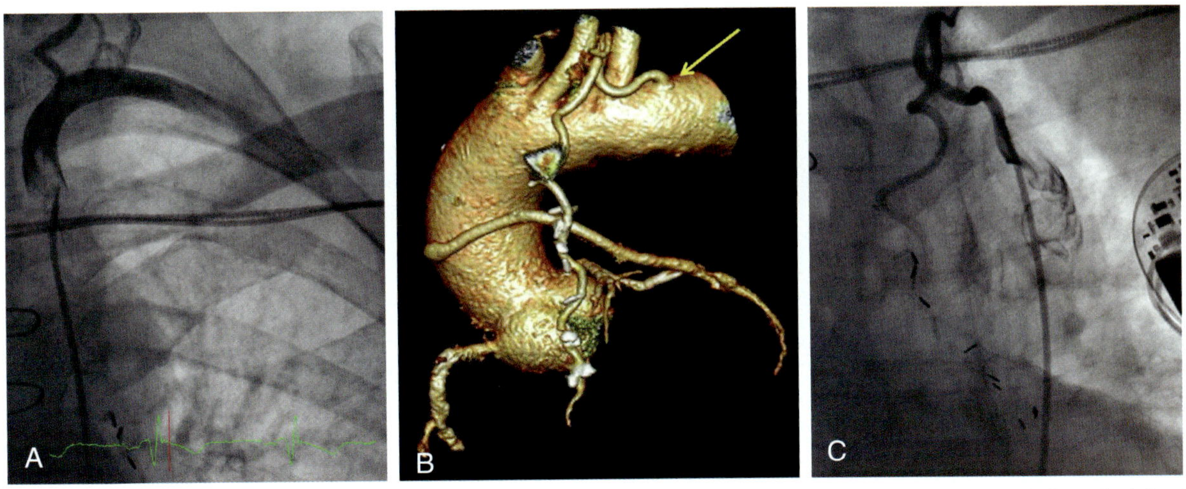

FIG. 1.8 Anomalous left internal mammary artery (LIMA). (A) LIMA (Online Video 1.11) could not be identified arising from the left subclavian artery with conventional catheterization. (B) Cardiac computed tomographic angiography (CCTA) demonstrated its origin from the aortic arch (*arrow*), as shown on CCTA reconstruction, and (C) (Online Video 1.12) selectively engaged on coronary angiography.

LIMAs have also been reported arising at the junction of the left subclavian and aorta or from an aberrant vertebral artery.[2,3] This case illustrates the potentially variable origin of the LIMA and the utility of CCTA in difficult graft studies. It also highlights the importance of looking for collaterals, as their absence in this case prompted further investigation for an anomalous vessel.

References

1. Henriquez-Pino JA, Gomes WJ, Prates JC, Buffolo E. Surgical anatomy of the internal thoracic artery. *Ann Thorac Surg*. 1997;64:1041-1045.
2. Chavez J, Osborn LA. Anomalous origin of left internal mammary artery from the lateral junction of the left subclavian artery and aorta. *Cathet Cardiovasc Diagn*. 1996;37:168-169.
3. Kirsch J, Williamson EE. Aberrant left internal mammary artery off an aberrant vertebral artery. *Eur Heart J*. 2008;29:1782.

Anomalous Origin of the Nonculprit Right Coronary Artery From the Left Anterior Descending Artery in a Patient With Anterolateral ST-Segment Elevation Myocardial Infarction

Mohammad Waleed, MBBS, MPH, Konstantinos Aznaouridis, MD, PhD

A 47-year-old man was admitted with anterolateral ST-segment elevation myocardial infarction (Fig. 1.9) and underwent emergency coronary angiography (Fig. 1.10) through the right radial artery. Attempts to cannulate the nonculprit right coronary artery (RCA) were unsuccessful, and subsequent contrast injection into the right sinus of Valsalva showed that the RCA did not arise from its usual position. Left coronary angiography showed a proximally occluded left anterior descending artery (LAD).

Coronary anomalies are usually found incidentally during coronary angiography, as the majority of these anomalies are benign and the patients remain asymptomatic.[1] We present a rare coronary anomaly of an RCA originating from the midsegment of the left LAD. Very few similar cases have been reported in the published data to date.[2,3] A recent study shows that the prevalence of an anomalous RCA arising from the LAD has been 0.018% in patients undergoing coronary angiography, which is only 6% of all anomalies of coronary artery origin and course.[3] In this anomaly the aberrant RCA usually has a course in front of the pulmonary artery and is associated with a good prognosis.[4]

To our knowledge, this is the first reported case of acute occlusion of an aberrant RCA arising from the LAD as the result of acute thrombosis of proximal LAD. However, our patient had codominant circulation with the anomalous RCA providing a small posterior descending branch, and therefore he had no evidence of acute inferior wall ischemia (no inferior ST-segment elevations, no inferior wall motion abnormality with quick bedside echocardiography before the procedure, and no hemodynamic instability).

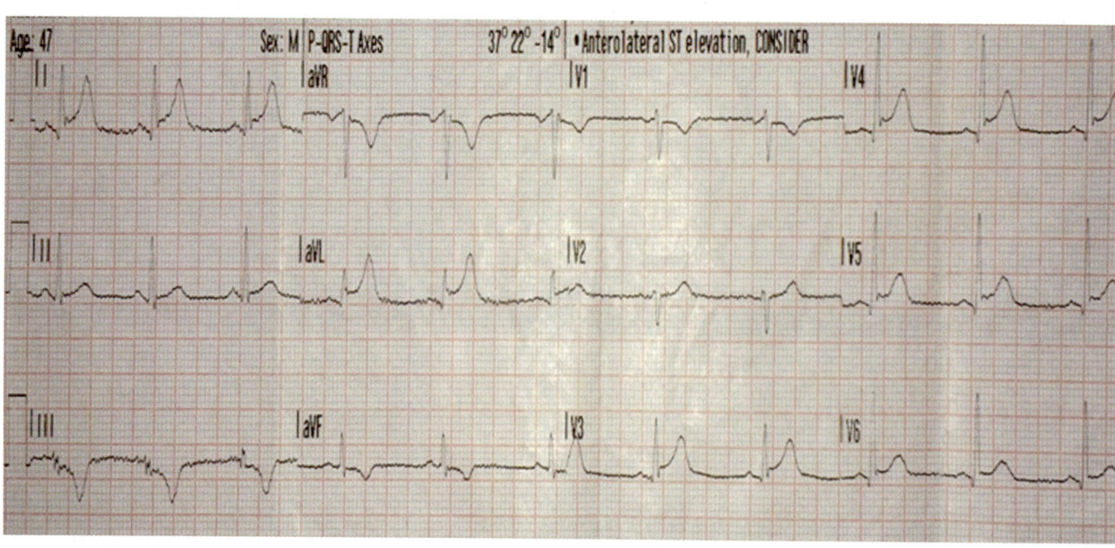

FIG. 1.9 Twelve-lead electrocardiogram shows ST-segment elevations on the anterolateral leads.

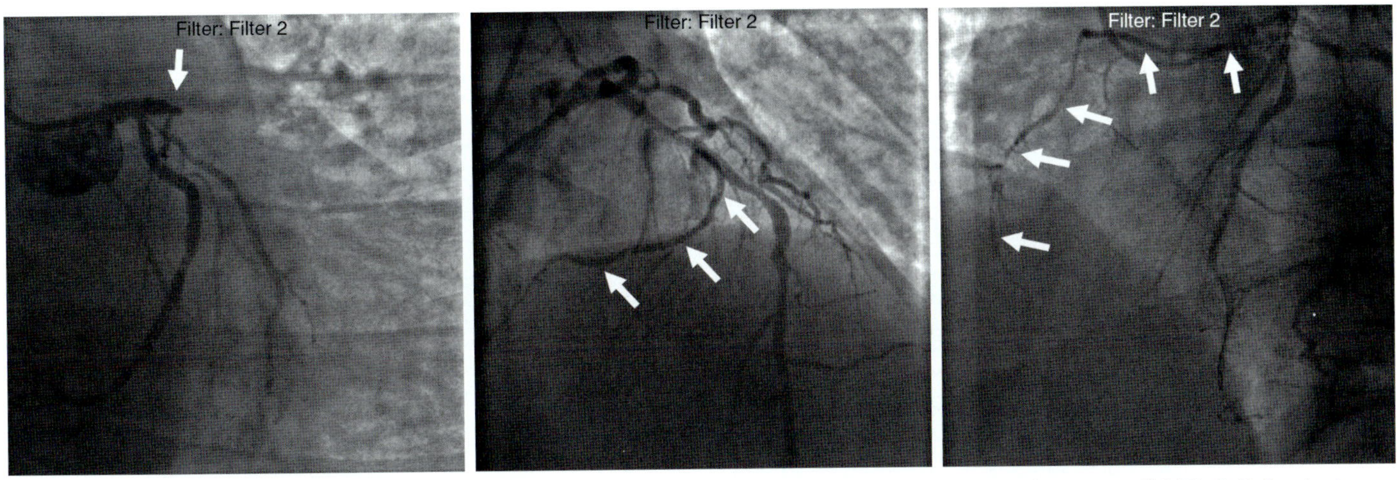

FIG. 1.10 Anomalous right coronary artery (RCA) from the midsegment of the left anterior descending artery (LAD). (*Left*) Proximal occlusion of the LAD (*arrow*) in anteroposterior caudal view. (*Center*) Origin of anomalous RCA from the mid-LAD (*arrows*) in anteroposterior cranial view. (*Right*) Course of anomalous RCA (*arrows*) in left anterior oblique view (Online Video 1.13–1.15).

Interventional cardiologists must be aware of this rare coronary anomaly. In a setting of emergency catheterization for ST-segment elevation myocardial infarction, revascularization of the culprit artery should be performed promptly if the nonculprit artery cannot be readily cannulated first. In rare cases, the nonculprit coronary artery may have an anomalous origin from the culprit artery.

References

1. Yamanaka O, Hobbs RE. Coronary artery anomalies in 126,595 patients undergoing coronary angiography. *Cathet Cardiovasc Diagn.* 1990;21:28-40.
2. Hourani R, Haddad N, Zughaib M. Anomalous origin of the RCA from the proximal LAD and a single coronary artery anomaly: two case reports of two rare coronary anomalies. *J Invasive Cardiol.* 2009;21:E216-E217.
3. Yuksel S, Meric M, Soylu K, et al. The primary anomalies of coronary artery origin and course: a coronary angiographic analysis of 16,573 patients. *Exp Clin Cardiol.* 2013;18:121-123.
4. Teragawa H, Okada K, Sueda T. Anomalous origin of the right coronary artery from the left anterior descending coronary artery. *Heart.* 2004;90:1492.

Concomitant Anomalous Right Coronary Artery and Iatrogenic Left Circumflex Artery Entrapment Treated Successfully With Percutaneous Coronary Intervention

Carrie Eshelbrenner, MD, S. Hinan Ahmed, MD

The incidence of anomalous coronary arteries is approximately 1% with heterogeneous clinical outcomes.[1] Left circumflex coronary artery (LCx) entrapment is an infrequently reported complication of mitral valve surgery and correlates to the dominance and the distance of the artery from the mitral annulus. Nearly all reported cases occur intraoperatively or immediately postoperatively.[2] Our patient was seen 14 years after mitral valve annuloplasty with longstanding chest pain and dyspnea on exertion. Myocardial perfusion imaging showed a large area of inferolateral ischemia. Computed tomography angiography revealed an anomalous right coronary artery arising from the left cusp and coursing between the great arteries with a narrowed proximal segment. It also showed a severe focal stenosis of the LCx with traction of the artery toward the mitral valve, suggestive of an iatrogenic entrapment (Fig. 1.11).

Cardiac catheterization confirmed the anomalous origin of the right coronary artery and the high-grade stenosis of the mid LCx (Fig. 1.12). Intravascular ultrasound imaging of the LCx revealed a highly fibrotic, high-grade stenosis of the mid vessel. This lesion was treated with serial low-pressure balloon inflations using a compliant balloon. Stent implantation was performed using a 4.5 × 15 mm bare-metal stent (Vision, Abbott Vascular, Abbott Park, Illinois) followed by postdilation with a noncompliant balloon. The patient is completely symptom free at 6-month follow-up.

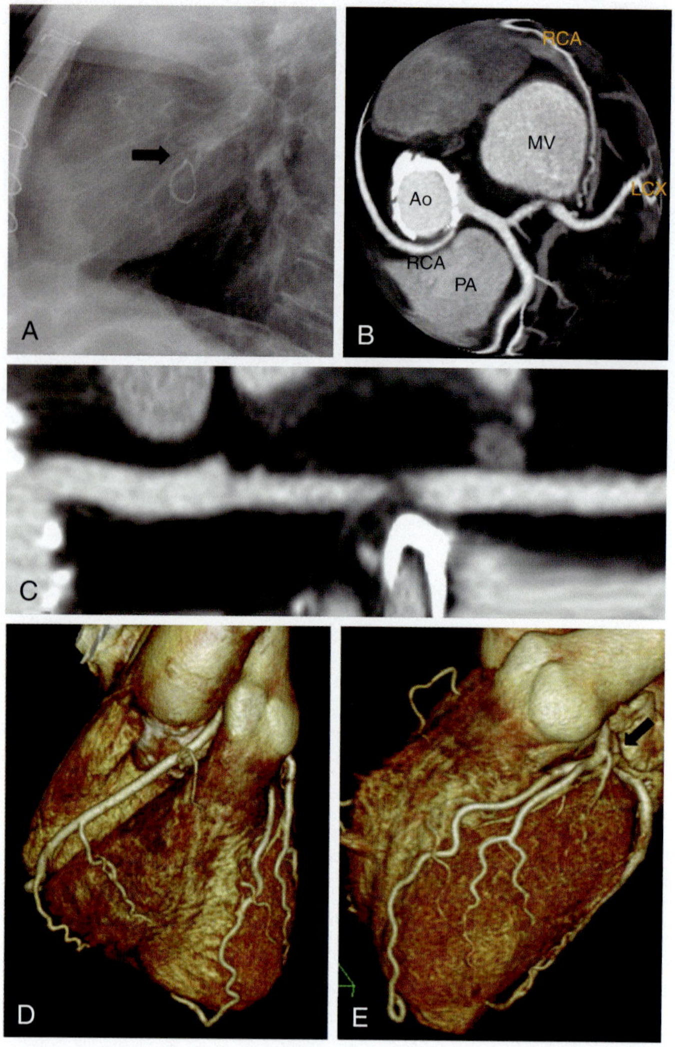

FIG. 1.11 Computed tomography (imaging of the coronary abnormalities. (A) Lateral chest radiograph shows focal protrusion (*arrow*) of the mitral annuloplasty ring. (B) Computed tomography angiography revealed the anomalous origin of the right coronary artery (*RCA*) from the left coronary cusp and taking an interarterial course between the aorta (*Ao*) and the pulmonary artery (*PA*) with proximal narrowing. The proximal left circumflex (*LCx*) artery coursing adjacent to the mitral valve (*MV*) with a focal segment of traction and significant stenosis is also visible. (C) Multiplanar reconstruction shows the mitral annuloplasty ring and proximal stenosis of the LCX, possibly as the result of entrapment. (D) Volume-rendered reconstruction images show the anomalous origin and the subsequent course of the right coronary artery and (E) the course of the LCX with focal narrowing (*arrow*) at the mitral annular area.

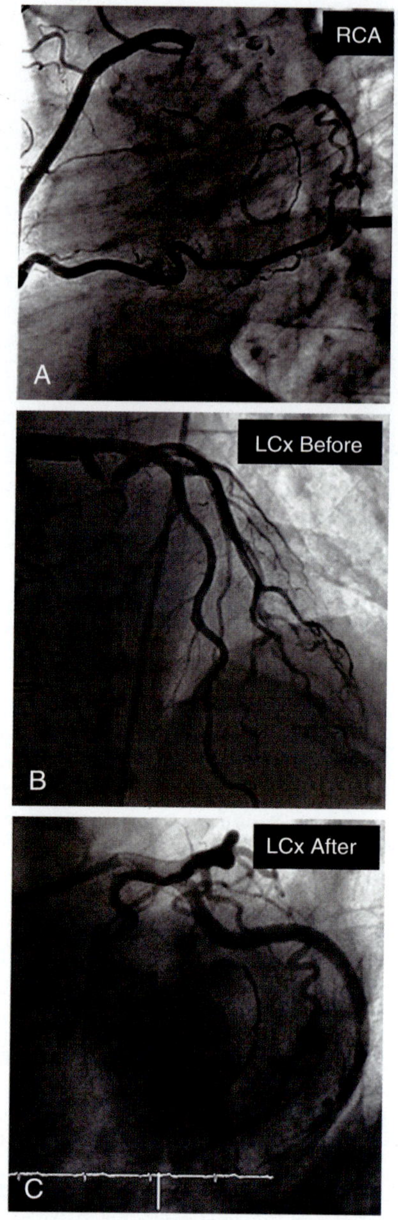

FIG. 1.12 Coronary angiography before and after intervention. (A) Coronary angiography shows the anomalous origin of right coronary artery (*RCA*) providing distal collaterals to the left circumflex coronary artery (*LCx*) (*arrow*), (B) the proximal subtotal stenosis of the LCx, and (C) no residual stenosis after stenting.

This is an unusual case of these two abnormalities occurring in the same patient with a late presentation, albeit with long-standing symptoms. In the literature, management of both conditions is largely anecdotal, and percutaneous coronary intervention is infrequently used.

References

1. Angelini P, Velasco JA, Flamm S. Coronary anomalies: incidence, pathophysiology, and clinical relevance. *Circulation.* 2002;105:2449-2454.
2. Grande AM, Fiore A, Massetti M, Viganò M. Iatrogenic circumflex coronary lesion in mitral valve surgery: case report and review of the literature. *Tex Heart Inst J.* 2008;35:179-183.

Dual Anomalous Origins of the Thyrocervical Trunk and Left Internal Mammary Artery

Abdulelah Nuqali, MD, Qaiser Shafiq, MD, Mujeeb Sheikh, MD

A 56-year-old man with diabetes and a history of triple coronary artery bypass graft surgery (left internal mammary artery [LIMA] to left anterior descending [LAD] artery, saphenous vein grafts to the posterior descending artery and the obtuse marginal artery) underwent coronary catheterization for unstable angina. Left main coronary artery angiography showed competitive follow in the distal left anterior descending coronary artery (Fig. 1.13, Online Video 1.16). However, the LIMA could not be visualized despite multiple angiographic images of the left subclavian artery. Aortic arch angiography showed an artery coming off the aortic arch just distal to the origin of the subclavian artery (Fig. 1.13, Online Video 1.17).

This artery appeared to be the anomalous origin of the thyrocervical trunk (Fig. 1.14), and selective engagement of this branch was performed. The LIMA was seen to arise as a branch from this thyrocervical trunk (Fig. 1.14, Online Video 1.18) and to supply the distal LAD. The right internal mammary artery was normal angiographically and arose from the proximal right subclavian artery (Fig. 1.14, Online Video 1.19). The thyrocervical trunk usually originates from the upper part of the first subclavian artery segment,[1] and the LIMA arises from the proximal part of the subclavian artery in 92% of cases, from the mid portion in 7% of cases, and from the distal part of the subclavian artery in 1% of cases. Anomalous origins of LIMA from the lateral junction of the left subclavian artery and aorta,[2] from an aberrant vertebral artery,[3] and from the aortic arch[4] have been reported.

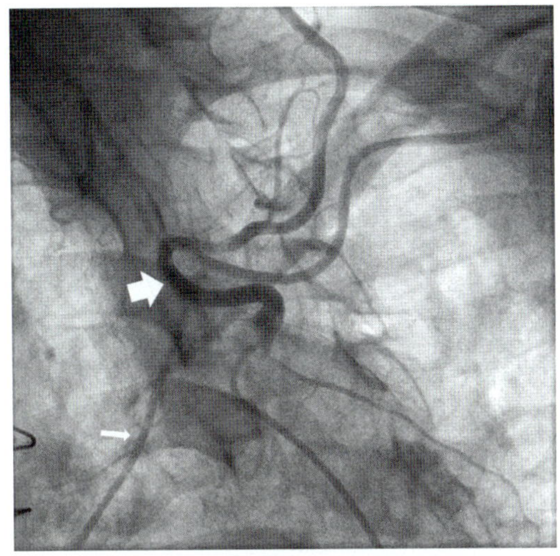

FIG. 1.14 Angiogram showing the anomalous origin of the left internal mammary artery. The angiogram of the thyrocervical trunk (*thick arrow*) shows the anomalous origin of the left internal mammary artery (*thin arrow*). See Online Videos 1.18 and 1.19.

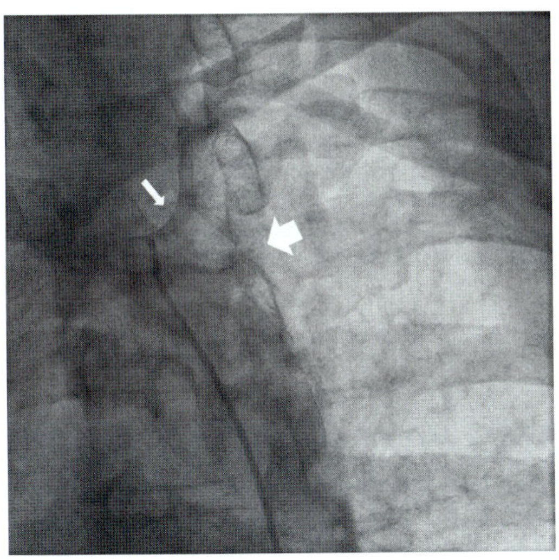

FIG. 1.13 Aortic arch angiogram showing the anomalous origin of the thyrocervical trunk. The aortic arch angiogram shows the anomalous origin of the thyrocervical trunk from the aortic arch (*thick arrow*) distal to the origin of the subclavian artery (*thin arrow*). See Online Videos 1.16 and 1.17.

To our knowledge, this dual anomalous origin of the thyrocervical trunk and origin of the LIMA from it has not been reported. These rare anomalies should be considered before concluding that this important vessel is occluded. Competitive flow in LAD was an important clue in our case that this vessel was patent, although anomalous.

References

1. Lischka MF, Krammer EB, Rath T, Riedl M, Ellböck E. The human thyrocervical trunk: configuration and variability reinvestigated. *Anat Embryol (Berl).* 1982;163:389-401.
2. Chavez J, Osborn LA. Anomalous origin of left internal mammary artery from the lateral junction of the left subclavian artery and aorta. *Cathet Cardiovasc Diagn.* 1996;37:168-169.
3. Kirsch J, Williamson EE. Aberrant left internal mammary artery off an aberrant vertebral artery. *Eur Heart J.* 2008;29:1782.
4. Hailan A, Obaid D, Zaidi A, Smith D. Anomalous origin of left internal mammary artery arising directly from the aortic arch. *BMJ Case Rep.* 2014. bcr2014206583.

Multimodality Imaging of an Anomalous Connection of the Right Coronary Artery With Aortic Intramural Course

Pierre Aubry, MD, Amir-Ali Fassa, MD, Ali Alshamsi, MD, Xavier Halna du Fretay, MD, Patrick Dupouy, MD, Jean-Michel Juliard, MD

A 47-year-old man underwent a medical examination. He was a professional firefighter, with no notable medical history, who regularly performed high-grade aerobic exercise. He denied any specific symptom at rest or during efforts. Results of his physical examination were unremarkable. An electrocardiogram showed nonspecific repolarization abnormalities in the lateral leads. Single-photon emission computed tomography revealed a small reversible defect in the inferolateral wall during stress. The workup was completed with a cardiac computed tomography, which showed a moderate stenosis of the distal left anterior descending artery and an anomalous connection of the right coronary artery from the left coronary sinus (Fig. 1.15A) with a narrowing of the initial segment through an aortic intramural course (Fig. 1.15B). The patient was referred for a coronary angiogram, which confirmed the anomalous connection of the right coronary artery and a typical nonatherosclerotic narrowing in right anterior oblique projection owing to the intramural course (Fig. 1.15C). Intravascular ultrasonography and optical coherence tomography demonstrated the oblong shape of the initial intramural lumen of the right coronary artery (Fig. 1.15D–E) with a 50% reduction in lumen surface compared with the proximal extramural

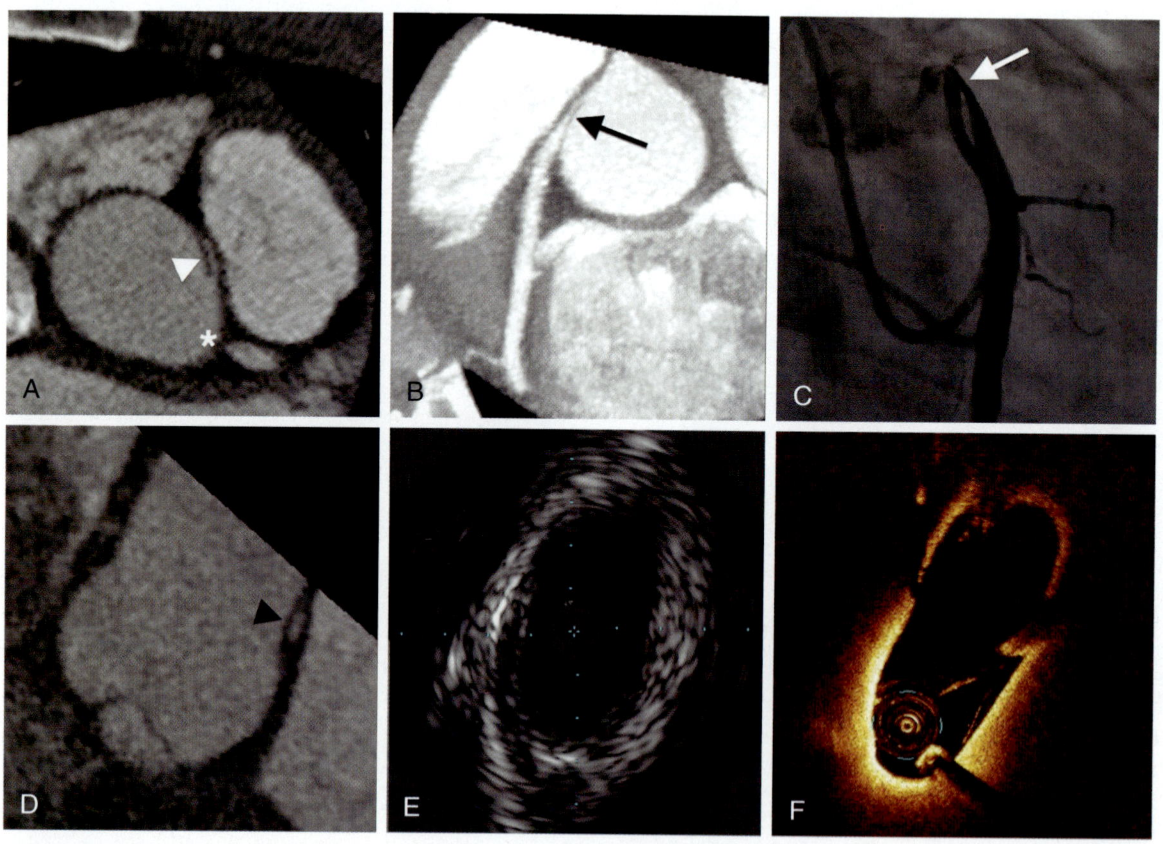

FIG. 1.15 Multimodality imaging of an anomalous connection of the right coronary artery. (A) Computed tomography angiography with an axial view showing an anomalous connection of the right coronary artery (*white arrowhead*) from the left sinus near the origin of the left coronary artery (*white star*). (B) Computed tomography angiography with a curved multiplanar reconstruction showing a narrowing (*black arrow*) of the initial coronary segment owing to an aortic intramural course. (C) Selective angiography in 30-degree right anterior oblique projection demonstrating a narrowing (*white arrow*) of the initial coronary segment. (D) Computed tomography angiography with a cross-sectional view showing an oblong shape (*black arrowhead*) of the intramural coronary lumen. (E) Intravascular ultrasound and (F) coherence tomography images demonstrating an oblong shape of the intramural coronary lumen.

lumen. The fractional flow reserve was 0.81 after administration of intravenous adenosine. Because of the evidence of an aortic intramural course associated with inducible ischemia and the potential risk for sudden cardiac death, it was decided to perform coronary bypass surgery of the right coronary artery with the right internal mammary artery.[1] The operation was uncomplicated and the recovery was uneventful.

This report illustrates the capability of multimodality imaging in providing essential anatomic information on coronary arteries with anomalous origin and, more specifically, to demonstrate the presence of an aortic intramural course, a well-known at-risk anatomy, which is often confused in the literature with a compression between the aorta and pulmonary artery

Reference

1. Warnes C, Williams R, Bashore T, et al. ACC/AHA 2008 guidelines for the management of adults with congenital heart disease: a report of the American College of Cardiology/American Heart Association Task Force on Practice Guidelines (Writing Committee to Develop Guidelines on the Management of Adults With Congenital Heart Disease). *J Am Coll Cardiol.* 2008;52:e143-e263.

Origin of Right and Left Coronary Arteries From the Right Sinus of Valsalva as a Common Coronary Trunk

Panagiotis Kariofillis, MD, Irene Mastorakou, MD, Vassilis Voudris, MD

A 71-year-old woman with a history of rheumatoid arthritis, pulmonary fibrosis, pericardiectomy, and a heavily calcified tricuspid aortic valve stenosis was referred for coronary angiography for preoperative evaluation for aortic valve replacement. The coronary angiogram demonstrated an anomalous coronary anatomy, with the origin of the right coronary artery and left main stem from the right sinus of Valsalva as a common coronary trunk (single coronary artery) (Fig. 1.16). Multislice computed tomography confirmed the presence of a single coronary artery arising from the right sinus of Valsalva, with a posterior course of the main stem that turns behind the aorta in an inferoposterior direction (Fig. 1.17). The coronary arteries were free of atherosclerotic disease. Because there was an unacceptable high surgical risk the patient was successfully treated with percutaneous aortic valve implantation.

The overall incidence of coronary anomalies in humans is 0.6% to 1.3%. An aberrant origin of the main stem from the right sinus of Valsalva represents one of the rarest forms of all coronary anomalies, and the situation of a single coronary artery is an extremely rare congenital anomaly that is seen in only 0.0024% to 0.044% of the population.

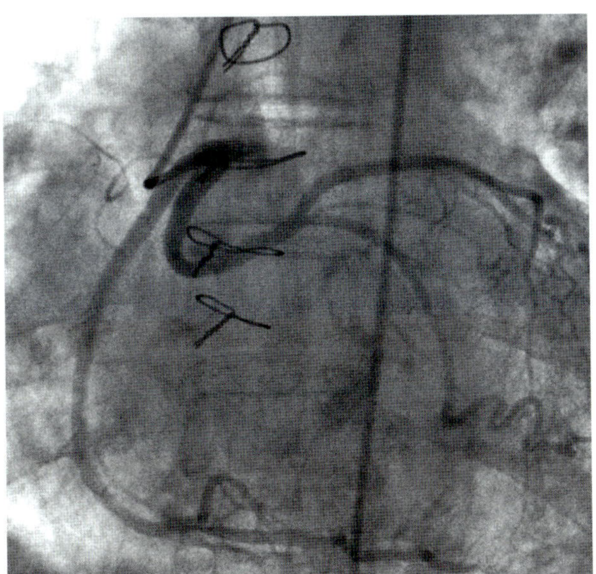

FIG. 1.16 Coronary angiography showing a single coronary artery arising from the right sinus of Valsalva, in left anterior oblique projection giving rise to right coronary artery and left main stem.

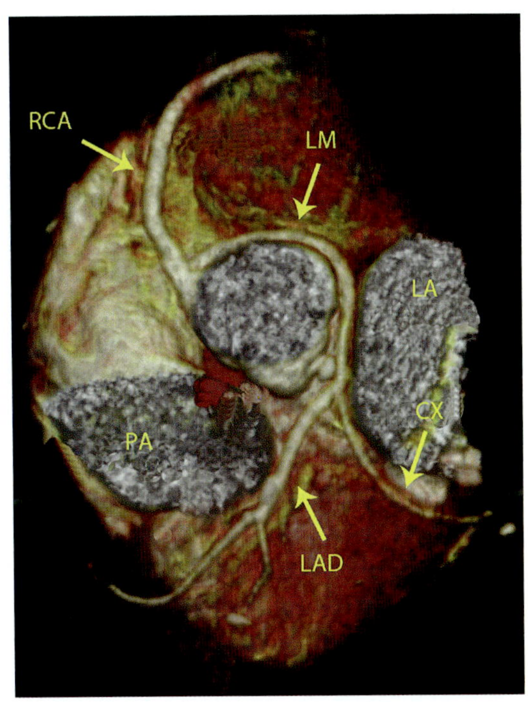

FIG. 1.17 Multislice spiral computed tomography showing the single coronary artery arising from the right sinus of Valsalva. The main stem turns posteriorly behind the aorta and divides into left anterior descending (*LAD*) and left circumflex (*CX*) coronary arteries. *LA*, *Left atrium; LM, left main; PA*, pulmonary artery; *RCA*, right coronary artery.

In the case of a single coronary artery arising from the right coronary sinus, the main stem takes one of four aberrant pathways to reach its proper vascular territory. These pathways are designated as type A (anterior to the right ventricular outflow tract), type B (between the aorta and pulmonary trunk), type C (cristal, coursing through the crista supraventricularis portion of the septum), and type D (dorsal or posterior to the aorta).[1-3]

References

1. Liberthon RR, Dinsmore RE, Bharati S, et al. Aberrant coronary artery origin from the aorta: diagnosis and clinical significance. *Circulation.* 1974;50:774-779.
2. Yamanaka O, Hobbs RE. Coronary artery anomalies in 126,595 patients undergoing coronary angiography. *Cathet Cardiovasc Diagn.* 1990;21:28-40.
3. Desmet W, Vanhaecke J, Vrolix M, et al. Isolated single coronary artery: a review of 50,000 consecutive angiographies. *Eur Heart J.* 1992;13:1637-1640.

Primary Percutaneous Intervention in a Patient With Anterior and Inferior Wall Myocardial Infarction Because of a Rare Coronary Artery Anomaly

Mohit D. Gupta, MD, DM, Girish MP, MD, DM, Bhagya N. Pandit, MD, Sanjay Tyagi, MD, DM

A 40-year-old male smoker had acute myocardial infarction involving the anterior and inferior walls at presentation. Electrocardiography showed ST-segment elevation in the anterior leads and the inferior leads, suggesting a probable occlusion of a type III left anterior descending coronary artery (LAD). Coronary angiography showed a single coronary artery originating from the left sinus of Valsalva. The LAD showed thrombus containing 95% long-segment stenosis after the first diagonal with thrombolysis in myocardial infarction (TIMI) flow grade 2 (Fig. 1.18). A large vessel originating from the mid LAD just after the stenosis and after the course of the right coronary artery (RCA) had a TIMI flow grade 2 (Fig. 1.18A). Percutaneous coronary intervention of the LAD was performed by implanting a drug-eluting stent. TIMI flow grade 3 was achieved in both the anomalous RCA and the LAD (Fig. 1.18B). A computed tomography coronary angiogram obtained later revealed the anomalous RCA originating from the mid LAD that coursed to the right, anterior to the pulmonary artery and the right ventricular outflow tract (Fig. 1.19). The anomalous origin of the RCA from the mid LAD is one of the rarest coronary anomalies reported to date.[1,2] Most anomalies of the RCA originating from the LAD are generally considered benign.[3] However, ischemia because of this anomaly may be caused by the acute angle made by the anomalous RCA to turn toward the right atrioventricular groove, thereby causing reduced flow velocity.[2] The course between the great arteries leading to compression of anomalous artery and atherosclerotic involvement of the vessels (jeopardizing a large amount of myocardium, as

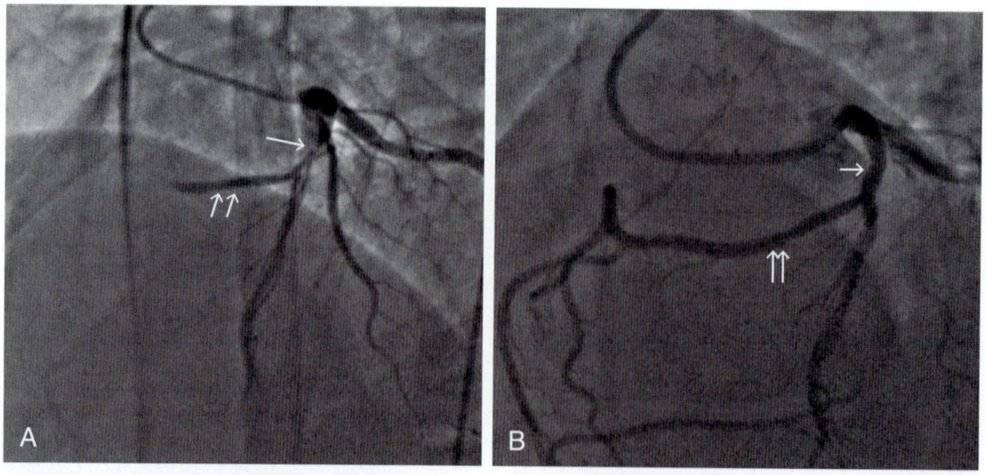

FIG. 1.18 Angiograms showing anomalous origin of the right coronary artery (RCA) from the stenosed mid left anterior descending coronary artery (LAD) before and after angioplasty. (A) Angiogram showing the anomalous origin of the RCA from the stenosed mid LAD. Coronary angiogram of the left main coronary artery engaged with a Judkins left F7 guide catheter in the left anterior oblique cranial view showing critical stenosis in the mid LAD (*single arrow*) and anomalous origin of the RCA from the mid LAD (*double arrows*). Poor opacification of the RCA and distal LAD is evident. (B) Angiogram showing good flow in the LAD and the anomalous RCA after angioplasty. Coronary angiogram of the left main coronary artery engaged with a Judkins left F7 guide catheter in the left anterior oblique cranial view after stent deployment in the LAD showing no residual stenosis in the LAD (*single arrow*) and restoration of good flow in the anomalous RCA (*double arrows*).

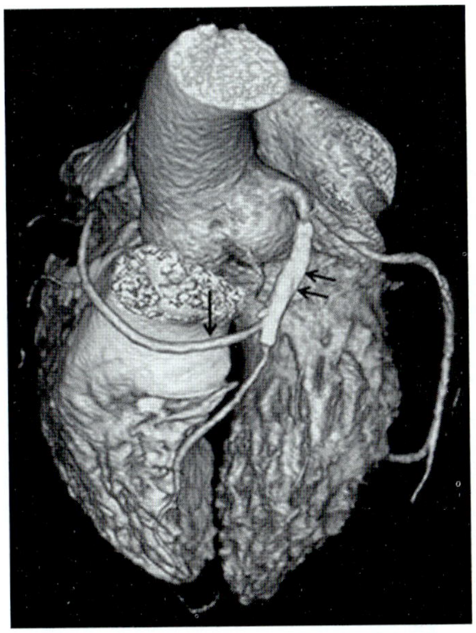

FIG. 1.19 Computed Tomogrpahy Coronary Angiogram (Post-Angioplasty) Showing the Anomalous Right Coronary Artery From the Mid Left Anterior Descending Coronary Artery. Computed tomography coronary angiogram of the left main coronary artery after deployment of the stent in the left anterior descending coronary artery showing the anomalous right coronary from the mid left anterior descending coronary artery coursing anterior to the pulmonary artery and entering the right atrioventricular groove.

in the present case) may also cause angina or infarction.[2] While performing primary percutaneous coronary intervention in such an anomaly, certain technical considerations such as protection of the anomalous RCA with a wire, use of a flexible and steerable wire (keeping in mind the angulated origin of the RCA), and mandatory kissing balloon technique despite good flow in the RCA, (this being a major epicardial artery and not a branch) should be kept in mind. This variant has not been listed in the classification of such an anomaly, but it resembles the IB1 category type of Shirani and Roberts' classification.[3]

References

1. Yiangou K, Georgiou G, Avraamides P, Kassianides M, Henein M. Anomalous origin of right coronary artery from the mid-left anterior descending artery. *Int J Cardiol.* 2008;129:e59-e60.
2. Amasyali B, Kursaklioglu H, Kose S, Iyisoy A, Kilic A, Isik E. Single coronary artery with anomalous origin of the right coronary artery from the left anterior descending artery with a unique proximal course. *Jpn Heart J.* 2004;45:521-525.
3. Shirani J, Roberts WC. Solitary coronary ostium in aorta in the absence of major congenital cardiovascular anomalies. *J Am Coll Cardiol.* 1993;21:137-143.

Right Aortic Arch With Left-Sided Arteria Lusoria: A Challenge for Radial Interventionalists

Nagaraja Moorthy, DM, Rajiv Ananthakrishna, DM, Dattatreya P.V. Rao, DM, Madhav Hegde, MD, Manjunath C. Nanjappa, DM

A 67-year-old male, hypertensive nonsmoker was admitted with unstable angina. He had a history of acute anterior wall myocardial infarction 4 months earlier for which he underwent primary percutaneous coronary intervention (PCI) with stenting of the left anterior coronary artery (LAD). During primary PCI, an incidentally isolated right aortic arch (Fig. 1.20A, Online Video 1.20) was noticed, and there was difficulty in hooking both right and left coronary arteries. However, the primary PCI with stenting of the culprit vessel LAD was performed by a transradial approach, and the left circumflex coronary artery (LCx) lesion was medically managed. During readmission, in view of the difficulties in the previous intervention owing to the right aortic arch, it was decided to perform coronary angiography by a left radial artery approach. Surprisingly, the guidewire was repeatedly entering the descending thoracic aorta, which was situated on the right of the spine. The TIG catheter (Terumo Corporation, Tokyo, Japan) was used to enter the arch and ascending aorta. With the M-shaped loop of the catheter (Fig. 1.20B, Online Video 1.21 and 1.22), it was realized that the left subclavian artery was arising anomalously from the descending thoracic aorta with a retroesophageal course. There was difficulty in hooking both right and left coronary arteries (Fig. 1.20C, Online Video 1.23) with the TIG catheter. Coronary angiography showed a patent stent in the mid LAD with progression of the LCx lesion. Using a 6F extra backup guide catheter with gentle manipulation using the reverse end of a 0.035-in (190-cm) guidewire, we were successful in engaging the left coronary artery. The culprit lesion in the distal LCx was stented using a 2.5 × 24-mm drug-eluting stent. A later esophagogram using diluted contrast showed a severe indentation on the posterior aspect of the esophagus (Fig. 1.20D, Online Video 1.24) caused by the retroesophageal course of the anomalous left subclavian artery. A computed tomography aortogram confirmed the right aortic arch (Fig. 1.20E) with an aberrant left subclavian artery arising from the descending thoracic aorta following a retroesophageal course (Fig. 1.20F), resulting in a prominent compression of the esophagus, a finding consistent with left-sided arteria lusoria. The sequential branching patterns of the arch of the aorta were left common carotid artery, right common carotid artery, and right subclavian followed by the anomalous left subclavian artery (Fig. 1.20G–H). A virtual computed tomography esophagogram showed significant compression of esophagus caused by the retroesophageal course of the left subclavian artery (Fig. 1.20). However, the patient had never experienced

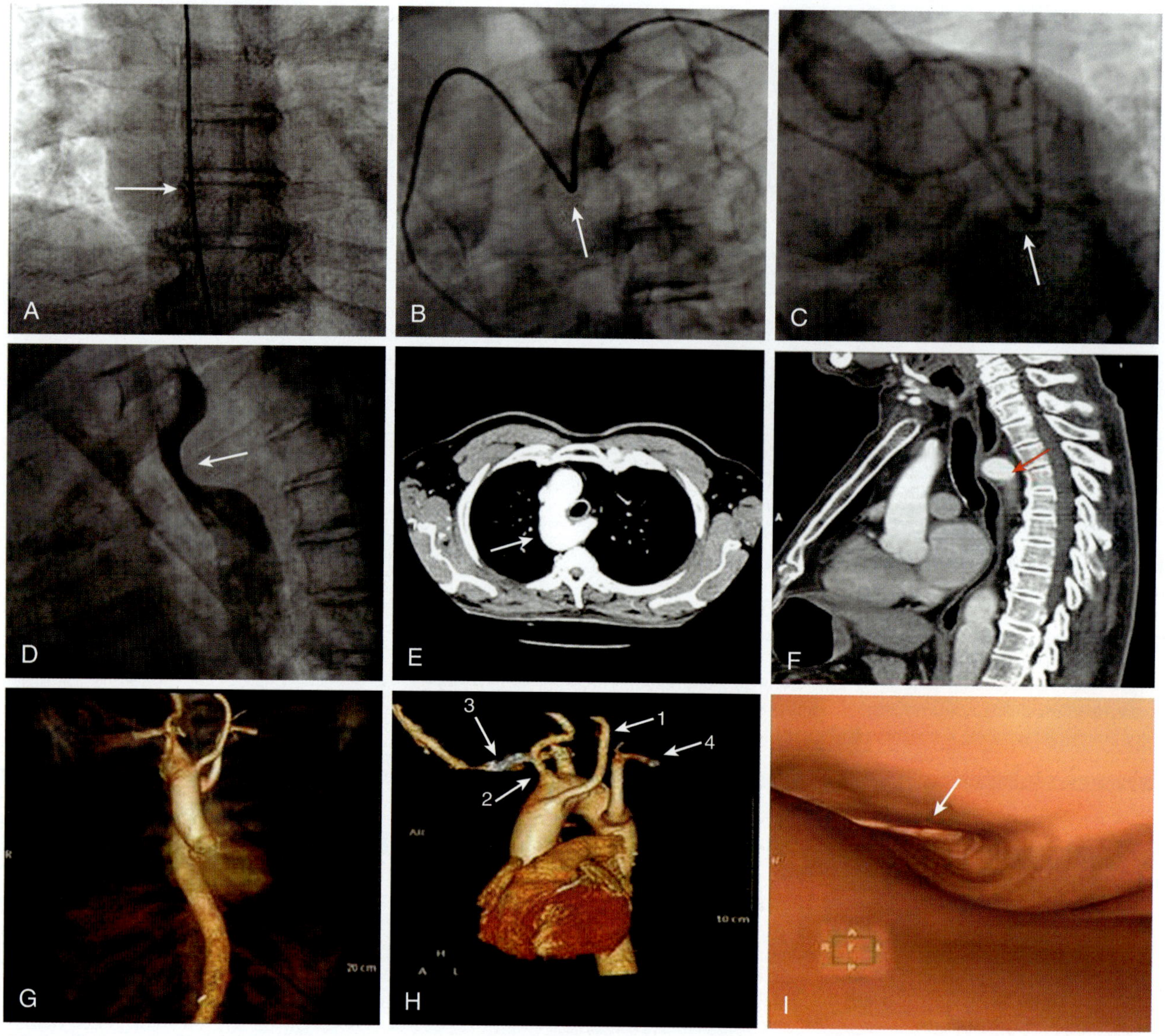

FIG. 1.20 Fluoroscopic and Computed Tomography Images Illustrating Right Aortic Arch With Left-Sided Arteria Lusoria. (A) Guidewire position (*arrow*) suggestive of a right aortic arch (Online Video 1.20). (B) M-shaped loop (*arrow*) of the TIG catheter suggesting arteria lusoria on the left side (Online Videos 1.21 and 1.22). (C) Left coronary injection done using the TIG catheter. Note the abnormal loop of the TIG catheter (*arrow*) (Online Video 1.23). (D) Contrast esophagogram showing indentation on the posterior aspect of the esophagus (*arrow*) caused by the retroesophageal course of the left subclavian artery (Online Video 1.24). (E) Computed tomography (CT) aortogram showing the right aortic arch (*arrow*). (F) CT aortogram showing severe posterior indentation of the esophagus by the retroesophageal course of the left subclavian artery (*arrow*). (G) Volume-rendered CT aortogram showing right aortic arch with abnormal branching pattern. (H) Volume-rendered CT aortogram showing the origins of the left common carotid artery (*1*), right common carotid artery (*2*), right subclavian artery (*3*), and left subclavian artery (*4*) in sequence from proximal to distal. (I) Virtual CT esophagogram showing significant stenosis of the esophagus owing to compression by the retroesophageal course of the left subclavian artery.

dysphagia in the past despite significant compression of the esophagus.

Most patients with an aberrant subclavian artery are asymptomatic, and with increasing use of transradial access to perform coronary angiography, arteria lusoria may be discovered as an incidental surprise. Transradial coronary angiography and interventions in patients with arteria lusoria, though challenging, are feasible. To our knowledge, this is the first description of incidental discovery of right aortic arch with left-sided arteria lusoria in an adult during a transradial intervention.

Right Coronary Artery With Anomalous Origin: The Role of Imaging Techniques

Maria Alejandra Restrepo-Cordoba, MD, Carlos Arellano-Serrano, MD, Susana Mingo-Santos, PhD

A 19-year-old woman with no relevant medical history came to the hospital with typical chest pain that had started while she was running. Her electrocardiogram showed significant ST-segment elevation in inferior and V_4 to V_6 leads (Fig. 1.21). In the transthoracic echocardiogram examination the left ventricle (LV) inferior segments were hypokinetic and the right ventricle (RV) systolic function was mildly impaired. Urgent coronary angiography was performed, revealing right coronary artery (RCA) arising from a single ostium in the left sinus of Valsalva (Fig. 1.21, Online Video 1.25). Computed tomography coronary angiography confirmed this finding, demonstrating a sharpened proximal RCA coursing between the aortic root and pulmonary artery (Fig. 1.22A–B). A significant increase

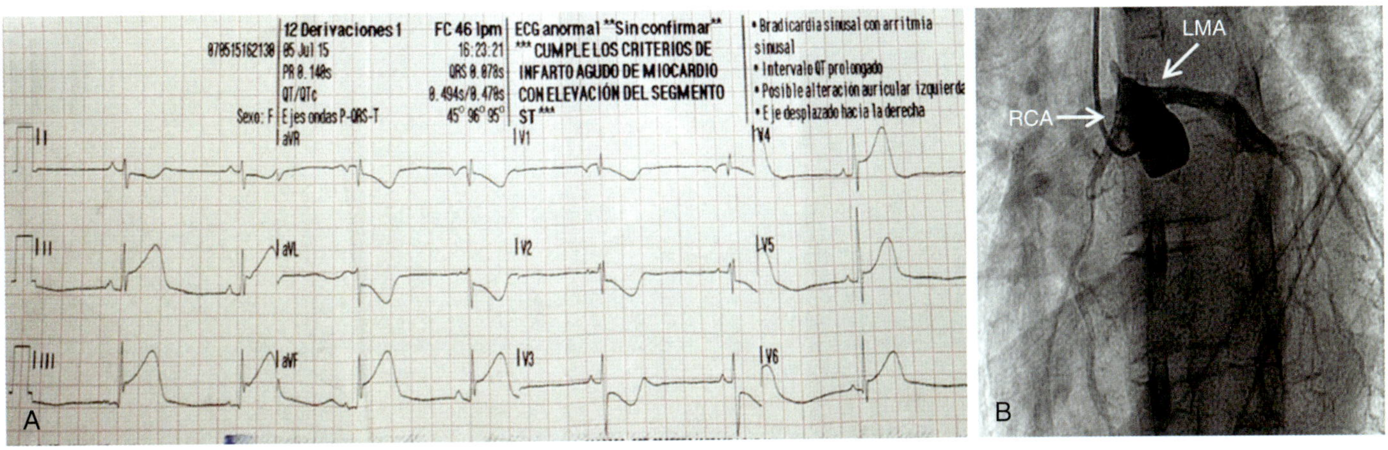

FIG. 1.21 Urgent Electrocardiogram and Coronary Angiography Findings. (A) Electrocardiogram showing signs of myocardial ischemia. (B) Coronary angiography reveals the anomalous origin of the right coronary artery (*RCA*) from the left sinus of Valsalva (Online Video 1.25). *LMA*, left main artery.

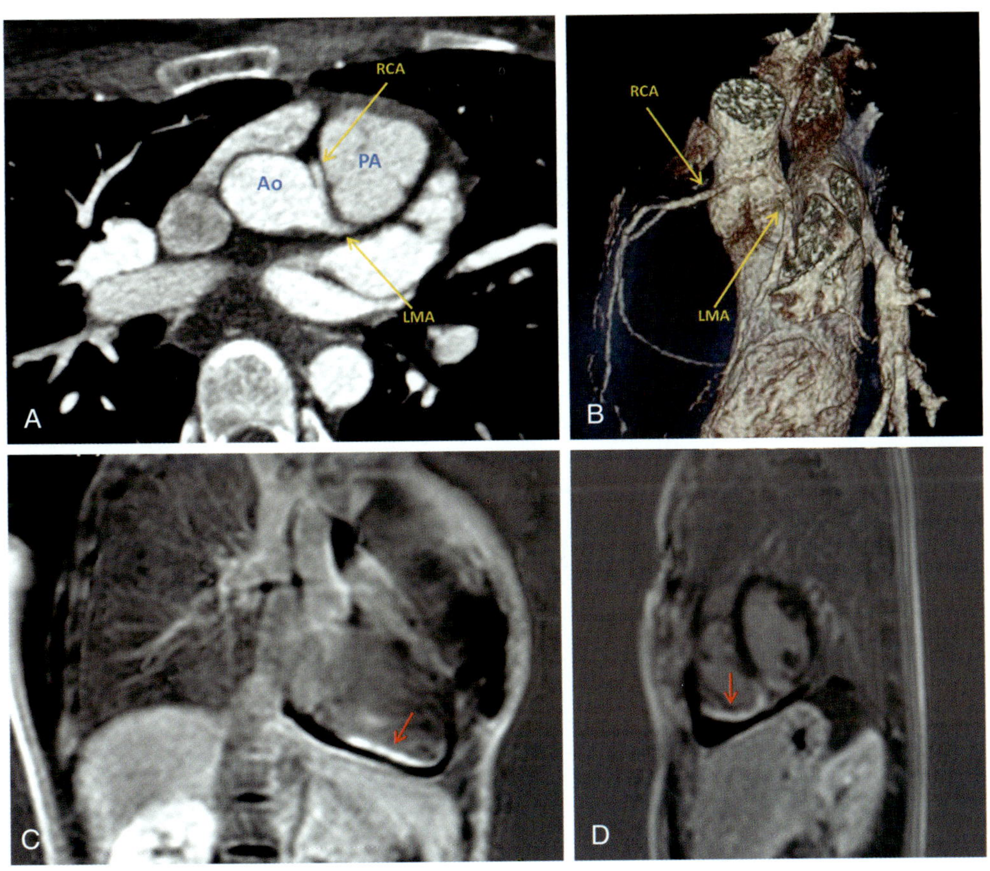

FIG. 1.22 Findings on the Imaging Studies: Computed Tomography Coronary Angiography and Cardiac Magnetic Resonance. (A and B) Computed tomography coronary angiography showing anomalous origin and course of the right coronary artery (*RCA*) between the aortic root (*Ao*) and pulmonary artery (*PA*). (C and D) Cardiac magnetic resonance views demonstrating subendocardial late gadolinium enhancement (*red arrows*). *LMA*, left main artery.

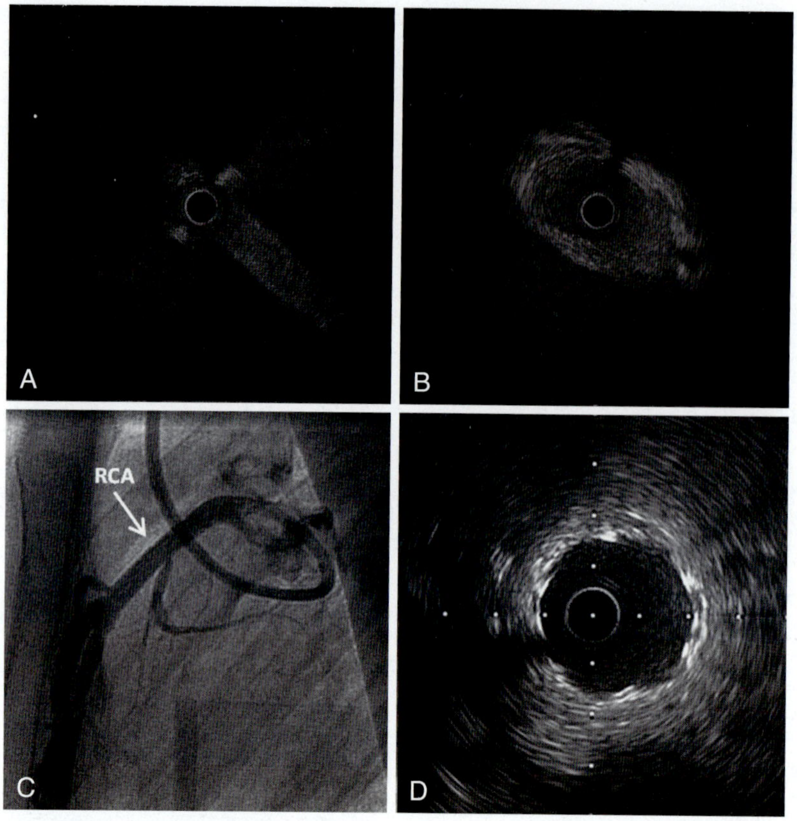

FIG. 1.23 Intravascular Ultrasound Image of the Proximal Right Coronary Artery (RCA). (A and B) Image of the systolic compression and diastolic decompression of the proximal 20 mm. (C) Implanted drug-eluting stent. (D) Intravascular ultrasound of the proximal RCA after stent angioplasty with the area expanded and optimal angiographic result (Online Videos 1.26–1.28).

of myocardial necrosis marker was observed (total creatine kinase 1207 IU/L, troponin I 271.73 μg/L). Cardiac magnetic resonance showed a subendocardial area of delayed gadolinium enhancement in the inferior LV wall and the RV (Fig. 1.22C–D).

Given these findings, intervention was justified; therefore, a complete evaluation was performed to establish the treatment options. A second coronary angiography with intravascular ultrasound (IVUS) was performed for further evaluation. The IVUS results proved systolic compression and diastolic decompression of the proximal 20 mm of RCA. A 3 × 28-mm drug-eluting stent was directly implanted in the site of the compression with optimal angiographic result and adequate expansion demonstrated by IVUS (Fig. 1.23, Online Videos 1.26–1.28). Before discharge, an exercise stress test result was normal and systolic LV and RV function was normalized on the echocardiogram. The patient was treated with instructions to take dual-antiplatelet therapy for at least 6 months. In symptomatic patients with anomalous origin of the RCA, intervention is indicated. In this case, integration of clinical presentation with the findings in imaging techniques was essential to decide the best management strategy.

Coronary Aneurysms

A Giant Coronary Artery Aneurysm Treated With a New-Generation Drug-Eluting Stent

Krysthel Engstrom, MD, Asaad A. Khan, MD, Gina LaRocca, MD, MHSC, Annapoorna S. Kini, MD, Samin K. Sharma, MD

A 40-year-old man came to our facility with progressive angina 1 month after an unsuccessful attempt at right coronary artery (RCA) revascularization after a non–ST-segment elevation myocardial infarction. Coronary angiography revealed a dominant RCA with a very large aneurysm in the mid segment that was totally occluded (Fig. 1.24). The distal vessel was large, with mild atherosclerotic disease filling via bridging collateral vessels. The left anterior descending and circumflex coronary arteries were ectatic and large vessels.

The RCA was treated with a Synergy (Boston Scientific, Natick, Massachusetts) 4.0/38-mm stent with excellent angiographic results. Computed tomography angiography confirmed the presence of a

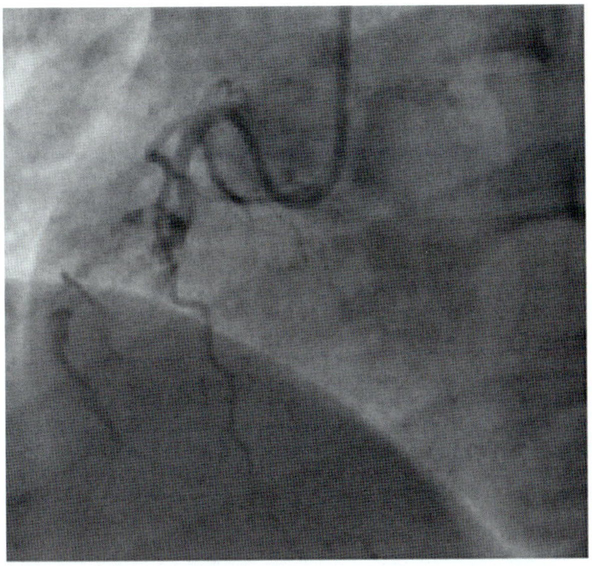

FIG. 1.24 Coronary Angiography of the Right Coronary Artery (RCA). The image shows a totally occluded RCA with a very large aneurysm in the mid segment.

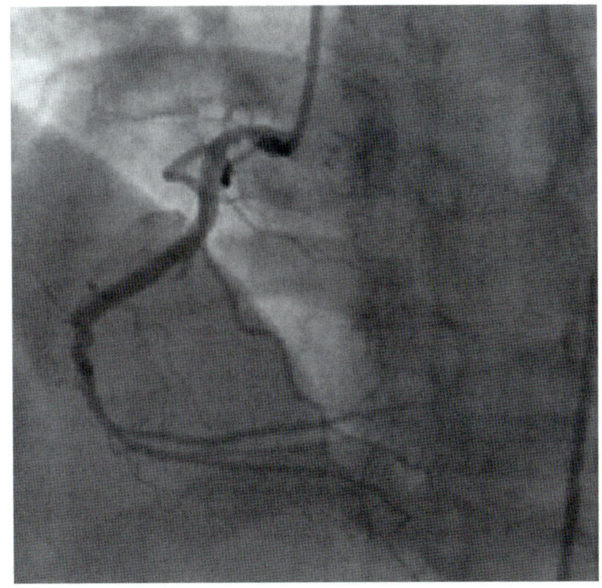

FIG. 1.26 Angiography at 6 Months. Angiography at 6 months showing a patent right coronary artery stent with good distal flow.

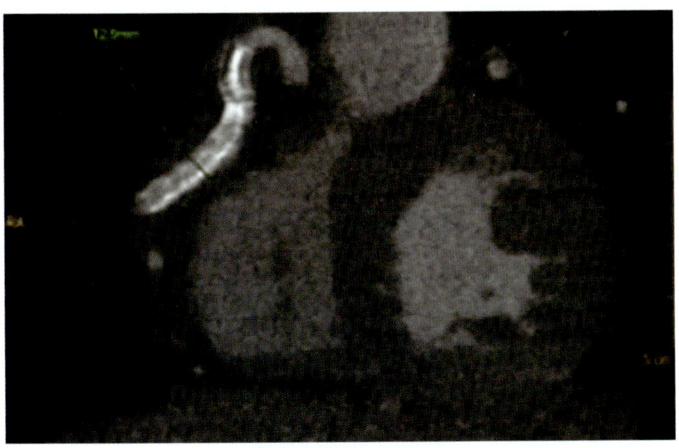

FIG. 1.25 Computed Tomography (CT) Angiography of the Aneurysm. CT angiography confirmed the presence of a giant aneurysm measuring 12.9 mm in diameter with a patent stent.

giant aneurysm measuring 12.9 × 19 mm (Fig. 1.25). Angiography at 6 months showed a patent stent with good distal flow and no flow into the aneurysm (Fig. 1.26).

Covered stents have been used for percutaneous treatment of coronary aneurysms despite poor short- and long-term outcomes.[1-3] In view of our patient's age, we decided to treat the thrombosed aneurysm with a drug-eluting stent. This novel use of a drug-eluting stent in symptomatic, young patients with a coronary aneurysm and complex anatomy proved to be a successful and relatively safe approach with potentially better long-term outcomes.

References

1. Boyer N, Gupta R, Schevchuck A, et al. Coronary artery aneurysms in acute coronary syndrome: case series, review, and proposed management strategy. *J Invasive Cardiol.* 2014;26:283-290.
2. Heuser RR, Diethrich EB, Papaoglou C, Reynolds GT. Endoluminal grafting for percutaneous aneurysm exclusion in an aortocoronary saphenous vein graft: the first clinical experience. *J Endovasc Surg.* 1995;2:81-88.
3. Heuser RR. Treatment for coronary aneurysms: twenty years of experience with covered stents. *J Invasive Cardiol.* 2015;27:E36.

Acute Myocardial Infarction Caused by Left Main Coronary Artery Compression as a Result of a Mycotic Aneurysm of the Sinus of Valsalva

Kenji Goto, MD, Hideo Takebayashi, MD, PhD, Shogo Mukai, MD, PhD, Hiroki Yamane, MD, Arata Hagikura, MD, Yoshimasa Morimoto, MD, Yuetsu Kikuta, MD, Katsumasa Sato, MD, Masahito Taniguchi, MD, Shigeki Hiramatsu, MD, PhD, Seiichi Haruta, MD

An 83-year-old woman with a history of fever had severe chest pain progressing to cardiogenic shock. Her electrocardiogram showed evidence of anteroseptal myocardial infarction (MI). Urgent coronary angiography, with intraaortic balloon pump support, indicated total occlusion of the left main trunk (LMT) (Fig. 1.27A). Drug-eluting stents were successfully implanted from the LMT into the proximal left anterior descending (LAD) coronary artery (Fig. 1.27C). Subsequently, computed tomography (CT) angiography was performed to understand the etiology of acute MI, because the LAD with no plaque was determined to be compressed from the outside, on the basis of preprocedural intravascular ultrasonography (Fig. 1.27B, a–d). CT demonstrated a 4 × 3 cm aneurysm with a 1-cm wide neck from the left sinus of Valsalva (SVA) causing external compression of the LMT (Fig. 1.28). Because subsequent SVA rupture may have led to acute hemodynamic instability, early elective surgical treatment of the SVA was considered. Surgery

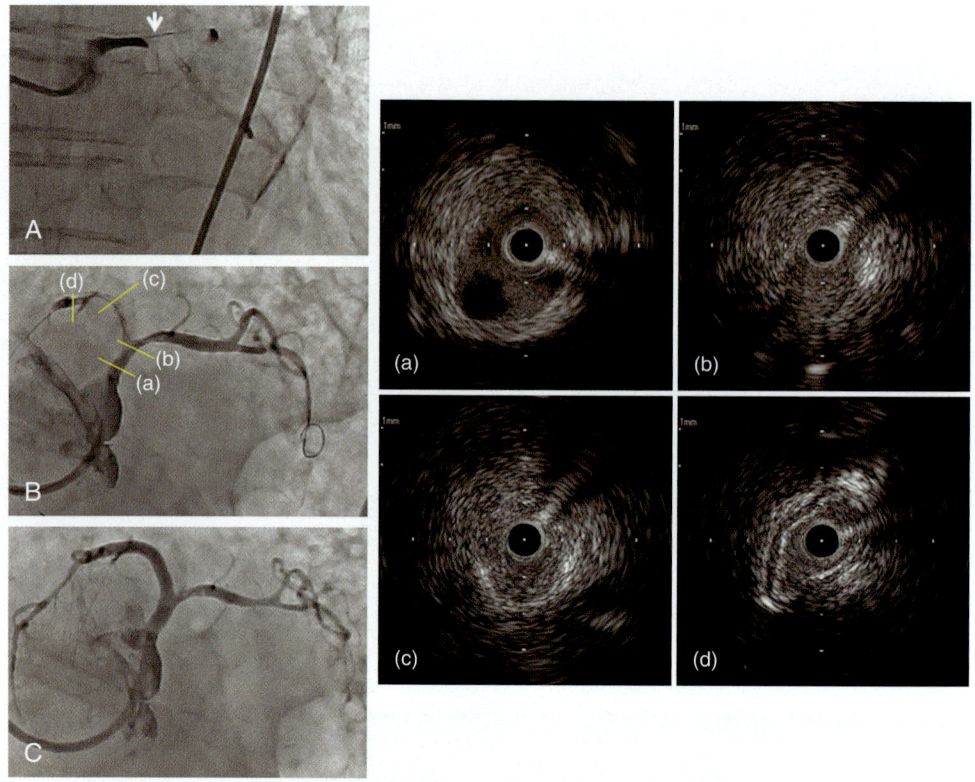

FIG. 1.27 Findings of Coronary Angiography and Intravascular Ultrasound. (A) Urgent coronary angiography showing total occlusion of the left main trunk (*white arrow*). (B) Coronary flow remained limited even after the guidewire crossed over the culprit lesion (spider view). Intravascular ultrasound showed that the distal left anterior descending coronary artery lumen was flattened, causing severe fusiform stenosis (d). Although the lumen of the left main trunk was not compromised (a), the proximal thorough midsection of the left anterior descending coronary artery was obstructed, as if compressed from the outside (b and c). (C) Thrombolysis in myocardial infarction flow grade 3 was obtained after stent implantation.

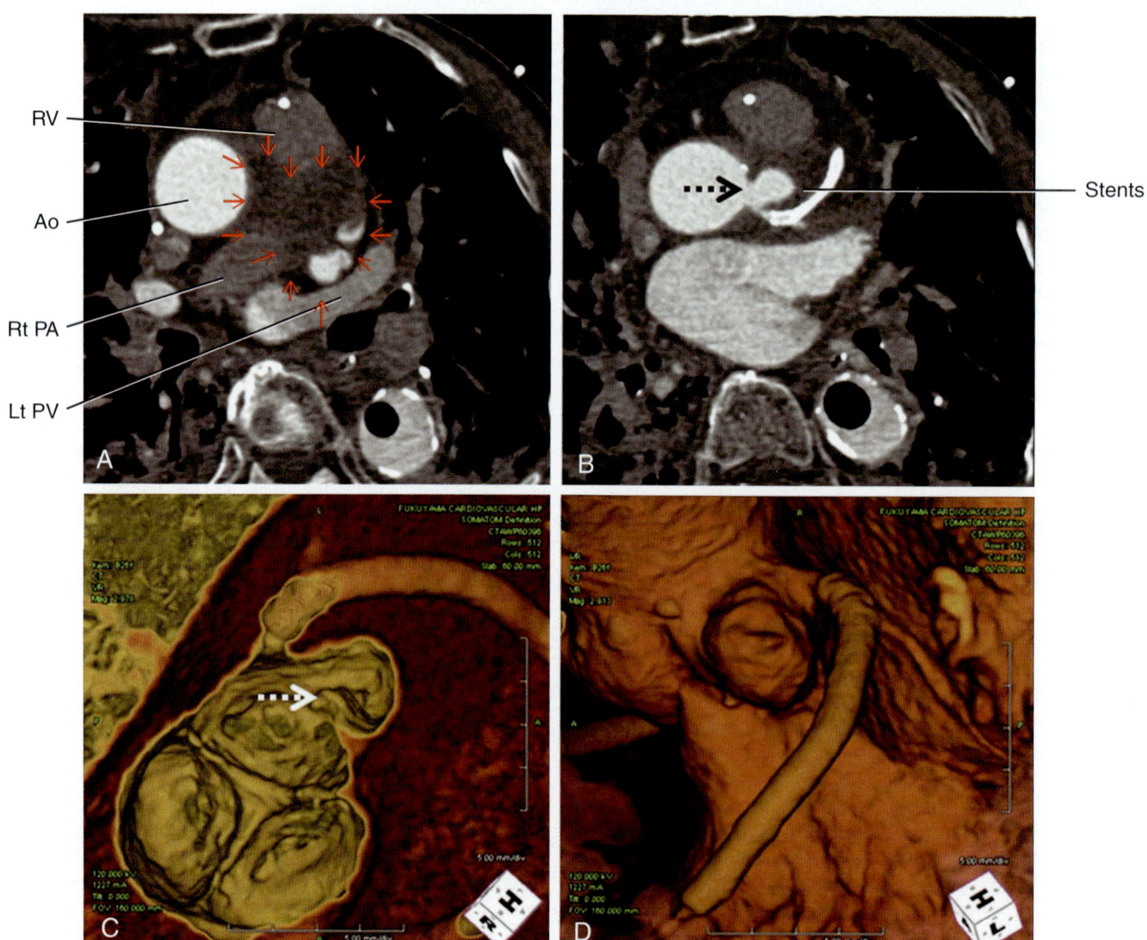

FIG. 1.28 Findings of Computed Tomography. Poststenting computed tomography (A and B: axial view; C and D: volume-rendered reconstruction) demonstrated a 3 × 4 cm aneurysm that protruded between the left atrium and pulmonary trunk and compressed the left main trunk (*red arrows* in [A]). The mouth of the aneurysm was located next to the left coronary ostium (*dotted arrow* B, C). *Ao,* aorta; *Lt PV,* left pulmonary vein; *Rt PA,* right pulmonary artery; *RV,* right ventricle.

(aortocoronary bypass surgery and aortic root reconstruction) was performed successfully and confirmed the presence of the SVA, which contained organized thrombus and pus and was directly compressing the LMT. Because antibiotics were administered before surgery, acquired etiologic factors were not detected. Echocardiography after the operation showed a normal aortic root with no aortic regurgitation, and left ventricular function had improved. The patient died as a result of deterioration of interstitial pneumonia 2 weeks after surgery.

Acute MI resulting from compression of the LMT associated with a left mycotic SVA is extremely rare and often carries a poor prognosis.[1-4] The proposed pathophysiologic mechanism in this case was that the infective aneurysm of the left coronary cusp in the SVA may have caused weakness in the tunica media layer, leading to rapid expansion. This, in turn, may have precipitated the MI, as well as the cardiogenic shock. Both intravascular ultrasound and CT can play an important role in achieving an accurate and rapid diagnosis.

References

1. Lijoi A, Parodi E, Passerone GC, Scarano F, Caruso D, Iannetti MV. Unruptured aneurysm of the left sinus of Valsalva causing coronary insufficiency: case report and review of the literature. *Tex Heart Inst J.* 2002;29:40-444.
2. Ott DA. Aneurysm of the sinus of Valsalva. *Semin Thorac Cardiovasc Surg Pediatr Card Surg Annu.* 2006;9:165-176.
3. Regueiro Abel M, Penas Lado M, López Ciudid V, Castro Beiras A. Sinus of Valsalva aneurysm as a cause of acute myocardial infarction [in Spanish]. *Rev Esp Cardiol.* 2002;55:77-79.
4. Hausinger P, Sasi V, Volford G, et al. Unruptured aneurysm of the left sinus of Valsalva compressing the left main coronary artery: successful percutaneous treatment. *Herz.* 2014;39:770-773.

Formation of Infectious Coronary Artery Aneurysms After Percutaneous Coronary Intervention in a Patient With Acute Myocardial Infarction as the Result of Septic Embolism

Nobuaki Kobayashi, MD, PhD, Yusaku Shibata, MD, Noritake Hata, MD, PhD, Wataru Shimizu, MD, PhD

A 68-year-old man who underwent aortic valve replacement (biological valve, Carpentier-Edwards Perimount Magna aortic bioprosthesis 21 mm, Edwards Lifesciences, Irvine, California) for aortic valve regurgitation without coronary artery disease 5 months earlier was admitted to our institution because of prolonged fever. Fifteen hours after admission, he suddenly experienced severe chest pain with ST-segment elevation in the lateral and aVR leads. Emergency coronary angiography (CAG) showed a contrast medium filling defect for the left main trunk (LMT), the proximal left anterior descending coronary artery (LAD), the ostial left circumflex coronary artery (LCx), and the ramus intermedius artery (RA) (Fig. 1.29, Online Video 1.29). Owing to insufficient intracoronary aspiration, a stent was implanted at the LMT and proximal LAD. After using the kissing balloon technique for the LAD and LCx, acceptable coronary flow for the LAD and LCx was obtained, although the RA was occluded (Fig. 1.30A–B, Online Videos 1.30 and 1.31). On the basis of the Duke criteria (i.e., more than two positive blood cultures [*Staphylococcus epidermidis*], predisposing heart condition, fever, and major arterial embolism), a diagnosis of prosthetic valve endocarditis and subsequent myocardial infarction as the result coronary artery septic embolism was made. The infection was controlled by intravenous vancomycin administration for more than 2 months. CAG performed 1 year later showed a giant aneurysm with coronary flow disturbance in the RA and a small aneurysm in the LMT (Fig, 1.30C–D, Online Videos 1.32 and 1.33). Repeated CAG performed after 5 years of careful clinical follow-up showed that the giant coronary artery disappeared in association with the RA occlusion, and the small aneurysm in the LMT remained unchanged (Fig. 1.30E–F, Online Videos 1.34 and 1.35).

Although some reports have previously described coronary embolization caused by infectious endocarditis,[1-4] none showed aneurysm formation in the culprit coronary artery during follow-up. The possible mechanism responsible for the aneurysm formation was infectious embolism. In the current case, long-term angiographic follow-up demonstrated that the infectious aneurysms did not deteriorate.

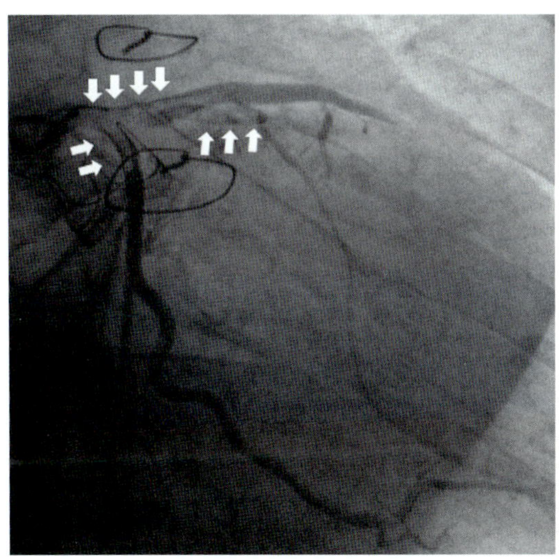

FIG. 1.29 Initial Coronary Angiography. Initial coronary angiography showing the contrast medium filling defect (*white arrows*) for the left main trunk, the proximal left anterior descending artery, the ramus intermedius artery, and the ostial left circumflex artery (Online Video 1.29).

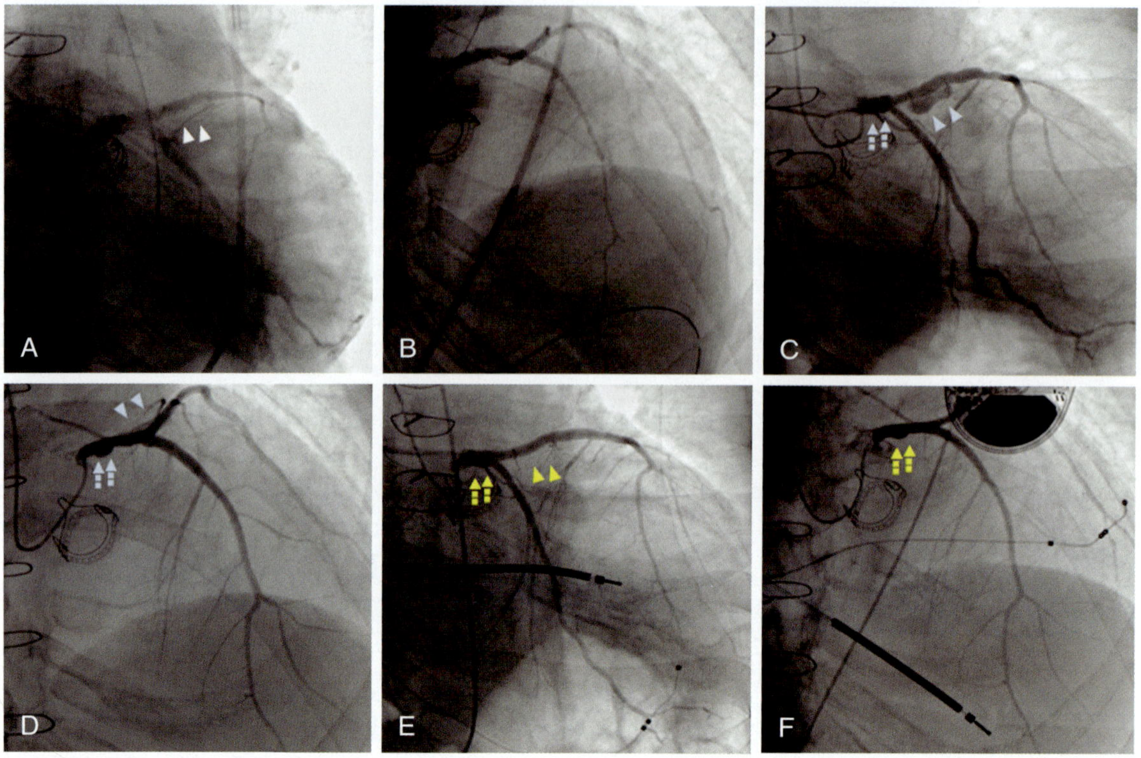

FIG. 1.30 Serial Coronary Artery Images Over 6 Years. (A and B) Poststenting coronary angiography (CAG) showing acceptable coronary flow for the left anterior descending coronary artery and left circumflex coronary artery and occluded ramus intermedius artery (RA) (*white arrowheads*) (Online Videos 1.30 and 1.31). (C and D) CAG performed 1 year after the intervention showing the giant coronary artery aneurysm with flow disturbance in the RA (*blue arrowheads*) and small aneurysm in the left main trunk (*blue dashed arrows*) (Online Videos 1.32 and 1.33). (E and F) Repeated CAG performed 6 years after the intervention showing the disappearance of giant coronary aneurysm in association with the RA occlusion (*yellow arrowheads*) and the small aneurysm in the left main trunk, which had not worsened (*yellow dashed arrows*) (Online Videos 1.34 and 1.35).

References

1. Jeremias A, Casserly I, Estess JM, Smedira NG, Topol EJ. Acute myocardial infarction after aortic valve endocarditis. *Am J Med.* 2001;110:417-418.
2. Bracco D, Noiseux N, Duong P, Prieto I, Basile F. Aortic vegetation and acute coronary embolism. *Can J Cardiol.* 2006;22:113.
3. Motreff P, Roux A, Souteyrand G. Aspiration therapy in septic coronary embolism complicating infectious endocarditis. *Heart.* 2010;96:809.
4. Roxas CJ, Weekes AJ. Acute myocardial infarction caused by coronary embolism from infective endocarditis. *J Emerg Med.* 2011;40:509-514.

Left Internal Mammary Artery Graft Decompression by Covered Stent Treatment of an Adjacent Saphenous Vein Graft Pseudoaneurysm

Richard Pearl, MD, Mustafa Hassan, MD, R. David Anderson, MD, MS

A 75-year-old man with a history of coronary artery bypass grafting and recent pacemaker site infection was transferred to our institution for treatment of a descending aortic pseudoaneurysm. A computed tomography scan performed on arrival also revealed a suspected mycotic aneurysm of the saphenous vein bypass graft to the circumflex coronary artery. After consultation with infectious disease specialists, the descending aortic pseudoaneurysm was treated with an endograft, and the patient underwent cardiac catheterization. This revealed not only the pseudoaneurysm of the saphenous vein bypass graft to the circumflex artery (Fig. 1.31), but also associated compression of the left internal mammary artery graft to the left anterior descending coronary artery (Fig. 1.32). Additionally, the patient was found to have an ischemic cardiomyopathy with an ejection fraction of 30% and anteroapical hypokinesis. Ventricular function had been normal just a few months earlier. The patient was deemed not to be a surgical candidate. After a complete course of antibiotic therapy for methicillin-susceptible *Staphylococcus aureus*, repeat discussion with infectious disease specialists, and institutional review board approval for their off-label use, two Jostent GraftMaster (Abbott Vascular, Abbott Park, Illinois) stents were implanted in the saphenous vein graft to the native circumflex coronary artery (Fig. 1.33). This excluded the pseudoaneurysm, restored normal flow to the distal native circumflex artery (Fig. 1.34), and within 1 week resulted in decompression of the left internal mammary artery to the left anterior descending artery (Fig. 1.35). The patient was discharged home using long-term dual-antiplatelet and suppressive antibiotic

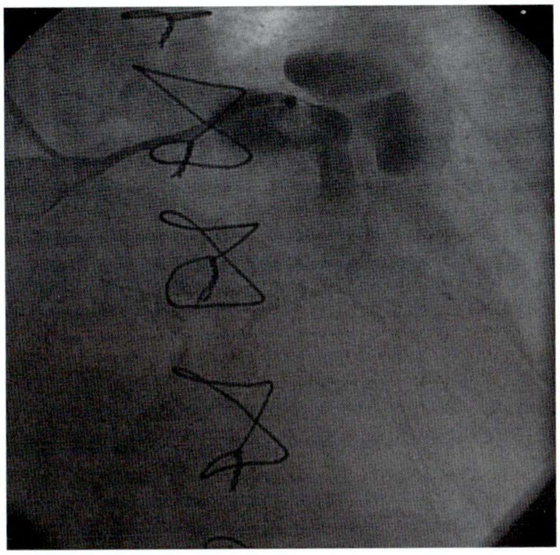

FIG. 1.31 Pseudoaneurysm of the Saphenous Vein Graft to the Obtuse Marginal Branch. A rapidly filling pseudoaneurysm of the saphenous vein graft to the obtuse marginal branch with poor distal filling was found on diagnostic coronary angiography.

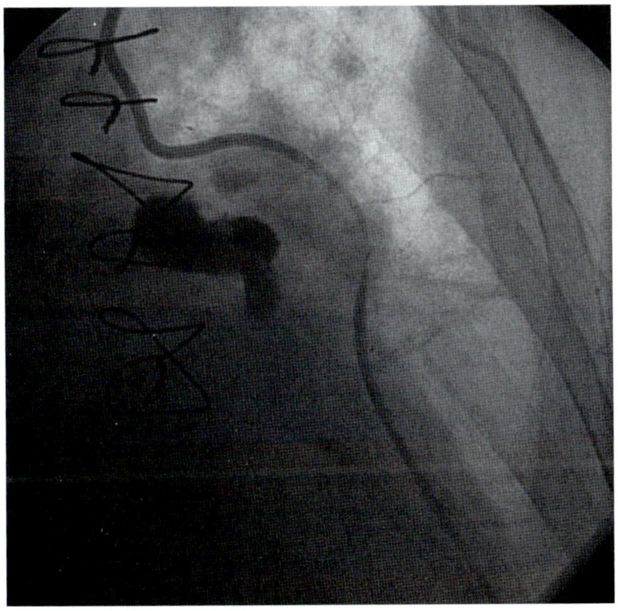

FIG. 1.32 Left Internal Mammary Artery Compressed by Large Pseudoaneurysm. The left internal mammary artery graft appeared to be compressed by the large pseudoaneurysm.

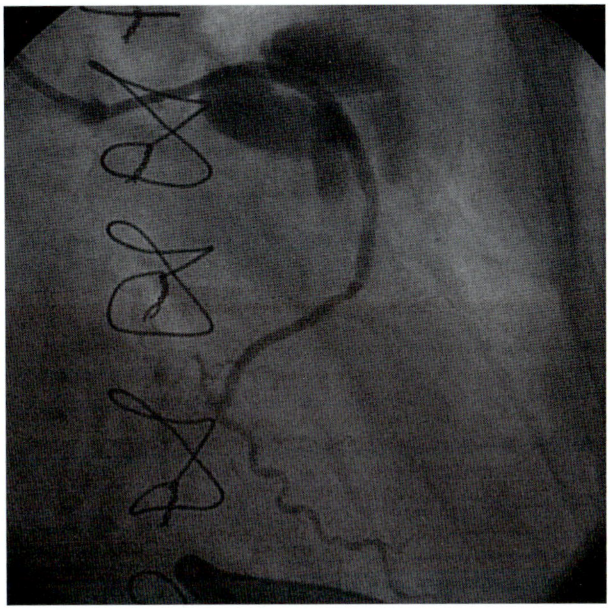

FIG. 1.33 Angiography of the Saphenous Vein Graft 5 Days After Intervention. Angiography of the saphenous vein graft to the circumflex marginal 5 days after the intervention. The pseudoaneurysm is no longer seen.

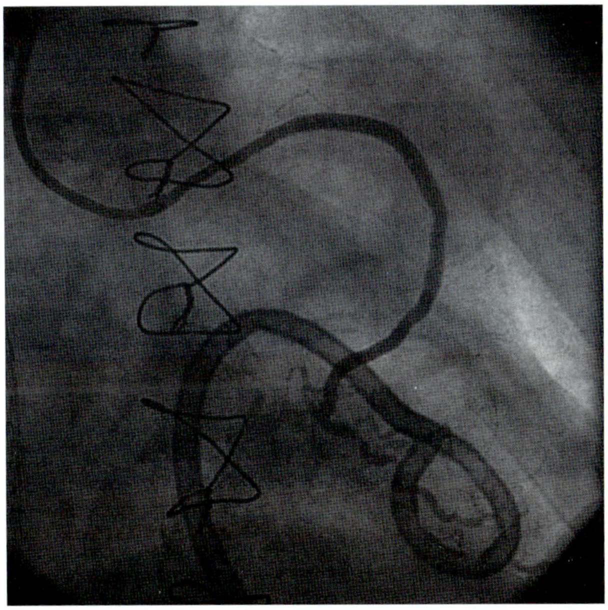

FIG. 1.34 PostIntervention Image Showing Restoration of Flow to the Obtuse Marginal. An immediate postintervention image of the saphenous vein graft showing restoration of the flow in the distal native circumflex marginal with residual contrast in the excluded cavity.

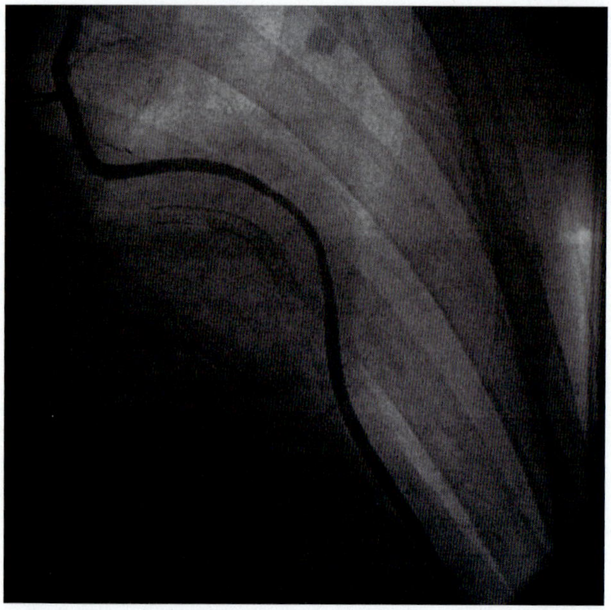

FIG. 1.35 Angiography of Left Internal Mammary Artery Graft 5 Days After Intervention. Angiography of the left internal mammary artery graft 5 days after the vein graft pseudoaneurysm was treated. The previously observed compression along the course of the left internal mammary artery is much improved.

therapy. Follow-up echocardiography revealed normal left ventricular function.

Mycotic aneurysms remain an uncommon clinical occurrence, usually in the setting of infective endocarditis or endovascular infections. There are only a few case reports of mycotic aneurysms of the native coronary arteries and fewer in bypass grafts.[1-4] Surgical treatment has been the mainstay of therapy but carries a high risk for those patients with multiple comorbidities. The percutaneous approach used in this patient offers a suitable alternative to surgery, but the long-term risk of recurrent infection is unknown.

References

1. Kapur NK, Conte JV, Wittstein IS. Successful management of an unruptured mycotic coronary aneurysm. *J Invasive Cardiol.* 2007;19: E366-368.
2. Le MQ, Narins CR. Mycotic pseudoaneurysm of the left circumflex coronary artery: a fatal complication following drug-eluting stent implantation. *Catheter Cardiovasc Interv.* 2007;69:508-512.
3. Geneidy AA, Weise WJ. Coronary artery bypass graft mycotic aneurysms in a dialysis patient. *Am J Kidney Dis.* 2005;46:962-926.
4. Hirsch GA, Johnston PV, Conte JV Jr, Achuff SC. Mycotic aortocoronary saphenous vein graft aneurysm presenting with unstable angina pectoris. *Ann Thorac Surg.* 2004;78:1456-1458.

Recurrent Myocardial Infarctions as a Result of Thrombosis of a Coronary Aneurysm in Neurofibromatosis Type 1: Is Antiplatelet Treatment Enough?

Javier Molina-Martin de Nicolas, MD, Alfonso Jurado Roman, MD, Belen Rubio Alonso, MD, Julio Garcia Tejada, MD

A 68-year-old woman was admitted for an anterolateral myocardial infarction (MI). She had neurofibromatosis type 1 and 2 previous hospitalizations for non–ST-segment elevation MI that was medically treated. In those episodes, aneurysmal coronary arteries with fresh thrombus in left anterior descending artery were described.

Emergent coronary angiography revealed a giant aneurysm in the mid left anterior descending artery with multiple small fresh thrombi (Fig. 1.36A–C, Online Videos 1.36–1.38). There was thrombolysis in myocardial infarction grade flow 3 and no significant stenosis. Aneurysmal dilations without significant stenosis were also observed in the right coronary and circumflex arteries (Fig. 1.36A–D). Triple-antiplatelet therapy (aspirin, clopidogrel, abciximab [intracoronary bolus and 12-hour perfusion]) and anticoagulation (enoxaparin 60 mg twice a day) medications were administered.

One week later, scheduled coronary angiography showed a complete angiographic resolution of the thrombus (Fig. 1.36E–F, Online Videos 1.39 and 1.40). No percutaneous coronary intervention was performed. Given that this episode was the third MI in aneurysmal coronary arteries, we decided to continue permanent anticoagulation and double-antiplatelet therapy for 1 year. Fourteen months later, the patient remains asymptomatic without any event.

Vascular manifestations of neurofibromatosis type 1 consist of aneurysmal and stenotic abnormalities that can affect different arterial territories.[1] Although effects on coronary arteries are extremely rare, coronary aneurysms have been described and can cause MI by thrombosis, vasospasm, and stenosis.[2] No consensus exists regarding the treatment, and several percutaneous coronary interventions (thromboaspiration, stent implantation) and

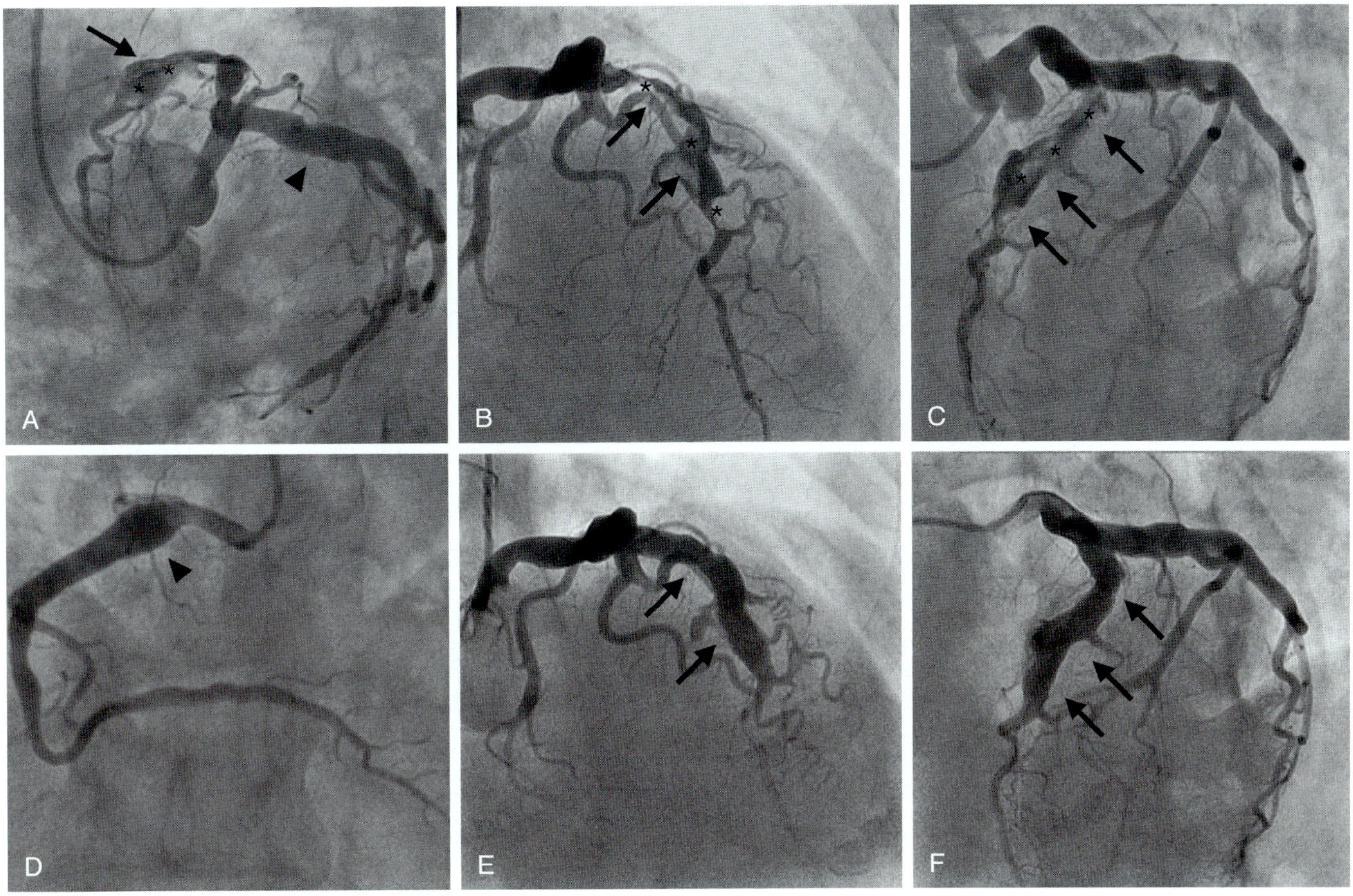

FIG. 1.36 Emergent and After Treatment Coronary Angiograms. Emergent coronary angiograms (A–C, Online Videos 1.36–1.38). Scheduled coronary angiography 1 week later (D–F, Online Videos 1.39 and 1.40). Arrows indicate the giant left anterior descending artery aneurysm. *Asterisks* indicate multiple small fresh thrombi. Arrowheads indicate aneurysmal dilations in the right coronary and circumflex arteries.

antithrombotic regimens have been used.[3] If thrombolysis in myocardial infarction grade flow 3 is preserved and no significant stenosis exists, a conservative management with antithrombotics and permanent anticoagulation may be the best option and could reduce further events.

References

1. Trevelyan J, Been M, Patel R. Multiple coronary aneurysms in a patient with neurofibromatosis type 1: case report and intravascular ultrasound of aneurysm. *Postgrad Med J*. 2001;77:45-47.
2. Syed M, Lesch M. Coronary artery aneurysm: a review. *Prog Cardiovasc Dis*. 1997;40:77-84.
3. Smith A, Araoz PA, Kirsch J. Coronary arterial aneurysms in neurofibromatosis 1: case report and review of the literature. *J Thorac Imaging*. 2009;24:129-31.

Salmonella enteritidis Mycotic Aneurysm of Stented Saphenous Vein Graft to Coronary Artery

Arka Chatterjee, MD, Jeremy S. White, MD, Benjamin Tuck, MD, James E. Davies, Jr, MD

A 67-year-old man with a history of hypertension and coronary artery disease (requiring aortocoronary bypass 18 years earlier and multiple percutaneous coronary interventions) came to a referring hospital with chief symptoms of fever, chills, and diaphoresis after a recent gastrointestinal illness. Blood cultures obtained revealed *Salmonella* bacteremia. Transesophageal echocardiography revealed no evidence of endocarditis and he was treated with intravenous ciprofloxacin.

One month after discharge, he returned with recurrent fevers with blood cultures revealing recurrent *Salmonella* growth. He started an outpatient course of intravenous ceftriaxone before developing increased shortness of breath prompting his return. His

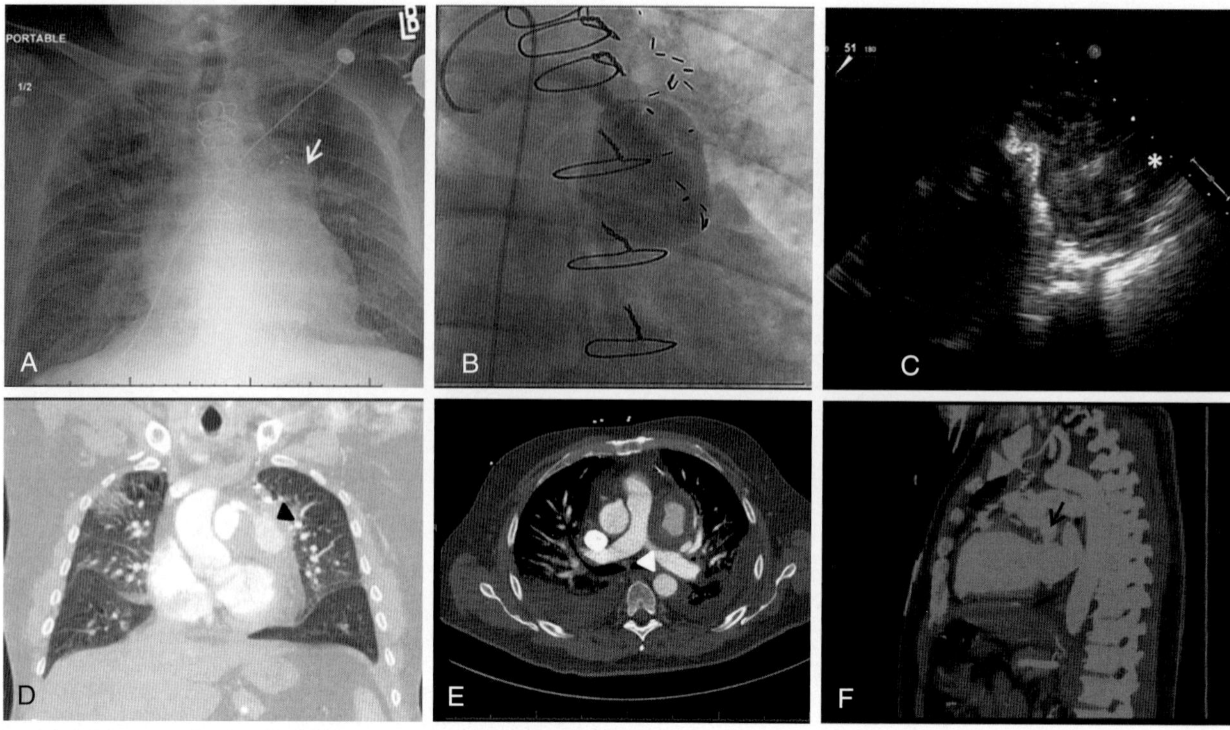

FIG. 1.37 Stent-Related Mycotic Aneurysm. (A) Chest radiograph showing pulmonary edema and enlargement of the left atrial shadow (*white arrow*). (B) Angiogram showing large aneurysm of stented saphenous vein graft (Online Video 1.41). (C) Transesophageal echocardiograph demonstrating echogenic mass/thrombus in the left atrial appendage (*asterisk*). (D) Computed tomography angiogram delineating origin of fistulous tract from aneurysm of the saphenous vein graft (*black arrowhead*). (E) Aneurysm abutting the main pulmonary artery (*white arrowhead*). (F) Rupture of aneurysm into left atrium/left atrial appendage (*black arrow*).

physical examination showed increased jugular venous pressure and marked crackles in both lungs; a chest radiograph showed pulmonary edema and enlargement of the left atrium (Fig. 1.37A). Troponin I was elevated at 63 ng/mL. A transthoracic echocardiogram revealed a reduced ejection fraction of 30% to 35%. Coronary angiography showed severe native 3-vessel disease with a patent left internal mammary graft to the left anterior descending artery, saphenous vein graft (SVG) to the right coronary artery, as well as an occluded vein graft to the diagonal. More notably, angiography of the SVG to the first obtuse marginal branch showed a large aneurysm (Fig. 1.37B) around a previously stented segment in the body that had ruptured into the left atrium/left atrial appendage (Online Video 1.41).

The patient was transferred subsequently to our institution for further evaluation and surgical treatment. Transesophageal echocardiography (Fig. 1.37C) revealed a 6.5 × 5 cm mass invading the left atrial appendage. A computed tomography angiogram of his chest (Fig. 1.37D–F) was obtained and showed a large thick-walled contrast collection along the left margin of the main pulmonary artery, which appeared to communicate with the left atrial appendage. Direct observation during surgery revealed a ruptured SVG aneurysm communicating with the pulmonary artery and left atrial appendage. The SVG aneurysm was resected successfully with repair of the left atrial appendage and the main pulmonary artery. Culture of his saphenous venous aneurysm identified *Salmonella enteritidis*. He had an uncomplicated postoperative course and was discharged 7 days after surgery receiving intravenous ceftriaxone for 6 weeks followed by chronic suppressive therapy with oral amoxicillin-clavulanic acid. A repeat computed tomography angiogram was performed 2 months after surgery, which showed no new signs of fluid collection or infection.

Coronary stent infection is a rare complication with only 17 documented cases from 1990 to 2012.[1] Nontyphoidal *Salmonella* is a rare cause of bacteremia and an even rarer cause of mycotic aneurysms in atherosclerotic vessel.[2] A stented vessel may be an additional risk factor for developing such a complication, and a high index of suspicion should be maintained for patients not clearing *Salmonella* bacteremia despite optimal antimicrobial therapy. Multiple imaging modalities may be needed to confirm a diagnosis of coronary stent infection. Transesophageal echocardiography may reveal an aneurysm, but coronary angiography/computed tomography angiography is almost always required to confirm the diagnosis and detect complications such as vessel aneurysm or pseudoaneurysm. Positron emission tomography computed tomography is an active area of interest in diagnosis because it may be used to reveal occult inflammation surrounding the stent. Surgical excision is almost always required, especially in stent-related infections that occur remotely after implantation.[3]

References

1. Elieson M, Mixon T, Carpenter J. Coronary stent infections: a case report and literature review. *Tex Heart Inst J.* 2012;39:884-849.
2. Wang JH, Liu YC, Yen MY, et al. Mycotic aneurysm due to nontyphi *Salmonella*: report of 16 cases. *Clin Infec Dis.* 1996;23:743-747.
3. Sekhar S, Vupputuri A, Nair RC, Palaniswamy SS, Natarajan KU. Coronary stent infection successfully diagnosed using 18F-flurodeoxyglucose positron emission tomography computed tomography. *Can J Cardiol.* 2016;32:1575.e1-1575.e3.

Sinus of Valsalva Aneurysm Causing Extrinsic Compression of the Left Main Coronary Artery

Vishal J. Dahya, MD, Prasad Chalasani, MD

An 84-year-old woman with aortic valve stenosis was seen after a month-long history of midsternal chest pain with exertion that was relieved with rest. Stress testing was performed and revealed possible ischemia in the anterior wall. She then underwent coronary angiography and was found to have a giant aneurysm of the left sinus of Valsalva (Fig. 1.38) causing critical left main coronary artery compression (Fig. 1.39). Computed tomographic angiography revealed similar findings, which led to the diagnosis of crescendo angina secondary to extrinsic compression of the left main coronary from the giant sinus aneurysm (Fig. 1.40). She was emergently taken to the operating room, and the aorta was opened obliquely with wide exposure of the aortic root and aortic valve leaflets. The "mouth" of the aneurysm was identified, and the rim of the aneurysm was noted to be involved with the annular segment of the left coronary leaflet, as well as with the bottom of the left coronary ostia (Fig. 1.41). A tailor patch of the native pericardium was sewn in to completely close the mouth of the aneurysm.

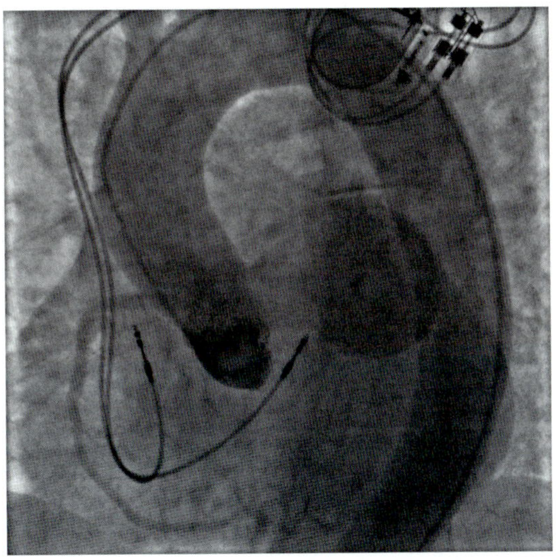

FIG. 1.38 Coronary Angiography of the Aneurysm. Preoperative imaging revealing a giant aneurysm of the left sinus of Valsalva.

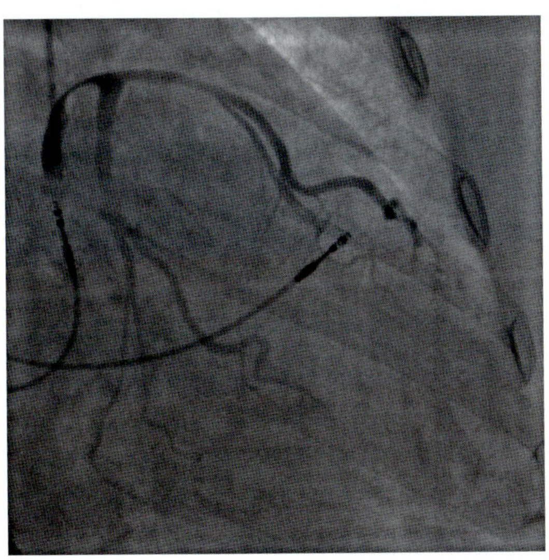

FIG. 1.39 Coronary Angiography of the Left Main Artery. Selective angiogram revealing extrinsic compression of the left main coronary artery by the giant aneurysm of the left sinus of Valsalva.

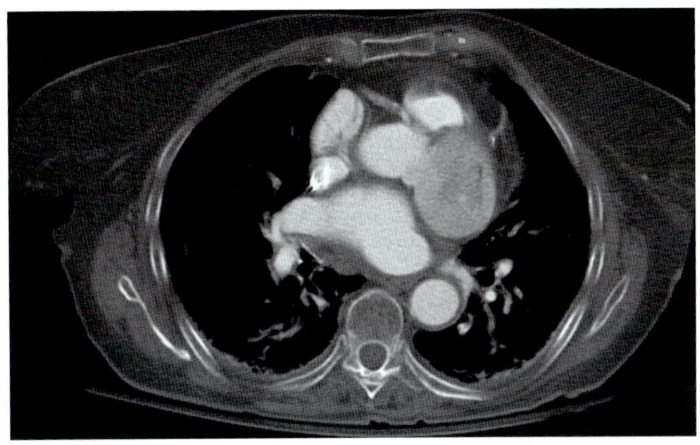

FIG. 1.40 Computed Tomographic Angiography. Preoperative imaging using computed tomographic angiography revealing the giant aneurysm of the left sinus of Valsalva.

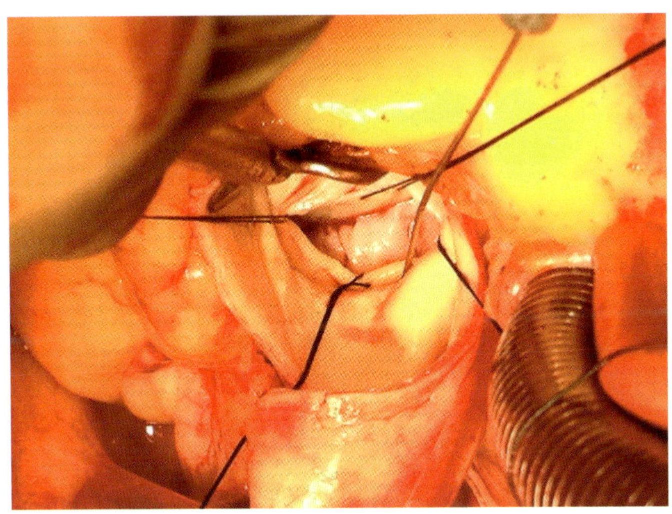

FIG. 1.41 Intraoperative Image. Image taken during surgery revealing the rim of the giant aneurysm marked off with black sutures and the metal probe paced in the left coronary artery ostium.

Aneurysms of the left sinus of Valsalva are extremely rare, and compression of the coronary artery causing coronary insufficiency and anginal symptoms is an uncommon complication.[1] These cases require an aggressive surgical approach once the diagnosis is made to prevent serious cardiac ischemia. Patients with this rare malformation who do not undergo prompt surgical correction are at risk for further aneurysmal dilation, malignant arrhythmias, left ventricular failure, and sudden death with rupture.[2,3]

References

1. Takach TJ, Reul GJ, Duncan JM, et al. Sinus of Valsalva aneurysm or fistula: management and outcome. *Ann Thorac Surg.* 1999;68:1573-1577.
2. Bjursten H, Harnek J, Cunha-Goncalves D, Koul B. Giant aneurysm in the sinus of Valsalva presenting as an acute coronary symptom. *Interact Cardiovasc Thorac Surg.* 2013;17:193-195.
3. Lijoi A, Parodi E, Passerone GC, Scarano F, Caruso D, Iannetti MV. Unruptured aneurysm of the left sinus of Valsalva causing coronary insufficiency: case report and review of the literature. *Tex Heart Inst J.* 2002;29:40-44.

Unusual Obstructions

A Beating Left Main Coronary Artery

Julien Wain-Hobson, MD, Calin Ivascau, MD, Vincent Roule, MD, Farzin Beygui, MD, PhD

A 37-year-old man with a history of active smoking and heroin addiction was admitted after successful prehospital intravenous fibrinolysis for ST-segment elevation myocardial infarction. Coronary angiography (Fig. 1.42) performed systematically after fibrinolysis showed a dynamic severe systolic compression (*black arrow*) of the left main coronary artery (LM) with a "milking effect" (Online Video 1.42) and a thrombotic lesion (*white arrow*) of the left circumflex artery. Intracoronary optical frequency domain imaging showed a thrombotic lesion of the left circumflex coronary artery (Fig. 1.43A) and an ovoid deformation of the LM (Fig. 1.43B) that was free of atherosclerosis. Cardiac multislice computed tomography (Fig. 1.44) showed that the LM originated near the right coronary artery with an initial course between the aorta and the pulmonary artery. Because of the assumed high risk for sudden

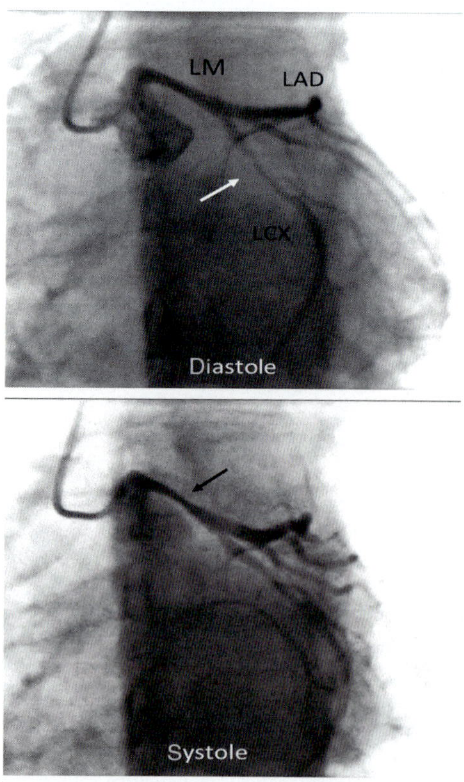

FIG. 1.42 Coronary Angiography. The left panel shows the thrombotic lesion of the left circumflex coronary artery (*LCX, white arrow*). The right panel shows the dynamic compression of the left main coronary artery (*LM*) during systole (*black arrow*). See Online Video 1.42. *LAD,* left anterior descending coronary artery.

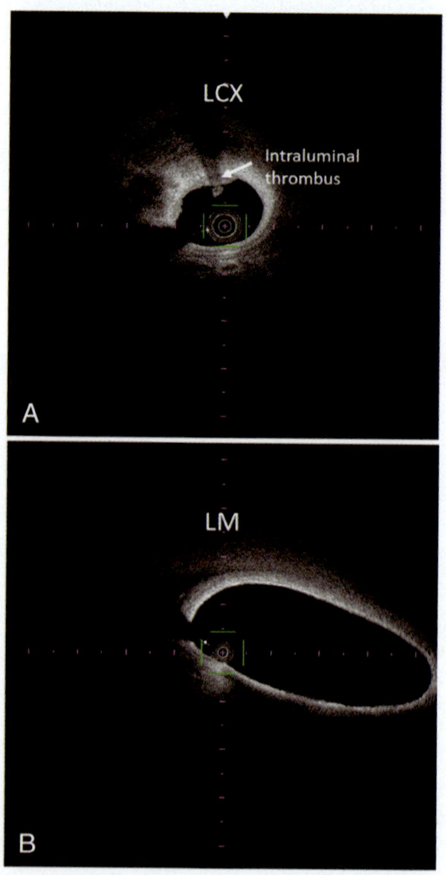

FIG. 1.43 Optical Frequency Domain Imaging. (A) Thrombotic lesion (*arrow*) of the left circumflex coronary artery (*LCX*). (B) Ovoid deformation of the left main coronary artery (*LM*).

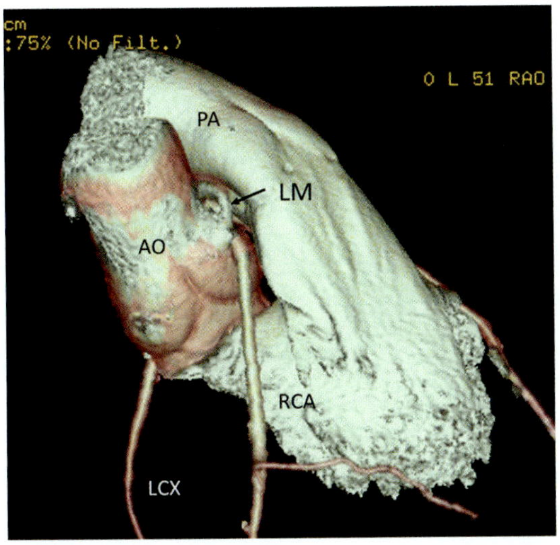

FIG. 1.44 Computed Tomography. The left main coronary artery (*LM*) has an initial course between the aorta (*AO*) and the pulmonary artery (*PA*). *LCX,* left circumflex coronary artery; *RCA,* right coronary artery.

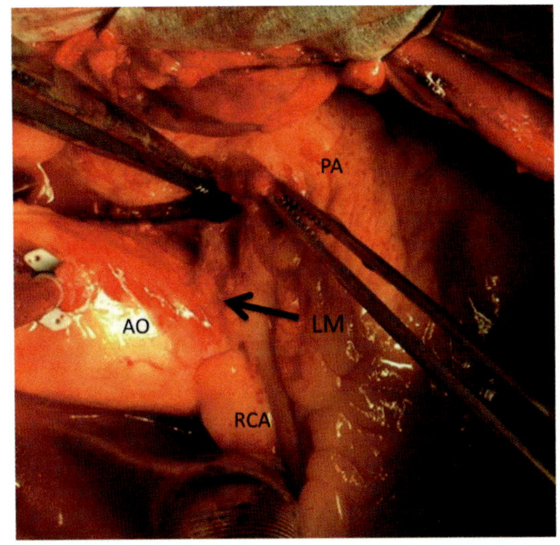

FIG. 1.45 Surgical View. The left main coronary artery (*LM*) has an initial course between the aorta (*AO*) and the pulmonary artery (*PA*). *RCA,* right coronary artery.

cardiac death,[1] the patient underwent coronary artery bypass surgery with native vessel ligation, confirming the ectopic course of the LM (Fig. 1.45).

Ectopic origin of the LM arising from the right aortic coronary sinus is a rare condition, found in 0.025% to 0.15% of patients undergoing coronary angiography.[2] The inter-aorticopulmonary course of the LM is associated with a high risk for sudden cardiac death and requires adequate correction. Surgical options are bypass grafting, pulmonary artery translocation, ostium reimplantation, or an unroofing technique in case of an intramural aortic segment.[3] LM stenting has also been performed as an alternative with a risk for stent compression.[4]

The unusual location of a milking effect on the LM should lead to adequate imaging modalities for the detection and correction of an ectopic inter-aorticopulmonary course of the LM.

References

1. Taylor AJ, Rogan KM, Virmani R. Sudden cardiac death associated with isolated congenital coronary artery anomalies. *J Am Coll Cardiol.* 1992;20:640-647.
2. Mery CM, Lawrence SM, Krishnamurthy R, et al. Anomalous aortic origin of a coronary artery: toward a standardized approach. *Semin Thorac Cardiovasc Surg.* 2014;26:110-122.
3. Krasuski RA, Magyar D, Hart S, et al. Long-term outcome and impact of surgery on adults with coronary arteries originating from the opposite coronary cusp. *Circulation.* 2011;123:154-162.
4. Doorey AJ, Pasquale MJ, Lally JF, et al. Six-month success of intracoronary stenting for anomalous coronary arteries associated with myocardial ischemia. *Am J Cardiol.* 2000;86:580-582.

A Freestyle Problem

Frederic De Vroey, MD, Tim Glenie, MD, Alex Cicovic, MD, Peter Raudkivi, MD, Sally Greaves, MD, Mark Webster, MD

A 77-year-old man had an acute inferior ST-segment elevation myocardial elevation. One year earlier, he underwent aortic valve replacement for moderate aortic regurgitation and a dilated proximal ascending aorta. A 27-mm Freestyle stentless porcine bioprosthesis (Medtronic, Minneapolis, Minnesota) with a 28-mm Dacron cuff was used. The native coronary artery and aortic buttons were implanted into the porcine prosthesis using standard techniques.

Immediate coronary angiography revealed moderate left coronary disease. The right coronary artery (RCA) was engaged with the catheter toward the cranial edge of a funnel-shaped coronary ostium. An angiogram showed normal flow down the RCA without significant downstream disease. Soon after coronary injection, the patient had resolution of his chest pain and ST-segment elevation. An ascending aortogram confirmed a pedunculated mass that appeared attached to the caudal aspect of the RCA ostium (Fig. 1.46), oscillating with the cardiac cycle and intermittently obstructing the RCA (Online Videos 1.43 and 1.44). A transesophageal echocardiogram confirmed normal bioprosthetic function and a 2.2 × 1.0 cm mass, with the echodensity of thrombus, in a dilated right coronary sinus.

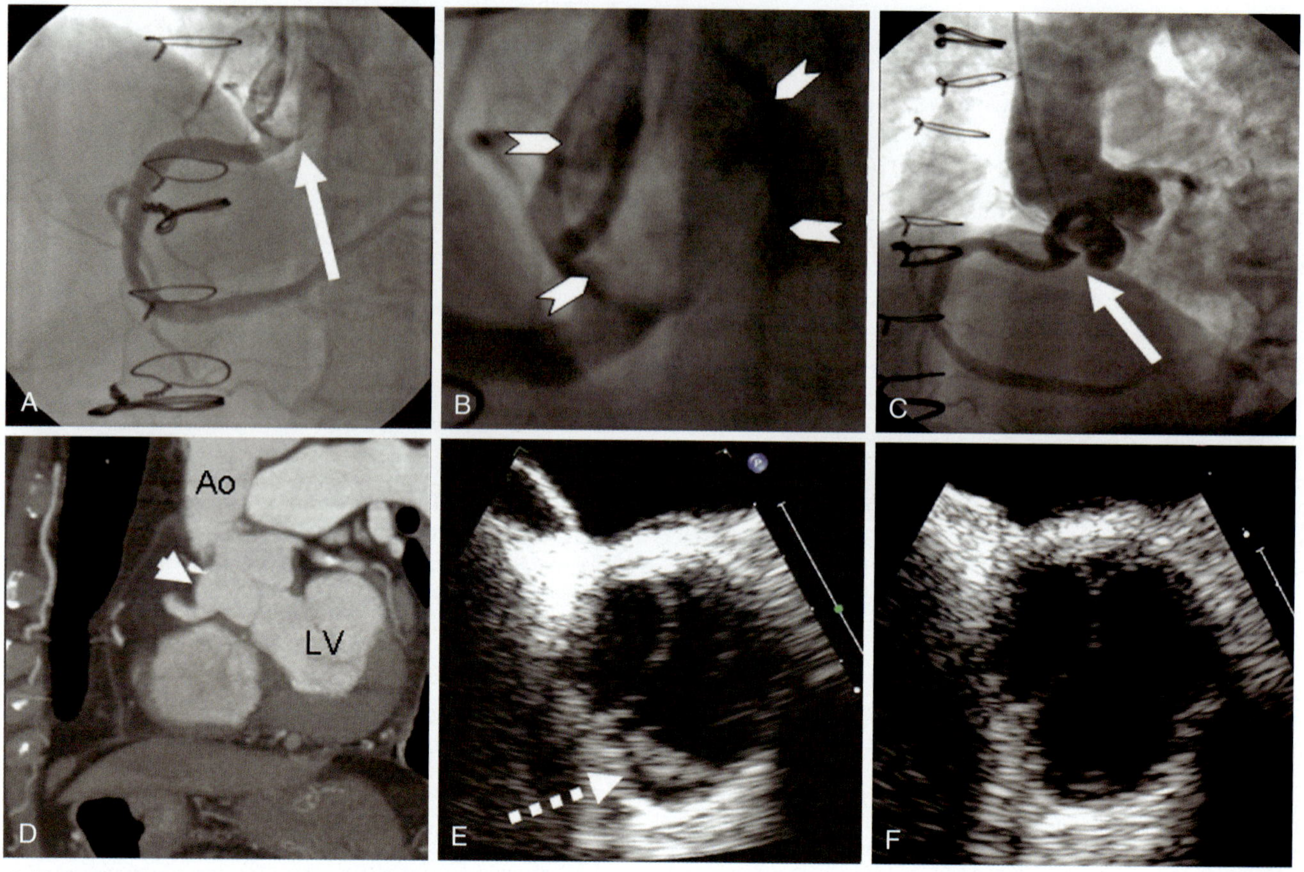

FIG. 1.46 Angiographic, Computed Tomography (CT), and Echocardiographic Images of a Mass in the Right Coronary Artery (RCA). Images (A), (B), and (C) show angiographic images of the RCA with a mass (*solid white arrows* and *arrowheads*) obstructing the funnel-shaped ostium. In (D), a CT aortogram 3 months later shows the funnel-shaped right coronary artery ostium (*short arrowhead*) without thrombus. Image (E) shows a short-axis transesophageal echocardiographic image of the mass (*dashed arrow*) in the right coronary sinus. In (F), it has cleared 5 days later. See Videos 1.43 and 1.44. *Ao,* aorta; *LV,* left ventricle.

Results of serial blood cultures were negative. The patient was treated conservatively with intravenous heparin and warfarin. A follow-up transesophageal echocardiogram 5 days later showed minimal residual thrombus in the RCA ostium. He remains well 3 months later.

A large pedunculated thrombus, presumably arising from the coronary anastomosis suture line, is a rare cause of ST-elevation myocardial infarction presenting late after aortic valve and root replacement.

Acute Coronary Syndrome Resulting From Systolic Compression of Left Main Coronary Artery Secondary to Aortic Subvalvular Aneurysm

Partha Sardar, MD, Evbu Enakpene, MD, James C. Fang, MD, Frederick G. P. Welt, MD

A 73-year-old man with acute decompensated heart failure was admitted to the hospital. He had a history of coronary artery bypass graft and aortic valve replacement (AVR) 12 years earlier, left anterior descending artery (LAD) stent, and repeat AVR and mitral valve replacement with bioprosthetic valves for endocarditis 5 years earlier. The echocardiogram showed aortic valve instability, significant subvalvular dilation with an aneurysmal left ventricular outflow tract (LVOT) (4.8 cm), and moderate paravalvular leak (Fig. 1.47A). A previous echocardiogram (1 year earlier) did not show any paravalvular leak and the LVOT diameter was 2.4 cm. During the hospital stay and presurgical planning for valve disease, severe recurrent anginal chest pain developed and the troponin level was elevated to 1.42 ng/mL, which was suggestive of non–ST-segment elevation myocardial infarction. Urgent coronary

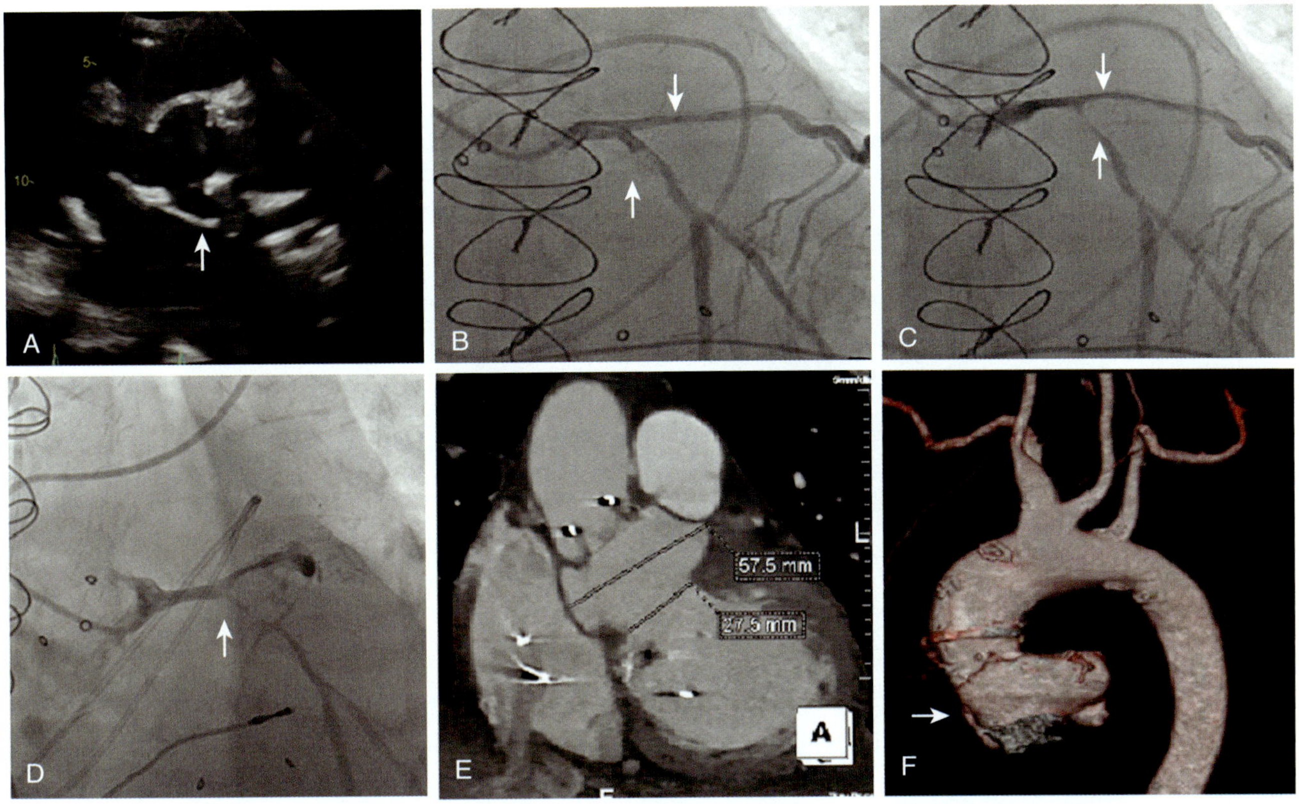

FIG. 1.47 Echocardiogram, Coronary Angiograms, and Computed Tomography. (A) Echocardiogram showing aneurysmal left ventricular outflow tract with significant aortic subvalvular dilation. The arrow indicates the edge of the aneurysm. (B) Left main coronary artery and proximal left circumflex artery during diastole. The upper arrow indicates the left anterior descending artery; the lower arrow indicates the left circumflex artery during diastole. (C and D) Compression of the left main coronary artery and proximal left circumflex artery during systole (Online Video 1.45). The upper arrow demonstrates the left anterior descending artery; the lower arrows in (C) indicate the left circumflex artery compression during systole. (E and F) Contrast-enhanced computed tomography shows a focal, well-defined dilation/pseudoaneurysm inferior to the level of the bioprosthetic aortic valve up to 5.7 cm in diameter compared with a 2.7-cm diameter at the neck of the left ventricular outflow tract. The arrow indicates the edge of the aneurysm.

angiography showed patent left main coronary artery (LMCA) but with significant systolic compression of both the LMCA and proximal left circumflex artery, likely secondary to an aortic subvalvular aneurysm (Fig. 1.47B–D, Online Video 1.45). He had 50% stenosis in the proximal LAD stent and 70% lesion in the proximal left circumflex artery and a known occluded right coronary artery with left to right collaterals. A bypass graft angiogram remained unchanged compared with a previous angiogram 8 years prior: patent left internal mammary artery to the diagonal with an occluded limb to the LAD, and a known occluded saphenous vein graft to the right posterior descending artery. Multidetector computed tomography showed focal dilation or pseudoaneurysm inferior to the level of the bioprosthetic aortic valve, up to 5.7-cm diameter compared with 2.7 cm diameter at the neck of the LVOT (Fig. 1.47E–F). The patient was referred for urgent repeat AVR, coronary artery bypass graft, and aortic root repair. This case illustrates a very unusual etiology of acute coronary syndrome in LMCA as the result of mechanical compression resulting from aortic subvalvular aneurysm secondary to prosthetic valve malfunction and paravalvular aortic regurgitation.

An Unusual Cause of ST-Segment Elevation Myocardial Infarction

Maria Ferré Vallverdú, MD, Tomás Heredia Cambra, MD, Jorge Sanz Sánchez, MD, José Luis Díez Gil, MD, PhD

A giant coronary artery aneurysm (CAA) is defined as dilation (more than 1.5 times the diameter of normal adjacent segments) of the coronary artery thrombosed giant right CAA, responsible for ST-segment elevation myocardial infarction. The most common cause of CAA in adults is atherosclerosis.

A 71-year-old woman with a history of arterial hypertension underwent urgent coronary angiography for inferior ST-segment elevation myocardial infarction. Angiography showed total occlusion of the mid right coronary artery. Several crossing attempts with a hydrophilic wire resulted in contrast extravasation to a cavity that initially seemed to be the pericardial space (Fig. 1.48A). At that moment, the procedure was stopped and echocardiography was performed, showing a cyst-like mass compressing the atrial and ventricular right chambers (Fig. 1.48B). Coronary computed

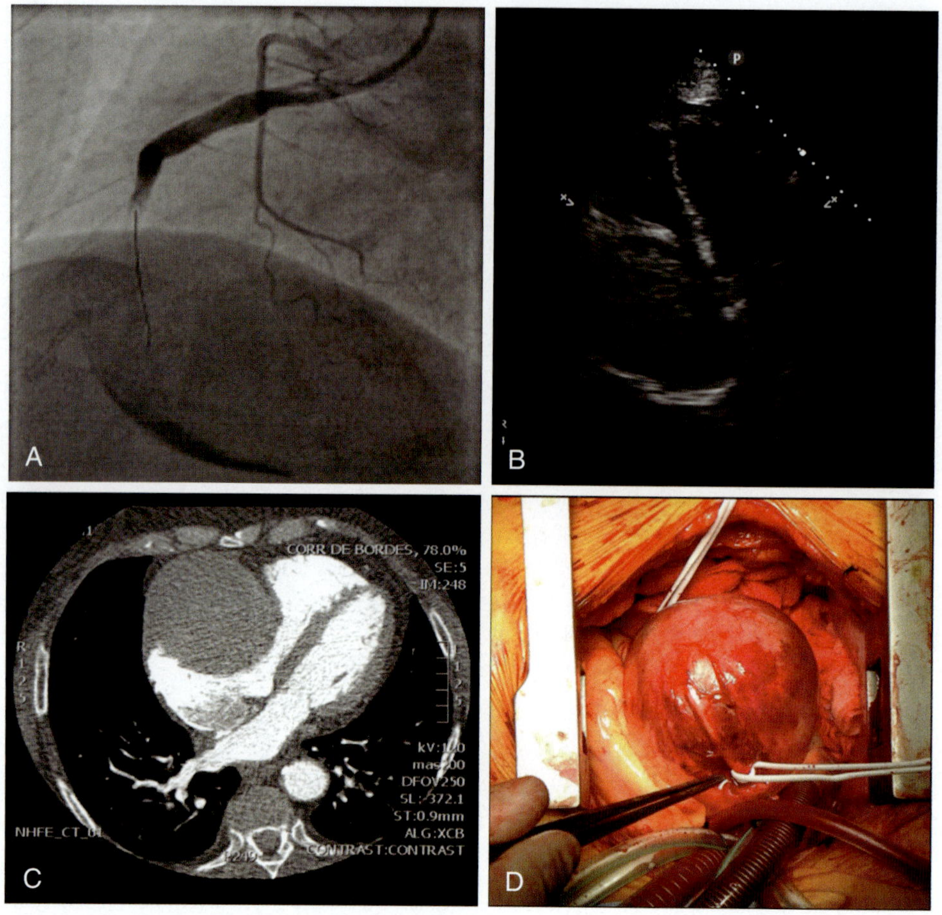

FIG. 1.48 Thrombosed Giant Coronary Artery Aneurysm Causing ST-Segment Elevation Myocardial Infarction. (A) Total occlusion of the mid right coronary artery and contrast extravasation. (B) Echocardiography showing a mass compressing the atrial and ventricular right chambers. (C) Coronary computed tomography revealed a 9 × 9 cm mass. (D) Giant artery aneurysm of right coronary artery. See Online Video 1.46.

tomographic angiography revealed a 9 × 9 cm mass, with no contrast capture in the arterial phase and with retention of contrast in the venous phase (Fig. 1.48C). It was described as a vascular mass with active bleeding; therefore urgent surgery was performed. The mass resulted in a thrombosed giant right CAA, which was responsible for the ST-segment elevation myocardial infarction (Fig. 1.48D, Online Video 1.46). Both the proximal and distal ends of the aneurysm were ligated after bypassing the distal right coronary artery. The patient progressed favorably during hospitalization, with no predischarge complications.

The majority of patients with giant CAAs are asymptomatic, but they may have angina pectoris, myocardial infarction, sudden death, or other complications at presentation. No optimal management strategy is established for patients with giant CAAs. Surgery is likely the preferred option in asymptomatic patients because of the risk for complications, as this case illustrates.

Cancer in the Left Anterior Descending Artery: A Therapeutic Aspect of Thrombus Aspiration?

Dieter Dauwe, MD, PhD, Nick Hiltrop, MD, Willem Schurmans, MD, Philippe Moerman, MD, PhD, Jan Bogaert, MD, PhD, Stefan Janssens, MD, PhD, Mark Coosemans, MD

A 49-year-old man was admitted for surgical resection of a solitary pulmonary metastasis. A mixed germ cell testis tumor (mature teratoma and seminoma) was diagnosed 1 year earlier and was treated with orchidectomy and adjuvant chemotherapy. Surgical resection of regional retroperitoneal disease progression during follow-up demonstrated transformation into a high-grade sarcoma. Four days after lung surgery, the patient experienced chest pain. An electrocardiogram showed anteroseptal ST-segment elevation. Transthoracic echocardiography confirmed anteroseptal hypocontractility and revealed a large mobile left ventricular mass (Fig. 1.49C, Online Video 1.47). Urgent coronary angiography demonstrated an occluded proximal left anterior descending coronary artery

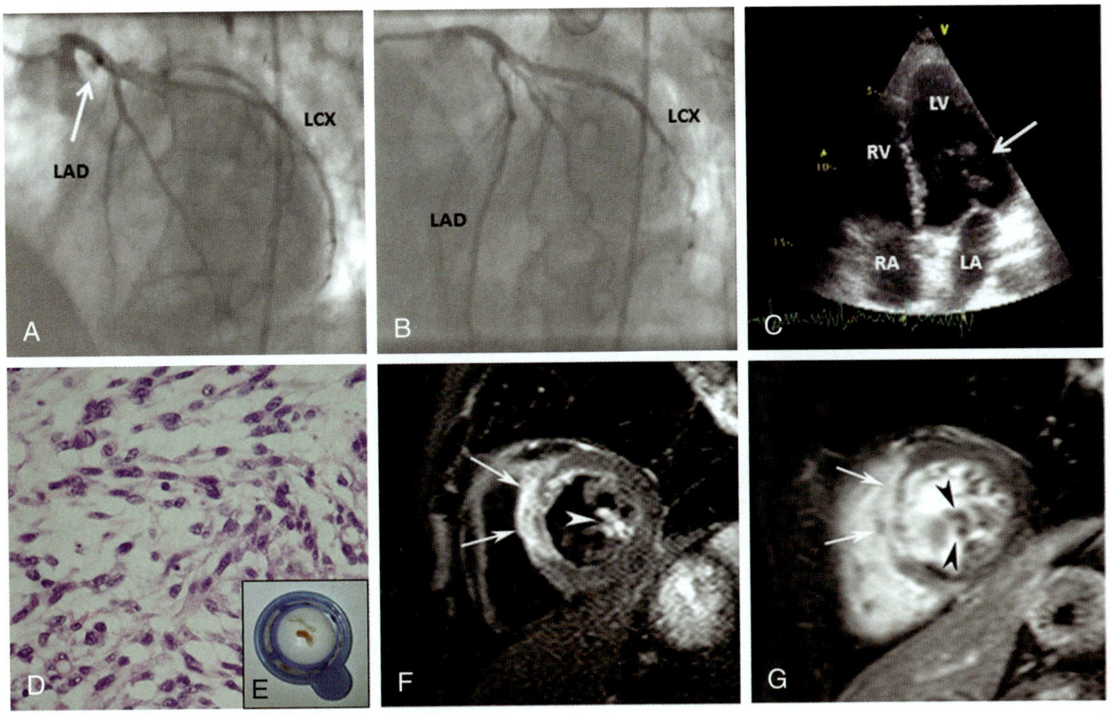

FIG. 1.49 Multimodality Imaging and Histopathology Confirming Malignant Etiology of Solid Tissue Coronary Thrombus. (A) Angiography demonstrated a total occlusion of the proximal left anterior descending artery (*arrow*), with reperfusion after thrombus aspiration (B). (C) Transthoracic echocardiogram (four-chamber view) revealed a mobile pedunculated intracardiac mass (*arrow*) (Online Video 1.47). (D) Cellular spindle cell proliferation in a myxoid background histopathologically documented high-grade sarcoma. (E) Thrombus aspirate. (F) Cardiac magnetic resonance showed myocardial edema in the infarct region (*white arrows*) and a hyperintense appearance of the intracavitary mass attached to the left ventricular lateral wall (*white arrowhead*) (G) T2-weighted short-T1 inversion recovery turbo spin-echo sequence short axis and transmural enhancement in the infarct region (*white arrows*) with irregular hypointense appearance of the intracavitary mass (*black arrowheads*). Late gadolinium enhancement sequence, short-axis. (Online Videos 48 and 49). *LA*, left atrium; *LAD*, left anterior descending; *LCX*, left circumflex; *LV*, left ventricle; *RA*, right atrium; *RV*, right ventricle.

(Fig. 1.49A). Evacuation of solid tissue during thrombus aspiration restored coronary perfusion with symptom relief and ST-segment normalization (Fig. 1.49B). Histopathology of the thrombus identified a high-grade sarcoma ex teratoma, suggesting embolization from an intracardiac metastasis (Fig. 1.49D–G). The patient died shortly afterward as the result of therapy-resistant cerebral edema and intracranial compression attributable to two new brain metastases.

Reported incidences of cardiac metastases are variable, ranging from 2.3% to 18.3% in patients dying of or with cancer.[1] Cardiac or pericardial metastases should be considered whenever patients with known malignancy in whom cardiovascular symptoms develop. Myocardial infarction is a rare but known complication of cardiac metastases.

Reference

1. Bussani R, De-Giorgio F, Abbate A, Silvestri F. Cardiac metastases. *J Clin Pathol.* 2007;60:27-34.

Chest Pain After Aortic Valve Surgery: Is It Serious?

Sandeep Basavarajaiah, MD, Anik Appaji, MD

A 65-year-old woman had symptoms of crescendo angina 7 months after bioprosthetic aortic valve replacement for stenosis of a previously placed prosthetic valve. She was initially reassured by her general physician after an echocardiogram that demonstrated a normally functioning prosthetic valve. In addition, a coronary angiogram before surgery had demonstrated normal arteries (Fig. 1.50). Because of her classic symptoms, the angiography was repeated, which exhibited tight ostial stenosis of the left main stem (LMS) (Fig. 1.51).

The patient subsequently underwent successful angioplasty with implantation of one drug-eluting stent (4.5 × 14 mm everolimus-eluting stent) (Figs. 1.52A–B and 1.53). The surgeon confirmed the cannulation of LMS during aortic valve surgery to induce cardioplegia.

Iatrogenic ostial LMS stenosis is a rare but life-threatening complication after valve surgery. It is attributed to a localized hyperplastic reaction secondary to antegrade cannulation of the coronary ostia to induce cardioplegia. Cannulation may lead to microinjuries as the result of perfusion pressure of cardioplegic fluid and overdilation of the vessel by the tip of the catheter.[1-3] In our case, because the LMS was at an acute angle from the aortic sinus, the cannulation might have caused a greater degree of intimal injury. One of the main

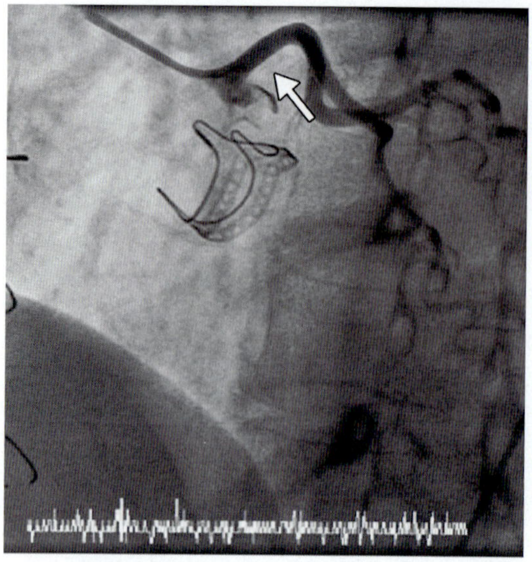

FIG. 1.50 Presurgery Coronary Angiogram. Coronary angiogram before aortic valve surgery exhibiting a smooth and unobstructed left coronary system (*arrow*).

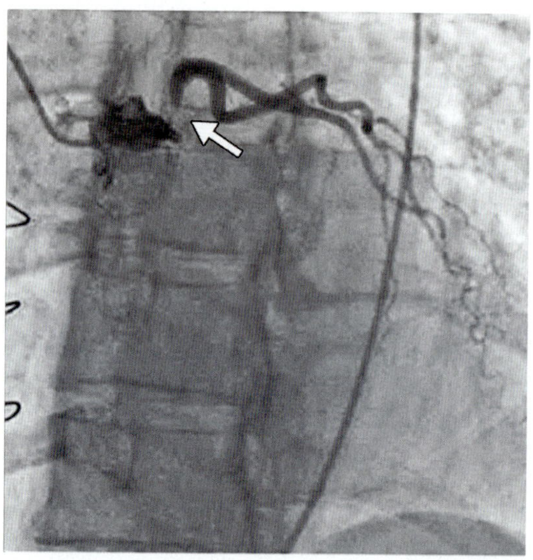

FIG. 1.51 Coronary Angiogram When Presented With Angina. Coronary angiogram 7 months after surgery exhibiting severe stenosis in the ostial left main stem (*arrow*).

challenges is the diagnosis because chest pain after aortic valve replacement AVR may be overlooked, especially in the absence of valve dysfunction and if the preoperative angiogram was normal. The condition is rapidly progressive, and without treatment, there is a risk of sudden death. Our patient was experiencing chest pain on minimal exertion and sometimes even at rest.

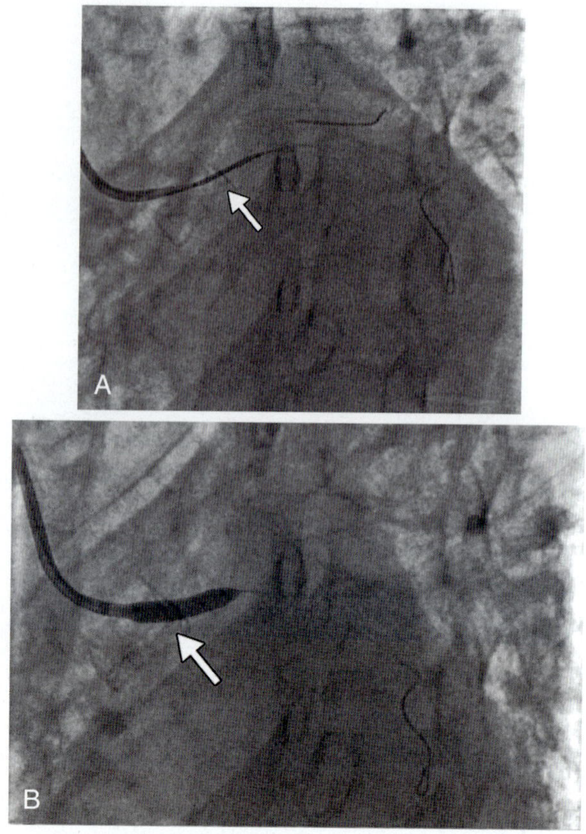

FIG. 1.52 Coronary Intervention. (A) Positioning and (B) deployment of a drug-eluting stent in the ostium of left main stem (*arrows*).

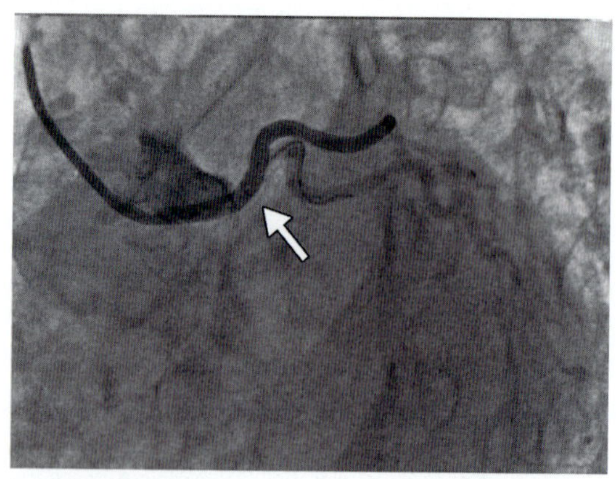

FIG. 1.53. Coronary Angiogram Postintervention. Angiogram after stent deployment exhibiting excellent final result (*arrow*).

References

1. Funanda A, Mizuno S, Ohsato K, et al. Three cases of iatrogenic coronary ostial stenosis after aortic valve replacement. *Circ J.* 2006;70:1312-1317.
2. Doenst T. Direct cannulation of the coronary ostia. *Multimed Man Cardiothorac Surg.* 2005;809. doi: 10.1510/mmcts.2004.000703.
3. Araszkiewicz A, Lesiak M, Urbanowicz T, Jankiewicz S, Grajek S. Acute coronary syndrome as a result of left main coronary artery stenosis after aortic valve replacement. A report of three cases. *Postepy Kardiol Interwencyjnej.* 2013;9:150-154.

Five-Year Follow-Up After Stenting for Iatrogenic Coronary Stenosis Owing to Mitral Annuloplasty: Insights With Multiple Imaging Modalities

Satoru Mitomo, MD, Toru Naganuma, MD, Koji Hozawa, MD, Kensuke Takagi, MD, Tatsuya Nakao, MD, PhD, Sunao Nakamura, MD, PhD

A 59-year-old woman with severe mitral regurgitation underwent mitral annuloplasty (MAP) with a 28-mm Carpentier-Edwards Physio II annuloplasty ring (Edwards Lifesciences, Irvine, California). On postoperative day 10, the patient reported chest oppression with ischemic changes on an electrocardiogram during rehabilitation therapy. Coronary angiography (CAG) showed severe focal stenosis in the middle of the left circumflex artery (LCx) that had not been detected by preoperative CAG (Fig. 1.54A–C). Preprocedural optical coherence tomography (OCT) showed severe narrowing (lumen area: 0.8 mm^2), with no evidence of hematoma, plaque, or thrombi. The vessel was compressed from the outside (Fig. 1.55A), with normal vessel structure of the three layers at the site of the culprit lesion. In addition, intravascular ultrasound (IVUS) showed that the vessel was bent with some force from the epicardial side (Fig. 1.55B). These intravascular images suggested that this new focal stenosis may have been caused by accidental ligation of the LCx during MAP.

Considering the high risk of repeat open surgery, the heart team opted for percutaneous revascularization. Predilation was performed gently with a 2.5-mm noncompliant balloon, followed by implantation of a 3.0 × 18 mm Driver stent (Medtronic CardioVascular, Santa Rosa, California) (Fig. 1.54D). Postprocedural OCT and IVUS showed good stent expansion and apposition (minimal stent area: 6.1 mm^2), with no evidence of coronary injury (Fig. 1.55C–E). At 5-year follow-up, CAG with aspirin alone (Fig. 1.54E), OCT, IVUS, and multidetector computed tomography showed no evidence of significant stent recoil (minimal stent area: 5.6 mm^2) (Fig. 1.55F–H). Furthermore, the echocardiogram showed no recurrent mitral regurgitation at that time.

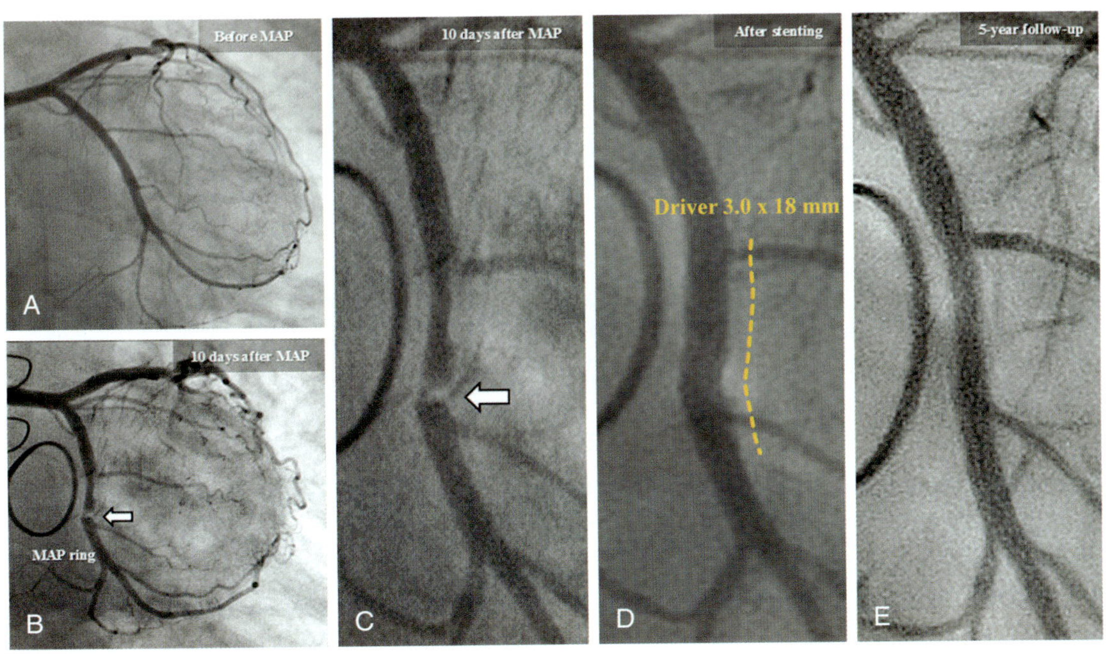

FIG. 1.54 Coronary Angiography (CAG) Images Showing Iatrogenic Coronary Stenosis in the Middle of the Left Circumflex Artery Caused by Accidental Ligation During Mitral Annuloplasty (*MAP*). (A) CAG before MAP showing no evidence of significant left circumflex artery stenosis. (B and C) CAG after mitral annuloplasty showing new severe focal stenosis in the middle of the left circumflex artery (*white arrow*). (D) CAG after implantation of a 3.0 × 18 mm bare-metal stent. (E) CAG at 5-year follow-up.

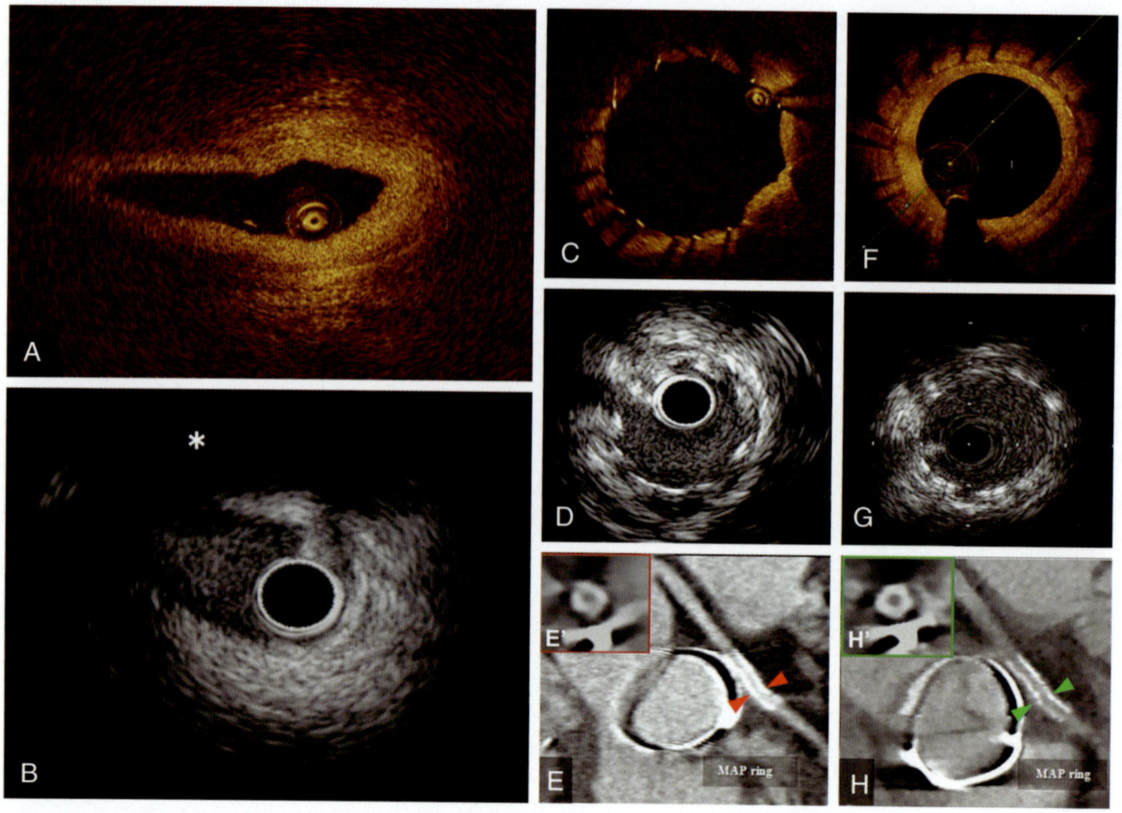

FIG. 1.55 Images of Iatrogenic Stenosis Due to Ligation During Mitral Annuloplasty (*MAP*) Before and After Stenting and at 5-Year Follow-Up. (A) Preprocedural optical coherence tomography (OCT) image showing a compressed vessel with THREE normal layers. (B) Preprocedural intravascular ultrasound (IVUS) image showing a vessel bent from the epicardial side (*asterisk*). (C and D) Postprocedural OCT and IVUS showing good stent expansion and apposition (minimal stent area 6.1 mm^2). (E) Postprocedural longitudinal multidetector computed tomography (MDCT) image showing a well-expanded stent adjacent to the MAP ring. E′ Postprocedural short-axis MDCT image showing a well-expanded stent adjacent to the *MAP* ring (*red arrowheads*). (F and G) Five-year follow-up OCT and IVUS images showing a stent covered with homogeneous neointima without significant stent recoil (minimal stent area: 5.6 mm^2) or stent fracture. (H) Five-year follow-up MDCT image showing a well-expanded stent adjacent to the MAP ring without deformation. H′ Five-year follow-up short-axis MDCT image showing a well-expanded stent adjacent to the MAP ring (*green arrowheads*).

To the best of our knowledge, there are no reports regarding long-term follow-up after stenting for iatrogenic coronary stenosi.[1] Our case suggests that bailout stenting with a bare metal stent for iatrogenic coronary stenosis may be associated with favorable long-term outcomes.

Reference

1. Grande AM, Fiore A, Massetti M, Viganò M. Iatrogenic circumflex coronary lesion in mitral valve surgery: case report and review of the literature. *Tex Heart Inst J.* 2008;35:179-183.

Left Anterior Descending Coronary Artery Occlusion During Transcatheter Pulmonary Valve Implantation: Successful Rescue Percutaneous Revascularization

Alban-Elouen Baruteau, MD, Jérôme Petit, MD, Philippe Brenot, MD, Jean-Yves Riou, MD, Claude-Yves Angel, MD

A 34-year-old woman was referred for transcatheter pulmonary valve implantation. She had been exposed to radiotherapy for Hodgkin disease and underwent a Ross procedure 16 years earlier for postendocarditis aortic regurgitation. Test balloon angioplasty with a 22 × 20 mm Atlas balloon (Bard Peripheral Vascular, Tempe, Arizona) inflated to 14 atm showed no coronary compression (Fig. 1.56A, Online Video 1.50). Prestenting of the right ventricular outflow tract with a 36-mm IntraStent LD-Max (EV3, Plymouth, Minnesota) mounted on a 22 × 45 mm BIB (balloon-in-balloon) catheter (NuMed, Hopkinton, New York) was uneventful, and

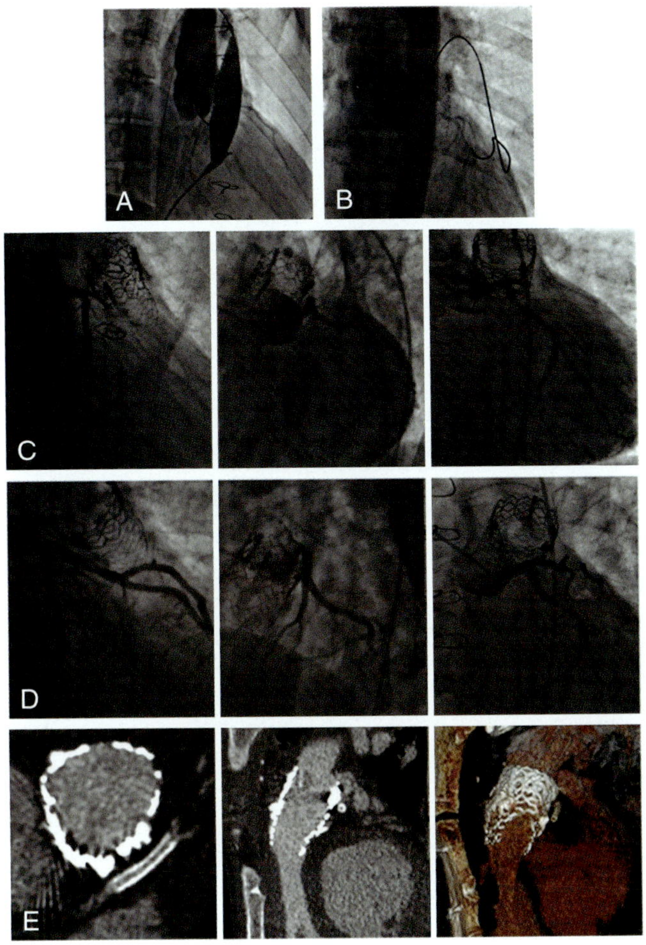

FIG. 1.56 Successful Recanalization of an Occluded Left Anterior Coronary Artery Occlusion During Transcatheter Pulmonary Valve Implantation. (A) Aortography during test balloon angioplasty (Online Video 1.50) and (B) after prestenting showed no coronary artery compression. (C) Pulmonary valve implantation was followed by occlusion of the proximal left anterior descending coronary artery at coronary angiography (Online Video 1.51). Coronary artery revascularization attested by coronary angiography and cardiac computed tomography (Online Video 1.52). (D) Successful coronary artery revascularization (coronarography). (E) Successful coronary artery revascularization (computed tomography scan).

a second aortography showed no coronary compression (Fig. 1.56B). A 23-mm Edwards Sapien pulmonic valve (Edwards Lifesciences, Irvine, California) was implanted, followed by intractable ventricular fibrillation that was caused by left anterior descending coronary artery occlusion (Fig. 1.56C, Online Video 1.51). Extrinsic compression was attributed to a mediastinal tissue block displacement during valve implantation. Under chest compressions, rescue percutaneous coronary revascularization was performed (Fig. 1.56D–E, Online Video 1.52) with implantation of a bare-metal stent in the proximal left anterior descending artery. After 2 years of follow-up, the patient is alive and her coronary angiography results are normal. Coronary artery compression may be observed in 5% of patients during test balloon angioplasty.[1] This complication is associated with abnormal coronary anatomy, especially in patients with tetralogy of Fallot or transposition of the great arteries.[1] According to our exceptional case, caution should also be applied in patients with a radiated chest, even with normal coronary anatomy and normal test balloon angioplasty.

Reference

1. Morray BH, McElhinney DB, Cheatham JP, et al. Risk of coronary artery compression among patients referred for transcatheter pulmonary valve implantation: a multicenter experience. *Circ Cardiovasc Interv.* 2013;6:535-542.

Left Main Coronary Artery Compression by an Enlarged Pulmonary Artery

Wassef Karrowni, MD, Gardar Sigurdsson, MD, Phillip A. Horwitz, MD

A 43-year-old woman with World Health Organization group 1 severe pulmonary hypertension, associated with systemic lupus erythematosus, was referred for cardiac catheterization as part of evaluation for lung transplantation. She was also having anginal symptoms during walking. Physical examination was significant for a loud P2 and right ventricular lift. Coronary angiogram revealed a tight ostial left main stenosis (Fig. 1.57A, Online Video 1.53) that was thought to be the result of compression by a markedly enlarged pulmonary artery

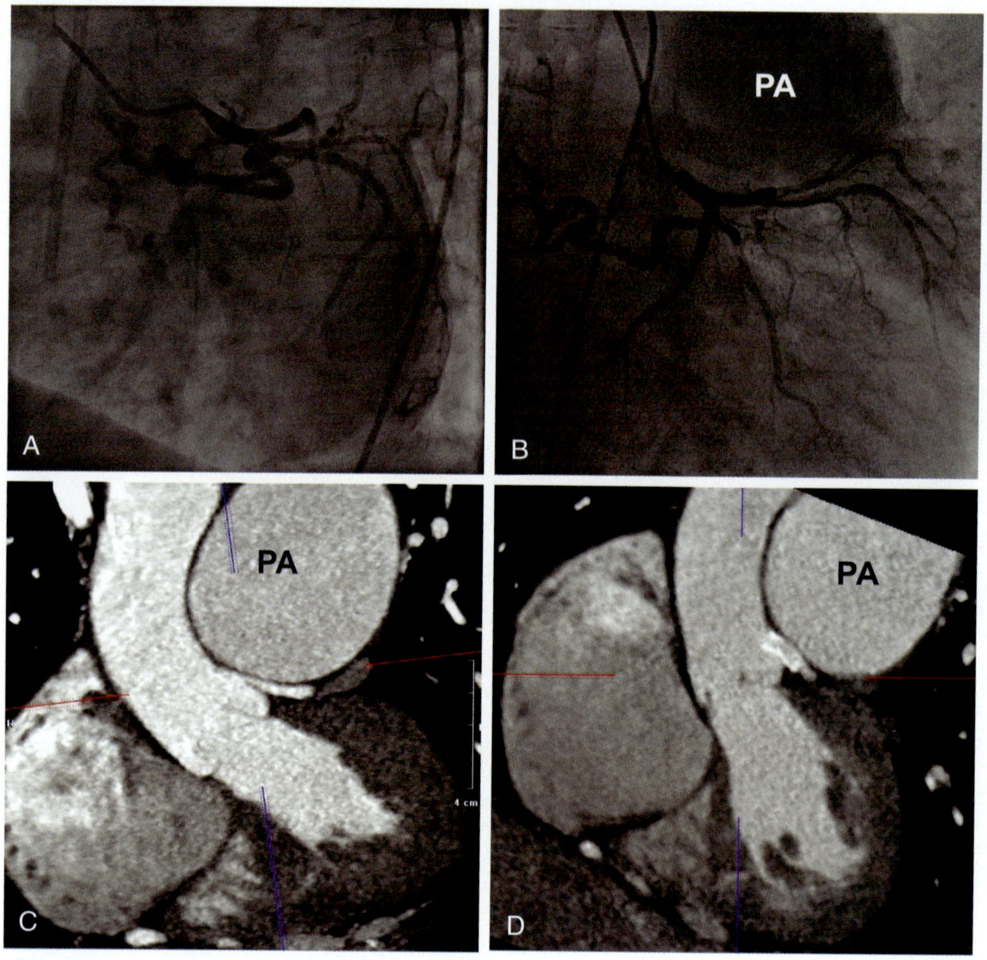

FIG. 1.57 Coronary Angiographic and Computed Tomography Findings at Presentation and Follow-Up. Angiography of the left coronary system at the index procedure demonstrating high-grade ostial left main stenosis (A) caused by compression by an enlarged pulmonary artery (*PA*). (B) Multidetector computed tomography confirmed the compression of the left main by the enlarged PA (C). (D) Repeat multidetector computed tomography 5 months after intervention revealed a widely patent stent.

(Fig. 1.57A–B, Online Video 1.53 and 1.54). This was confirmed by a coronary 64-slice multidetector computed tomography (Fig. 1.57C). The patient underwent successful left main stenting with a 4 × 15 mm bare-metal stent. Since that time she has had no recurrence of the angina. Follow-up coronary multidetector computed tomography was done at 5 months and confirmed patency of the stent (Fig. 1.57D). Given the severity of the underlying disease, the patient continues to be evaluated for lung transplantation.

Left Main Coronary Artery Occlusion Caused by Thrombus Embolization From a Prosthetic Mitral Valve

Ronen Jaffe, MD, Avinoam Shiran, MD, Ronen Rubinshtein, MD

A 46-year-old woman with a history of rheumatic heart disease and mitral and aortic valve replacement with mechanical bileaflet prosthesis was admitted with acute anterior wall ST-segment elevation myocardial infarction and cardiogenic shock after discontinuation of anticoagulant therapy. She underwent emergency coronary catheterization. Fluoroscopy confirmed normal motion of the prosthetic valve leaflets. Coronary angiography revealed a large filling defect within the left main coronary artery (Fig. 1.58) with TIMI (thrombolysis in myocardial infarction) grade flow 1 in the left anterior descending artery (Online Video 1.55). Intravenous heparin and intracoronary eptifibatide were administered. Multiple aspirations via a 7F guide catheter and two aspiration thrombectomy catheters (Pronto V3 and Pronto LP, Vascular Solutions, Minneapolis, Minnesota), which were advanced over a distal

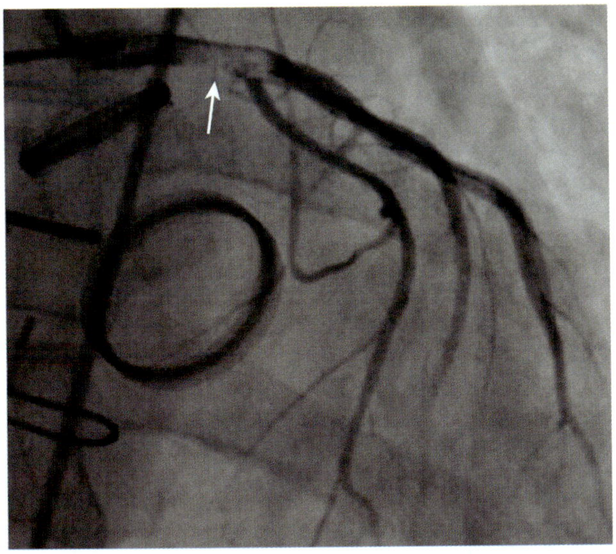

FIG. 1.58 Initial Coronary Angiogram. Coronary angiography revealed a large filling defect within the left main coronary artery (*arrow*).

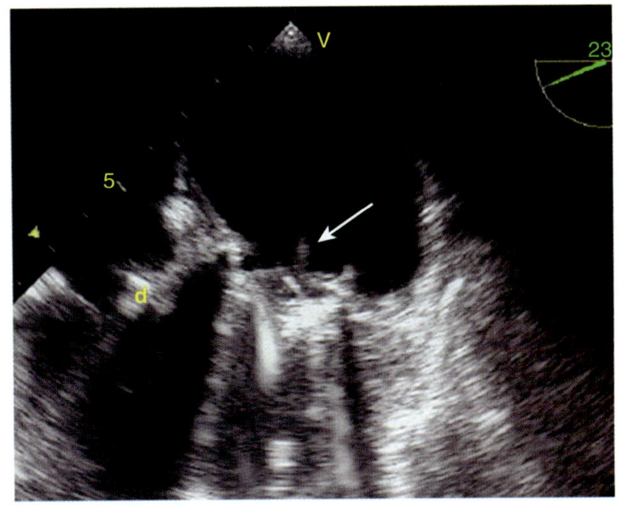

FIG. 1.60 Transesophageal Echocardiogram. Postprocedural transesophageal echocardiography revealed a 5 × 15 mm mobile object on the atrial aspect of the prosthetic mitral valve (*arrow*) compatible with thrombus.

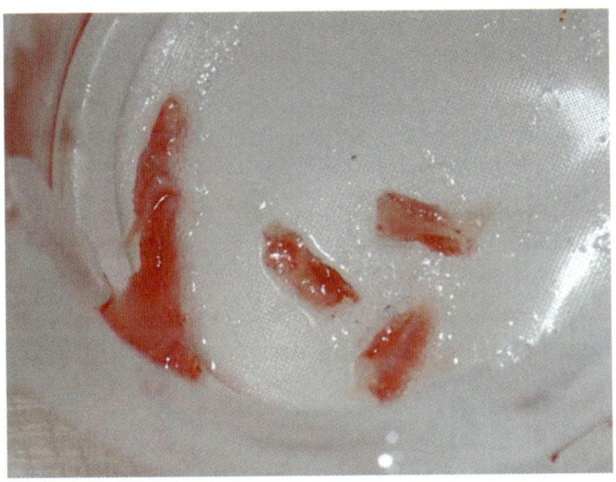

FIG. 1.59 Aspirated Thrombus. Multiple aspirations retrieved a large thrombus load.

embolic protection device (FilterWire EZ, Boston Scientific, Natick, Massachusetts), retrieved a large thrombus load (Fig. 1.59). At the end of the procedure normal coronary flow was achieved (Online Video 1.56).

Postprocedural transesophageal echocardiography revealed a 5 × 15 mm mobile thrombus attached to the atrial aspect of the prosthetic mitral valve (Fig. 1.60, *arrow*; Online Video 1.57). The patient made a full hemodynamic recovery, and warfarin therapy was reinstated. Predischarge transesophageal echocardiography revealed normal left ventricular function and resolution of the thrombus on the prosthetic mitral valve.

This case highlights the risk of thrombus formation on prosthetic heart valves in the absence of adequate anticoagulation and the potential for severe ischemic complications in the event of thrombus embolization to the coronary arteries.

Left Main Coronary Embolization After Direct Current Cardioversion for Persistent Atrial Flutter in the Absence of Detectable Intracardiac Thrombi

Daniel Garcia, MD, Mohammad Ansari, MD, Jaffid S. Majjul, MD, Elman M. Urbina, MD, Alexandre C. Ferreira, MD, Cesar E. Mendoza, MD

We report a case of left main coronary embolization after direct current cardioversion in the absence of detectable intracardiac thrombi by preprocedure comprehensive transesophageal echocardiographic assessment.[1] Although it is considered a rare event, in patients with postcardioversion acute coronary syndrome, the possibility of coronary thromboembolism must be considered.[2]

A 57-year-old man with a history of active smoking and persistent atrial flutter was admitted to the hospital because of atrial flutter with rapid ventricular response, progressive dyspnea on exertion, paroxysmal nocturnal dyspnea, orthopnea, and bilateral ankle edema. A transthoracic echocardiogram showed normal left ventricular dimensions, mild left atrial enlargement, severe left

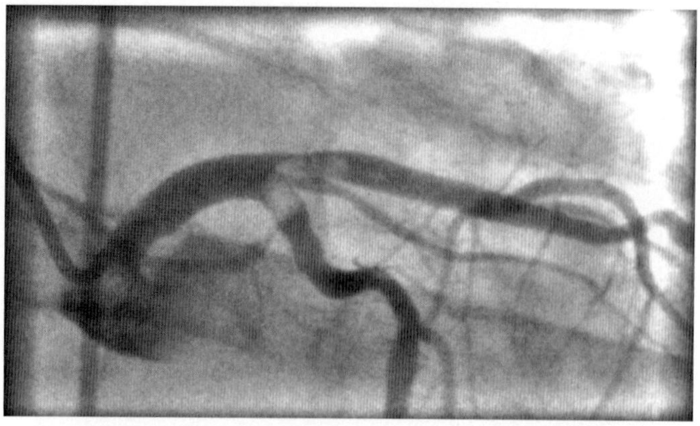

FIG. 1.61 Large riding thrombus on the left main coronary bifurcation.

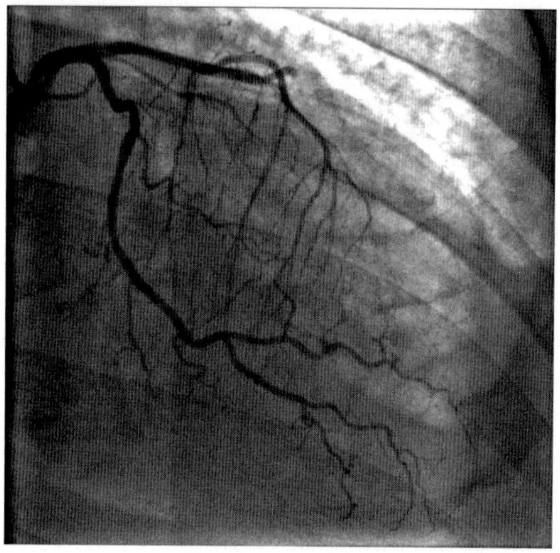

FIG. 1.62 Postangiography migration of the left main thrombus.

ventricular systolic dysfunction with an ejection fraction of 10%, severe left ventricular global hypokinesis, and no evidence of left ventricular thrombus. The patient underwent optimal anticoagulated with intravenous unfractionated heparin and was then referred for transesophageal echocardiography and direct current cardioversion. After ruling out the presence of thrombi within cardiac chambers, he underwent successful cardioversion with normalization of his heart rhythm. Postprocedure anticoagulation was continued

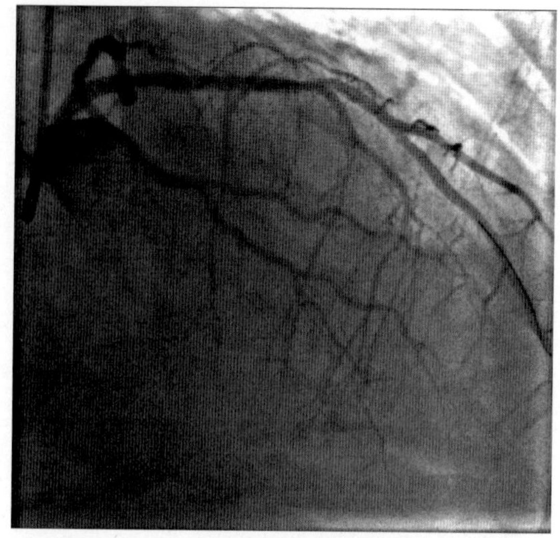

FIG. 1.63 Prompt manual coronary thombectomy restored normal coronary flow in the left anterior descending artery.

without any changes. Two hours after the procedure, severe retrosternal chest pain developed with new inverted T waves diffusely distributed in the anterior and lateral leads. He underwent emergent coronary angiography, which revealed the presence of a riding left main bifurcation thrombus (Fig. 1.61). His anticoagulation level was rechecked and found to be within the therapeutic range. Shortly after and while the interventional team prepared for coronary thrombectomy, the thrombus migrated downstream into the left anterior descending coronary artery, causing a total occlusion of the vessel in its midsegment (Fig. 1.62). His chest pain worsened, and his electrocardiographic tracing revealed ST-segment elevation in the monitored leads. Percutaneous coronary intervention of the left anterior descending coronary artery was performed with successful manual thrombectomy. Postprocedural angiography showed excellent results with reestablishment of a normal coronary blood flow (Fig. 1.63).

References

1. Manning WJ, Weintraub RM, Waksmonski CA, et al. Accuracy of transesophageal echocardiography for identifying left atrial thrombi. A prospective, intraoperative study. *Ann Intern Med.* 1995;123:817-822.
2. Nan YY, Chang JP, Lu MS, Kao CL. Mediastinal hematoma and left main dissection following blunt chest trauma. *Eur J Cardiothorac Surg.* 2007; 31:320-321.

Percutaneous Intervention of an Acute Left Main Coronary Occlusion Secondary to Dissection of the Aortic Root

Amir Ravandi, MD, PhD, William F. Penny, MD

An 86-year-old man came to the hospital with 4 hours of retrosternal chest pain and had an anterior ST-segment elevation myocardial infarction on electrocardiogram. His medical history included pulmonary sarcoidosis, a bioprosthetic aortic valve implanted in 1997, and long-standing aortic root dilation that had been followed clinically because of high reoperative risk.

He was taken to the cardiac catheterization laboratory for emergent percutaneous coronary intervention but diagnostic coronary angiography was difficult because of the enlarged aortic root. With a 5F multipurpose catheter, the left coronary artery was engaged, revealing a total occlusion of the ostial left main coronary artery (LMCA) (Fig. 1.64A, Online Video 1.58A). Subsequent angiography

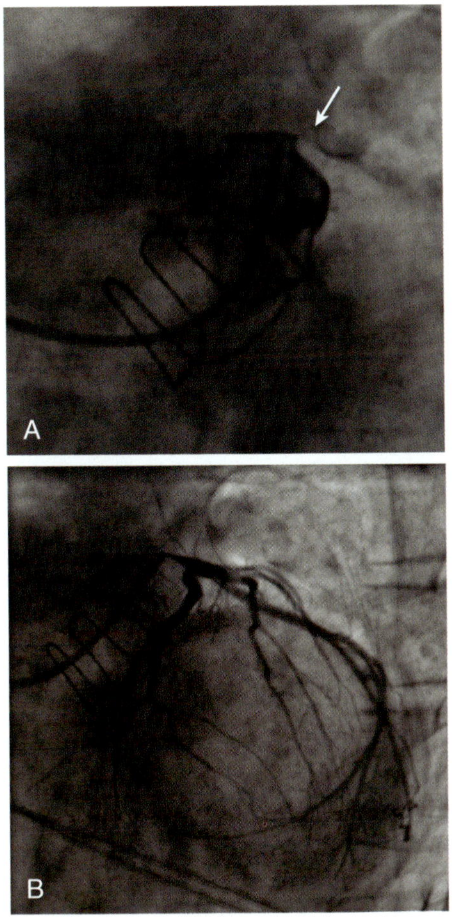

FIG. 1.64 Occlusion of the Left Main Ostium Due to Aortic Root Dissection Resulting in an Anterior ST-Elevation Myocardial Infarction. Diagnostic coronary angiogram of the left main coronary artery (LMCA) showing ostial occlusion (*arrow*) of the LMCA (A), then subsequently a 99% slitlike lesion of the ostial LMCA with minimal other obstructive coronary artery disease (B). See Online Videos 1.58A and 1.58B.

produced transient TIMI (Thrombolysis In Myocardial Infarction) grade flow 1 and then TIMI grade flow 2 through a 99% slitlike lesion of the ostial LMAC with minimal other obstructive coronary artery disease (Fig. 1.64B, Online Video 1.58B). The right coronary artery was normal. An aortogram was then performed, demonstrating a dissection flap adjacent to the LM ostium and 2+ aortic insufficiency (Fig. 1.65, Online Video 1.59). During diagnostic imaging, the patient had become hemodynamically unstable, requiring inotropic support and multiple rounds of defibrillation because of pulseless ventricular tachycardia; intraaortic balloon pump support was contraindicated by the aortic dissection and insufficiency. The cardiothoracic surgical team was consulted urgently, but a surgical approach was deemed not feasible because of the patient's age, hemodynamic instability, and comorbidities.

A percutaneous approach to revascularization was thus undertaken. A 6F multipurpose guide was placed and the lesion was crossed into the left anterior descending artery with a 0.014-inch balanced middle-weight wire (Abbott Vascular, Santa Clara, California). The ostial and proximal LM were predilated with a 2.0 mm × 15 mm compliant balloon, followed by deployment of a 3.5 mm × 13 mm Cypher drug-eluting stent (Cordis Corp., Bridgewater, New Jersey) at 14 atm, resulting in TIMI grade flow 3 (Fig. 1.66, Online Video 1.60). The patient became hemodynamically stable after stent placement and was transferred to the critical care unit for post–ST-segment elevation myocardial infarction care.

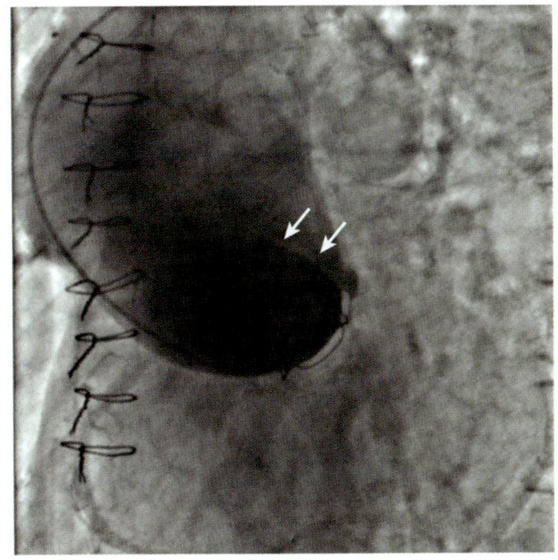

FIG. 1.65 Ascending Root Aortogram. Ascending root aortogram demonstrating an enlarged aortic root and evidence of a dissection flap at the left sinus of Valsalva (*arrows*) (Online Video 1.59).

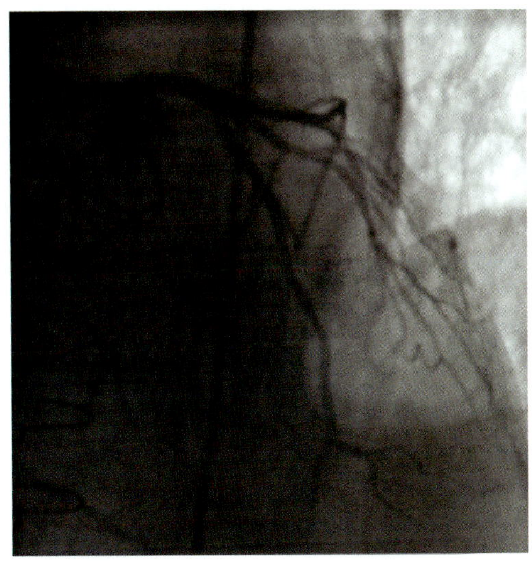

FIG. 1.66 Thrombolysis in Myocardial Infarction Flow Grade 3 After Stent Deployment in the Proximal Left Main. Coronary angiography of the left main coronary artery (LMCA) showing TIMI grade flow 3 after stent deployment in the proximal LMCA (Online Video 1.60).

After the procedure, a 64-slice computed tomography scan of the thorax was performed that showed that the origin of the dissection was the sinus of Valsalva at the LM, with the stent traversing into the aorta at the false lumen (Fig. 1.67).

Aortic root dissection involving the LM is a rare cause of ST-segment elevation myocardial infarction. The standard approach in treating patients with a type A dissection and LM involvement is surgical. The role of preoperative diagnostic angiography is still

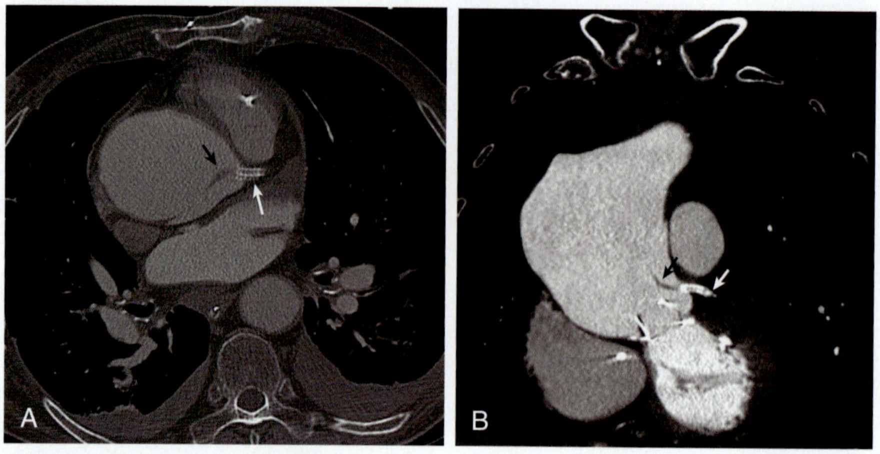

FIG. 1.67 Computed Tomography (CT) of the Ascending Aorta After Stent Placement at the Ostium of the Left Main. CT demonstrating that the origin of the dissection (*black arrow*) was at the sinus of Valsalva with the stent (*white arrow*) traversing into the aorta at the false lumen. (A) Axial view. (B) Coronal view.

controversial in that elucidating the coronary anatomy before surgery can potentially increase mortality, but a recent large case series has suggested that prior cardiac catheterization does not have an impact on mortality. However, in cases such as this case, in which the patient is excluded from surgical repair by hemodynamic instability or comorbid conditions, a percutaneous interventional approach of stenting of the LMCA can be considered an alternative.

Simultaneous Coronary and Pulmonary Angiography to Diagnose Critical Left Main Coronary Artery Stenosis Secondary to Dilated Pulmonary Artery

Abdul Rahman Ihdayhid, MBBS, Muhammad Asrar ul Haq, MBBS, Lawrence Dembo, MBBS, Gerald Yong, MBBS

A 68-year-old woman with long-standing severe pulmonary arterial hypertension was referred for coronary catheterization for investigation of worsening exertional dyspnea associated with angina. Coronary angiography revealed critical ostial left main coronary artery (LMCA) stenosis. Given the history of severe pulmonary arterial hypertension, simultaneous angiography of the LMCA and main pulmonary artery (MPA) was performed, which suggested a severely dilated MPA compressing the ostial to mid LMCA, causing a critical stenosis (Fig. 1.68A). This correlated well with coronary computed tomography, which confirmed a severely dilated MPA with a diameter of 60 mm compressing the LMCA against the sinus of Valsalva (Fig. 1.68B). No atheromatous plaque was seen in this region.

The patient underwent percutaneous coronary intervention with stenting to the LMCA using a 3.5 × 16 mm Promus Premier drug-eluting stent (Boston Scientific, Natick, Massachusetts) (Fig. 1.68). Adequate stent expansion and ostial coverage was confirmed with intravascular ultrasound. Repeat computed tomographic coronary angiography 1 week after the procedure revealed a widely patent LMCA stent with good ostial coverage in the proximity of the dilated

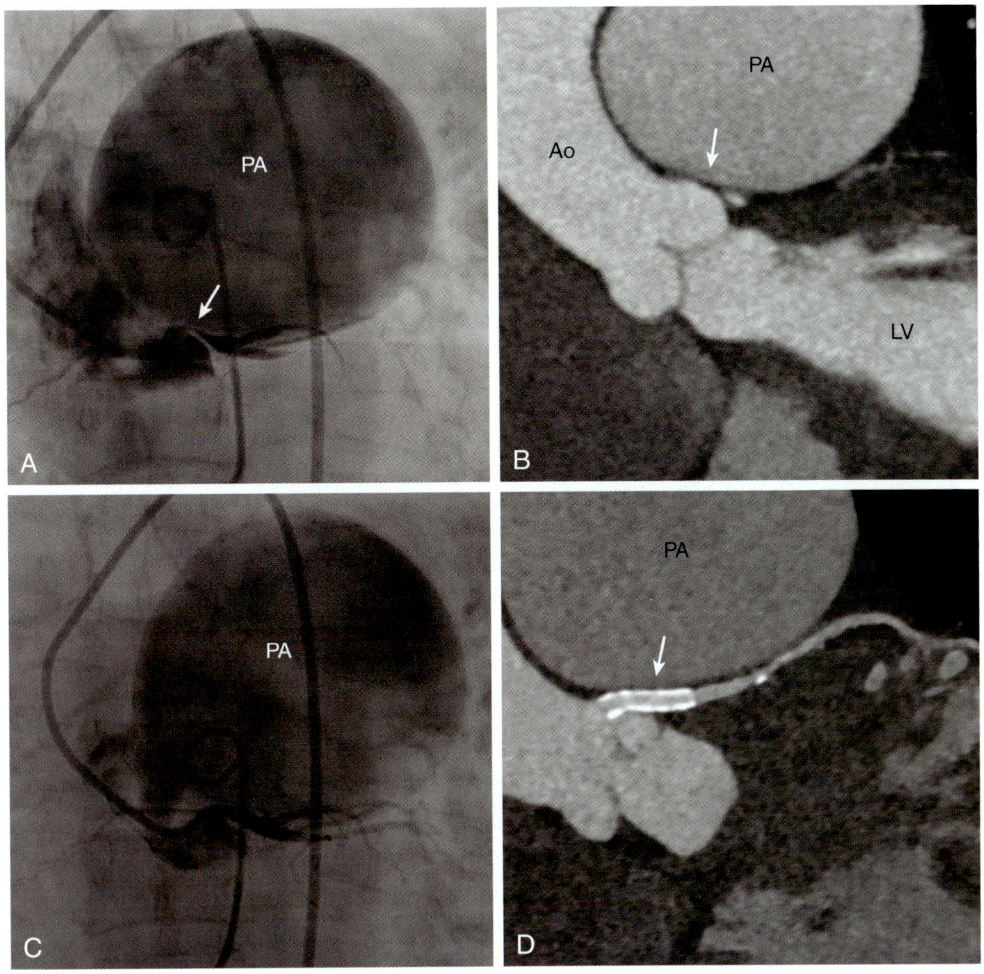

FIG. 1.68 Simultaneous Coronary Angiography of the Left Main Coronary Artery (LMCA) and Main Pulmonary Artery. (A) Simultaneous angiography showing a severely dilated main pulmonary artery (*PA*) compressing and causing a severe stenosis of LMCA as indicated by the *arrow*. (B) Coronary computed tomography (CTCA) showing similar findings of the PA compressing the LMCA (*arrow*). (C) After successful stenting to the LMCA (3.5 × 16 mm Promus Premier). (D) CTCA 1 week after the procedure showing a widely patent stent with ostial coverage. *Ao*, aorta; *LV*, left ventricle.

MPA (Fig. 1.68D). At 1-month follow-up, the patient's symptoms of angina had resolved.

Extrinsic compression of the LMCA should be considered as a cause of angina in patients with pulmonary hypertension. Simultaneous angiography of the LMCA and MPA was performed for diagnosis in our case, which correlated well with computed tomographic coronary angiographic findings. Treatment with percutaneous coronary intervention is safe and feasible.

Spontaneous Aortic Thrombosis Causing Left Main Coronary Occlusion in a Man With Secondary Polycythemia

Nimit C. Shah, MD, Shahzad M. Munir, BSc, MD, Nicholas J. Alp, PhD, DM

A 25-year-old man had ST-segment elevation myocardial infarction and cardiogenic shock. He was brought immediately to the cardiac catheter laboratory. The angiogram showed a large filling defect in the left coronary sinus that extended into the left main coronary artery (Fig. 1.69, Online Video 1.61). The coronary arteries were otherwise angiographically normal. The patient's condition deteriorated with cardiac arrest requiring emergency intubation and ventilation, followed by multiple external cardioversions for recurrent episodes of ventricular tachycardia and ventricular fibrillation. After aspiration of thrombus, the left main coronary artery was directly

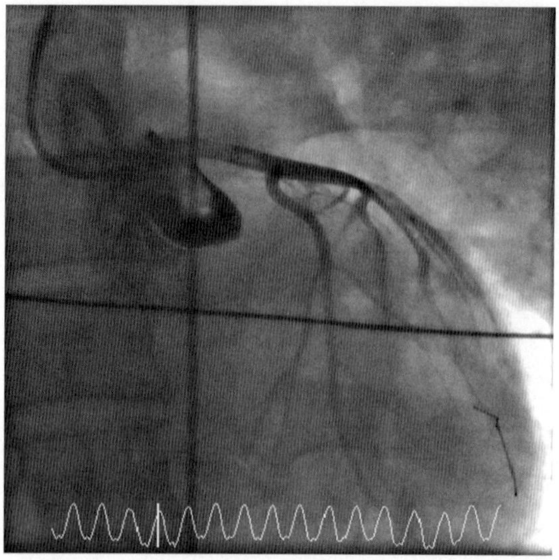

FIG. 1.69 Image acquisition of the left coronary artery injection showed a large filling defect in the left coronary sinus of the aortic root extending into the left main stem. The guidewire can be seen in the left anterior descending artery, and the accompanying electrocardiogram trace revealed broad complex tachycardia. See Online Video 1.61.

stented with a 4.0 × 15 mm bare-metal stent, leading to improvement in the hemodynamic status and cardiac rhythm of the patient. Subsequent transesophageal echocardiography with bubble contrast firmly excluded a patent foramen ovale.

The patient was known to have secondary polycythemia owing to excess alcohol consumption and heavy smoking. He denied the use of any recreational drugs, such as cocaine, and a drug screen was not performed. After his deep vein thrombosis in 2007, he was investigated for clotting abnormalities and was found to be polycythemia with an initial hemoglobin level of 21.1 g/dL and hematocrit of 0.57. The result for genetic testing for the Janus kinase 2 mutation was negative, and a diagnosis of secondary polycythemia was made. The hemoglobin of the patient during this admission was 18.7 g/dL, hematocrit of 0.51, with normal platelet and white blood cell counts. The patient was discharged after 2 weeks with normal results for computed tomography scan of his brain, no neurologic deficit, and only minor impairment of left ventricular function.

Acute thrombosis of major arterial vessels can be life-threatening.[1] Myocardial infarction and sudden death are more common in older patients with polycythemia and underlying coronary artery disease.[2] Cases have been reported with thrombus involving the descending aorta.[1] We now describe a case of spontaneous thrombus formation in the aortic root occluding the left main coronary artery in a young patient with otherwise normal coronaries. Immediate percutaneous coronary intervention is an accepted treatment for acute ST-segment elevation myocardial infarction with hemodynamic compromise,[3] and in this case led to a satisfactory outcome.

References

1. Josephson GD, Tiefenbrun J, Harvey J. Thrombosis of the descending thoracic aorta: a case report. *Surgery.* 1993;114:598-600.
2. Rossi C, Randi ML, Zerbinati P, Rinaldi V, Girolami A. Acute coronary disease in essential thrombocythemia and polycythemia vera. *J Intern Med.* 1998;244:49-53.
3. Venegoni P, Cyprus G. Polycythemia and the heart. A review. *Tex Heart Inst J.* 1994;21:198-201.

Intravascular Ultrasound-Diagnosed Acute Aortic Dissection Involving Left Main Closure

Kayo Takahashi, MD, Shinji Inaba, MD, Kenji Kikuchi, RT, Hiroe Aisu, MD, Toru Morofuji, MD, Makoto Saito, MD, Takumi Sumimoto, MD

A 72-year-old man was admitted to our hospital with cardiogenic shock after chest pain. A prehospital 12-lead electrocardiography showed lead aVR ST-segment elevation with widespread ST-segment depression, suggesting acute left main artery (LMA) obstruction. Therefore, we decided to perform coronary angiography immediately after admission for release from broad myocardial ischemia. Emergent coronary angiography revealed severe LMA obstruction (Fig. 1.70A, Online Video 1.62), consistent with electrocardiography findings. First, we performed dilatation using a 2.5-mm balloon to open the LMA obstruction. After the balloon procedure, we performed intravascular ultrasonography to investigate the cause of the LMA closure. Intravascular ultrasonography clearly showed a dissecting hematoma in the LMA that extended from the aorta (Fig. 1.70B, Online Video 1.63). We thus concluded

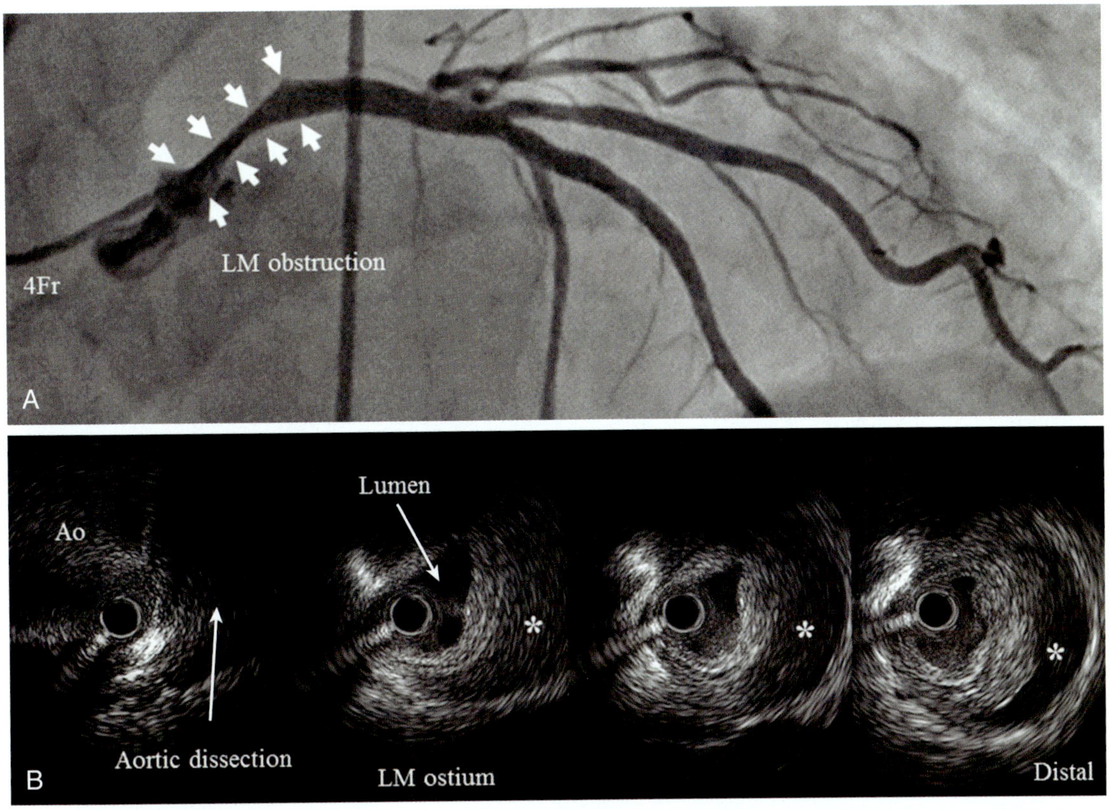

FIG. 1.70 Coronary Angiography and Intravascular Ultrasonography. (A) Angiography showing severe left main artery (*LM*) obstruction (*white arrows*) (Online Video 1.62). (B) Intravascular ultrasonography showing a dissecting hematoma (*asterisk*) in the left main artery that extended from the aorta (*Ao*) (Online Video 1.63).

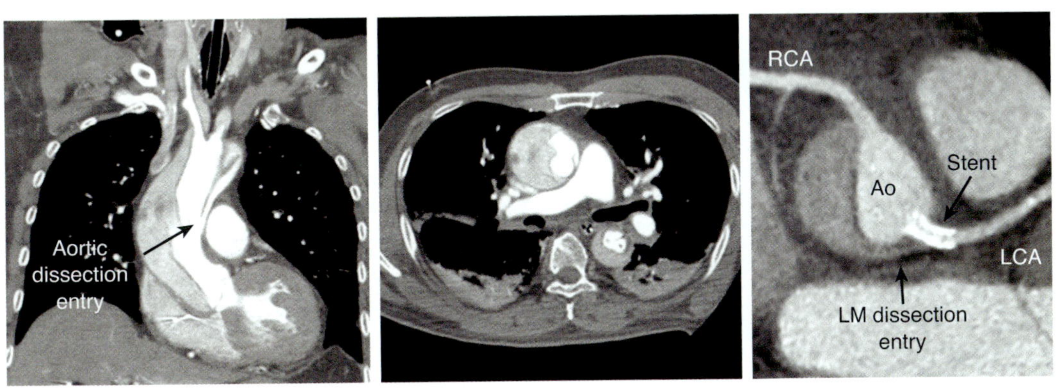

FIG. 1.71 Postprocedure Computed Tomogrpahy (CT). CT showing type A aortic dissection involving the left coronary artery (*LCA*). *Ao*, aorta; *LM*, left main; *RCA*, right coronary artery.

that the cause of the LMA closure was acute type A aortic dissection. Bailout stenting with a 4.0 × 15 mm bare-metal stent to the dissected LMA was needed for the bridge to the cardiac operation because reclosure of the LMA was observed by balloon angioplasty alone. Postprocedure computed tomography confirmed type A aortic dissection involving the LMA (Fig. 1.71). The patient was transferred to another hospital for cardiac surgery. Intravascular ultrasound observation could provide reliable information for diagnosis of life-threatening acute aortic dissection involving LMA closure.

Native Aortic Valve Thrombosis Leading to ST-Segment Elevation Myocardial Infarction

Ali Dogan, MD, Yelda Saltan, MD, Behzat Ozdemir, MD, Kenan Sever, MD, Emrah Ozdemir, MD, Denyan Mansuroglu, MD, Payam Hacisalihoglu, MD, Nuri Kurtoglu, MD

A 54-year-old man with no history of left bundle branch block was admitted to the emergency department with chest pain lasting for 1 hour. Electrocardiography demonstrated newly developed left bundle branch block indicating ST-segment elevation myocardial infarction. He was immediately taken to the catheterization laboratory. Coronary angiography and aortography revealed three-vessel disease and a huge thrombus in the left sinus of Valsalva protruding into the left main coronary artery (Fig. 1.72A, Online Video 1.64). He had neither atrial fibrillation nor an enlarged left atrium at presentation or by history. His hemodynamic status deteriorated quickly and cardiopulmonary arrest developed. The patient was transferred to the operating room to undergo emergent coronary bypass grafting and thrombus removal surgery under cardiopulmonary resuscitation. During surgery the thrombus was extracted from the left sinus of Valsalva (Fig. 1.72B). The surgeons noted that the thrombus was adherent to the aortic valve with a small pedicle, suggesting in situ thrombosis rather than embolization. The valve was involved with the thrombotic process. The mass was subsequently histopathologically proven to be a thrombus (Fig. 1.72C–D). Afterward, the patient was followed up for 1 week and unfortunately died in the intensive care unit as the result of multiorgan failure.

Coronary artery embolism from native aortic valve thrombus is an exceptional, yet possible, case during primary percutaneous coronary intervention.

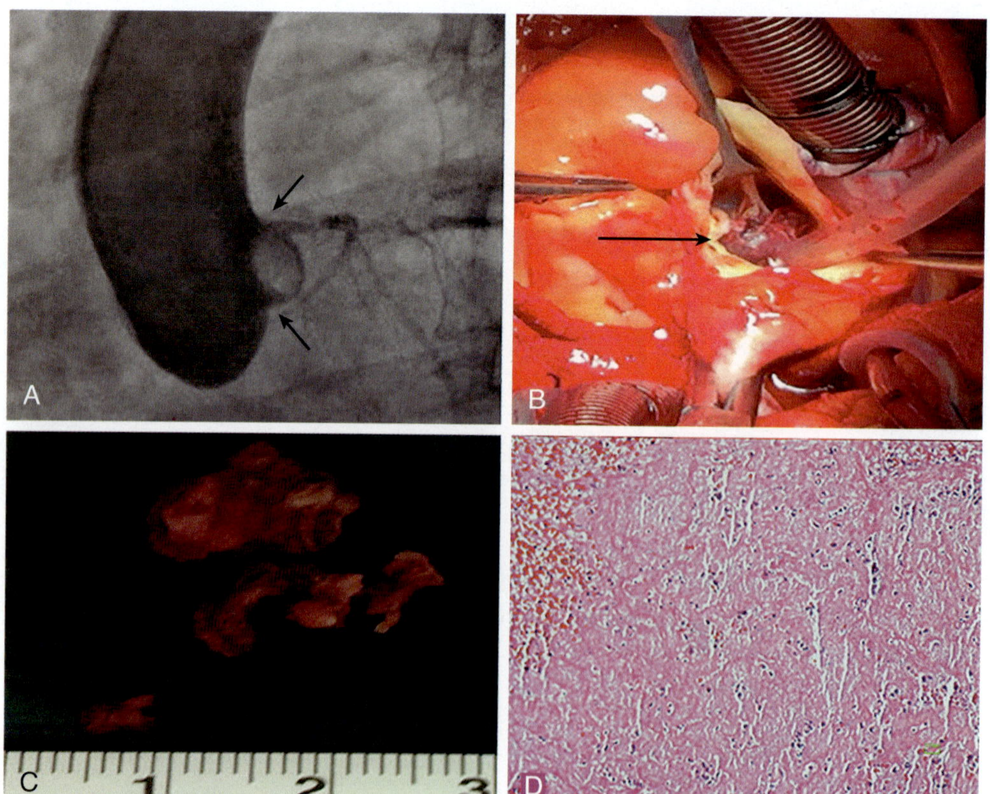

FIG. 1.72 Thrombus in Native Aortic Valve Causing ST-Segment Elevation Myocardial Infarction. (A) Aortographic imaging showing thrombus formation in the left sinus of Valsalva (*arrows*) (Online Video 1.64). (B) Thrombus appearance during emergent operation (*arrow*). (C) Gross appearance of thrombus. (D) Thrombus formation with scattered neutrophil leukocyte infiltration is seen on hematoxylin and eosin–stained pathology slides (×400).

Coronary Spasm

Cocaine-Induced Coronary Vasospasm Using Optical Coherence Tomography Imaging to Guide Management

Matthew W.P. Jackson, MBCHB, Paul D. Williams, BM, CHB, MA, MD

A 47-year-old male smoker had an inferior ST-segment myocardial infarction (STEMI) 4 hours after taking cocaine. Emergency coronary angiography demonstrated a large-caliber proximally occluded right coronary artery (Fig. 1.73A) and similarly large smooth left coronary arteries. Aspiration thrombectomy was performed directly via the guide catheter, and large volumes of red thrombus were removed (Fig. 1.73B). Flow was restored, revealing a tight proximal stenosis (Fig. 1.73C) that, after administration of copious intracoronary nitrates, completely resolved, suggesting cocaine-induced vasospasm (Fig. 1.73D).

Optical coherence tomography (OCT) was performed (Online Video 1.65), demonstrating only mild midvessel atheroma at the site of vasospasm (Fig. 1.73E) and extensive proximal residual thrombus (Fig. 1.73F). A small dissection was noted, possibly related to aspiration thrombectomy, but it was not thought to be clinically significant. Repeat OCT (Online Video 1.66) after 2 days of intravenous tirofiban and heparin showed that the laminar thrombus was still present (Fig. 1.73G–H).

Vasospasm should be considered in all cases of STEMI in which there has been recent cocaine use; it was likely the major contributing factor in our patient's presentation. Intracoronary imaging is important to exclude plaque rupture and erosion as alternative diagnoses, although it was not completely possible in this case owing to the large caliber of the artery and residual thrombus preventing the vessel wall from being fully imaged. Finally, this case demonstrates that aspiration thrombectomy continues to have an important role in selected STEMI cases despite recent evidence showing no benefit from routine use.[1]

References

1. Jolly SS, Cairns JA, Yusuf S, et al. Randomized trial of primary PCI with or without routine manual thrombectomy. *N Engl J Med.* 2015; 372:1389-1398.

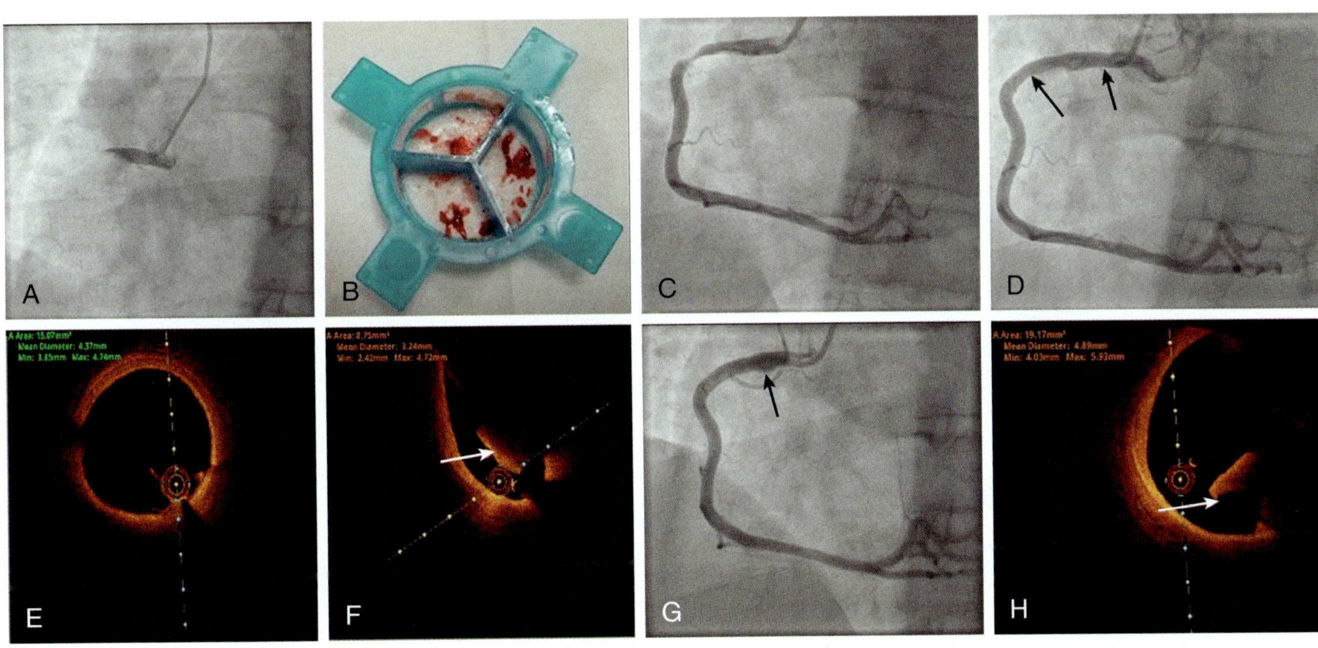

FIG. 1.73 Angiography and Optical Coherence Tomography (OCT) Findings. (A) Proximally occluded right coronary artery. (B) Aspirated thrombus. (C) Tight proximal stenosis and aneurysmal proximal vessel after thrombectomy. (D) Angiogram after administration of intracoronary glyceryl trinitrate; the distal arrow shows location of the image in (E), and the proximal arrow shows location of the image in (F). (E) Intracoronary OCT at the site of previous stenosis. (F) OCT showing proximal aneurysmal segment with extensive thrombus (*arrow*). (G) Repeat angiography after 48 hour; the arrow shows the location of the image in (H). (H) Repeat OCT showing that laminar thrombus is still present (*arrow*). See Online Videos 1.65 and 1.66.

Coronary Spasm Induced by Graves Disease

Naddi Marah, MD, Keisha Bryant, MD, Salman Haq, MD, Muhammad Khan, MD

A 51-year-old woman came to the emergency department with a 3-week history of intermittent palpitations, dyspnea, and substernal chest pain lasting up to 10 minutes with spontaneous resolution. She remained hemodynamically stable, and an electrocardiogram showed a 1.5-mm ST-segment elevation in lead V_2 along with sinus tachycardia. Given the persistence of her symptoms, she underwent diagnostic angiography. Upon coronary vessel engagement with the coronary catheter, there was severe left main and right coronary ostial vasospasm, with dampening of the blood pressure tracings; both subsequently relieved with the administration of sublingual and intracoronary nitroglycerin (Fig. 1.74).

Further investigation revealed an elevated serum-free thyroxine level of 7.22 ng/dL (range 0.76-1.46 ng/dL), suppressed thyroid-stimulating hormone of <0.005 μIU/mL (range 0.36-3.74 μIU/mL), elevated thyroid peroxidase antibody titer of 87 IU/mL (normal value is <9 μIU/ml), and thyroid-stimulating immunoglobulin of 341 IU/mL (normal value is <140 IU/mL), confirming the diagnosis of Graves disease. Although her clinical assessment, supported by a Burch-Wartofsky score of 20, indicated a low likelihood of thyrotoxicosis, she started taking methimazole and propanolol. Euthyroidism was restored thereafter, as well as symptomatic relief with the attenuation of her adrenergic drive.

Multiple hypothetical pathophysiologic pathways have been proposed for the mechanism of thyroid hormone–induced coronary vasospasm. In a Korean study of 6923 subjects undergoing coronary angiography for evaluation of chest pain, the incidence of coronary vasospasm was 5%, with 29% of cases occurring in women younger than 50 years of age.[1] During a thyrotoxic state, hypersensitivity to vasoconstrictive agents, decreased vasodilation, and a general hypermetabolic state precipitate an imbalance between blood supply and oxygen demand.[2] Controlling thyroid activity is in itself curative, obviating the need for unnecessary mechanical interventions and further antianginal therapy.

References

1. Choi YH, Chung JH, Bae SW, et al. Severe coronary artery spasm can be associated with hyperthyroidism. *Coron Artery Dis.* 2005;16:135-139.
2. Jung CH, Rhee EJ, Shin HS, et al. Higher serum free thyroxine levels are associated with coronary artery disease. *Endocrine J.* 2008;55:819-826.

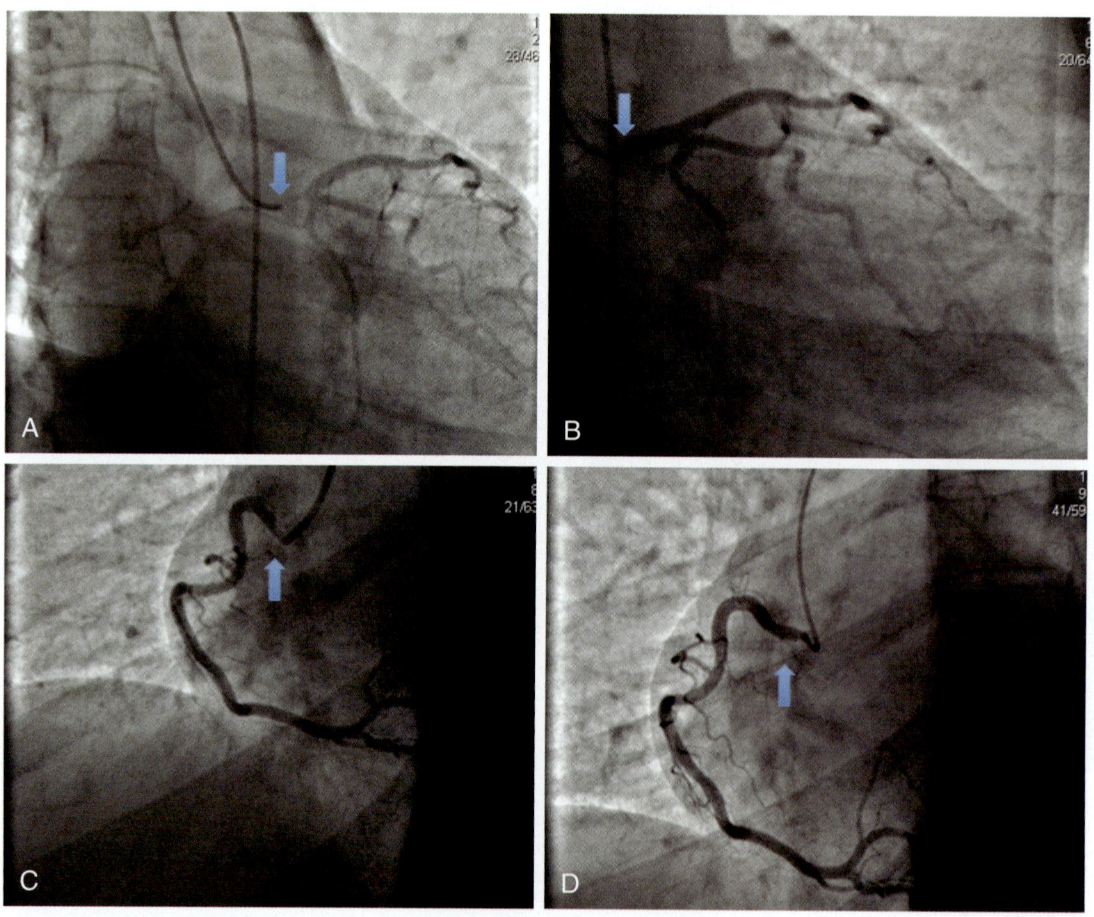

FIG. 1.74 Diagnostic Left Heart Catheterization of the Left and Right Coronary Vessels. (A) Left main coronary artery vasoconstriction (*blue arrow*). (B) Left main coronary vasodilation after intracoronary and sublingual nitroglycerin. (C) Right coronary artery vasoconstriction. (D) Right coronary artery vasodilation after intracoronary and sublingual nitroglycerin.

Severe Generalized Resistant Spasm of the Right Coronary Artery Causing Hemodynamic Collapse After Stenting

Ajit Bhagwat, MD, DM, Sachin Mukhedkar, MD, DM

A long-term male smoker (45 years of age) had substernal chest pain on and off for 2 days. His coronary angiogram revealed the presence of a discrete 80% stenosis in the mid right coronary artery (RCA) (Fig. 1.75A) and a normal left coronary system. Direct stenting with a 3.0 × 15 mm drug-eluting stent was performed at nominal pressure. Chest pain with ST-segment elevation occurred immediately. The angiogram showed severe coronary spasm involving the entire RCA before and after the stented segment, giving it a "threadlike" appearance (Fig. 1.75B). Intracoronary injection of nitroglycerin (200 mg) had no effect, and a repeat angiogram showed no flow in the RCA (Fig. 1.75C). Hypotension (systolic blood pressure, 40 mm Hg) and complete heart block ensued. Intravenous fluids and atropine were administered. Further administration of intracoronary vasodilators was deferred given the patient's hemodynamic instability. Ventricular fibrillation occurred that was cardioverted with a single DC shock. Immediate stenting of the ostioproximal segment of the RCA was performed with 3 × 18 mm drug-eluting stent to "break" the spasm. This resulted in restoration of flow in the artery, but persistent severe spasm of the nonstented segments of the artery was seen (Fig. 1.75D). However, partial restoration of flow resulted in immediate hemodynamic improvement (systolic blood pressure, 70 mm Hg) and disappearance of the heart block. Two more intracoronary doses of nitroglycerin (200 mg each) were given without any angiographic improvement. Intracoronary diltiazem was then administered with relief of coronary spasm and Thrombolysis In Myocardial_Infarction III flow in the artery (Fig. 1.75E–F). Blood pressure was restored after 15 minutes, and the patient was moved to the cardiac care unit in a stable condition. He was discharged after 48 hours taking oral diltiazem along with dual-antiplatelet therapy and a statin. He has been doing well during the 13 months after the procedure.

Life-threatening spasm of the coronary artery after stenting is very rare. Usually the spasm is restricted to a short segment at the edge of the stent and is generally responsive to intracoronary vasodilators. In this case, the spasm was resistant to drugs and caused serious arrhythmias and hemodynamic collapse. Mechanically breaking the spasm by stent implantation remains one of the quickest methods to tide over the crisis in a situation in which the spasm is responsible for life-threatening hemodynamic compromise.

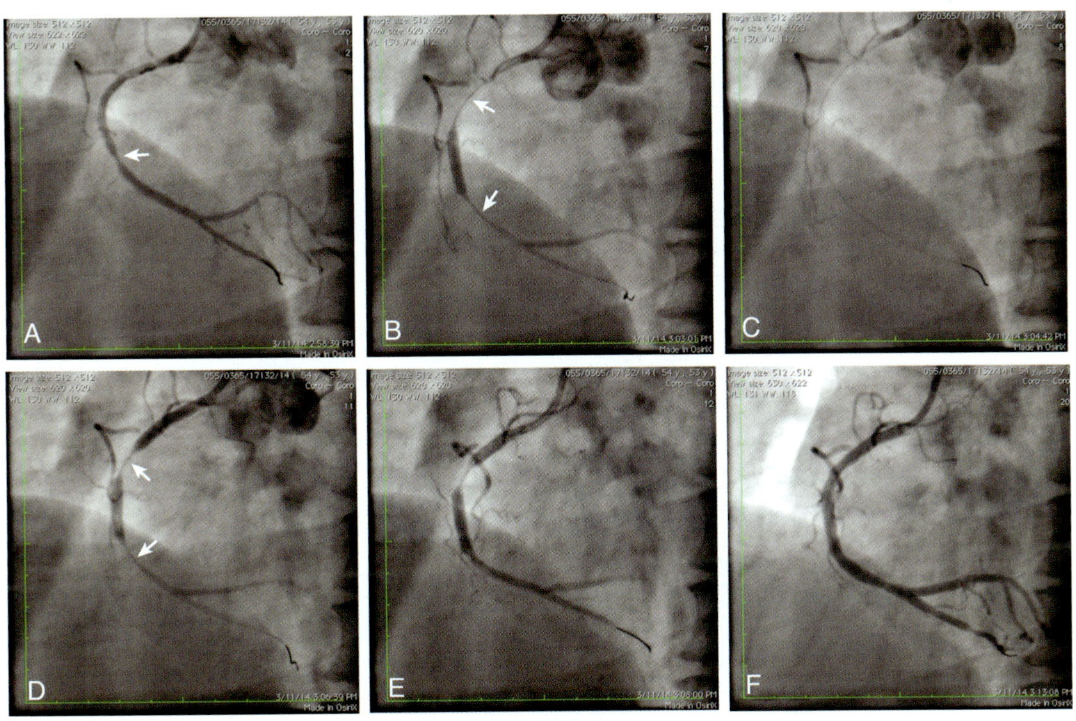

FIG. 1.75 Serial Angiograms of the Righ Coronary Artery (RCA) During the Procedure. (A) Discrete lesion in the mid-RCA (*arrow*). (B) Severe spasm of the entire RCA (*arrows*) before and after the stented segment. (C) No flow in the RCA. (D) Persistent spasm in the nonstented RCA (*arrows*) after proximal stenting. (E) Relief of spasm in the distal RCA after intracoronary diltiazem. (F) Normal RCA at the end of the procedure.

Diffuse Coronary Spasm in a Patient With a Recent Stent

Rabih R. Azar, MD, MSc

A 65-year-old man reported chest pain induced by heavy exercise but sometimes occurring at rest. An exercise stress test was mildly positive electrically (1 mm ST-segment depression at 9 minutes of exercise and at a heart rate of 92% of the maximally predicted heart rate for age). The patient was treated medically. A few months later, he came to the outpatient clinic with more severe and more frequent chest pain occurring mainly at rest. He was referred for coronary angiography, which revealed a 70% stenosis in the mid left anterior descending artery (LAD) (Fig. 1.76A–B). The lesion did not significantly improve with intracoronary nitroglycerin and was treated by implantation of a Liberté 3.5 × 16 mm bare-metal stent (Boston Scientific, Natick, Massachusetts), which was redilated in its proximal segment by a 4 × 10 mm noncompliant balloon at 18 atm. The result was excellent, with a negative residual stenosis and a normal flow (Fig. 1.77). The patient continued to experience chest pain occurring mainly in early morning and awakening him from sleep. The pain was described as more severe than before stenting. Repeat coronary angiography was performed 3 days after the initial procedure (see Online Video 1.67 for the first 2 runs) and revealed diffuse spasm involving all the left coronary circulation (including the left main artery), except in the segment of the LAD where the stent was present (Fig. 1.78, Online Video 1.67). After intracoronary nitroglycerin, the spasm resolved (Fig. 1.79, Online Video 1.67). The patient began taking oral nitroglycerin and a calcium channel blocker and remains pain-free more than 8 months after follow-up.

The stenosis in the LAD of the patient was, in retrospect, not the cause of the symptoms, which were caused by spasm. These images demonstrate that spasm can be diffuse and can involve all the coronary circulation including the left main. They also demonstrate that spasm can occur either proximal or distal to a stented segment, which explains the "inefficacy" of stenting in the treatment of spastic angina.

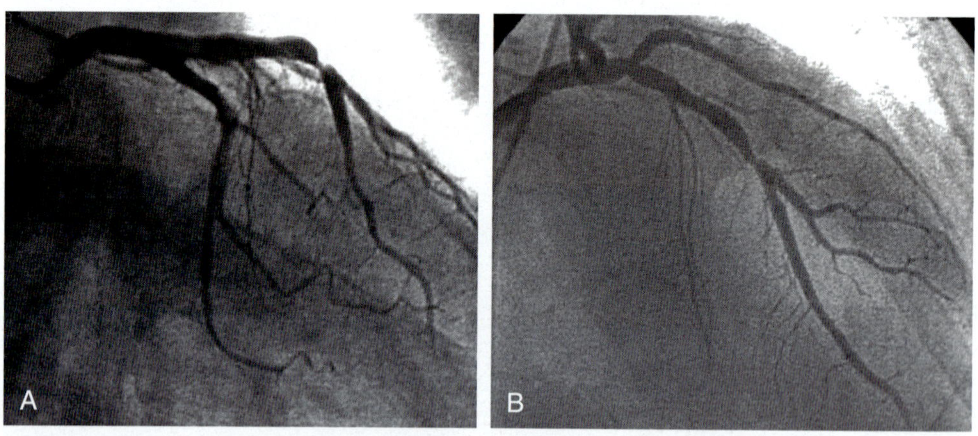

FIG. 1.76 Baseline Angiographic Views. Right caudal oblique view before administration of nitroglycerin. (A) Right cranial oblique view after intracoronary nitroglycerin (B) during the initial procedure showing a tight mid left anterior descending artery stenosis.

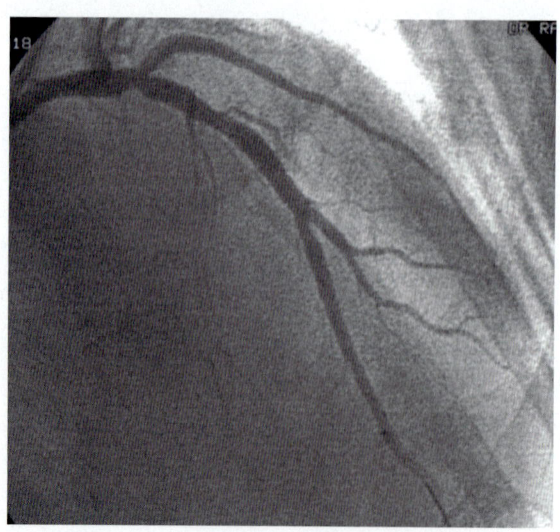

FIG. 1.77 Final Result After Stent Implantation. Right cranial oblique view showing the final angiographic result after implantation of a bare-metal stent (Liberté, Boston Scientific, Natick, Massachusetts), 3.5 × 16 mm in the mid left anterior descending artery. The stent was postdilated at 18 atm with a 4-mm noncompliant balloon.

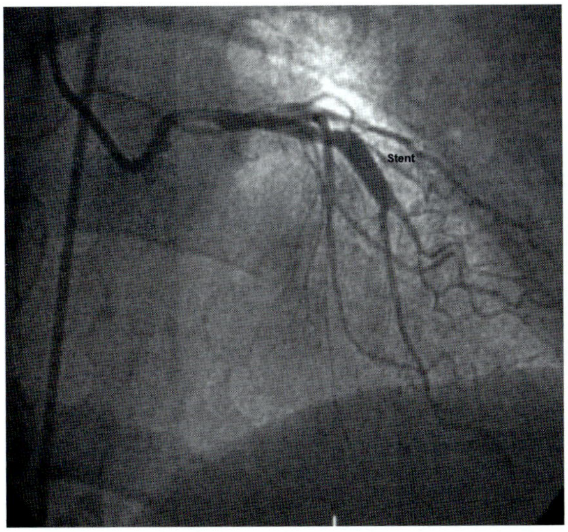

FIG. 1.78 Diffuse Coronary Spasm Except in the Stented Segment. Initial right oblique view during the follow-up procedure 3 days later, showing diffuse coronary spasm occurring proximal and distal to the stented segment and involving the left main artery (Online Video 1.67).

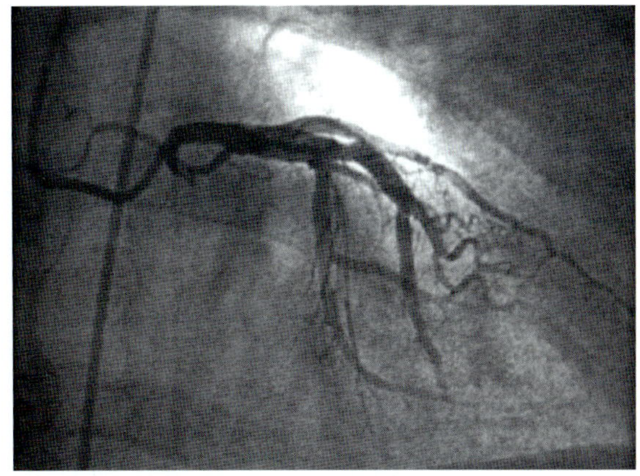

FIG. 1.79 Spasm Resolution. Same right-oblique view after injection of 200 mg of intracoronary nitroglycerin. The spasm has resolved.

Spontaneous Dissection/Hematoma

Three-Dimensional Intravascular Optical Coherence Tomography Rendering Assessment of Spontaneous Coronary Artery Dissection Concomitant With Left Main Ostial Critical Stenosis

Sunki Lee, MD, Chang-Soo Kim, BS, Dong Joo Oh, MD, PhD, Hongki Yoo, PhD, Jin Won Kim, MD, PhD

A 47-year-old man was emergently referred from another tertiary care center for percutaneous coronary intervention to the left main coronary artery (LMCA). Diagnostic coronary angiography indicated a critical stenosis at the LMCA ostium (Fig. 1.80A, *arrow*) and haziness in the proximal to mid left anterior descending coronary artery (LAD) (Fig. 1.80A, *dotted line*). Intravascular ultrasonography showed a heavy plaque burden at the LMCA ostium (Fig. 1.80B). Emergent stent implantation was performed with a Resolute Integrity 4.0 × 12 mm stent (Medtronic Vascular, Santa Rosa, California) from the ostium to the mid body of the LMCA. Because the chest pain was not relieved after stenting, optical coherence tomography (OCT) (C7-XR system, C7 Dragonfly catheter, LightLab Imaging, St. Jude Medical, Minneapolis, Minnesota) was performed to more accurately assess the thrombotic lesion in the proximal to mid LAD. Longitudinal OCT images clearly showed the intimal-medial dissection in the thrombotic LAD lesion. In cross-sectional OCT images, the true lumen was separated from the false lumen with the "entry" and the "reentry door" sites, which strongly suggested spontaneous coronary artery dissection (SCAD) in the proximal LAD. The three-dimensional (3D)-rendered OCT imaging on a stack of the color-coded 2D images using a Digital Imaging and Communications in Medicine (DICOM) viewer and OsiriX software (version 3.9.1; OsiriX Foundation, Geneva, Switzerland) clearly revealed the SCAD morphology (Fig. 1.81A and C), showing a proximal entry tear, dissection flap (Fig. 1.81B, *arrow*), and reentry tear to the true lumen in the distal part (Fig. 1.81D, *arrowhead*). Because of the sustained flow limitation in the LAD, a Resolute Integrity 3.0 × 30 mm stent (Medtronic Vascular) was implanted in the LAD SCAD lesion. Final angiogram and poststenting 3D-rendered OCT image showed optimal results, with Thrombolysis In Myocardial Infarction grade flow 3 (Figs. 1.80C and D). Because the intravascular OCT 3D-rendered images can identify coronary structures more accurately,[1,2] automatic 3D OCT rendering technology under development could be helpful to guide an optimal therapeutic strategy for patients with SCAD.

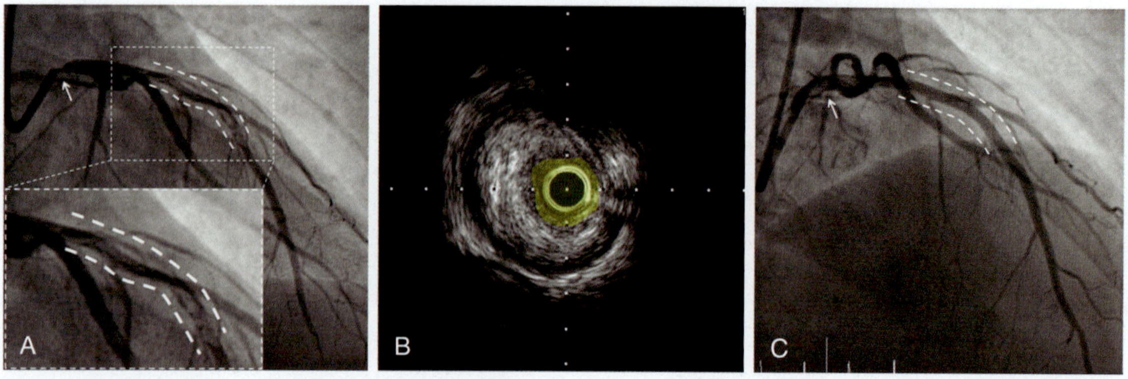

FIG. 1.80 Coronary Angiography and Intravascular Ultrasonography (IVUS). (A) Coronary angiography showed a critical stenosis of the left main coronary artery (LMCA) ostium (*arrow*). A long spiral with a hazy appearance suspicious of a spontaneous coronary artery dissection (SCAD) was identified at the proximal left anterior descending coronary artery (LAD) (*dashed line*). (B) Large fibrofatty plaque burden (*yellow* indicates the minimal luminal area) with tightly compacted guiding catheter at the LMCA ostium was shown by intravascular ultrasound. (C) Final angiogram showed optimal results at the LMCA (*arrow*) and at the SCAD lesion in the LAD (*dashed line*).

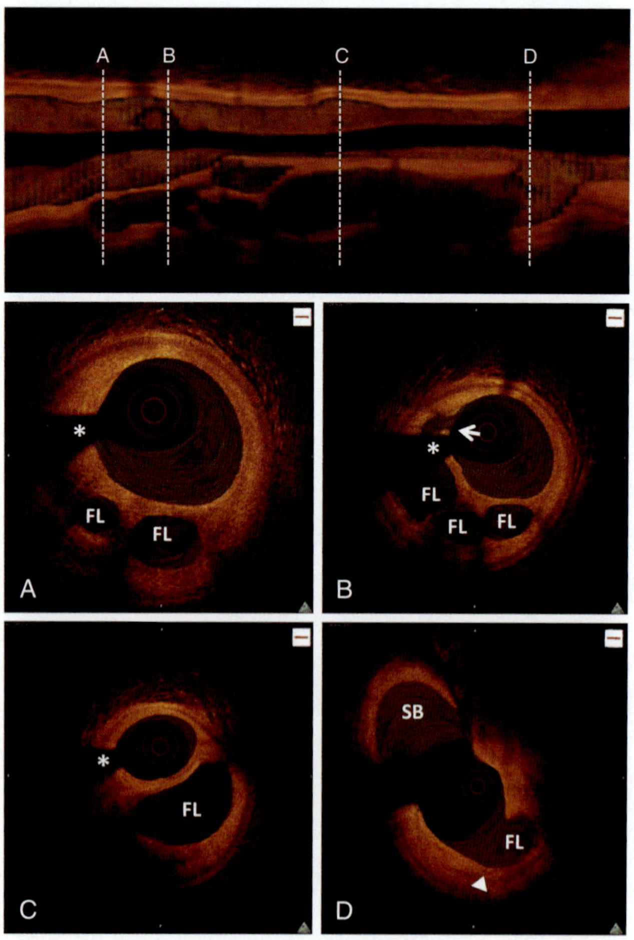

FIG. 1.81 Three-Dimensional–Rendered Optical Coherence Tomography Images. Axial three-dimensional–rendered images confirmed the existence of a spontaneous coronary artery dissection. Corresponding cross-sectional images clearly identified the true lumen separated from the false lumen (*FL*). The dashed white lines labeled A, B, C, and D indicate the entry door; the arrowhead shows the reentry door, and the asterisk shows a shadow artifact caused by the guidewire. SB, side branch.

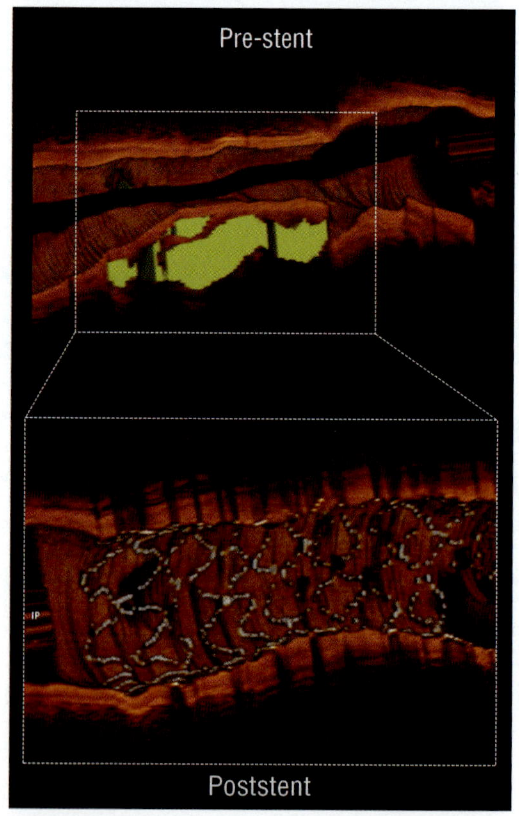

FIG. 1.82 Pre- and Poststenting Three-Dimensional Optical Coherence Tomography Reconstruction Imaging. The three-dimensional reconstruction images showed the morphology of the spontaneous coronary artery dissection lesion in detail. The false lumen is indicated by yellow. The poststenting three-dimensional–rendered image revealed a complete sealing of the false lumen by the stent.

ACKNOWLEDGMENTS

The authors thank Byoung Won Cheon and Woong Seo for their excellent technical assistance.

REFERENCES

1. Cordone S, Ghione M, Foin N, et al. Endovascular imaging and 3D reconstruction of spontaneous coronary artery dissection. *J Am Coll Cardiol.* 2013;62:350.
2. Lowe HC, Narula J, Fujimoto JG, Jang IK. Intracoronary optical diagnostics: current status, limitations, and potential. *J Am Coll Cardiol Intv.* 2011;4:1257-1270.

A Rare Case of Spontaneous Dissection in a Left Internal Mammary Artery Bypass Graft in Acute Coronary Syndrome

Kohei Koyama, MD, PhD, Kihei Yoneyama, MD, PhD, Maya Tsukahara, MD, Shingo Kuwata, MD, Takanobu Mitarai, MD, Ryo Kamijima, MD, Yuki Ishibashi, MD, PhD, Yasuhiro Tanabe, MD, Ken Kongoji, MD, PhD, Tomoo Harada, MD, PhD, Yoshihiro J. Akashi, MD, PhD

A 47-year-old man came to our hospital after he was successfully resuscitated from ventricular fibrillation. He had experienced chest pain while seated at home. He had undergone successful sequential coronary artery bypass grafting 17 months previously, by the use of left internal mammary artery (LIMA) grafts to the left anterior descending artery and the left circumflex artery and a saphenous vein graft to the right coronary artery. Angiography showed dissection with severe stenosis at the middle body of the LIMA (Fig. 1.83A). Intravascular ultrasound and optical coherence tomography revealed dissection at the LIMA (Fig. 1.83B, Online Video 1.68). Two stents were implanted to cover the entire lesion. A few cases of internal mammary artery dissection after physical movement have been reported[1]; however, to our knowledge, no previous report has described spontaneous dissection in a LIMA graft causing acute coronary syndrome without an external factor.

References

1. Freixa X, Gallo R. Internal thoracic artery dissection: a proposed mechanistic explanation. *J Am Coll Cardiol Intv.* 2013;6:533-534.

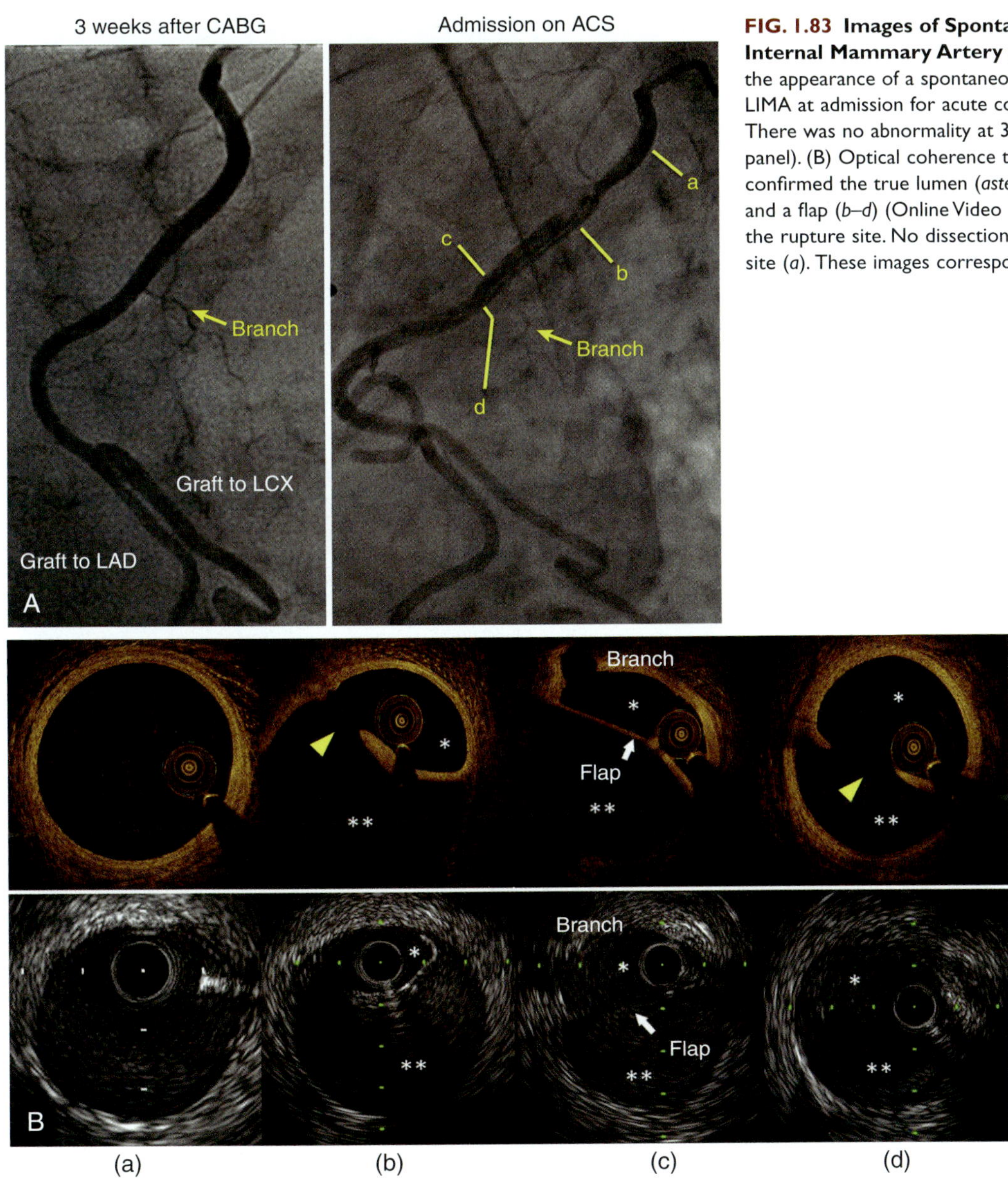

FIG. 1.83 Images of Spontaneous Dissection at the Left Internal Mammary Artery (LIMA). (A) The angiogram revealed the appearance of a spontaneous dissection at the middle body of the LIMA at admission for acute coronary syndrome (right panel; *b–d*). There was no abnormality at 3 weeks after bypass graft surgery (left panel). (B) Optical coherence tomography and intravascular ultrasound confirmed the true lumen (*asterisk*), false lumen (*double asterisk*), and a flap (*b–d*) (Online Video 1.68). The yellow arrowheads indicate the rupture site. No dissection was observed at the proximal site (*a*). These images correspond to the angiogram in (A).

Acute Coronary Syndrome With Clear Coronary Artery: The Case for Concealed Coronary Hematoma

Chiara Fraccaro, MD, Giambattista Isabella, MD, Giuseppe Tarantini, MD, PhD

A 67-year-old obese woman with a history of hypertension and dyslipidemia was admitted at our institution because of non–ST-segment elevation myocardial infarction. Electrocardiography at admission showed flat T waves in inferolateral leads. Two-dimensional transthoracic echocardiography revealed inferolateral wall hypokinesia. The troponin I level peaked at 18 J.g/L. Coronary angiography showed patent coronary arteries without significant stenoses and with Thrombolysis In Myocardial Infarction (TIMI) grade flow 3. Indeed, an intermediate tubular lesion with smooth shape and endoluminal haziness was present at the distal left circumflex artery (LCX) (segment marked in yellow in Fig. 1.84). There was no lumen thrombosis, but contrast density along the course of LCX was inhomogeneous. At intravascular ultrasound (Volcano Therapeutics, Rancho Cordova, California) evaluation, a crescent-shaped lesion (false lumen) through the LCX was visible (Fig. 1.84A–E), lined by the internal elastic membrane (*white arrows* in Fig. 1.84). Moreover, an echogenic mass was evident within the vessel wall (intramural hematoma).

No atherosclerotic lesions were visible. The backscatter intensity of blood increased from the proximal to the distal part of the crescent-shaped area as a consequence of partial thrombosis of the false lumen. The other coronaries appeared normal. The patient was discharged 1 week later with dual-antiplatelet therapy and remained asymptomatic at 1-year follow-up.

Intramural hematoma after spontaneous dissection is not exceptional and should always be suspected and confirmed by intravascular ultrasound in case of acute coronary syndrome without overt severe coronary lesions at angiography. The presence of intermediate, tubular coronary lesions with a smooth shape or the evidence of abrupt loss of the vessel size, in the absence of thrombosis or intimal flail, should prompt suspicion of intramural hematoma.[1,2] Of note, when a patient is clinically stable with TIMI grade flow 3, percutaneous treatment is not mandatory because of the risk of hematoma progression and the likelihood of spontaneous healing.[3]

References

1. Mintz GS, Nissen SE, Anderson WD, et al. ACC clinical expert consensus document on standards for the acquisition, measurement and reporting of intravascular ultrasound studies: a report of the American College of Cardiology Task Force on Clinical Expert Consensus Documents (Committee to Develop a Clinical Expert Consensus Document on Standards for Acquisition, Measurement and Reporting of Intravascular Ultrasound Studies [IVUS]). *J Am Coll Cardiol.* 2001;37:1478-1492.
2. Maehara A, Mintz GS, Castagna MT, et al. Intravascular ultrasound assessment of spontaneous coronary artery dissection. *Am J Cardiol.* 2002;89:466-468.
3. Sanchez-Recalde A, Moreno R, Jiménez-Valero S. Stenting of spontaneous intramural coronary haematoma: long-term consequences. *Eur Heart J.* 2008;29:1593.

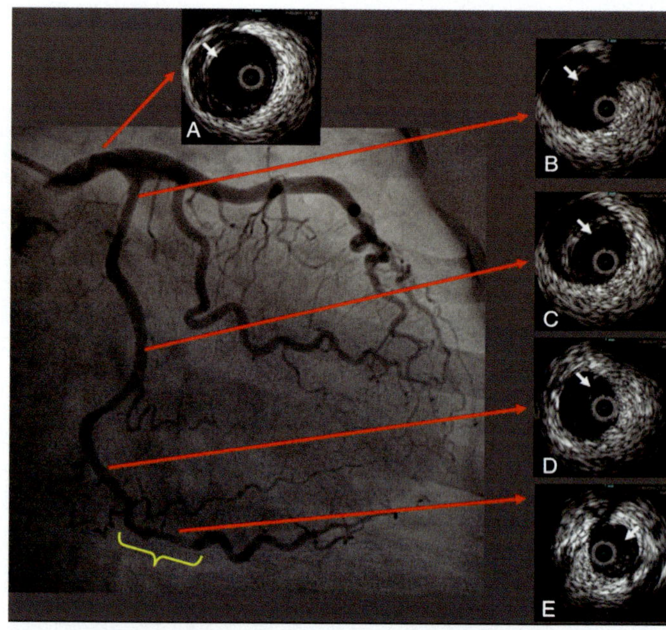

FIG. 1.84 Angiographic Appearance of Left Coronary Artery. Five slices (A–E) obtained by intravascular ultrasound, taken throughout the left circumflex coronary artery (*LCX*), show the presence of false lumen occupied by an echogenic mass (intramural hematoma). The true lumen is compressed and distorted and appears narrowed. No atherosclerosis was visible. *ACS*, acute coronary syndrome; *CABG*, coronary artery bypass grafting.

Cocaine-Induced Coronary Artery Dissection

Alexander Ijsselmuiden, MD, PhD, Stefan Verheye, MD, PhD

A 54-year-old woman came to our hospital with angina pectoris, negative precordial T waves, and normal cardiac enzyme levels. After medical stabilization, coronary angiography showed a focal nonsignificant (fractional flow reserve 0.95) narrowing in the proximal left anterior descending artery (Fig. 1.85A, *arrow*). Subsequent optical coherence tomography (OCT) showed a 1.13-mm long intimal flap (Fig. 1.85B, *arrow*). Because her symptoms had developed shortly after cocaine abuse, we suspected a subintimal tear resulting in a spontaneous dissection as the result of increased endothelial shear stress caused by the inotropic, chronotropic, and vasoconstrictive effects of cocaine. The patient was treated with aspirin, statin, and angiotensin-converting enzyme inhibition. The remainder of her course was uneventful.

The diagnosis of coronary artery dissection is generally based on coronary angiography or intravascular ultrasonography. OCT is a novel diagnostic tool using short-pulse lasers allowing high-quality micrometer resolution images of the coronary artery wall. Thus, OCT could be instrumental in diagnosing cocaine-induced coronary artery dissection.

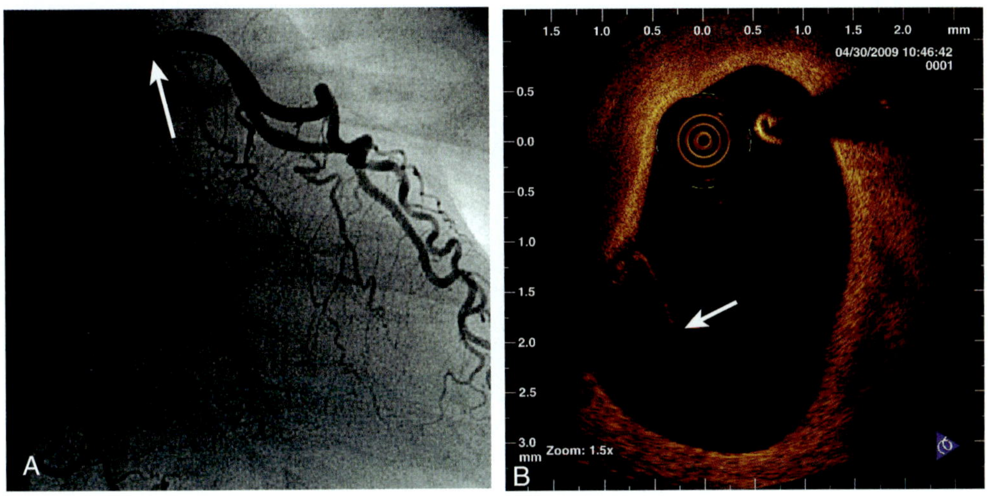

FIG. 1.85 Optical Coherence Tomography (OCT) Reveals Coronary Artery Dissection. Image (A) (*arrow*) shows an angiographic image of a focal nonsignificant (fractional flow reserve 0.95) narrowing in the proximal left anterior descending artery. Image (B) (*arrow*) shows a subsequent OCT image of the same narrowing in the proximal left anterior descending artery and reveals a 1.13-mm-long intimal flap. OCT is a novel diagnostic tool using ultrashort-pulse lasers allowing high-quality micrometer resolution images of the coronary artery.

Complete Healing of Spontaneous Coronary Artery Dissection Demonstrated by Optical Coherence Tomography in a Young Postpartum Female With Acute Coronary Syndrome

Periklis Davlouros, MD, PhD, Ioanna Xanthopoulou, MD, PhD, Grigorios Tsigkas, MD, PhD, Virginia Mplani, MD, Stefanos Despotopoulos, MD, George Hahalis, MD, PhD

Twenty days after a cesarean section, a 27-year-old primigravida had chest pain, ST-segment elevation in electrocardiogram leads I, aVL, and V_1 to V_6, positive troponin I level, and apical hypokinesia with a left ventricular ejection fraction of 45%. The patient was a smoker with no other risk factors for coronary artery disease. Coronary angiography disclosed a long, smooth-bordered proximal stenosis of the left anterior descending coronary artery (LAD), starting at the ostium of the vessel, without any filling defects (Fig. 1.86A), and with Thrombolysis In Myocardial Infarction (TIMI) grade flow 3. The patient subsequently had an optical coherence tomography (OCT) study with the C7-XR FD-OCT system (LightLab, St. Jude Medical, St. Paul, Minnesota) and the Dragonfly Duo optical fiber. The latter

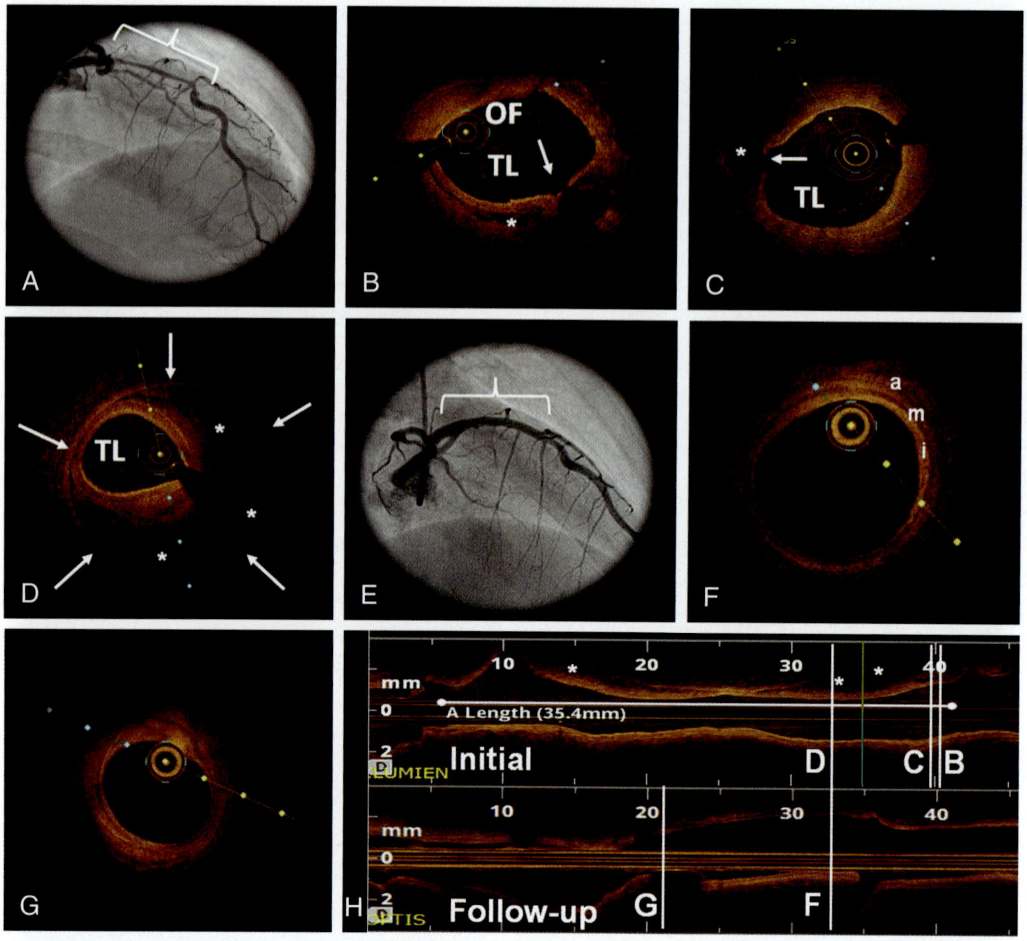

FIG. 1.86 Acute and Chronic Angiographic and Optical Coherence Tomography (OCT) Findings of Spontaneous Coronary Dissection. (A) Coronary angiography, right anterior oblique projection showing a long, smooth-bordered stenosis of the left anterior descending artery (LAD) extending from the very proximal part of the vessel, up to its middle part (*white square bracket*). (B) OCT cross section corresponding to line *B* of the initial longitudinal recording in (H) showing the proximal part of dissection with narrowing of the true lumen (*TL*). The arrow points to an area of thinning adventitia just before rupture. The asterisk denotes rupture of the media creating the false lumen. (C) OCT cross section corresponding to line C of the initial longitudinal recording in (H) showing the point of spontaneous rupture of the intima (*arrow*), creating communication with the false lumen. (D) OCT cross section corresponding to line D of the initial longitudinal recording in (H) showing severe narrowing of the TL. The asterisks denote the false lumen, and the arrows point to the perimeter of the adventitia. (E) Coronary angiography, right anterior oblique projection (similar to A), at 4 months of follow-up. Complete restoration of the angiographic anatomy of the LAD (*white square bracket*). (F) OCT cross section corresponding to line *F* of the follow-up longitudinal recording in (H) showing complete disappearance of dissection (compared with D). Restoration of the vessel wall with normal intima (*i*), media (*m*), and adventitia (*a*). (G) OCT cross section corresponding to line G of the follow-up longitudinal recording in (H) shows the absence of dissection with a 20% residual diameter stenosis. (H) Longitudinal OCT recordings from the distal (*left*), toward the proximal (*right*) LAD. The initial recording shows the dissected part of the vessel (approximately 35 mm in length), corresponding to the bracketed segment of (A) Follow-up recording of the same segment is presented at the bottom. Asterisks denote the false lumen, which has disappeared at 4-month follow-up.

disclosed rupture of the intima of the LAD (Fig. 1.86B–C), with two clearly oriented lumens (true and false), representing spontaneous coronary artery dissection, at a length of 35 mm (Fig. 1.86D and H). A conservative approach was decided on because the patient was stable without evidence of ongoing ischemia and with normal TIMI grade flow.[1-3] She was discharged at 4 days taking aspirin 100 mg once daily, rosuvastatin 20 mg once daily, and metoprolol 25 mg twice daily.[3] At 4 months, follow-up angiography was performed showing complete restoration of the angiographic anatomy (Fig. 45.1E); OCT imaging showed disappearance of the dissection with minimal residual diameter stenosis distally (Fig. 1.86F–H). OCT should be the preferred intravascular imaging modality for diagnosing and planning therapy of spontaneous coronary artery dissection.[1,3,4]

References

1. Tweet MS, Gulati R, Williamson EE, Vrtiska TJ, Hayes SN. Multimodality imaging for spontaneous coronary artery dissection in women. *J Am Coll Cardiol Img.* 2016;9:436-450.
2. Lettieri C, Zavalloni D, Rossini R, et al. Management and long-term prognosis of spontaneous coronary artery dissection. *Am J Cardiol.* 2015;116:66-73.
3. Saw J, Mancini GB, Humphries KH. Contemporary review on spontaneous coronary artery dissection. *J Am Coll Cardiol.* 2016;68:297-312.
4. Alfonso F, Paulo M, Gonzalo N, et al. Diagnosis of spontaneous coronary artery dissection by optical coherence tomography. *J Am Coll Cardiol.* 2012;59:1073-1079.

Endovascular Imaging of Angiographically Invisible Spontaneous Coronary Artery Dissection

Fernando Alfonso, MD, Manuel Paulo, MD, Jaime Dutary, MD

Spontaneous coronary artery dissection (SCD) is a rare clinical entity.[1,2] Clinical diagnosis is challenging and classically relies on the angiographic demonstration of an intimomedial "flap" leading to a double lumen appearance.[1,2] Angiography, however, is unable to visualize the coronary wall. New intracoronary diagnostic tools provide comprehensive, tomographic, high-resolution insights on vessel wall pathology, allowing a precise diagnosis of SCD.[3,4]

A 58-year-old woman had a non–ST-segment elevation inferior myocardial infarction. Angiography (Fig. 1.87A) revealed a normal right coronary artery with just minor lumen irregularities. Intravascular ultrasound (IVUS) (Fig. 1.87B) (resolution 150 μm) disclosed a large intramural hematoma along the entire right coronary artery. The coronary lumen was fully preserved, the coronary wall was readily recognized, and the abluminal hematoma (*asterisks*) had a heterogeneous pattern suggesting recent bleeding and ongoing thrombus formation. Optical coherence tomography (OCT) (Fig. 1.87C) (resolution 15 1-m) identified a confined proximal entry tear (*arrow*) leading to a large distal intramural hematoma (Fig. 1.87D). The clinical course was uneventful with conservative medical management.

Intravascular diagnostic techniques provide novel insights into the pathophysiology of SCD.[3,4] Currently, illnesses in many patients with negative angiographic findings are readily diagnosed with these tools if the level of clinical suspicion is adequate. This case clearly illustrates their potential complementary value in selected patients. OCT provides uniquely high-resolution images of the intimomedial "flap" and is able to accurately identify the "entry door." However, most of the outer boundary of the vessel is not visualized (especially in large vessels), and the presence of red thrombus (or thrombin-rich intramural hematoma) produces dorsal shadowing, preventing visualization of posterior structures in the coronary wall. Alternatively, IVUS has a lower axial resolution but better depicts the complete vessel wall, even in patients with intraluminal red thrombus and in those with large coronary vessels.

References

1. Pretty H. Dissecting aneurysms of coronary artery in woman aged 42: rupture. *BMJ.* 1931;1:667.
2. DeMaio SJ Jr., Kinsella SH, Silverman ME. Clinical course and long-term prognosis of spontaneous coronary artery dissection. *Am J Cardiol.* 1989;64:471-474.
3. Maehara A, Mintz GS, Castagna MT, et al. Intravascular ultrasound assessment of spontaneous coronary artery dissection. *Am J Cardiol.* 2002;89:466-468.
4. Alfonso F, Canales E, Aleong G. Spontaneous coronary artery dissection: diagnosis by optical coherence tomography. *Eur Heart J.* 2009;30:385.

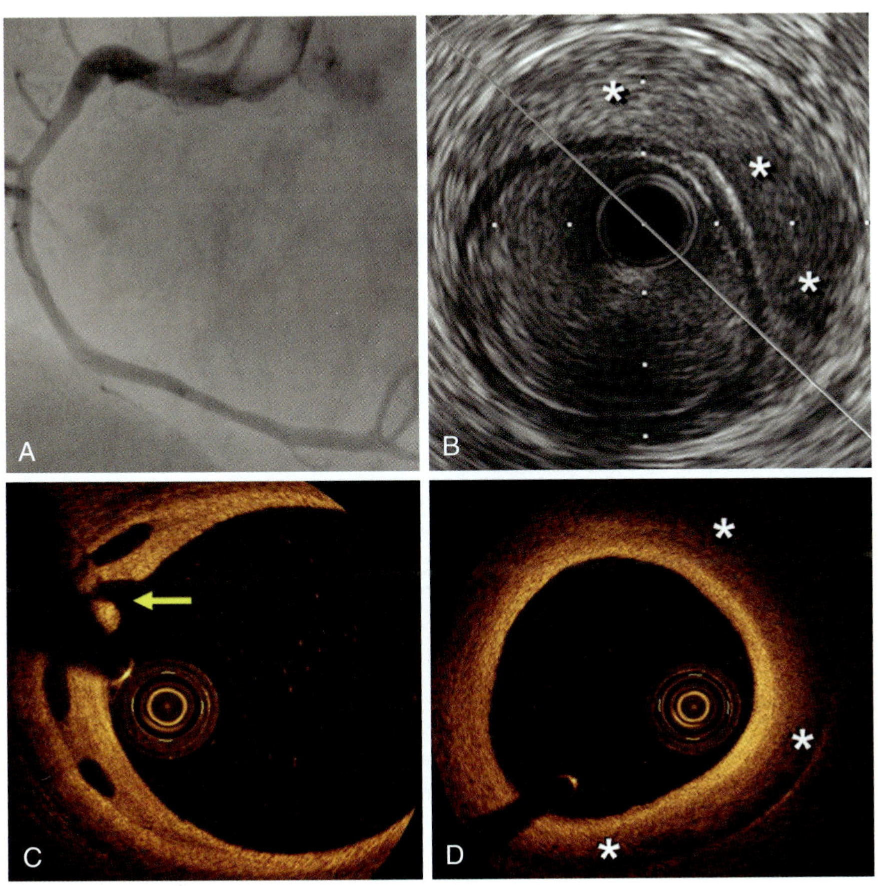

FIG. 1.87 Combined Use of Intravascular Ultrasonography and Optical Coherence Tomography (OCT) in Spontaneous Coronary Artery Dissection. (A) Coronary angiography showing a right coronary artery without significant coronary stenosis. (B) Intravascular ultrasonography imaging disclosing the presence of a large space (*asterisks*) separating the intimomedial membrane from the external elastic membrane. The coronary lumen was largely preserved (minimal lumen diameter 3.5 mm). (C) OCT unraveling (*arrow*) the intimal tear in the proximal right coronary artery with an anfractuous entrance into the coronary vessel wall. (D) An image of intramural hematoma (*asterisks*) was demonstrated in the mid and distal segments of the vessel. In most segments, the outer boundaries of the vessel were not visualized.

Fibromuscular Dysplasia Presenting With Spontaneous Dissection of the Left Main Artery

Mahmoud Abdelghany, MD, Puneet Bansal, MD, Hani Kozman, MD

A 31-year-old woman with a history of trisomy 10, subarachnoid hemorrhage, and previous myocardial infarction was seen with asystolic cardiac arrest preceded by chest pain and shortness of breath. After return of spontaneous circulation, electrocardiogram showed ST-segment elevation in the anteroseptal leads. Cardiac biomarker levels were elevated. Coronary angiogram showed spontaneous dissection of the left main artery extending into proximal left anterior descending and left circumflex arteries. The mid segment of the left anterior descending artery had an aneurysm, and the obtuse marginal artery showed smooth narrowing of the distal segment (Fig. 1.88, Online Video 1.69). The right coronary artery was normal. An intraaortic balloon pump was placed for hemodynamic support, but the patient died during the cardiac catheterization after multiple episodes of asystolic cardiac arrest. Coronary fibromuscular dysplasia (FMD) was suspected and confirmed by the finding of beading of the cavernous internal carotid arteries on a computed tomography angiogram of the head obtained 8 years earlier (Fig. 1.89).

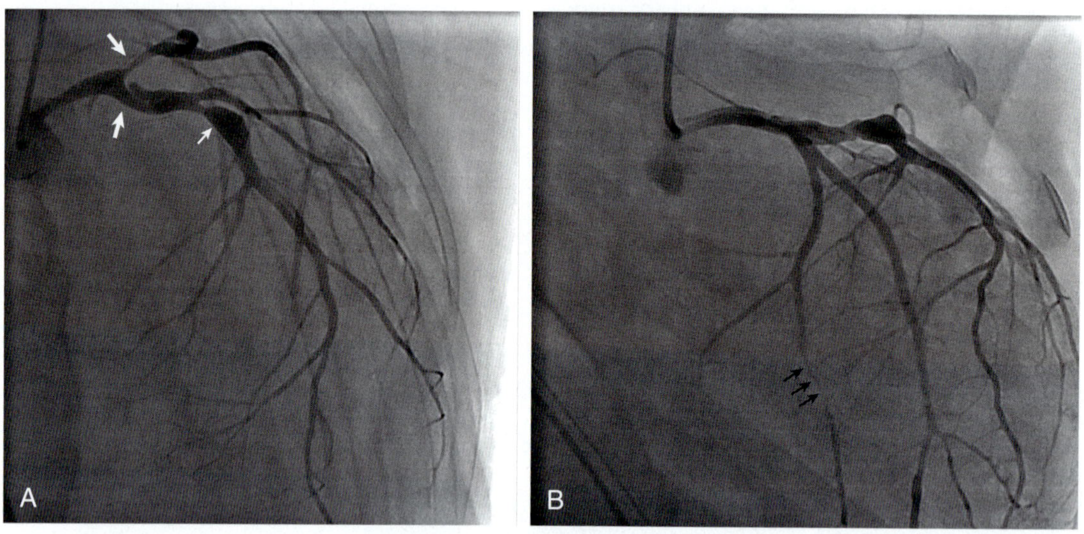

FIG. 1.88 Left Coronary Angiography. Left coronary angiography showing (A) dissection of the left main artery (Online Video 1.69) extending into the proximal left anterior descending and left circumflex arteries (*white thick arrows*). The mid segment of the left anterior descending artery had an aneurysmal dilatation (*white thin arrow*). (B) The obtuse marginal artery showed smooth narrowing of the distal segment (*black arrows*).

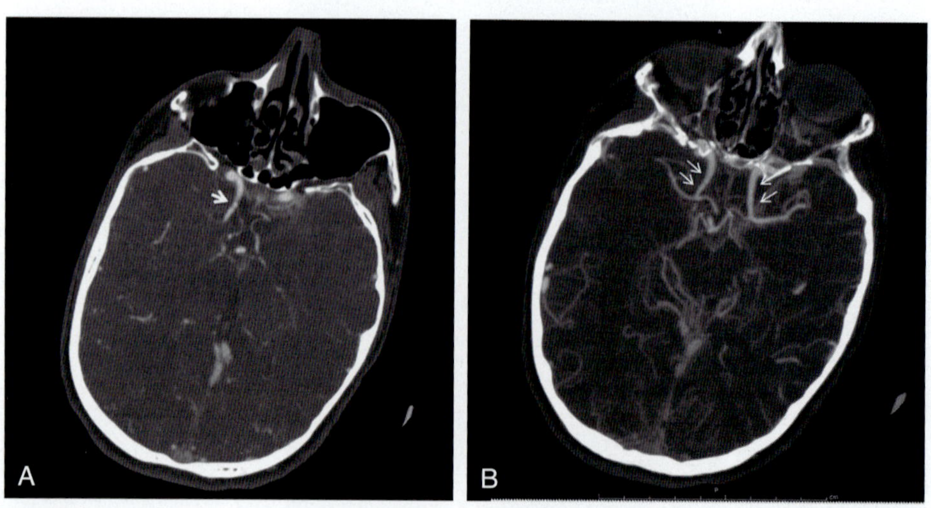

FIG. 1.89 Computed Tomography Angiogram of the Head. Computed tomography angiogram of the head showing (A) mild beading of the right cavernous internal carotid artery (*arrow*). (B) Computed tomography angiogram of the head, reconstruction image, showing mild beading of both right and left cavernous internal carotid arteries (*arrows*).

An FMD is an arteriopathy that predominantly affects middle-aged women.[1] The etiology of FMD is still unknown, although genetic predisposition is likely. The renal and cervicocranial arteries are most commonly involved, whereas the coronary arteries are rarely affected in FMD.[2] The classic angiographic "string of beads" that may be observed in the renal artery rarely occurs in coronary arteries. Spontaneous coronary arteries dissection (SCAD) is the most common manifestation of coronary FMD; FMD presents in most patients with SCAD.[1] Other angiographic findings include aneurysmal dilation, smooth narrowing, or distal tapering, typically with intramural hematoma, spasm, and tortuosity.[2] SCAD may be initiated by an intimal tear that leads to propagating medial dissection, or by a dissecting medial hematoma, initiated by rupture of the vaso vasorum.[1] In patients in hemodynamically stable condition with SCAD, conservative therapy, with aspirin and β-blockers, is preferred. Patients with symptoms of ongoing ischemia or hemodynamic compromise should be considered for revascularization, which can be technically challenging and associated with higher complications.[3]

References

1. Saw J, Ricci D, Starovoytov A, Fox R, Buller CE. Spontaneous coronary artery dissection: prevalence of predisposing conditions including fibromuscular dysplasia in a tertiary center cohort. *J Am Coll Cardiol Intv.* 2013;6:44-52.
2. Saw J, Bezerra H, Gornik HL, Machan L, Mancini GB. Angiographic and intracoronary manifestations of coronary fibromuscular dysplasia. *Circulation.* 2016;133:1548-1559.
3. Saw J, Aymong E, Sedlak T, et al. Spontaneous coronary artery dissection: association with predisposing arteriopathies and precipitating stressors and cardiovascular outcomes. *Circ Cardiovasc Interv.* 2014;7:645-655.

Is This Spontaneous Coronary Intramural Hematoma or Fibrotic Plaque? An Inconsistent Finding Between Optical Coherence Tomography and Intravascular Ultrasonography

Wei Liu, MD, Yu-Jie Zhou, MD, Yu-Yang Liu, MD, Dong-Mei Shi, MD

A 29-year-old woman (gravida 2, para 2) 3 months after an uneventful cesarean delivery had a non–ST-segment elevation myocardial infarction. The patient was healthy and not a smoker. Laboratory test results were unremarkable except for a white blood cell count of 7.46 g/L with 5% eosinophils. Both computed tomography and coronary angiography showed severe ostial left anterior descending artery (LAD) stenosis (Fig. 1.90A–B). Because of the lesion's critical lesion, intervention was deferred. Repeat coronary angiography 2 weeks later showed that the severe stenosis in the ostial LAD had greatly resolved (Fig. 1.90C–D). Intravascular ultrasound (IVUS) examination showed a small localized (7-mm) dense lesion resembling thick fibrotic plaque (Fig. 1.91A–B). Subsequently, optical coherent tomography (OCT) was performed showing that the lesion had an integrated intima and well-defined adventitia, separated by a healing residual intramural hematoma (Fig. 1.91C). No intervention of the LAD was performed.

A spontaneous intramural hematoma is a subset of spontaneous coronary dissection in which the dissection is commonly located between the medial and adventitial layer without an intimal tear or atherosclerosis.[1] Thus, it may be difficult to visualize the dissection with coronary angiography or CT angiography, and the real frequency may be underestimated.[2] An intramural hematoma can only be diagnosed by OCT or IVUS.[3]

There are no previous data describing how an intramural hematoma can be depicted by using virtual histology. However, this technique tends to depict an intramural thrombus as green

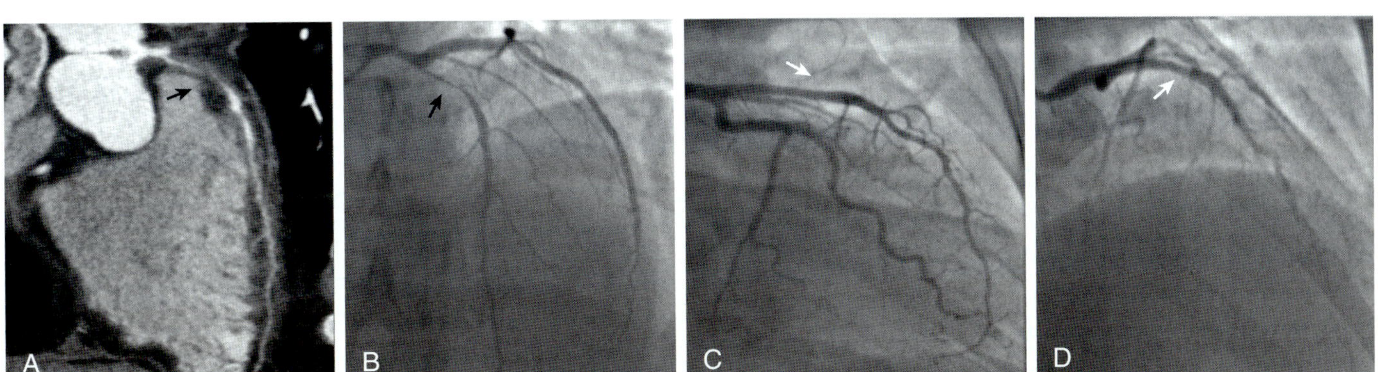

FIG. 1.90 Computed Tomography Angiography (CTA) and Coronary Angiography (CAG). (A and B) Both initial tomography angiography (CTA) and CAG were performed 3 months postpartum showing severe stenosis of ostial left anterior descending artery (LAD, *black arrow*). CTA and CAG were performed 1 day apart; intracoronary nitroglycerin was administered to rule out vasospasm; thus the lesion was unlikely caused by coronary spasm. (C and D) Repeat coronary angiography 2 weeks later showed that the LAD lesion had greatly resolved (*white arrow*).

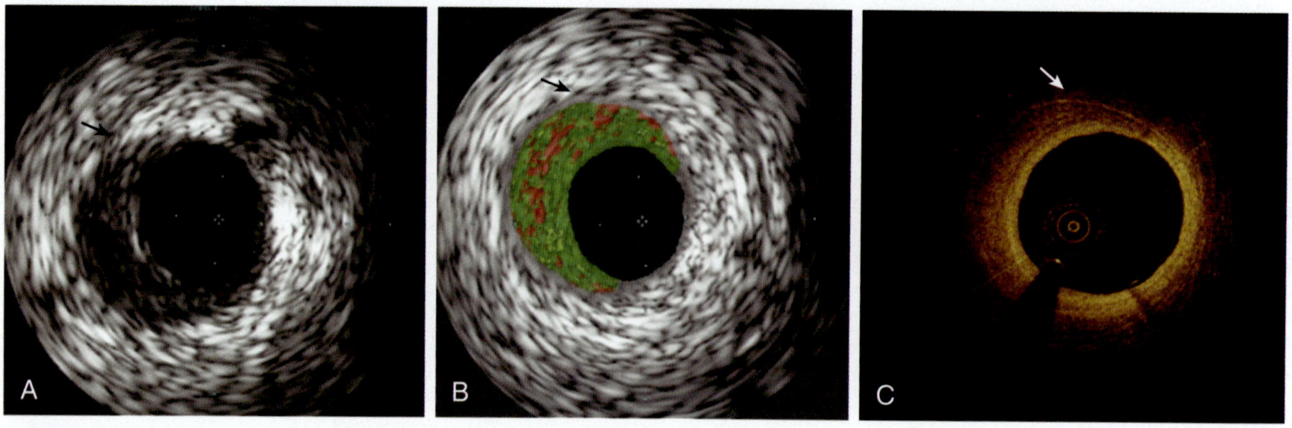

FIG. 1.91 Intravascular Ultrasonography and Optical Coherent Tomography (OCT). (A and B) Both gray-scale and virtual histology intravascular ultrasonography showed a lesion resembling thick fibrotic plaque (*black arrow*). (C) OCT showed that the intima was intact, and there was a healing intramural hematoma (*white arrow*) separating the media and adventitia from the 6- to 12-o'clock positions (*red dots*). The adventitia was clearly seen; there was no shadowing by OCT.

(masquerading as fibrotic or fibrolipid plaque).[4] Without consideration of the clinical setting, the IVUS images of a healing intramural hematoma in this case were also likely to be mistakenly interpreted as fibrotic plaque. A higher-resolution imaging system such as OCT may give a correct diagnosis by better characterization of intramural abnormalities.

References

1. Vrints CJ. Spontaneous coronary artery dissection. *Heart.* 2010;96:801-808.
2. Sheikh AS, O'Sullivan M. Pregnancy-related spontaneous coronary artery dissection: two case reports and a comprehensive review of literature. *Heart Views.* 2012;13:53-65.
3. Johnson TW, Smith D, Strange JW, Bucciarelli-Ducci C, Lowe R, Baumbach A. Spontaneous multivessel coronary intramural hematoma: an insight with OCT. *J Am Coll Cardiol Intv.* 2012;5:1070-1071.
4. Nasu K, Tsuchikane E, Katoh O, et al. Impact of intramural thrombus in coronary arteries on the accuracy of tissue characterization by in vivo intravascular ultrasound radiofrequency data analysis. *Am J Cardiol.* 2008; 101:1079-1083.

Multivessel Spontaneous Coronary Artery Dissection Mimicking Atherosclerosis

Mathieu Lempereur, MD, Kenneth Gin, MD, Jacqueline Saw, MD

A 54-year-old overweight postmenopausal woman with hypertension was admitted with prolonged (>12 hours) chest pain after a stressful work week of litigation. An electrocardiogram showed T-wave inversion anterolaterally, with a peak troponin I level of 1.67 mg/L. Coronary angiography the next day showed multivessel disease resembling atherosclerosis. She had severe diffuse disease in the first diagonal, first obtuse marginal, and right posterior descending artery (PDA), and moderate diffuse disease in the mid left anterior descending (LAD) artery (Fig. 1.92, Online Videos 1.70–1.72). Given the clinical suspicion of spontaneous coronary artery dissection (SCAD), optical coherence tomography (OCT) was performed. Surprisingly, this showed SCAD with intramural hematoma associated with a thickened and bright intima in the LAD (Fig. 1.92). An intramural hematoma was also seen in the first obtuse marginal, diagonal, and posterior descending artery stenoses. Classic "string-of-beads" fibromuscular dysplasia (FMD) was visualized in both the renal and external iliac arteries (Fig. 1.93). Blurred right vision also developed in the hospital and she was found to have spontaneous right vertebral artery dissection, with cerebrovascular FMD. Her case was managed conservatively and she was discharged in good condition.

This case highlights the challenge of diagnosing SCAD on coronary angiography alone, which explains the underdiagnosis and underappreciation of SCAD in women with myocardial infarction. Even though her coronary angiogram (especially the LAD) was compatible with an atherosclerotic appearance, a high clinical index of suspicion in this case (young woman, significant emotional stress, and presence of FMD) led to the use of OCT, which showed simultaneous four-vessel SCAD (first-ever report to our knowledge). In addition, she had simultaneous dissection in a noncardiac artery (vertebral) also related to FMD. We stress that a large proportion of SCADs have the angiographic appearance of diffuse and typically smooth stenosis that is due to intramural hematoma (as previously described by our group and others[1,2]), and they do not have the pathognomonic multiple radiolucent wall stains. Interventionists should strongly consider adjunctive intracoronary imaging for suspected SCAD.

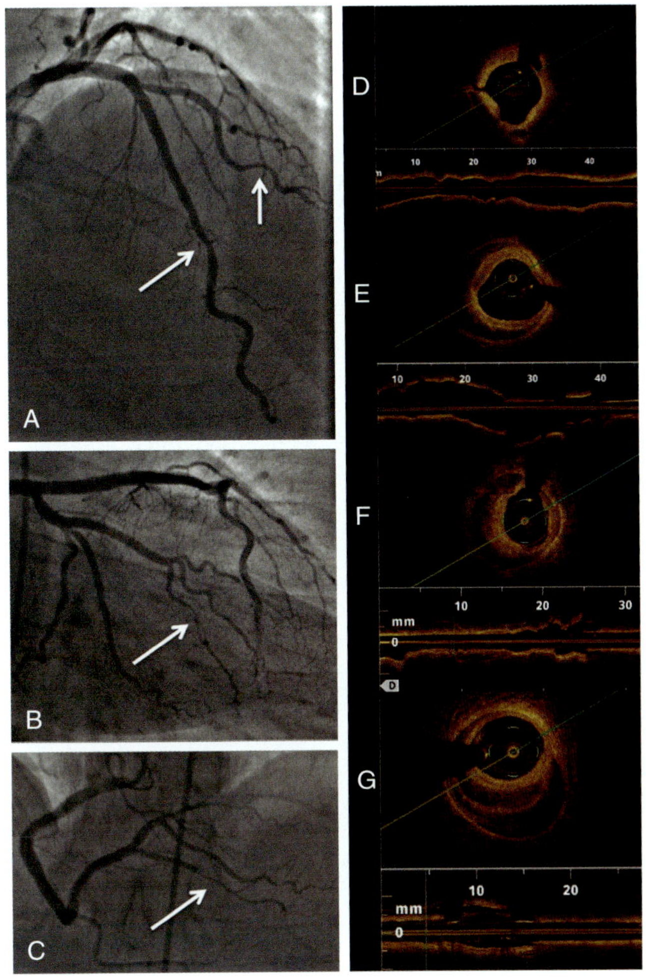

FIG. 1.92 Coronary Angiogram and Optical Coherence Tomography (OCT) Images. (A) Cranial projection showing moderate stenosis in the mid left anterior descending coronary artery (LAD) (*arrow*) and severe stenosis in the first diagonal artery (*arrow*). This is best seen on Online Video 1.70. B, Right anterior oblique caudal projection showing severe stenosis of the first obtuse marginal branch (*arrow*). See Online Video 1.71. (C) Left anterior oblique cranial projection showing severe stenosis of the right posterior descending artery (*arrow*). See Online Video 1.72. (D) OCT of the LAD (*arrow* in [A]) showing intramural hematoma. (E) OCT of the first diagonal artery (*arrow* in [A]) showing intramural hematoma. (F) OCT of the first obtuse marginal artery (*arrow* in [B]) showing intramural hematoma. (G) OCT of the right posterior descending artery (*arrow* in [C]) showing intramural hematoma.

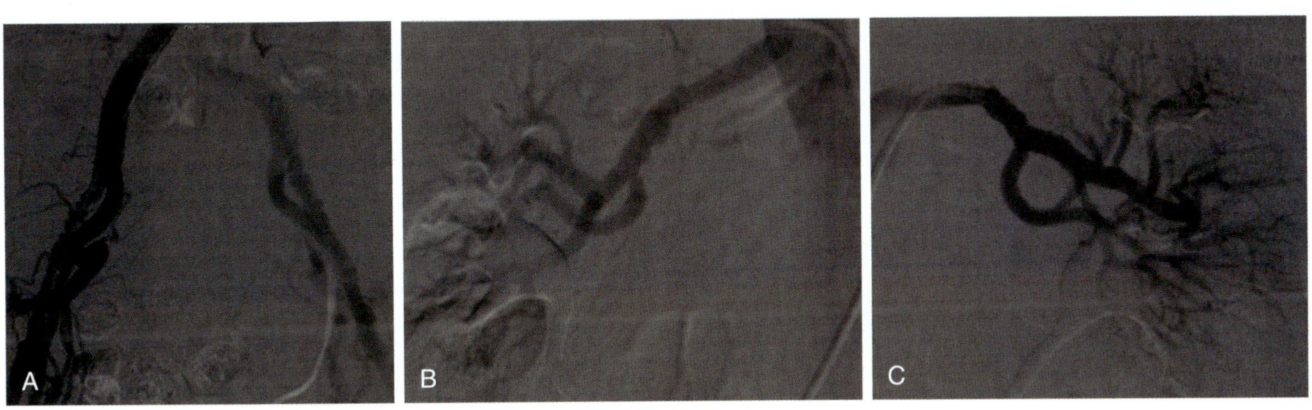

FIG. 1.93 Pelvic and Renal Angiograms. (A) Pelvic angiogram with digital subtraction showing string-of-beads fibromuscular dysplasia (FMD) changes of both iliac arteries. The patient also has FMD of the (B) right renal artery and (C) left renal artery.

References

1. Saw J, Ricci D, Starovoytov A, Fox R, Buller CE. Spontaneous coronary artery dissection: prevalence of predisposing conditions including fibromuscular dysplasia in a tertiary center cohort. *J Am Coll Cardiol Intv.* 2013;6:44-52.
2. Alfonso F, Paulo M, Gonzalo N, et al. Diagnosis of spontaneous coronary artery dissection by optical coherence tomography. *J Am Coll Cardiol.* 2012;59:1073-1079.

Spontaneous Coronary Artery Dissection: Failure of the Conservative Strategy Because of the Predominance of the False Lumen

Felipe Díez-Delhoyo, MD, Ricardo Sanz-Ruiz, MD, Fernando Sarnago-Cebada, MD, Enrique Gutiérrez-Ibañes, MD, PhD, Allan Rivera-Juárez, MD, Jaime Elízaga, MD, PhD, Francisco Fernández-Avilés, MD, PhD

A 50-year-old woman with an inferior ST-segment elevation myocardial infarction was transferred to our institution. Urgent coronary angiography demonstrated several intraluminal filling defects in the proximal segment of the right coronary artery (RCA) (Fig. 1.94A, Online Video 1.73), eventually interpreted as thrombi. However, after aspiration, multiple radiolucent lumens together with arterial wall contrast staining were observed. Optical coherence tomography imaging confirmed a type 1 spontaneous coronary artery dissection (SCAD), with the true arterial lumen (TL) compressed by the false lumen (FL) at several points (Fig.1.94B–C). Interestingly, the intimo-medial layers were severely fragmented and exposed to the blood flow. Because the patient was asymptomatic, with normalized ST-segment elevation and normal RCA flow, a conservative management with dual-antiplatelet therapy was decided according to general consensus.[1]

Four days later a routine angiography confirmed normal epicardial flow (Fig. 1.94D, Online Video 1.74). An intraluminal flap was evident, and optical coherence tomography revealed that the FL had completely obstructed the TL (Fig. 1.94E). Again, conservative treatment was decided for the same aforementioned reasons.

Twenty-four hours later, chest pain and inferior ST-segment elevation suddenly developed. An acute occlusion of the RCA was demonstrated on emergent angiography (Fig. 1.94F, Online Video 1.75), and three drug-eluting stents were implanted, eventually crushing the TL (Fig. 1.94G–H, Online Video 1.76). The patient's clinical course afterward and 1 year later has been uneventful.

Percutaneous coronary intervention is recommended in patients with SCAD when high-risk features are present.[1] Significant media exposure and massive intima dissection are not traditionally recognized as indications for stenting despite their prothrombotic potential. Because definitive indications of a conservative strategy in patients with SCAD remain unsettled, we hereby hypothesize that predominance of the FL may warrant a more aggressive strategy with stent implantation, if technically feasible.

Reference

1. Saw J, Mancini GB, Humphries KH. Contemporary review on spontaneous coronary artery dissection. *J Am Coll Cardiol.* 2016;68:297-312.

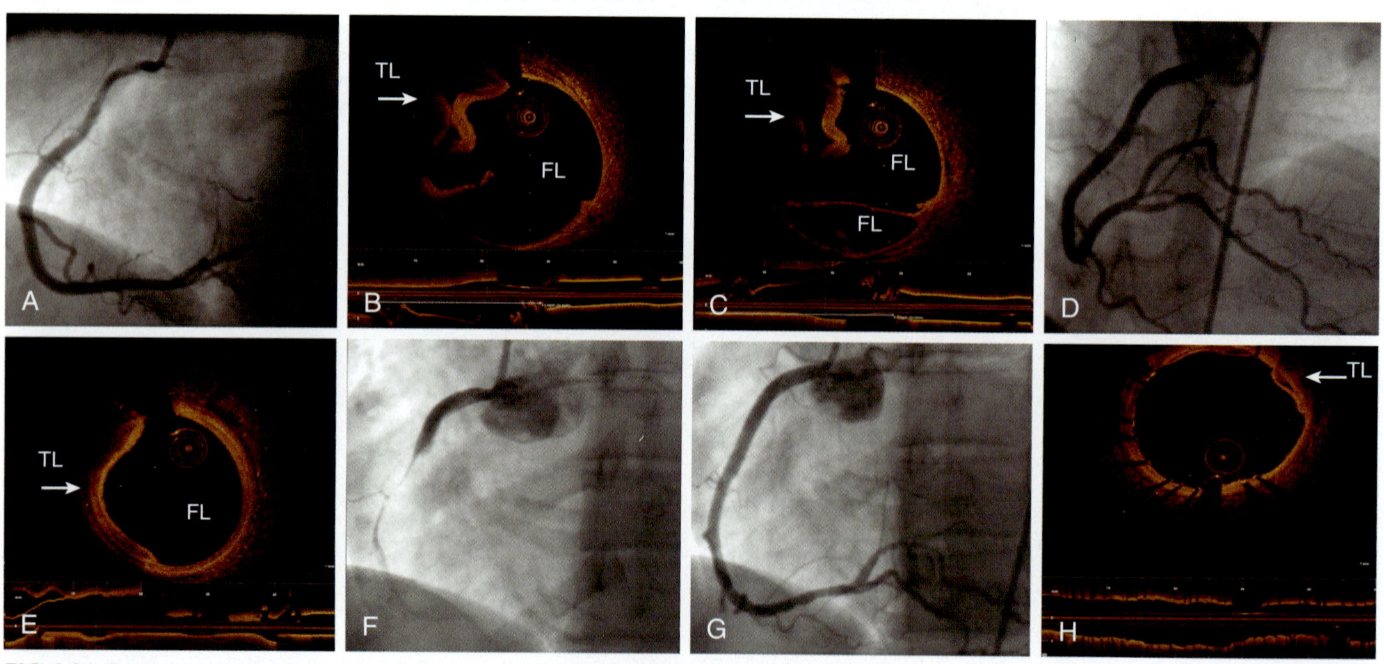

FIG. 1.94 Evolution of the Dissection During the First 5 Days by Invasive Imaging. Angiographic and optical coherence tomography findings in the right coronary artery at the three time points. (A–C) Admission findings (Online Video 1.73). (D and E) Day 4 findings (Online Video 1.74). (F–H) Day 5 findings (Online Videos 1.75 and 1.76). The white arrows show the true lumen (*TL*). FL, *false lumen.*

Coronary Pathology

Acute Inferior Myocardial Infarction Complicated by a Large Ventricular Septal Rupture and Cardiogenic Shock

Nishant Patel, MD, MBBS, Talhat Azemi, MD, Faisal Zaeem, MD, Daniel Fram, MD

A 71-year-old female ex-smoker was seen with a history of 6 hours of progressive dyspnea with an electrocardiogram that showed ST-segment elevation and Q waves in inferior leads. Upon arrival, she was in cardiogenic shock with a systolic blood pressure of 60 mm Hg. Left and right cardiac catheterization demonstrated total occlusion of a dominant right coronary artery (Fig. 1.95A, Online Video 1.77) with elevated filling pressures and a significant oxygen saturation step-up in the right ventricle (RV) (Table 1.1). Transthoracic echocardiography revealed a large inferior ventricular septal rupture (VSR) associated with a left-to-right shunt (Fig. 1.95B and 1.95C, Online Videos 1.77–1.80) with elevated filling pressures and a significant oxygen saturation step-up in the right ventricle (RV) (Table 1.1). Transthoracic echocardiography revealed a large inferior VSR associated with a left-to-right shunt (Figs. 1.95B and 1.95C, Online Videos 1.78–1.81). She was immediately taken to the operating room, where she died as the result of multiple irreparable rupture sites at the right ventricle. VSR is associated with risk factors including advanced age, female sex, tobacco use, first infarction, and a lack of collaterals. Historically, inferior VSRs have been associated with a poor prognosis.

TABLE 1.1 Hemodynamic Data Derived From Right and Left Heart Catheterization

Parameter	Value
RA pressure	24 mm Hg
RV pressure	49/29 mm Hg
PA pressure	38/25 mm Hg
Pulmonary capillary wedge pressure	25 mm Hg
RA oxygen saturation	29%
RV oxygen saturation	99%
PA oxygen saturation	97%
AO oxygen saturation	99%

AO, aorta; *PA*, pulmonary artery; *RA*, right arterial; *RV*, right ventricular.

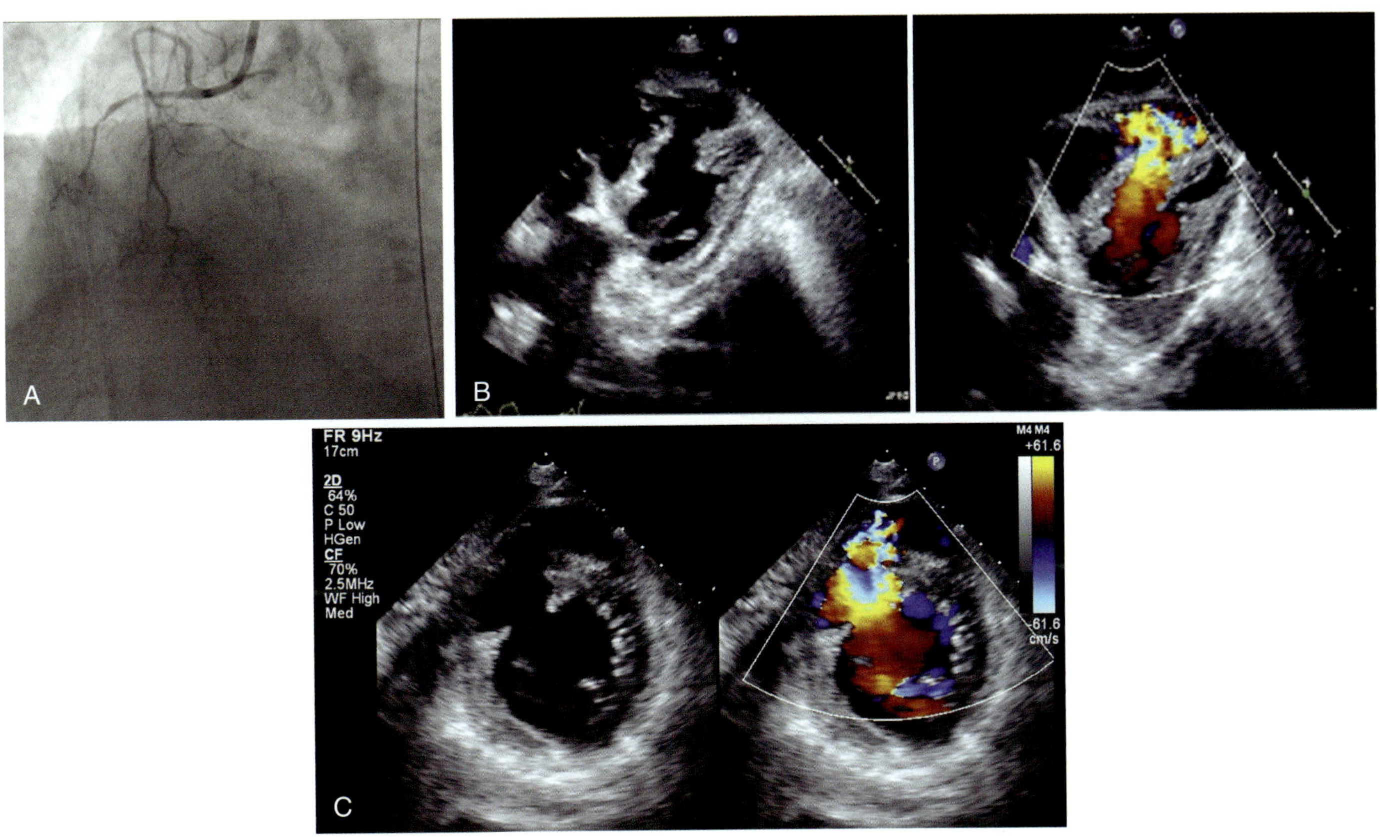

FIG. 1.95 Coronary Angiography of Right Coronary Artery (RCA) and Echocardiogram in an Elderly Female Ex-Smoker With Ventricular Septal Rupture. (A) Coronary angiogram of RCA showing proximal total occlusion. (B) Subcostal view on two-dimensional electrocardiography. (C) Short-axis view of the left ventricle on two-dimensional echocardiogram, with and without color Doppler, showing large direct ventricular septal rupture. See Online Videos 1.77 through 1.81.

Plaque Erosion: In Vivo Diagnosis and Treatment Guided by Optical Coherence Tomography

Sining Hu, MD, Haibo Jia, MD, PhD, Rocco Vergallo, MD, Farhad Abtahian, MD, PhD, Jinwei Tian, MD, PhD, Tsunenari Soeda, MD, PhD, Kenneth Rosenfield, MD, Ik-Kyung Jang, MD, PhD

A 60-year-old man was transferred to the catheterization laboratory after a witnessed ventricular fibrillation arrest. The electrocardiogram was remarkable for ST-segment elevations in leads II, III, aVF, and V_6, with reciprocal ST-segment depression in leads V_1 to V_4 and aVL (Fig. 1.96). The coronary angiogram showed total occlusion of the distal right coronary artery (RCA) (Fig. 1.97A, *white arrow*). After aspiration thrombectomy, anterograde flow was restored (Fig. 1.97B), and optical coherence tomography (OCT) imaging showed nonobstructive plaque with residual white (platelet-rich) thrombus (Fig. 1.97C, *white arrows*) overlying a fibrocalcific plaque. There was no evidence of plaque rupture. Low-pressure balloon angioplasty was performed with intracoronary administration of abciximab. Repeat OCT imaging demonstrated a smooth luminal surface without evidence of plaque rupture (Fig. 1.97D). Plaque erosion was suspected. The patient was treated with aspirin, clopidogrel, and high-dose atorvastatin. His hypercoagulation workup was negative. His stress test result at 3 months was negative for ischemia, and the patient remained asymptomatic at 6-month follow-up.

Acute coronary syndrome is caused by 3 different underlying mechanisms, including plaque rupture, plaque erosion, and calcific nodules.[1,2] Plaque erosions are responsible for one-third of patients who experience sudden cardiac death.[3] Despite the different pathophysiology, patients with acute coronary syndrome are uniformly treated with stenting in current clinical practice. This case demonstrates that differentiation of different underlying mechanisms has become possible with OCT. Given the minimal disruption to the vessel wall, the relatively preserved underlying vascular structure, and the relatively large lumen,[2,4] it is possible that effective antithrombotic therapy, by promoting thrombus resolution and preventing further thrombus formation, will allow for healing of the eroded surface and abrogating the need for stenting.

References

1. Falk E, Nakano M, Bentzon JF, Finn AV, Virmani R. Update on acute coronary syndromes: the pathologists' view. *Eur Heart J.* 2013;34:719-728.
2. Jia H, Abtahian F, Aguirre AD, et al. In vivo diagnosis of plaque erosion and calcified nodule in patients with acute coronary syndrome by intravascular optical coherence tomography. *J Am Coll Cardiol.* 2013;62:1748-1758.
3. Virmani R, Kolodgie FD, Burke AP, Farb A, Schwartz SM. Lessons from sudden coronary death: a comprehensive morphological classification scheme for atherosclerotic lesions. *Arterioscler Thromb Vasc Biol.* 2000;20:1262-1275.
4. Farb A, Burke AP, Tang AL, et al. Coronary plaque erosion without rupture into a lipid core: a frequent cause of coronary thrombosis in sudden coronary death. *Circulation.* 1996;93:1354-1363.

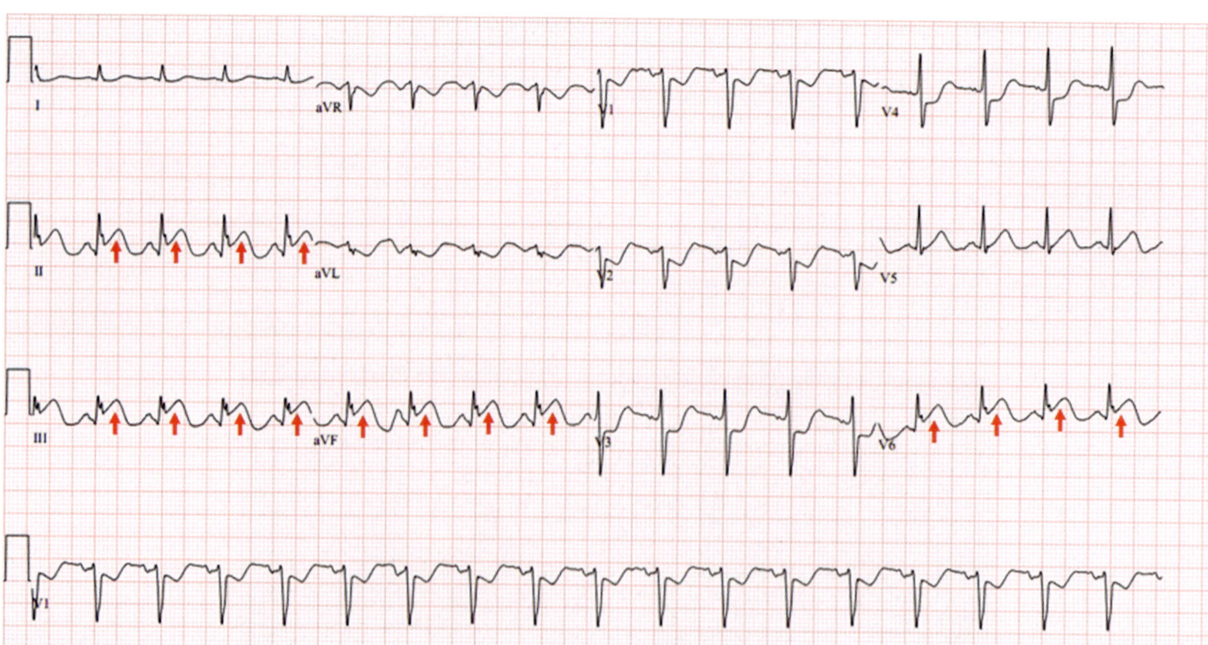

FIG. 1.96 Electrocardiogram. An electrocardiogram on admission showed ST-segment elevation in leads II, III, aVF, and V_6 (*red arrows*) with reciprocal ST-segment depression in leads V_1 to V_4 and aVL.

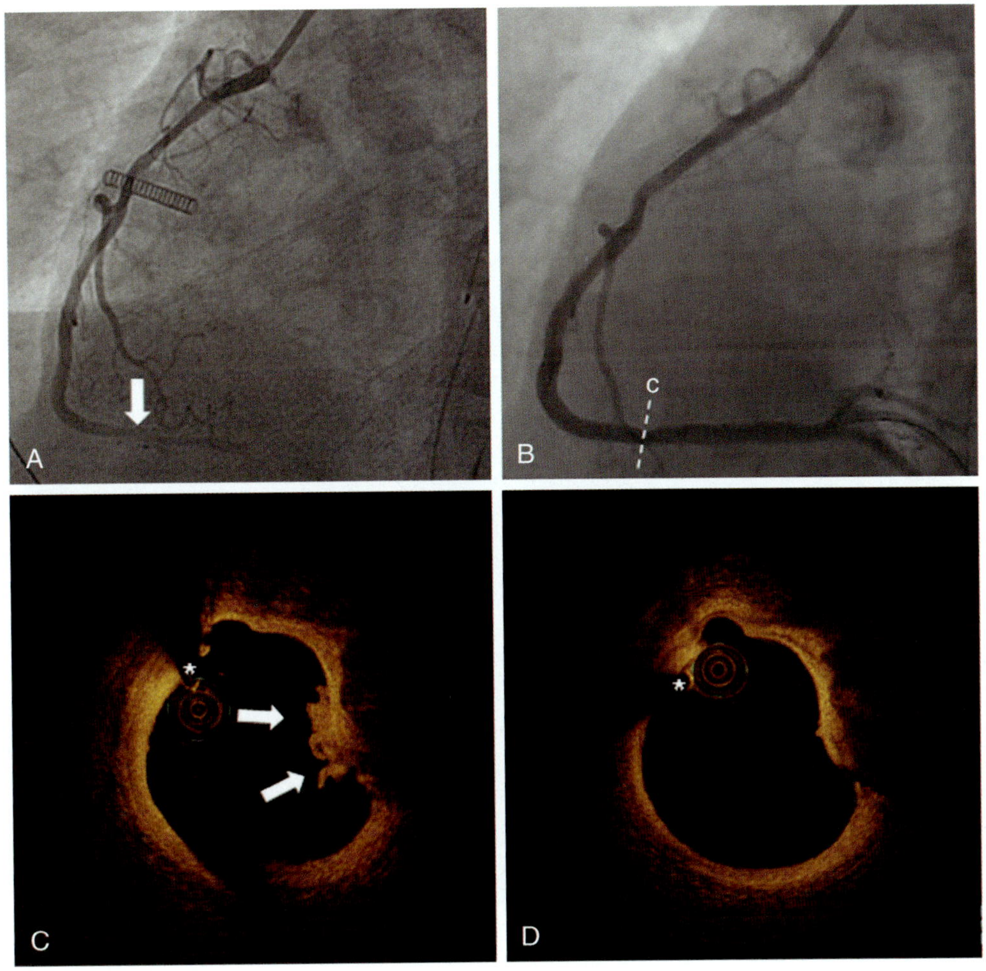

FIG. 1.97 Coronary Angiography and Optical Coherence Tomography (OCT). (A) A coronary angiogram revealed total occlusion of the distal right coronary artery (*white arrow*). (B) Anterograde flow was restored after successful aspiration thrombectomy. No severe residual stenosis was shown on the angiogram. (C) OCT image after thrombectomy demonstrated white thrombus (*white arrows*) overlying a fibrocalcific plaque. (D) Repeat OCT imaging immediately after low-pressure balloon angioplasty with intracoronary administration of abciximab demonstrated a smooth luminal surface without evidence of plaque rupture. (C and D) The *asterisk* indicates a guidewire artifact.

Recanalized Thrombus Treated With a Paclitaxel-Coated Balloon: Insights from Optical Coherence Tomography

Yusuke Watanabe, MD, Yusuke Fujino, MD, PhD, Hisaaki Ishiguro, MD, PhD, Sunao Nakamura, MD, PhD

A 56-year-old man with a medical history of hypertension and diabetes was referred by his primary care physician to our hospital for an electrocardiographic abnormality. An echocardiogram showed moderately reduced left ventricular function (ejection fraction 45%). Coronary angiography revealed a lesion with a contrast filling defect and an irregular lumen border at the mid segment of the left anterior descending coronary artery (Fig. 1.98A and 1.98A′). Optimal coherence tomography (OCT) was performed on this lesion, revealing multiple honeycomb-like channels (Fig. 1.98a–d). After OCT, angioplasty was performed with a paclitaxel-coated balloon (PCB) (SeQuent Please, B. Braun, Melsungen, Germany). The final angiographic result obtained was satisfactory (Fig. 1.99A). OCT revealed adequate expansion without a subliminal hematoma and intimal dissection (Fig. 1.99a′–d′). Follow-up angiography 8 months later revealed excellent results in the PCB-treated segment (Fig. 1.99B). OCT demonstrated a smooth lumen surface and acceptable lumen areas (Fig. 1.99a″–d″).

A previous study reported that multiple honeycomb-like channels represent spontaneous recanalization of the coronary artery after thrombotic occlusion.[1] The acceptable outcomes of treatment with a

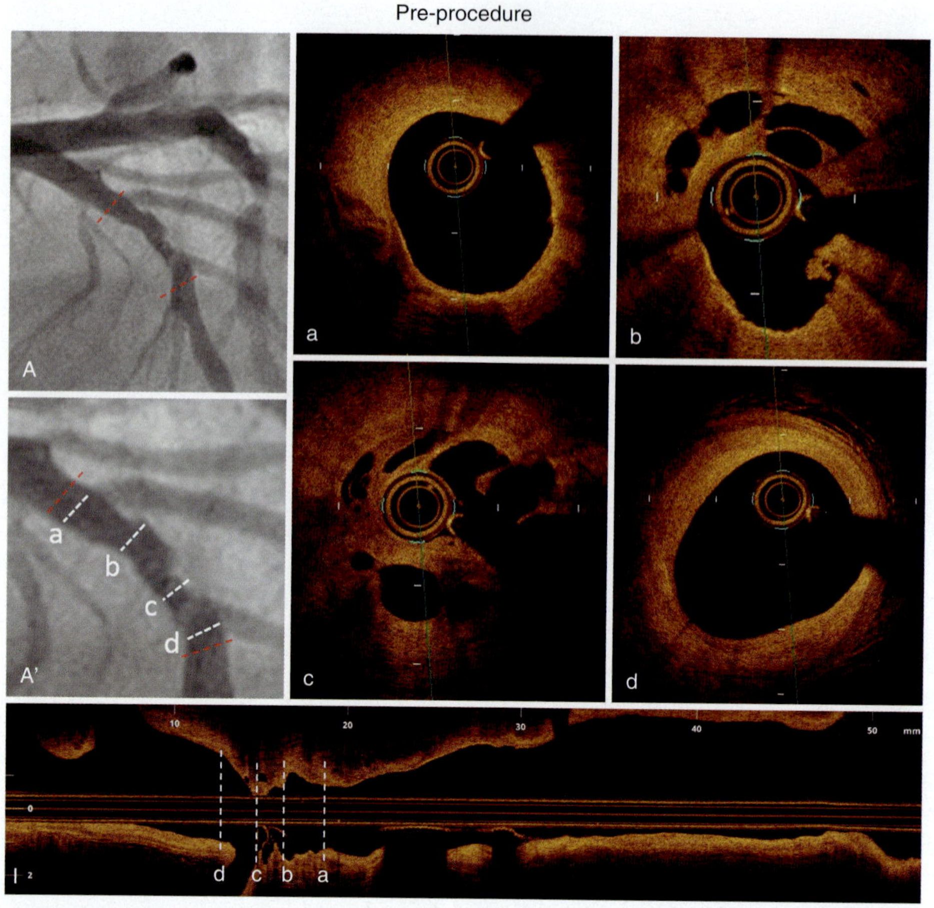

FIG. 1.98 Angiography and Optimal Coherence Tomography (OCT) Before the Procedure. (A) Initial coronary angiography showing a lesion with a contrast filling defect and haziness at the mid segment of the left anterior descending artery. Image (A) identifies segments corresponding to OCT images (a), (b), (c), and (d). Images a and d are OCT images showing multiple honeycomb-like channels. Images (a) and (d) correspond to the proximal and distal segments and image (I) is a longitudinal OCT image.

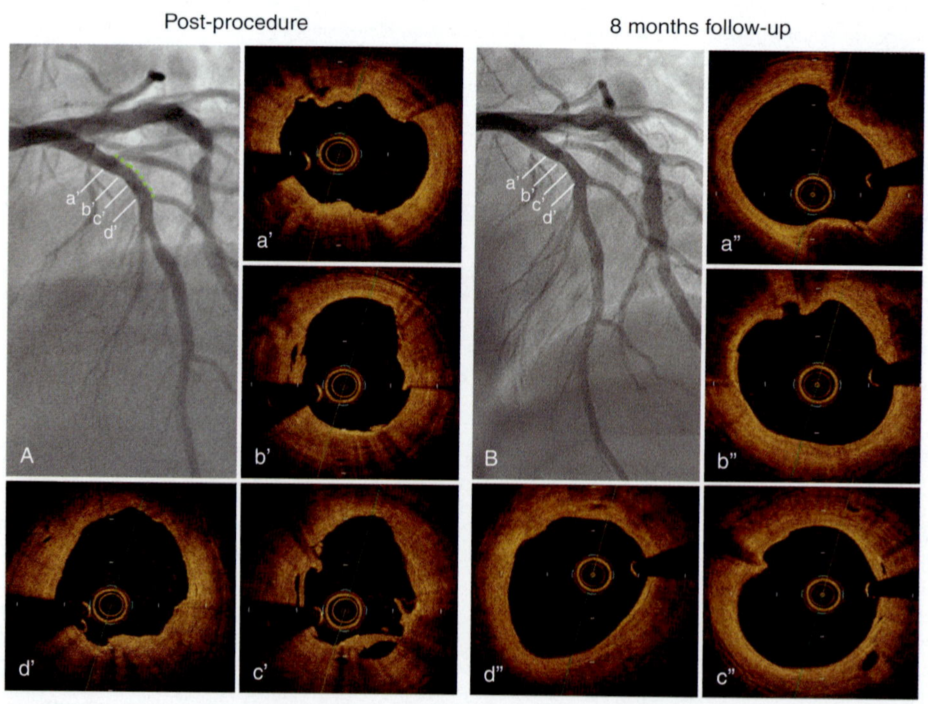

FIG. 1.99 Angiography and Optimal Coherence Tomography (OCT) After the Procedure and at Follow-Up. (A) Coronary angiography after angioplasty. The angioplasty was performed with a paclitaxel-coated balloon (PCB). The segment treated with the paclitaxel-coated balloon is indicated by the green dotted line. Images (a′) to (d′) OCT after procedure. OCT showed adequate expansion without a subliminal hematoma and intimal dissection. (B) Follow-up coronary angiography after 8 months. Images (a″) to (d″) show OCT at follow-up coronary angiography. OCT showed a smooth lumen surface and acceptable lumen areas.

drug-eluting stent and a bioresorbable vascular scaffold for these lesions were reported.[2,3] To the best of our knowledge, this is the first report of acceptable outcomes of treatment with PCB for such lesions evaluated through OCT. PCB might be a therapeutic alternative in percutaneous treatment of such lesions.

References

1. Cho JM, Raffel OC, Stone JR, Kim CJ, Jang IK. Spontaneous recanalization of a coronary artery after thrombotic occlusion: in vivo demonstration with optical coherence tomography. *J Am Coll Cardiol.* 2010;55:1274.
2. Toutouzas K, Karanasos A, Stathogiannis K, et al. A honeycomb-like structure in the left anterior descending coronary artery: demonstration of recanalized thrombus by optical coherence tomography. *J Am Coll Cardiol Intv.* 2012;5:688-689.
3. Gomez-Monterrosas O, Regueiro A, Santos A, et al. Recanalized thrombus treated with bioresorbable vascular scaffold: insights from optical coherence tomography. *J Am Coll Cardiol Intv.* 2014;7:1453-1455.

Rescue Percutaneous Coronary Intervention Revealing Impending Left Ventricle Rupture

Benoit Plourde, MD, Olivier F. Bertrand, MD, PhD

A 53-year-old woman was seen in a referring hospital and received intravenous tenecteplase for anterolateral myocardial infarction (Fig. 1.100A). Because her condition did not improve, she was transferred for rescue percutaneous coronary intervention. Successful percutaneous coronary intervention was performed on the left anterior descending artery, although persisting slow flow was noted (Fig. 1.100B–C, Online Video 1.82). Diffuse narrowing of the distal left anterior descending artery was also observed, suggesting external compression of the vessel.

Left ventriculography showed anterolateroapical akinesis with aneurysmal dilation of the left ventricle and an apical thrombus. Surprisingly, extravasation of contrast within the myocardium was visible in the anterior free wall (Fig. 1.100D, Online Video 1.83). Impeding left ventricular rupture was suspected. After repeat interrogation, the patient mentioned that chest pain had begun 3 weeks before admission and that she had been treated with nonsteroidal antiinflammatory drugs without improvement. Minutes after transfer to the intensive care unit, electromechanical dissociation developed and she died. During cardiopulmonary resuscitation, the echocardiogram revealed cardiac tamponade.

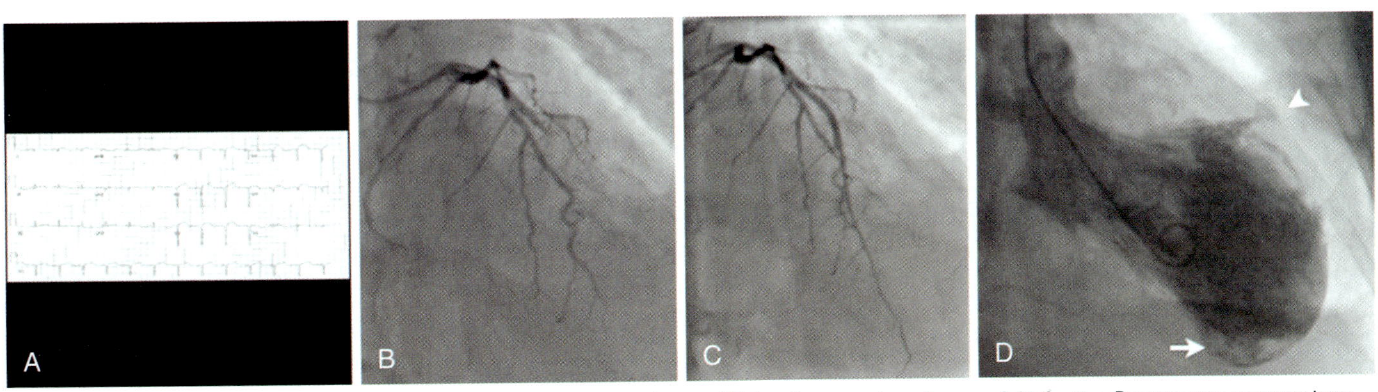

FIG. 1.100 Impending Left Ventricle Rupture. (A) Electrocardiogram showing ST-elevation anterolateral myocardial infarction. Percutaneous coronary intervention was performed ([B and C], Online Video 1.82). Extravasation of contrast within the myocardium is visible in the anterior free wall ([D], Online Video 1.83).

Cardiovascular Interventions in the Modern Age: The Million Dollar Man

Elliott M. Groves, MD, MEng, Matthew J. Price, MD

Images for this chapter were obtained from an 84-year-old man with a history of diabetes, heart failure, coronary artery disease, severe mitral regurgitation, sick sinus syndrome, and atrial fibrillation. A single fluoroscopic still image of the patient's left chest illustrates the extent of his procedural treatment (Fig. 1.101; the left and right panels are unannotated and annotated, respectively; annotations are listed in chronologic order of implantation). Owing to sick sinus syndrome, the patient underwent implantation of a dual-chamber pacemaker with a passive fixation lead. Later, because of lead fracture the atrial lead was replaced with an active fixation lead (Fig. 1.101A).

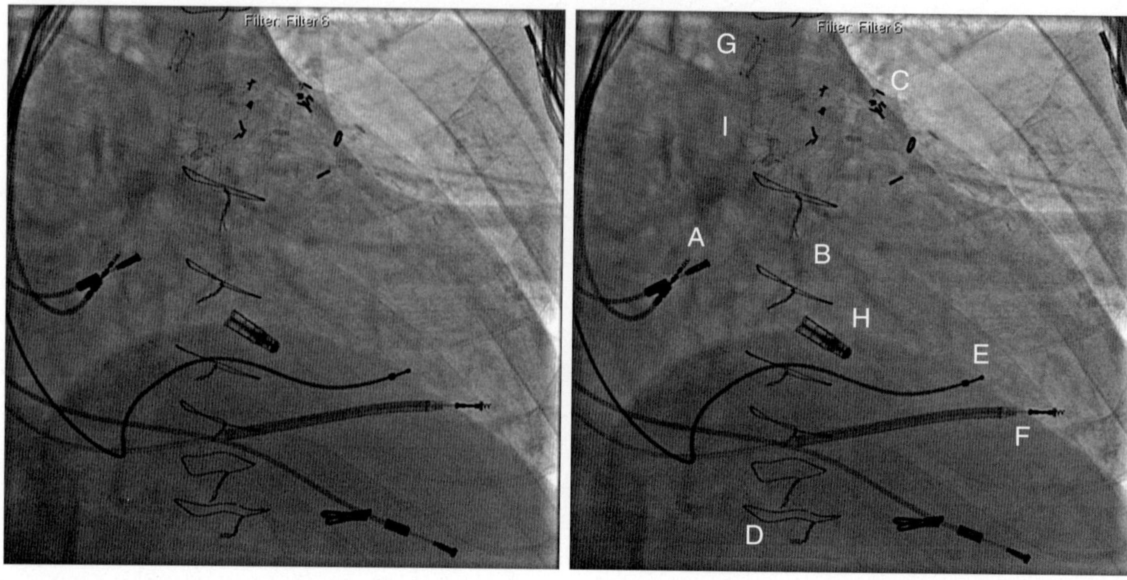

FIG. 1.101 Cardiovascular Interventions in the Modern Age. (A) Active and passive fixation right atrial pacemaker leads. (B) Right coronary artery stent. (C) Surgically placed vascular clips. (D) Sternal wires with fracture. (E) Coronary sinus lead. (F) A right ventricular lead with defibrillation capabilities. (G) CardioMEMS device (St. Jude Medical). (H) MitraClip (Abbott Vascular). (I) Watchman (Boston Scientific) left atrial appendage exclusion device.

Percutaneous coronary intervention to the right coronary artery was performed because of the development of symptomatic coronary artery disease (Fig. 1.101B). Subsequently, because of disease progression the patient underwent coronary artery bypass graft surgery during which vascular clips (Fig. 1.101C) and sternotomy wires (Fig. 1.101D) were placed with wire fracture. A bundle branch block developed in the setting of a decline in left ventricular ejection fraction, and the pacemaker was upgraded to a biventricular implantable cardioverter defibrillator with a coronary sinus lead (Fig. 1.101E) and a right ventricular lead with defibrillation capability (Fig. 1.101F). The patient eventually was seen with heart failure requiring hospitalization, and a CardioMEMS device (St. Jude Medical, St. Paul, Minnesota) was implanted within the left pulmonary artery (Fig. 1.101G).[1] The patient continued to have symptomatic heart failure despite aggressive management, thought to be due in part to worsening severe mitral regurgitation as a result of a combination of degenerative and functional etiologies. He was deemed to be at prohibitive risk for open repair, and underwent transcatheter mitral valve repair with a MitraClip (Abbott Vascular, Abbott Park, Illinois) (Figure 1.101H).[2] Finally, he was intolerant of oral anticoagulation and given his thromboembolic risk and rationale to seek a nonpharmacologic approach to stroke prevention, his left atrial appendage was closed using a Watchman occlusion device (Boston Scientific, Marlborough, Massachusetts) (Fig. 1.101I).[3]

References

1. Abraham WT, Adamson PB, Bourge RC, et al. Wireless pulmonary artery haemodynamic monitoring in chronic heart failure: a randomised controlled trial. *Lancet.* 2011;377:658-666.
2. Glower DD, Kar S, Trento A, et al. Percutaneous mitral valve repair for mitral regurgitation in high-risk patients: results of the EVEREST II study. *J Am Coll Cardiol.* 2014;64:172-181.
3. Price MJ, Valderrabano M. Left atrial appendage closure to prevent stroke in patients with atrial fibrillation. *Circulation.* 2014;130:202-212.

Detection of Angioscopic Yellow Plaque by Intracoronary Near-Infrared Spectroscopy

Yasunori Ueda, MD, PhD, Koshi Matsuo, MD, Yuji Nishimoto, MD, Ryuta Sugihara, MD, Mayu Nishio, MD, PhD, Akio Hirata, MD, PhD, Mitsutoshi Asai, MD, PhD, Takayoshi Nemoto, MD, Ayaka Murakami, BS, Kazunori Kashiwase, MD, PhD, James E. Muller, MD, Kazuhisa Kodama, MD, PhD

Angioscopy can detect vulnerable, lipid-rich coronary plaques (LRPs), but it requires removal of blood plus expert technique and interpretation.[1,2] We studied the use of a near-infrared spectroscopy (NIRS) intravascular ultrasound (IVUS) catheter,[3] which does not require blood removal, to detect an LRP identified by angioscopy.

An angiogram (Fig. 1.102A) shows the mid left anterior descending artery with a stent. Angioscopy shows a proximal, yellow LRP with a white fibrotic plaque under the stent. Through blood NIRS detected the LRP (yellow halo on the IVUS image), and IVUS detected the stent. Throughout the artery angioscopy (Fig.1.102B, Online Video 1.84) detected yellow plaque at locations 2, 3, and 4, with white thrombus at location 3. NIRS-IVUS (Fig. 1.102C, Online Video 1.85) and a chemogram (Fig. 1.102D) detected LRP (*yellow*) at locations 2, 3, and 4, with no LRP (*red*) at location 1 and 5, coinciding with angioscopic findings.

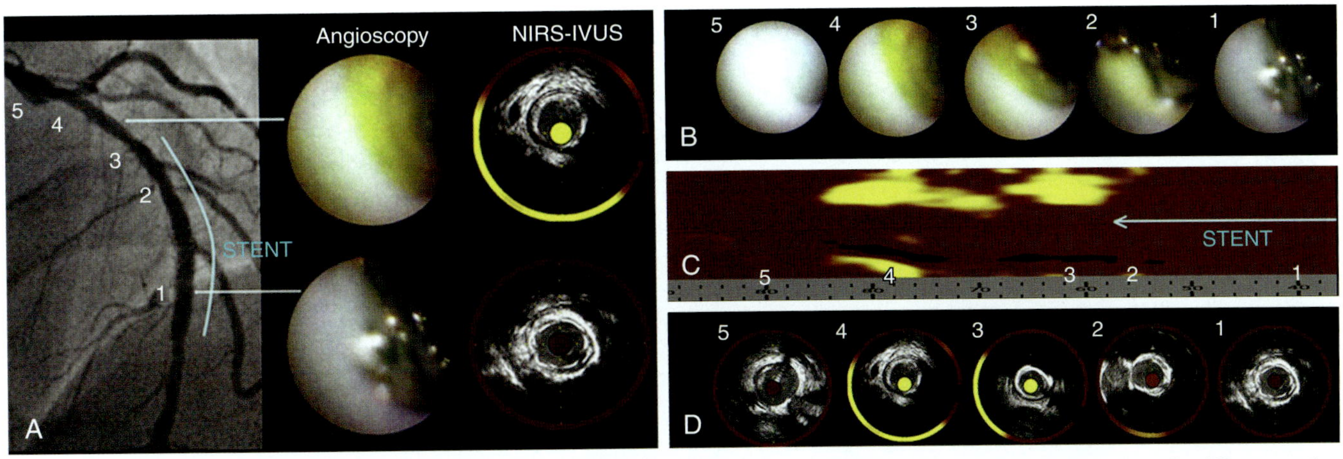

FIG. 1.102 Detection of Lipid-Rich Plaque (LRP) by Angioscopy and Near-Infrared Spectroscopy (NIRS)–Intravascular Ultrasound (IVUS). (A) The target lesion evaluated by angiography, angioscopy, and near-infrared spectroscopy (NIRS). The angiogram shows the target lesion in the mid left anterior descending coronary artery where the stent was implanted. Angioscopy shows a proximal yellow LRP with a white fibrotic plaque under the stent. NIRS detected the LRP (*yellow halo* on the intravascular ultrasound IVUS image), and IVUS detected the stent. (B) Angioscopic images throughout the vessel detected yellow plaque at locations 2, 3, and 4 with white thrombus at 3 (Online Video 1.84). (C) Chemogram of the vessel shows an LPR as a yellow area at locations 2, 3, and 4, with no LRP (shown as a *red* area) at locations 1 and 5, coinciding with the angioscopic findings. (D) NIRS-IVUS images throughout the vessel detected an LRP (*yellow*) at locations 2, 3, and 4, with no LRP (*red*) at locations 1 and 5, coinciding with angioscopic findings (Online Video 1.85). NIRS-IVUS images also show the direction of the LPR on the IVUS image. The numbers in (B–D) show the locations on the angiogram in (A).

The NIRS-IVUS catheter, which is easy to use and quantitative, might be a valuable tool to detect vulnerable plaques.

References

1. Ueda Y, Ohtani T, Shimizu M, Hirayama A, Kodama K. Assessment of plaque vulnerability by angioscopic classification of plaque color. *Am Heart J.* 2004;148:333-335.
2. Ohtani T, Ueda Y, Mizote I, et al. Number of yellow plaques detected in a coronary artery is associated with future risk of acute coronary syndrome: detection of vulnerable patients by angioscopy. *J Am Coll Cardiol.* 2006;47:2194-2200.
3. Madder RD, Goldstein JA, Madden SP, et al. Detection by near-infrared spectroscopy of large lipid core plaques at culprit sites in patients with acute ST-segment elevation myocardial infarction. *J Am Coll Cardiol Intv.* 2013;6:838-846.

Distinct Pattern of Constrictive Remodeling in Radiotherapy-Induced Coronary Artery Disease

Menno van Gameren, MD, PhD, Jurgen M.R. Ligthart, RT, Tjebbe W. Galema, MD, PhD, Koen Nieman, MD, PhD, Nicolas M. Van Mieghem, MD, PhD

A 31-year-old woman with a history of chemotherapy and mediastinal radiation therapy for Hodgkin lymphoma had stable angina followed by a positive stress test result. A coronary computed tomography scan revealed a high-grade ostial right coronary artery stenosis without calcium (Agatston score 0) (Fig. 1.103A). Invasive coronary angiography confirmed a focal tight ostial lesion with no further lesions or signs of atherosclerosis (Fig. 1.103B–C). Lesion characterization by intravascular ultrasonography and optical coherence tomography identified an eccentric fibrous and fibrofatty plaque (Fig. 1.103D–E) with extraordinary constrictive remodeling (Fig. 1.104). The patient was successfully treated with a drug-eluting stent.

The presence of fibrous and fibrofatty plaques and lack of calcium has been described previously in patients who had undergone radiation therapy for Hodgkin lymphoma.[1-4] The constrictive remodeling revealed by intravascular ultrasound analysis in our patient provides further insights into the distinct pattern of radiation-induced coronary plaque formation compared with typical atherosclerotic coronary artery disease.

References

1. Krzesinski P, Piotrowicz K, Horszczaruk GJ, Kowal J. Unstable angina in a young woman with Hodgkin's lymphoma. *Cardiol J.* 2013;20:90-93.
2. Caro-Codon J, Jimenez-Valero S, Galeote G, Sanchez-Recalde A, Moreno R. Radiation-induced coronary artery disease: useful insights from OCT. *Int J Cardiol.* 2016;202:535-536.
3. Dunsmore LD, LoPonte MA, Dunsmore RA. Radiation-induced coronary artery disease. *J Am Coll Cardiol.* 1986;8:239-244.
4. Veinot JP, Edwards WD. Pathology of radiation-induced heart disease: a surgical and autopsy study of 27 cases. *Hum Pathol.* 1996;27:766-773.

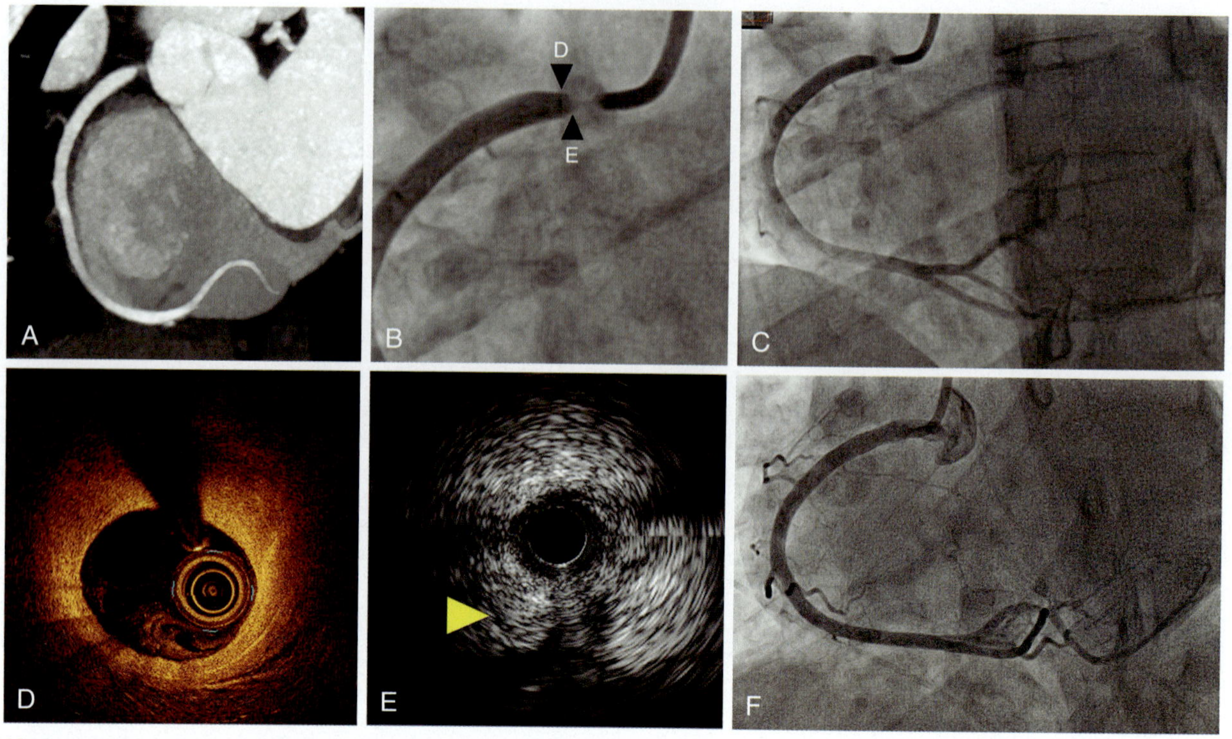

FIG. 1.103 Ostial Right Coronary Artery Stenosis Visualized Using Noninvasive and Invasive Imaging Modalities. (A) A thin-slab maximum intensity projection from coronary computed tomography angiography. (B) The arrowheads indicate the locations of the cross sections presented in (D) and (E) near and at the ostium of the right coronary artery. (C) Full right coronary artery, left anterior oblique view. (D) Optical coherence tomography shows eccentric fibrous and fibrofatty plaque. (E) Intravascular ultrasonography shows eccentric fibrous plaque at the ostium indicated by the yellow arrowhead. (F) Left anterior oblique view after intervention (direct stenting after dilation with noncompliant balloon).

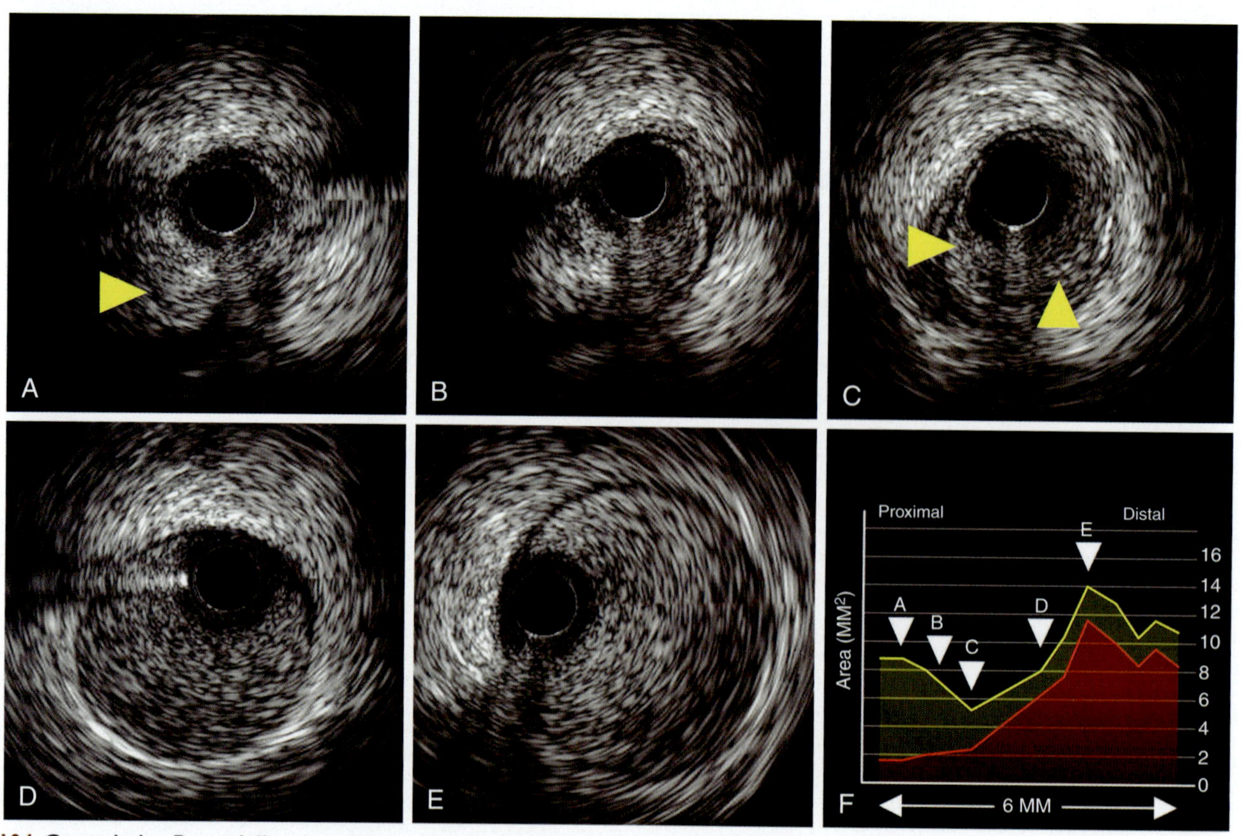

FIG. 1.104 Constrictive Remodeling. Intravascular ultrasound cross sections presented in images (A) to (E) range from (A) the ostium to (E) 6 mm into the right coronary artery. Cross sections (A) and (B) show eccentric fibrous plaque at the 7-o'clock position (*arrowhead* in [A]); (C) reveals soft, lossy tissue (*arrowheads*). No calcifications were found. Constrictive remodeling is visualized by the graph in image (F) (QCU-CMS Research, Leiden University Medical Center, Leiden, Netherlands). The red line represents the lumen area and the yellow line represents the total vessel area (both in mm^2). Arrowheads mark the locations of the corresponding cross sections (A) to (E).

Quantitative Optical Coherence Tomography Tissue–Type Imaging for Lipid-Core Plaque Detection

Evelyn Regar, MD, PhD, Muthukaruppan Gnanadesigan, MSC, Antonius F. W. Van der Steen, PhD, Gijs van Soest, PhD

Tissue type in the coronary artery wall is an important parameter with significant clinical implications in interventional cardiology. Lipid-rich necrotic lesions may cause periprocedural complications, stent failure, and acute coronary events. Analysis of the optical properties of a lesion imaged by optical coherence tomography (OCT) can serve as a tool to discriminate different tissue components. A necrotic core has a higher attenuation coefficient than calcified and fibrous tissues.[1] In this case description, we compare in vivo OCT-derived attenuation with independent lipid-core plaque detection by a combined near-infrared reflection spectroscopy–intravascular ultrasonography (IVUS) device.[2]

A 59-year-old man was referred to our center for cardiac catheterization because of non–ST-segment elevation acute coronary syndrome with positive cardiac enzyme levels (troponin T) and dynamic electrocardiographic changes in the anterior leads. Invasive imaging with OCT (St. Jude Medical C7-XR, C7 Dragonfly catheter, St. Paul, Minnesota) and near-infrared reflection spectroscopy/IVUS (Infraredx TVC system and catheter, Burlington, Massachusetts) before intervention revealed a high plaque burden in the proximal left anterior descending artery with marked lumen narrowing (Fig. 1.105). We matched three locations in both pullbacks, based on anatomic landmarks. OCT data of plaques in the images were analyzed to quantify the local attenuation coefficient.[1]

The sites selected for analysis are shown in Fig. 1.106. The sectors identified as containing lipid-core plaque by near-infrared reflection spectroscopy (*yellow*) have OCT features that are highly attenuating, confirming our in vitro findings that a necrotic core has a high attenuation coefficient. In addition, calcium is analyzed as having low attenuation, suggesting a possible method to discriminate between these tissue types, which are sometimes difficult to classify in the OCT image.[3,4]

This observation is the first confirmation in a clinical setting, with independent invasive imaging control, that quantitative analysis of the OCT signal may assist in tissue-type identification. As our insight into the interaction between intervention and vessel wall biology grows, intravascular imaging of plaque composition can acquire a role in procedure planning and treatment decisions.

References

1. van Soest G, Goderie T, Regar E, et al. Atherosclerotic tissue characterization in vivo by optical coherence tomography attenuation imaging. *J Biomed Opt.* 2010;15:011105.
2. Garg S, Serruys PW, van der Ent M, et al. First use in patients of a combined near infra-red spectroscopy and intra-vascular ultrasound catheter to identify composition and structure of coronary plaque. *EuroIntervention.* 2010;5:755-756.
3. Manfrini O, Mont E, Leone O, et al. Sources of error and interpretation of plaque morphology by optical coherence tomography. *Am J Cardiol.* 2006;98:156-159.
4. Goderie TP, van Soest G, Garcia-Garcia HM, et al. Combined optical coherence tomography and intravascular ultrasound radio frequency data analysis for plaque characterization: classification accuracy of human coronary plaques in vitro. *Int J Cardiovasc Imaging.* 2010;26:843-850.

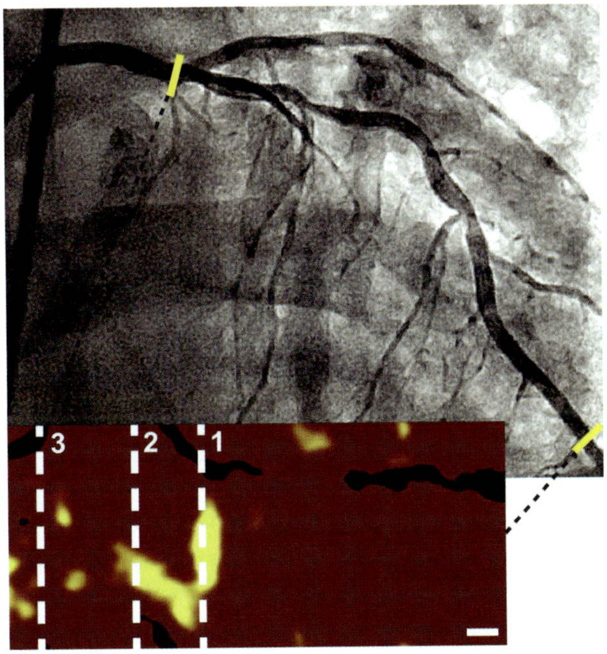

FIG. 1.105 Angiogram of the Left Anterior Descending Artery Prior to Intervention and Chemogram Acquired by Near-Infrared Spectroscopy. In the chemogram, yellow indicates the presence of a lipid-core plaque in a two-dimensional map. The white lines indicate the locations of cross sections in Fig. 1.106.

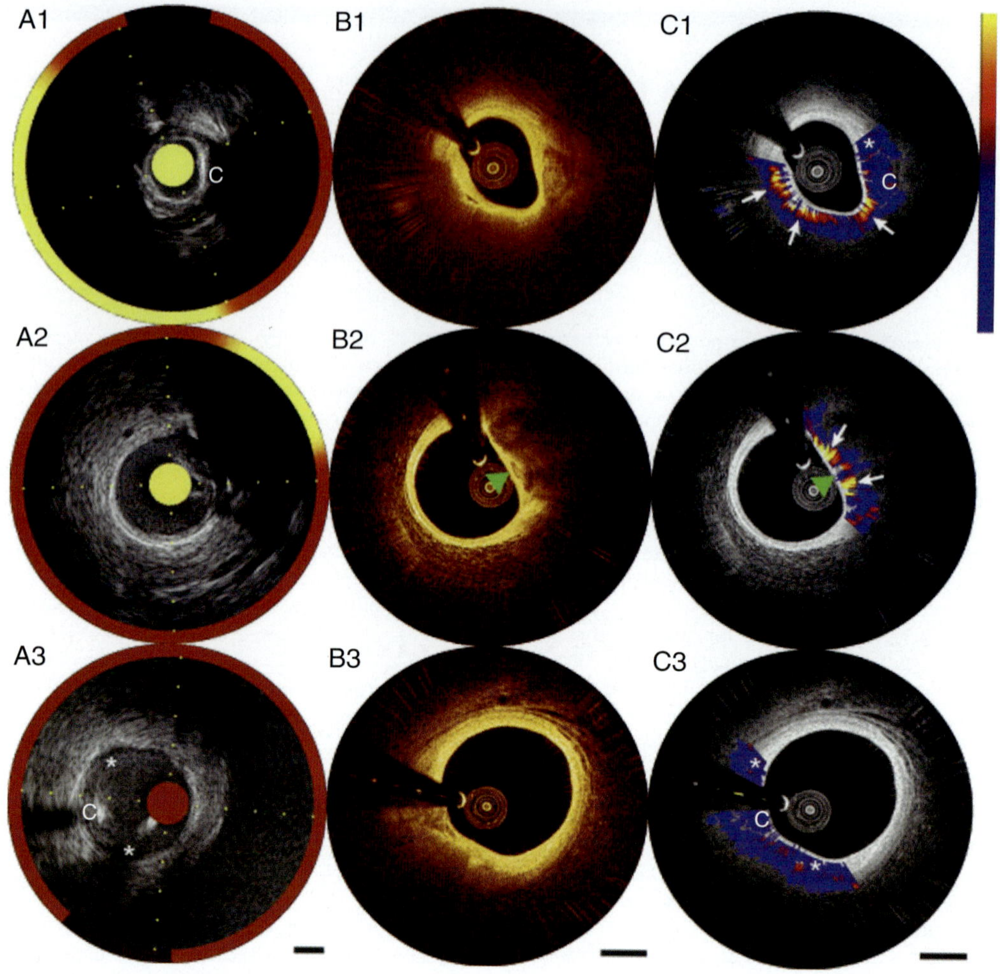

FIG. 1.106 Comparison Between Optical Coherence Tomography (OCT) Attenuation Imaging and Near-Infrared Reflection Spectroscopy (NIRS) for Three Sites. (A) NIRS–intravascular ultrasonography (IVUS) images. (B) OCT and (C) attenuation coefficient analyzed from the OCT data (color-coded 0 to 12 mm^{-1}). Scale bars are 1 mm. Site 1 (refer to Fig. 1.105) shows a mixed lesion containing calcifications (bright echoes on IVUS with dorsal shadowing at the 3- to 5-o'clock position) and lipid-rich tissue (at 5- to 10-o'clock position). High attenuation (*red-orange-yellow*) in the plaque (*white arrow*) coincides with the yellow in the NIRS data. The calcification (marked by *c*) identified on IVUS and OCT has low attenuation (*blue*). Site 2 shows an eccentric lipid-core plaque (*yellow* at the 1- to 3-o'clock position) that contains small calcifications (dorsal shadowing in the same sector). High attenuation (*white arrows*) coincides with the yellow in the NIRS data. A small calcification (marked by the *green arrow*) may be identified by a local lower attenuation coefficient. Site 3 shows an eccentric fibrous (*asterisk*) lesion with calcification (*c*). This fibrocalcific plaque is characterized by the absence of high-attenuation areas, in accordance with the red appearance of the NIRS image.

Stiff Coronary Stenosis in a Young Female With Pseudoxanthoma Elasticum

Harue Sasai, MD, Kenichi Sakakura, MD, Hiroshi Wada, MD, Yoshitaka Sugawara, MD, Junya Ako, MD, Shin-ichi Momomura, MD

Pseudoxanthoma elasticum (PXE), which is caused by mutation in the *ABCC6* gene, is a heritable systemic disorder affecting elastic fibers, most markedly in skin, retina, and blood vessels.[1] To date, there is one case report of a percutaneous coronary intervention (PCI) performed in a patient with PXE.[2] In that case, the stenosis was successfully treated by the conventional techniques. However, lesion pathology in PXE is reported to be different from that in atherosclerosis.[3]

A 26-year-old Japanese woman had a diagnosis of PXE. She had typical skin involvement (yellow cobblestone appearance of the neck and elastofibroma on skin histopathology) and eye involvement (angioid streak). She was referred to our cardiology division for examination of coronary artery disease. The multidetector computed tomography (MDCT) images revealed significant stenoses of the mid left anterior descending coronary artery and the left circumflex

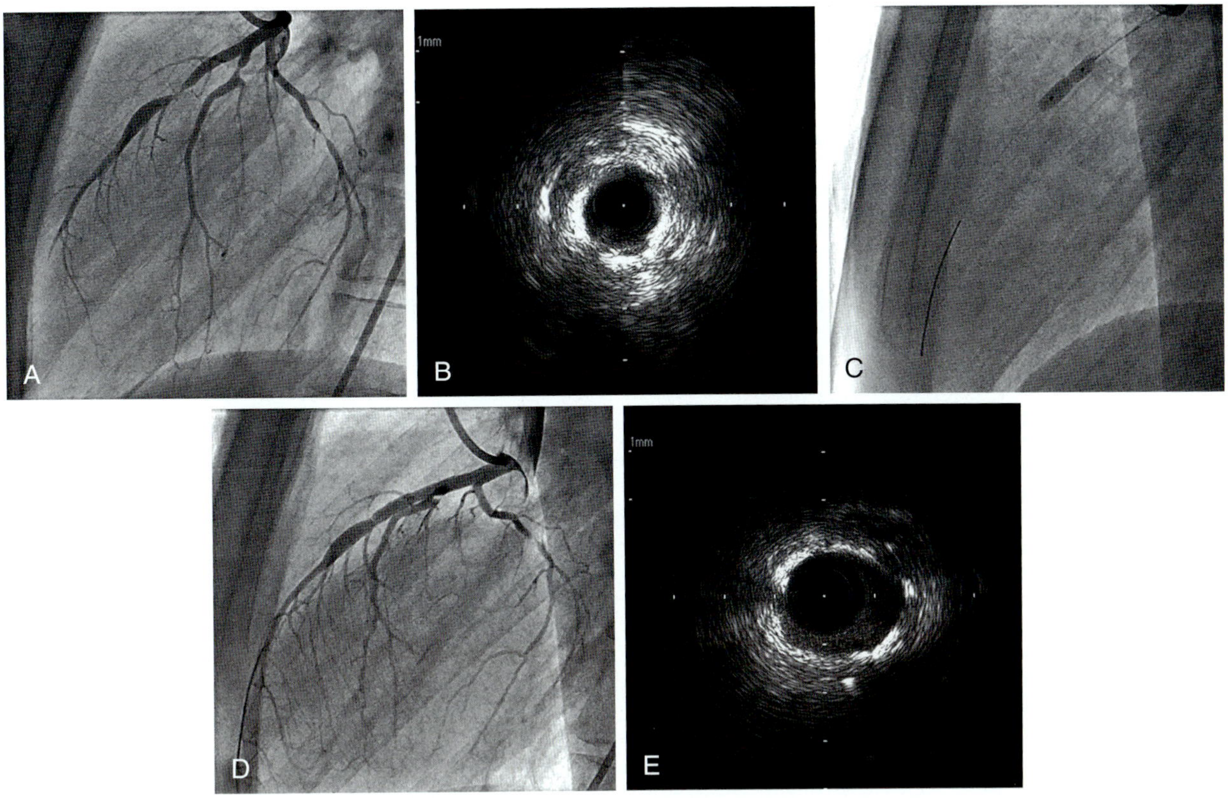

FIG. 1.107 Findings of the Left Anterior Descending Coronary Artery. (A) Coronary angiogram revealed severe stenoses without visible calcification. (B) Intravascular ultrasound (IVUS) revealed a superficial high-echoic component with several breaches around the vessel. (C) After postdilation using a large noncompliant balloon (3.75-mm Quantum Maverick), optimum stent expansion could not be achieved. (D) Final angiography showed stent underexpansion of the lesion. (E) Final IVUS finding of the underexpanded lesion.

coronary artery. However, no coronary calcification was visible. Coronary angiography revealed severe stenoses without visible calcification, consistent with the findings on MDCT (Fig. 1.107A).

Transfemoral PCI was tried to treat the stenosis in the left anterior descending coronary artery. Intravascular ultrasonography (IVUS) (View It, Terumo Medical, Tokyo, Japan) revealed a superficial high-echoic component around vessels without acoustic shadowing (Fig. 1.107B). A 3.0 × 18 mm bare-metal stent (Driver, Medtronic, Minneapolis, Minnesota) was implanted (maximum inflation pressure of 16 atm). Postdilations using several noncompliant balloons, such as the 3.75-mm Quantum Maverick (Boston Scientific, Massachusetts), were performed (maximum inflation pressure of 24 atm) (Fig. 1.107C). Unfortunately, the final angiogram showed stent underexpansion (Fig. 1.107D). The minimum stent area of the lesion was 4.4 cm^2 (Fig. 1.107E). We added bisoprolol for the treatment of other nondilated vessels.

Intimal calcification in the coronary artery is one of the characteristics of atherosclerosis. By contrast, intimal fibrosis in the coronary artery is an idiopathic change with PXE.[3,4] Although there was no visible calcification on both MDCT and angiography, IVUS suggested the presence of dense intimal fibrosis. This dense fibrosis might impede the stent expansion. Our case suggests the necessity of taking a cautious approach in PCI of lesions in patients with PXE, because the presence of dense fibrosis, which is invisible by angiogram or MDCT, may inhibit the vessel expansion. Cautious and aggressive predilation before stenting may be needed to prevent stent underexpansion.

References

1. Plomp AS, Toonstra J, Bergen AA, van Dijk MR, de Jong PT. Proposal for updating the pseudoxanthoma elasticum classification system and a review of the clinical findings. *Am J Med Genet A.* 2010;152A:1049-1058.
2. Baglini R, Sesana M, Capuano C, Danzi GB. Intracoronary ultrasound guided percutaneous coronary angioplasty using a drug eluting stent in a patient with pseudoxanthoma elasticum. *Atherosclerosis.* 2005;180:205-207.
3. Miki K, Yuri T, Takeda N, Takehana K, Iwasaka T, Tsubura A. An autopsy case of pseudoxanthoma elasticum: histochemical characteristics. *Med Mol Morphol.* 2007;40:172-177.
4. Sakata S, Su JC, Robertson S, Yin M, Chow C. Varied presentations of pseudoxanthoma elasticum in a family. *J Paediatr Child Health.* 2006;42:817-820.

A Honeycomb-Like Structure in the Left Anterior Descending Coronary Artery: Demonstration of Recanalized Thrombus by Optical Coherence Tomography

Konstantinos Toutouzas, MD, Antonios Karanasos, MD, Konstantinos Stathogiannis, MD, Andreas Synetos, MD, Eleftherios Tsiamis, MD, Dimitrios Papadopoulos, MD, Christodoulos Stefanadis, MD

A 41-year-old man had atypical chest pain in another hospital with an electrocardiogram-negative finding for ischemia, but the patient had slightly elevated troponin I levels (0.12 ng/mL). The patient underwent cardiac catheterization within 24 hours. Coronary angiography revealed two nonsignificant lesions at the proximal left anterior descending (LAD) coronary artery and angiographic haziness in the middle LAD, but with Thrombolysis In Myocardial Infarction grade flow 3. The patient was referred to our institution for intravascular lesion assessment.

Coronary angiography (Fig. 1.108) was repeated in our institution 3 days later. The haziness was still present, so we assessed the segment between the lines in Fig. 1.108 by optical coherence tomography (OCT). Image analysis (Fig. 1.109, Online Video 1.86) revealed a honeycomb-like structure with multiple intraluminal channels, separated by tissue with high signal intensity and low signal attenuation, consistent with white thrombus. We concluded that this appearance was compatible with intraluminal thrombus recanalization. Interestingly, the vascular wall had normal vessel intima morphology without evidence of atheromatic changes. The site was then treated with an everolimus-eluting stent (Promus Element Monorail, 2.75 × 20 mm, Boston Scientific, Natick, Massachusetts).

In this case, OCT was used for the assessment of angiographic haziness because it is the best method for intracoronary thrombus evaluation. Recanalized thrombus is a rare finding in patients undergoing coronary angiography, and by using OCT, we demonstrated in vivo a honeycomb-like structure composed of multiple microchannels, separated by bridges of organized thrombus. Interestingly, the underlying vascular wall was nonatheromatic, suggesting either the possibility of plaque erosion or proximal embolism as the cause of thrombus formation.

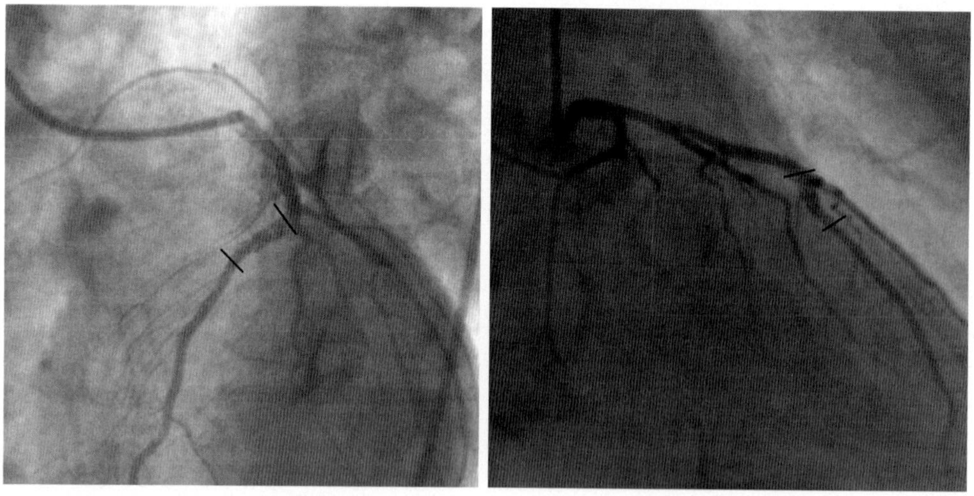

FIG. 1.108 Coronary Angiography of the Left Coronary Artery. Optical coherence tomography image acquisition was performed in the segment between the lines.

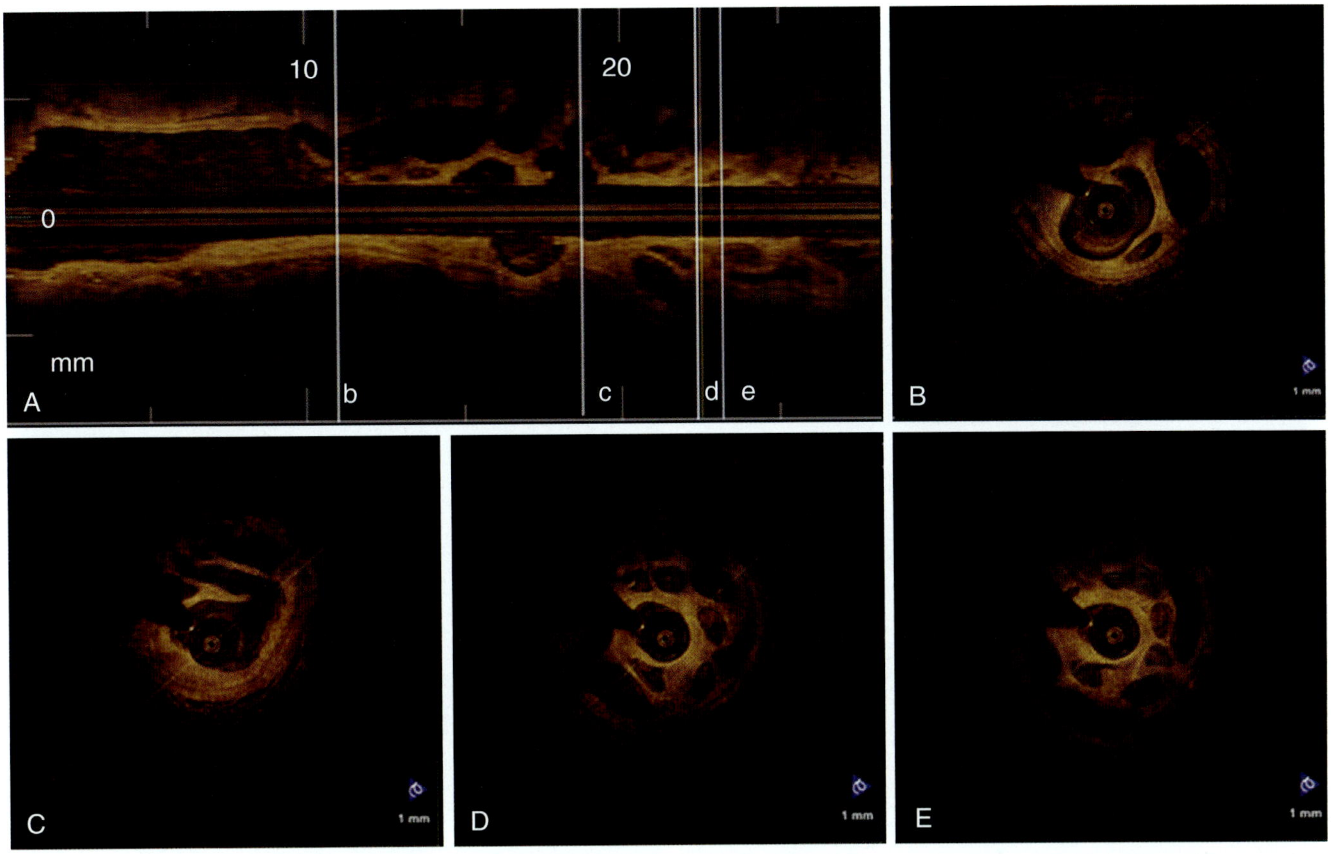

FIG. 1.109 Longitudinal and Cross-Sectional Morphology of the Microchannels. (A) L-mode image showing the longitudinal morphology of the microchannels. (B–E) Optical coherence tomography cross-sectional images acquired from the sites corresponding to the lines (b–e) in (A). See Online Video 1.86.

DVT of the Heart: A Novel Treatment for an Old Problem

Naga Venkata Pothineni, MD, Amit Bahia, MD, Freij Gobal, MD, Zubair Ahmed, MD, Barry F. Uretsky, MD, Abdul Hakeem, MD

Thrombotic lesions of saphenous venous grafts (SVGs) are frequently encountered, and interventions may be technically fraught with embolic complications. The following two cases suggest the potential role in selected cases of novel oral anticoagulants (NOACs) in the treatment of SVG thrombosis to obviate the need for percutaneous intervention (PCI).

Case 1. A 62-year-old man with four-vessel coronary artery bypass graft surgery performed 9 years earlier was seen with a non–ST-segment elevation myocardial infarction. Angiography showed the SVG to right posterior descending artery had a large thrombus in its mid segment with Thrombolysis In Myocardial Infarction grade flow 3, but it was otherwise without significant graft disease (Fig. 1.110A). All other grafts were patent. The patient was treated with low-molecular-weight heparin for 1 week, followed by dabigatran etexilate 150 mg twice a day for 1 week. Repeat angiography after 2 weeks showed complete thrombus resolution (Fig. 1.110B).

Case 2. A 67-year-old woman with three-vessel coronary artery bypass graft surgery 5 years earlier had unstable angina. Angiography showed subtotal occlusion of the SVG to an obtuse marginal branch with a large layered thrombus and minimal atherosclerotic obstruction elsewhere in the graft (Fig. 1.111A). All other grafts were patent. The patient began taking rivaroxaban 20 mg daily. Angiography 4 weeks later revealed thrombus resolution and normalization of coronary flow (Fig. 1.111B).

Acute SVG thrombosis frequently presents as acute coronary syndrome (ACS). PCI has traditionally been the treatment of choice for abrupt SVG thrombotic occlusions. It carries the risk of distal embolization, no reflow, and periprocedural myocardial infarction. Among pharmacologic alternatives for acute SVG thrombosis, glycoprotein IIb/IIIa antagonists[1] and warfarin[2] have been successfully used as pre-PCI thrombus reduction strategies. We report the use of NOACs as "destination therapy" without the need for PCI for acute

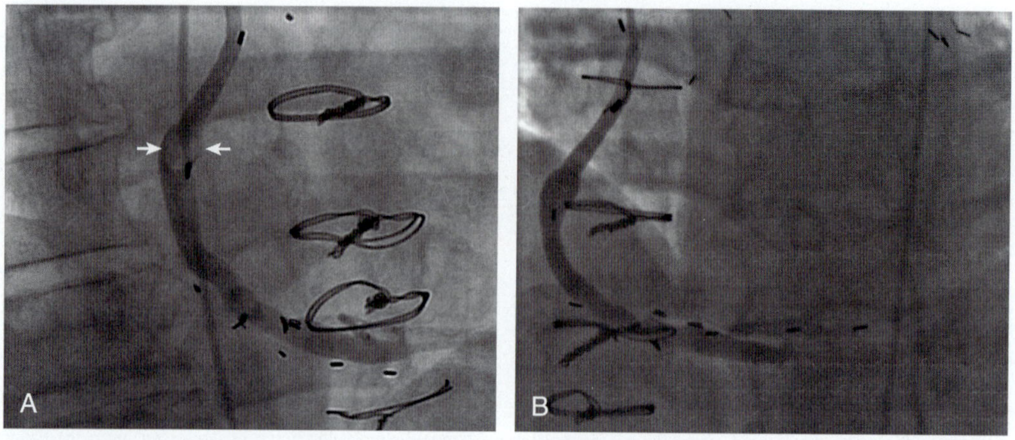

FIG. 1.110 Right Anterior Oblique Projections of Case 1. Case 1. (A) Right anterior oblique projection showing a thrombus (*arrows*) in the mid portion of the saphenous venous graft (SVG). (B) Right anterior oblique projection with resolution of SVG thrombus and widely patent saphenous venous graft.

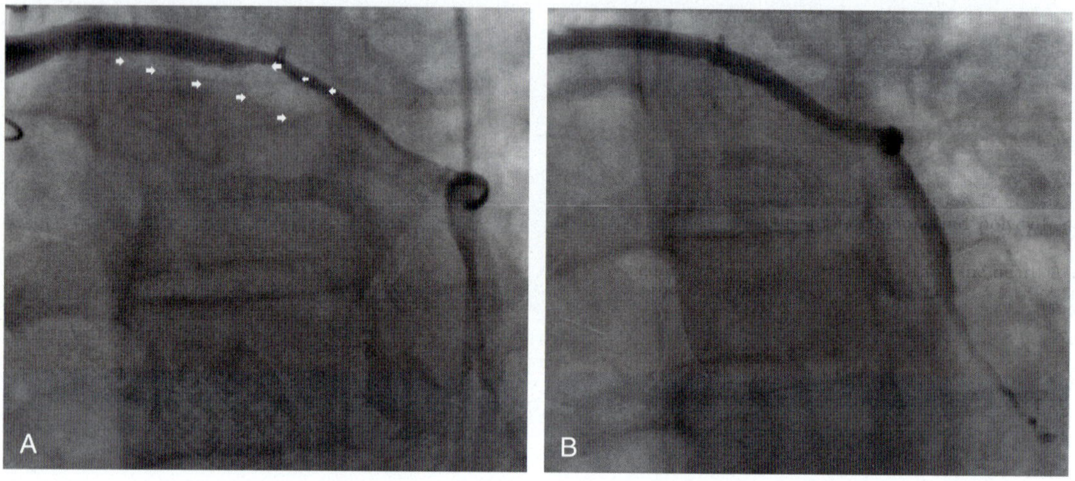

FIG. 1.111 Anteroposterior Projections of Case 2. Case 2. (A) Anteroposterior projection with a large layered thrombus (*arrows*) in a saphenous venous graft (SVG). (B) Anteroposterior projection with resolution of thrombus and patent SVG.

SVG thrombosis in the setting of ACS. It is unclear if the thrombus resolution was spontaneous with time or secondary to NOACs. We are also uncertain about the success rate and patient selection for this approach. Factors that might influence success rate include thrombus burden, age of the graft, and presence or absence of graft degeneration. In summary, we report the first use of NOACs for the treatment of acute SVG thrombosis in the setting of ACS. This noninvasive approach may be safe and effective in selected patients who have focal non–flow-limiting thrombotic SVG occlusions in the absence of significant angiographic graft disease.

References

1. Senturk T, Aydin Kaderli A, Aydin O, Yesilbursa D, Akin Serdar O. Successful treatment of saphenous venous graft thrombus by tirofiban infusion. *Heart Lung.* 2010;39:237-239.
2. Chow WH, Hon PH. Successful stenting after Coumadin therapy and thrombus resolution in a stenotic saphenous vein graft. *Cathet Cardiovasc Diagn.* 1996;39:438-439.

Thrombocytosis and Coronary Occlusion

Amit Nanavati, MD, Nainesh Patel, MD, James Burke, MD, PhD

The differential diagnosis for ST-segment elevation myocardial infarction in young patients without traditional risk factors for coronary artery disease often includes coronary artery vasospasm, dissection, and pericarditis. However, in the setting of focal, sustained arterial closure, one must revisit a platelet-mediated mechanism. We report a case of platelet-mediated occlusion as the result of essential thrombocytosis.

A 33-year-old white man with a recent diagnosis of essential thrombocytosis (platelet count 684,000/μL) and *JAK-2* mutation was seen with acute severe chest pain, preceded by two weeks of

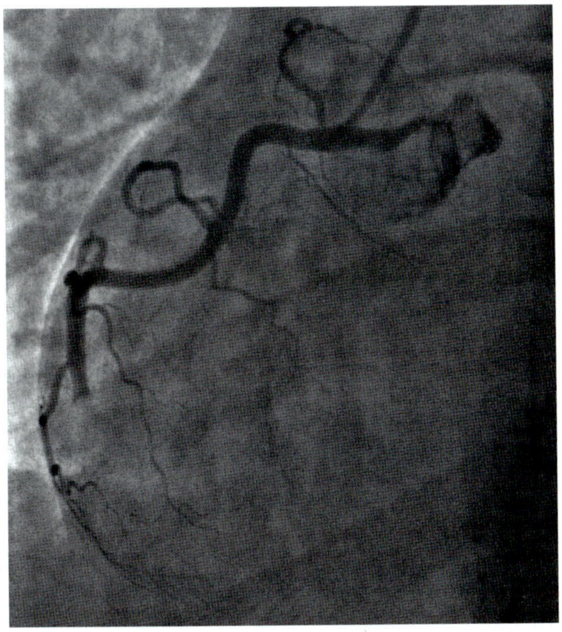

FIG. 1.112 Acute Occlusion of the Right Coronary Artery. A right coronary artery angiography left anterior oblique view shows occlusion in the mid segment with thrombus and thrombolysis in myocardial infarction (TIMI) grade flow 0. A Promus 4.0 × 28 mm everolimus-eluting coronary stent was then placed across this occlusion with restoration of TIMI grade flow 3.

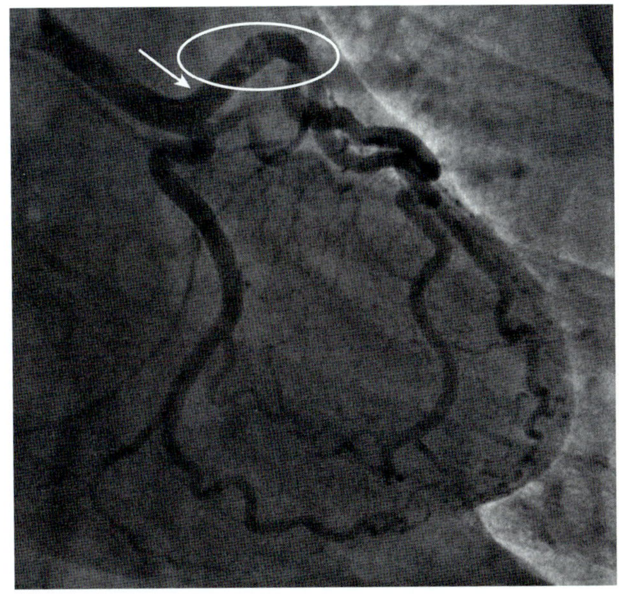

FIG. 1.113 Thrombus in the Left Anterior Descending Coronary Artery. A left coronary artery angiography right anterior oblique caudal view shows the left anterior descending coronary artery (*arrow*) with a large nonocclusive thrombus (*circled*) in the proximal segment with Thrombolysis In Myocardial Infarction grade flow 3.

intermittent pain. Inferior ST-segment elevation myocardial infarction was diagnosed, and coronary angiography was emergently performed. An occlusive mid right coronary artery lesion was seen (Fig. 1.112) and a Promus 4.0 × 28 mm everolimus-eluting stent (Boston Scientific, Natick, Massachusetts) was placed after thrombectomy. Distal embolization was noted in the posterior descending artery. Additionally, a large nonocclusive thrombus was seen in the left anterior descending artery (Fig. 1.113) and was treated with 18 hours of eptifibatide. Clopidogrel and aspirin therapy was started, and the patient was discharged 3 days later in stable condition. No further therapy was recommended specifically for the essential thrombocytosis.

Essential thrombocytosis, typified by abnormal megakaryocyte proliferation[1] is rare, with an incidence of approximately 2.5 to 7 cases per 1,000,000 people.[1,2] It can be associated with both thrombosis and hemorrhage.[3] Even rarer is coronary artery thrombosis, especially in those without traditional risk factors, with few reported cases.[1,3] Thrombosis in the left anterior descending coronary artery was most common, with fewer reports of multivessel thrombosis.[3] Proposed management strategies include coronary artery bypass grafting, intracoronary thrombolysis, and primary percutaneous intervention.[2] However, randomized or definitive retrospective data are not available. Although a first episode of thrombosis may predispose individuals to additional episodes,[4] the efficacy of long-term dual-antiplatelet agents in prevention is unknown. A particular *JAK-2* mutation has been associated with an increased risk of thrombosis, although data are inconclusive.[4] Also noteworthy as seen in these case reports is that thrombosis can occur without a severely abnormal platelet count.

References

1. Bildirici U, Celikyury U, Ural E. Essential thrombocythemia: a case of acute ST-segment elevation myocardial infarction in a young female. *Clin Cardiol.* 2009;32:104-105.
2. Tekin M, Gokaslan S, Diker E, et al. Development of acute coronary syndrome in three patients with essential thrombocythemia or polycythemia vera. *Arch Turk Soc Cardiol.* 2008;36:35-38.
3. Ozben B, Ekmekci A, Bugra Z, et al. Multiple coronary thrombosis and stent implantation to the subtotally occluded right renal artery in a patient with essential thrombocytosis: a case report with review. *J Thromb Thrombocytosis.* 2006;22:79-84.
4. Ziakas PD. Effect of JAK2 V617F on thrombotic risk in patients with essential thrombocythemia: measuring the uncertain. *Haematologica.* 2008;93:1412-1413.

Stent Pathology

In-Stent Thin-Cap Fibroatheroma After Drug-Eluting Stent Implantation: Ex Vivo Evaluation of Optical Coherence Tomography and Intracoronary Angioscopy

Kenichi Fujii, MD, Hiroyuki Hao, MD, Takahiro Imanaka, MD, Taro Kawano, MD, Tadateru Takayama, MD, Atsushi Hirayama, MD, Tsutomu Yamada, PhD, Hatsue Ishibashi-Ueda, MD, Seiichi Hirota, MD, Tohru Masuyama, MD

A 57-year-old man died of sepsis and an autopsy was performed. He had previously undergone percutaneous coronary intervention of the middle left anterior descending coronary artery, with two sirolimus-eluting stents implanted 61 months before death. Post mortem ex vivo optical coherence tomography (OCT) (LightLab Imaging, Westford, Massachusetts), coronary angioscopy (CAS) (FiberTech, Tokyo, Japan) imaging, and pathologic examination were performed in the stented segments. OCT images showed in-stent eccentric intimal growth of moderate intimal hyperplasia with rapid attenuation of the signals with diffuse border, such as a thin-cap fibroatheroma (TCFA) in native coronary arteries (Fig. 1.114A). Corresponding CAS images revealed that stent struts were covered by intensive yellow neointima (Fig. 1.114B). Corresponding histopathologic images demonstrated a large, lipid-rich necrotic core covered with a thin fibrous cap infiltrated by lipid-laden macrophages with few smooth muscle cells (Fig. 1.114C–D).

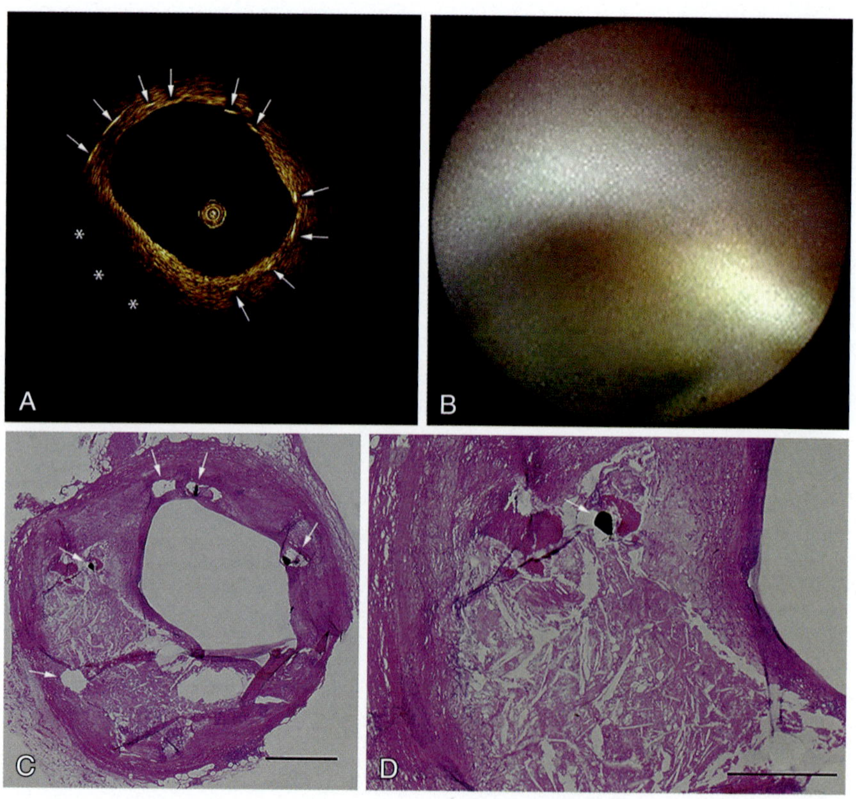

FIG. 1.114 Histopathology and Intravascular Images of In-Stent Thin-Cap Fibroatheroma. (A) A cross-sectional image of optical coherence tomography clearly showed an eccentric intimal growth with the appearance of rapid attenuation of the signals (*asterisks*) with a diffuse border. The signal-poor area was located inside the stent struts (*arrows*). In this cross section, the stent struts behind the signal-poor mass (6- to 9-o'clock positions) were completely invisible because of attenuation of the signal, and the thickness of the fibrous cap overlying the signal-poor area was 60 μm by optical coherence tomography image. (B) Coronary angioscopy showed intensive yellow plaque, and there were no visible stent struts. (C) Corresponding histology from the same section of the lesion in (A) showed a thin fibrous cap overlying a large, lipid-rich, eccentric necrotic core, indicating a thin-cap fibroatheroma–like appearance within the stent. (Hematoxylin and eosin stain, scale bar = 1 mm, allows the identification of stent struts [*arrows*].) The minimal thickness of the fibrous cap by histology was 52 μm. (D) Higher magnification of the neointima within the stent struts demonstrated necrotic debris with cholesterol clefts. The thin fibrous cap was infiltrated by lipid-laden macrophages. (Hematoxylin and eosin stain, scale bar = 500 μm, allows the identification of the stent struts.)

Based on recent pathologic study, rupture of a TCFA-like lesion within the neointima has been reported in the long term after stent implantation and has been proposed as being responsible for very late stent thrombosis.[1] To the best of our knowledge, this is the first case found by autopsy specimen of ex vivo interrogation of in-stent TCFA containing neointima after drug-eluting stent implantation with OCT and CAS. On OCT images, the lipid-rich necrotic core appears as a low-signal-intensity mass because of the strong optical absorption and scattering of lipids at light wavelengths around 1000 nm.[2] Therefore stent struts cannot be visualized by OCT if there is a lipid-rich necrotic core within the neointima. Conversely, stent struts behind organized fibrin thrombus can be visualized because OCT signals are not attenuated by this material.[3] Therefore it is important to identify the in-stent TCFA-like neointima whether stent struts behind a low-signal-intensity area are visible or invisible.

ACKNOWLEDGMENTS

The authors thank Mrs. Mayumi Oka and Mr. Gen Satoh for their technical assistance.

REFERENCES

1. Nakazawa G, Otsuka F, Nakano M, et al. The pathology of neo-atherosclerosis in human coronary implants: bare-metal and drug-eluting stents. *J Am Coll Cardiol.* 2011;57:1314-1322.
2. Allen TJ, Hall A, Dhillon AP, Owen JS, Beard PC. Spectroscopic photoacoustic imaging of lipid-rich plaques in the human aorta in the 740 to 1400 nm wavelength range. *J Biomed Opt.* 2012;17:061209.
3. Nakano M, Vorpahl M, Otsuka F, et al. Ex vivo assessment of vascular response to coronary stents by optical frequency domain imaging. *J Am Coll Cardiol Img.* 2012;5:71-82.

BIOMECHANICAL ASSESSMENT OF FULLY BIORESORBABLE DEVICES

Bill D. Gogas, MD, Spencer B. King III, MD, Lucas H. Timmins, PhD, Tiziano Passerini, PhD, Marina Piccinelli, PhD, Alessandro Veneziani, PhD, Sungho Kim, PhD, David S. Molony, PhD, Don P. Giddens, PhD, Patrick W. Serruys, MD, PhD, Habib Samady, MD

The use of bioresorbable technologies for the treatment of coronary artery disease is a novel approach with potential advantages over the use of metal stents.[1] Several devices have undergone First-In-Man studies; however, the Absorb bioresorbable vascular scaffold (BVS) (Abbott Vascular, Santa Clara, California) is the only bioresorbable platform approved for clinical use in Europe (CE mark). The BVS platform is made of poly-L-lactide that is shown to completely resorb over a 2- to 3-year period. Insights from the ABSORB Cohort B trial (NCT00856856) suggest that the scaffold is more conformable than metal stents (Xience everolimus-eluting stent, Abbott Vascular), resulting in less vascular straightening and greater retention of the original angulation and curvature. Although the polymeric struts of the Absorb BVS are thicker (150 μm) compared with those of second-generation metal stents, the hemodynamic effects change over time as the scaffold resorbs. Therefore the overall biomechanical footprint of the bioresorbable scaffold compared with metal stents is transient with different effects on local vessel and strut level wall shear stress (WSS). We have proposed that such detailed biomechanical evaluation of the Absorb BVS will add critical mechanistic insights into its potential beneficial effects, particularly in angulated and curved vessels.[2]

In this report we illustrate the assessment of biomechanical properties by two methods in two selected patients who underwent implantation of the Absorb BVS from the ABSORB Extend study (NCT01023789). The evaluation used three-dimensional (3D) angiographic reconstruction techniques and computational fluid dynamics (CFD) to calculate the WSS before and after BVS deployment (Fig. 1.115A–D) for vessel-level analysis. The second method used optical coherence tomography imaging data to reconstruct the 3D geometry and CFD to visualize flow streamlines over the polymeric struts for more detailed strut-level analysis (Fig. 1.115E–E′). Fusion of angiographic data with optical coherence tomography data has been previously shown to be a feasible approach to calculate WSS by CFD simulations,[3] and biomechanical analyses by these methods may yield important insights into potential advantages of bioresorbable technologies over metal stents.

ACKNOWLEDGMENTS

Dr. Gogas acknowledges the American College of Cardiology Foundation for the International Society of Cardiovascular Translational Research Scholarship. Dr. Timmins and Dr. Passerini acknowledge the American Heart Association for their Postdoctoral Fellowships. The authors thank Prof. Didier Carrie from the Hôpital de Rangueil, Toulouse, France; Prof. Stephen Lee, from the Queen Mary Hospital, Hong Kong; and Christos Bourantas from the Thoraxcenter, Erasmus University Medical Center, Rotterdam, for their valuable comments.

REFERENCES

1. Serruys PW, Garcia-Garcia HM, Onuma Y. From metallic cages to transient bioresorbable scaffolds: change in paradigm of coronary revascularization in the upcoming decade? *Eur Heart J.* 2012;33:16-25b.
2. McDaniel MC, Samady H. The sheer stress of straightening the curves: biomechanics of bioabsorbable stents. *J Am Coll Cardiol Intv.* 2011;4:800-802.
3. Tu S, Holm NR, Koning G, et al. Fusion of 3D QCA and IVUS/OCT. *Int J Cardiovasc Imaging.* 2011;27:197-207.

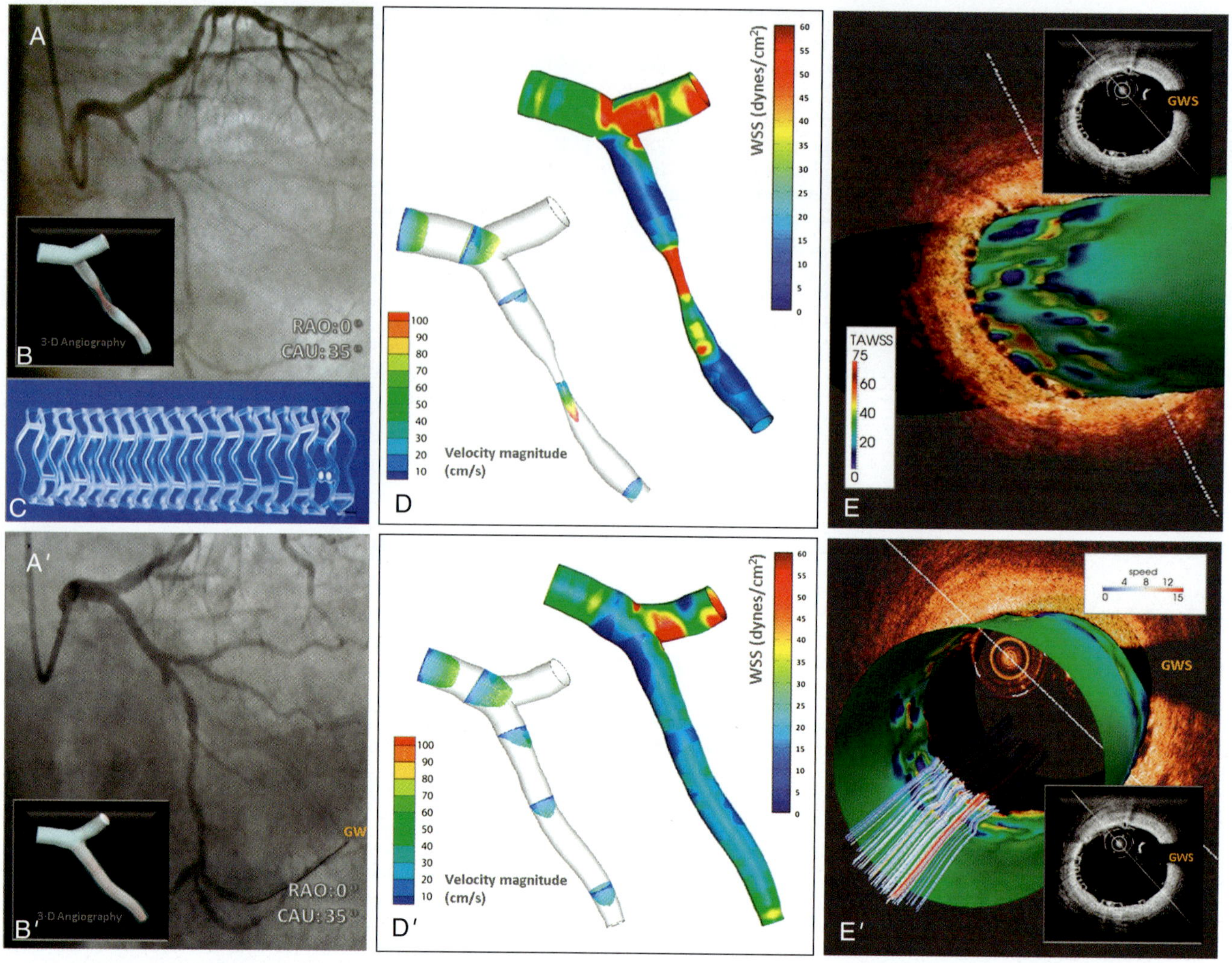

FIG. 1.115 Presentation of WSS Derived From Angiographic and OCT Imaging Data Projections Using CFD Modeling Techniques After Implantation of the Absorb Bioresorbable Vascular Scaffold (BVS). (A and A′) Two-dimensional (2D) angiographic views of the significant proximal left circumflex artery lesion (A) and (A′) the scaffolded segment after implantation of the 3.0 × 18 mm BVS. (B and B′), Three-dimensional (3D) angiographic views before (B) and after (B′) scaffold implantation. (C) The Absorb BVS. (D), (D′) Time-averaged wall shear stress (*TAWSS*) magnitude distribution from angiographically derived 3D geometries before (D) and after (D′) scaffold deployment. Velocity profiles before and after implantation of the Absorb BVS are superimposed. (E) 2D OCT cross section with embedded polymeric struts demonstrating in a 3D pattern the distribution of TAWSS between the polymeric struts. The quantified color coding demonstrates low-WSS regions (*blue color*). The matched OCT cross section is superimposed. (E′), Reconstructed streamlines of the velocity field at the systolic peak demonstrating altered flow patterns in the proximity of the arterial wall induced by the polymeric struts. *GWS*, guidewire shadow; *WSS*, wall stress shear.

Coronary Artery Aneurysm After Everolimus-Eluting Bioabsorbable Vascular Scaffold Implantation

Swaroop Varghese, MBBS, Bernward Lauer, MD, Marc-Alexander Ohlow, MD

Among the rare complications after percutaneous coronary intervention, coronary artery aneurysms (CAAs) reportedly have an incidence of 0.3% to 6.0%. The detection of CAAs varies from 3 days to up to 4 years after drug-eluting stent (DES) and from 6 days to up to 6 years after bare-metal stent (BMS) implantation. Associated factors include residual dissection and deep arterial wall injury caused by oversized balloons or stents, high-pressure balloon inflations, atherectomy, and laser angioplasty.[1,2] Although the pathogenesis of CAA after DES, as well as after BMS, implantation, has been studied, there seems to be neither sufficient literature nor adequate evidence of CAA after a bioabsorbable stent implantation.

A 59-year-old male patient with exertional angina underwent percutaneous coronary intervention of the first obtuse marginal branch. After predilation with a regular balloon, a 3.0 × 18 mm

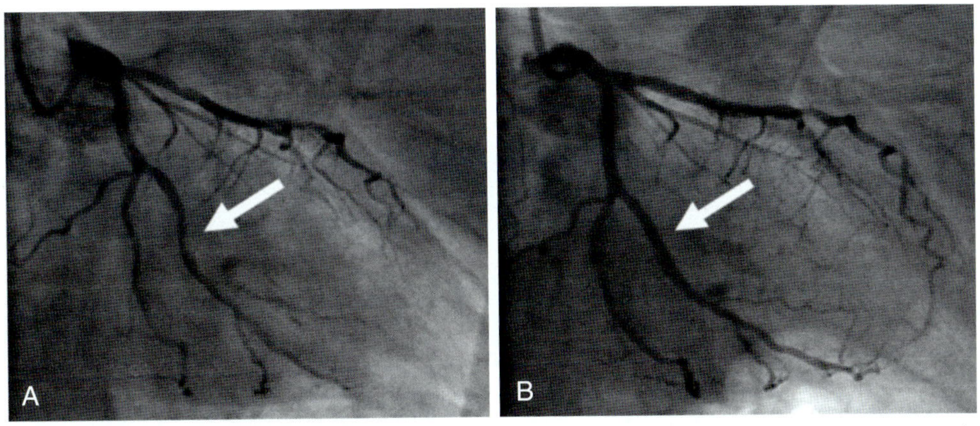

FIG. 1.116 Coronary Angiography of the Obtuse Marginal Branch. (A) Stenosis of the obtuse marginal branch (*white arrow*). (B) Result immediately after implantation of a bioabsorbable vascular scaffold. The white arrow shows the repaired stenosis of the obtuse marginal branch after implantation of a bioabsorbable stent.

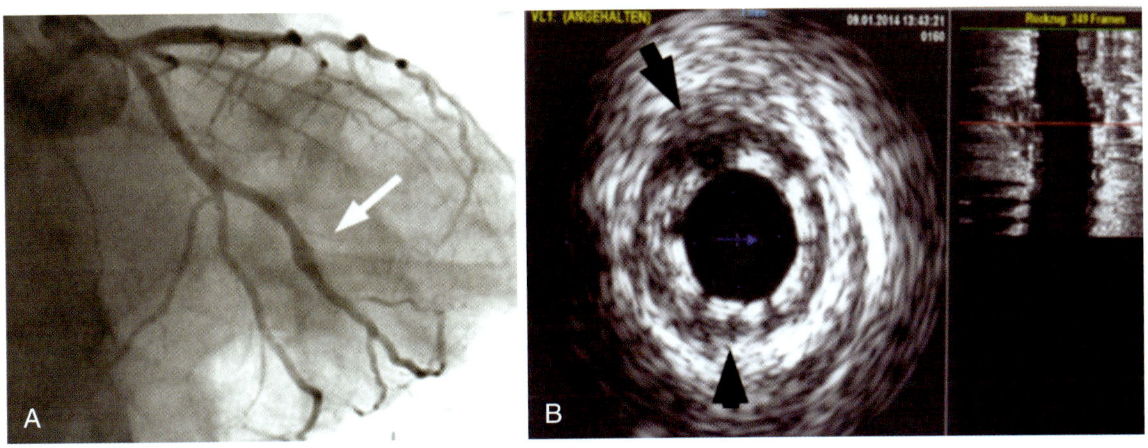

FIG. 1.117 Coronary Angiography and Intravascular Ultrasound (IVUS) After 6 Months. (A) Coronary angiography after 6 months. The white arrow show the aneurysmatic structure in the stented segment of the obtuse marginal branch. (B) IVUS image visualizing the aneurysmatic structure (*black arrows*).

bioabsorbable vascular scaffold (BVS) (Absorb, Abbott Vascular, Santa Clara, California) was positioned with good immediate results (Fig. 1.116). An angiographic and intravascular ultrasound (IVUS) follow-up at 6 months revealed an aneurysm in the stented segment (Fig. 1.117). Because of the patient's atypical symptoms, an angiographic and IVUS follow-up was recommended. At 1 year, the aneurysm had significantly increased in size (Fig. 1.118), and a covered stent (3.0 × 18 mm BeGraft (Bentley Innomed, Hechingen, Germany) was implanted to exclude the aneurysm (Fig. 1.119). It could be hypothesized that the distinct morphologic attributes of the BVS stent such as relatively thicker struts and the slower expandability requiring higher pressures of balloon inflations (thereby causing deep arterial wall injury) during implantation and inflammatory/hypersensitivity changes (occurring in the vessel wall) after implantation could play a multifactorial role in the pathogenesis of a CAA.[2] Further studies are needed to comprehensively study the incidence and understand the underlying pathomechanisms of CAAs after implantation of bioabsorbable stents.

References

1. Slota PA, Fischman DL, Savage M, Rake R, Goldberg S. Frequency and outcome of development of coronary artery aneurysm after intracoronary stent placement and angioplasty. *J Am Coll Cardiol.* 1997;79:1104-1106.
2. Aoki J, Kirtane A, Leon MB, Dangas G. Coronary artery aneurysms after drug-eluting stent implantation. *J Am Coll Cardiol Intv.* 2008;1:14-21.

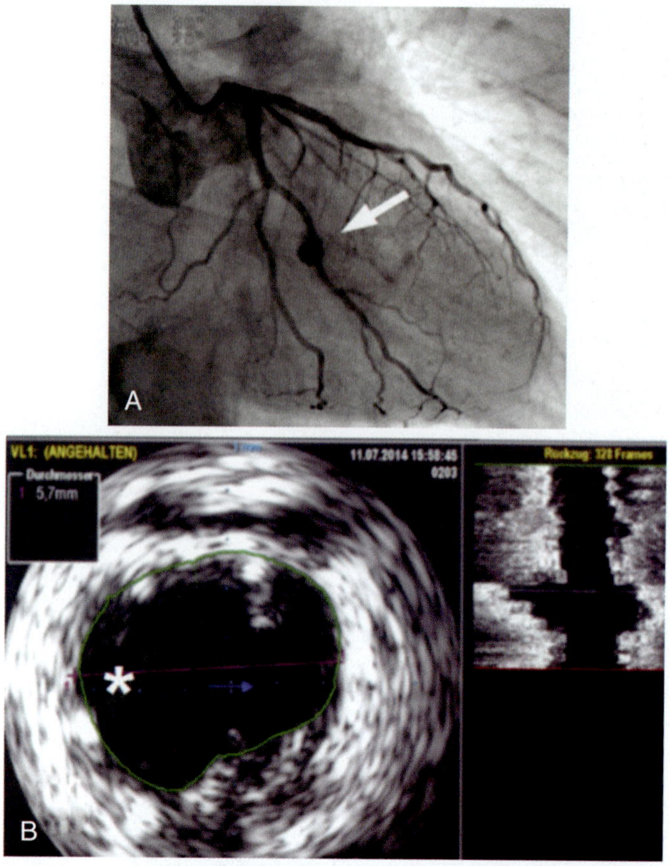

FIG. 1.118 Coronary Angiography and Intravascular Ultrasound (IVUS) After 12 Months. (A) Coronary angiography after 12 months. The white arrow shows a large aneurysmatic structure in the stented segment of the obtuse marginal branch. (B) IVUS visualizing the aneurysmatic structure (*asterisk*).

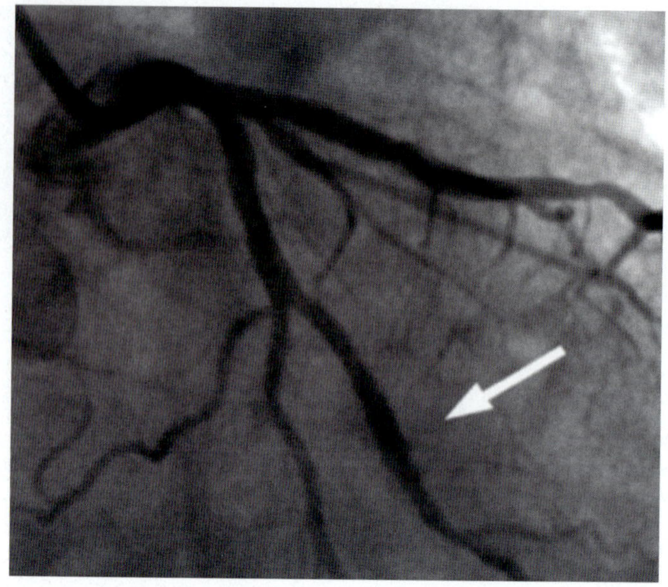

FIG. 1.119 Coronary Angiography: Final Result. Coronary angiography shows the final result of the obtuse marginal branch after implantation of a covered stent in the aneurysmatic region (*white arrow*).

Extremely Late Catch-Up Phenomenon After First-Generation Sirolimus-Eluting Stent in the Left Main Stem: Insights From Optical Coherence Tomography

Toru Naganuma, MD, Yusuke Fujino, MD, PhD, Satoko Tahara, MD, PhD, Satoru Mitomo, MD, Sandeep Basavarajaiah, MD, Sunao Nakamura, MD, PhD

A 72-year-old man had undergone angioplasty of the left main stem (LMS) with implantation of a first-generation drug-eluting stent (DES) (3.5 × 18 mm Cypher stent, Cordis—Johnson & Johnson, Bridgewater, New Jersey) (Fig. 1.120A). Postprocedural intravascular ultrasonography (IVUS) had shown a well-expanded stent (Fig. 1.120 A′ and 1.120Aa–c). Four years later both angiography and IVUS exhibited no significant in-stent restenosis (ISR) or stent recoil (Fig. 1.120B–B′, Ba′–c′). At 7 years, he was seen with acute coronary syndrome (ACS) while still using long-term dual-antiplatelet therapy. A subsequently obtained coronary angiogram exhibited severe ISR at the mid shaft of the LMS (Fig. 1.120C). Preprocedural optical coherence tomography (OCT) showed a massive low-intensity neointimal plaque including microvessels, indicating neoatherosclerosis within the stent (Fig. 1.120C″, a″–g″). In addition, a plaque rupture was noted at the distal shoulder of the plaque with white thrombi (Fig. 1.121A). There was no evidence of malapposed struts. Successful revascularization was performed using a new-generation DES.

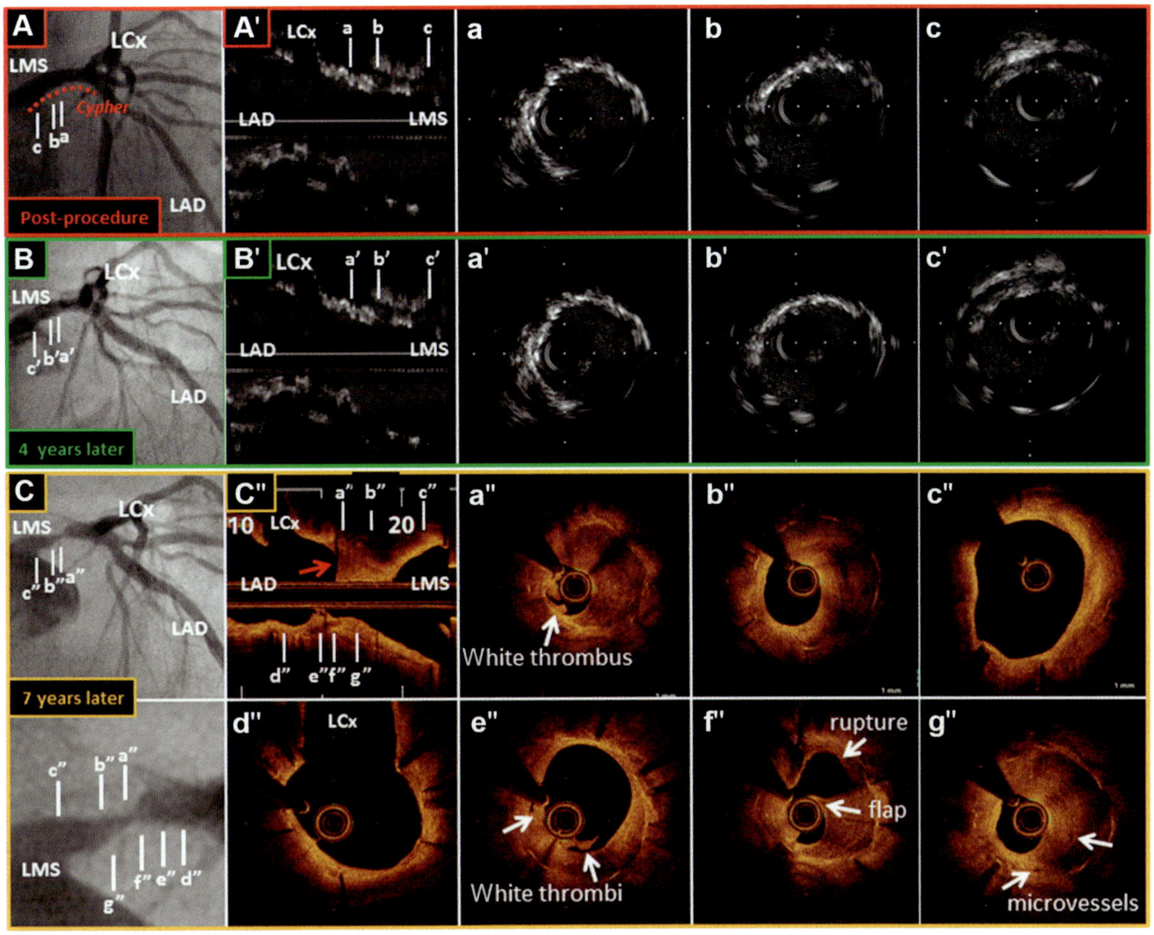

FIG. 1.120 Serial Assessments of Left Main Stem (*LMS*) With Angiography, Intravascular Ultrasound (IVUS), and Optical Coherence Tomography (OCT). (A) Postprocedural angiography showing an excellent result after a 3.5 × 18 mm Cypher stent (Cordis—Johnson & Johnson, Bridgewater, New Jersey) implantation followed by postdilation with a 4.0-mm noncompliant balloon. (A′), Postprocedural IVUS longitudinal view (a–c) showing a well-expanded stent (stent area, 10.3 mm^2; stent diameter, 3.3 × 4.0 mm [a]). (B) Angiography at 4 years with no restenosis. (B′), IVUS longitudinal view at 4 years. (a′–c′), IVUS showing adequate lumen and stent areas (stent diameter and area were quite similar to the postprocedural ones). (C) Angiography at 7 years showing a focal severe in-stent restenosis at the LMS midshaft. (C″), OCT longitudinal view at 7 years (a rupture site in the distal shoulder of the in-stent neointimal plaque is indicated with a *red arrow*). (a″), OCT showing a low-intensity neointimal plaque with a few white thrombi at the site with minimal lumen area (stent area 8.0 mm^2; stent diameter 3.2 × 3.4 mm; lumen area 1.3 mm^2). (b″), OCT showing a low-intensity neointimal plaque with no evident uncovered and/or malapposed stent struts as well as stent fracture. (c″), OCT showing the proximal part of the left main stem with adequate lumen and stent areas. (d″) OCT showing a left anterior descending artery/left circumflex artery bifurcation site. (e″) OCT showing white thrombi (indicated by *white arrows*). (f″) OCT showing a neointimal plaque rupture in the distal shoulder with a thin flap. (g″) OCT showing microvessels within the neointimal plaque (indicated by *white arrows*).

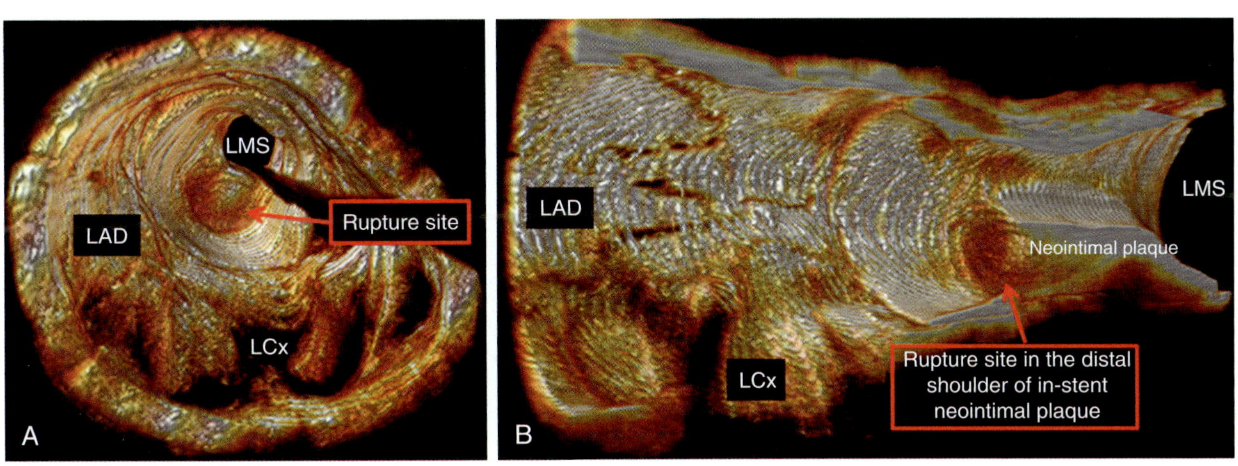

FIG. 1.121 Optical Coherence Tomography (OCT) Three-Dimensional (3D) Reconstruction Images. (A) OCT 3D reconstruction image confirming a neointimal plaque rupture as a cavity in its distal shoulder (a view from the left anterior descending artery toward the left main stem). (B) OCT 3D reconstruction image confirming a neointimal plaque rupture as a cavity in its distal shoulder (a vertical section). *LAD,* left anterior descending artery; *LCx,* left circumflex artery; *LMS,* left main stem.

Although late catch-up is a well-known complication after first-generation DES implantation,[1,2] our case demonstrates that this unfavorable phenomenon can occur even at an extremely late phase after stenting. Approximately 30% of ISR presents as ACS,[3] and, as seen in our case, it might be due to plaque rupture from neoatherosclerosis within the stent illustrated by some excellent OCT images. A previous IVUS study on ACS demonstrated that rupture at the distal shoulder of plaque is associated with less dramatic electrocardiographic changes and a relatively higher grade of Thrombolysis In Myocardial Infarction grade flow.[4] The plaque rupture at the distal shoulder in our case might explain why our patient could survive with ACS of the LMS.

References

1. Park DW, Hong MK, Mintz GS, et al. Two-year follow-up of the quantitative angiographic and volumetric intravascular ultrasound analysis after nonpolymeric paclitaxel-eluting stent implantation: late "catch-up" phenomenon from ASPECT Study. *J Am Coll Cardiol.* 2006;48:2432-2439.
2. Wessely R, Kastrati A, Schomig A. Late restenosis in patients receiving a polymer-coated sirolimus-eluting stent. *Ann Intern Med.* 2005;143:392-394.
3. Latib A, Mussardo M, Ielasi A, et al. Long-term outcomes after the percutaneous treatment of drug-eluting stent restenosis. *J Am Coll Cardiol Intv.* 2011;4:155-164.
4. Tanaka A, Shimada K, Namba M, et al. Relationship between longitudinal morphology of ruptured plaques and TIMI flow grade in acute coronary syndrome: a three-dimensional intravascular ultrasound imaging study. *Eur Heart J.* 2008;29:38-44.

Multiple Interstrut Cavities: A Potential Mechanism for Very Late Stent Thrombosis? Insights From Optical Coherence Tomography

Abdi Jama, MD, Abhiram Prasad, MD

A 48-year-old man who had had a 3.5 × 33 mm sirolimus-eluting stent (Cypher, Cordis, Warren, New Jersey) implanted 46 months earlier for unstable angina was seen with a 1-hour history of chest pain owing to an anterior ST-segment elevation myocardial infarction. He was taken to the cardiac catheterization laboratory for primary percutaneous coronary intervention. Coronary angiography demonstrated a filling defect, consistent with thrombus, within a stent in the proximal left anterior descending artery with Thrombolysis In Myocardial Infarction grade flow 3 (Fig. 1.122A). Successful thrombectomy was performed with an Expressway (Atrium Medical, Hudson, New Hampshire) catheter. Postthrombectomy angiography demonstrated minimal thrombus, but there was contrast staining outside the stent margins (Fig. 1.122B). Optical coherence tomography imaging showed multiple cavity-like structures between the struts that corresponded to the regions of contrast staining on the angiogram (Fig. 1.123A–C). There was some residual thrombus in the proximal stent, adjacent to an interstrut cavity (Fig. 1.123A). The stent was adequately expanded and well apposed. There was mild neointimal hyperplasia without plaque rupture and no uncovered struts.

The annual incidence of very late stent thrombosis (VLST) (occurring more than 1 year after implantation) is approximately 0.4% to 0.6%.[1] Proposed stent-related risk factors for VLST include incomplete neointimal stent coverage, late stent malapposition as the result of positive remodeling, neointimal plaque rupture, and stent fracture.[2] Our case illustrates the novel observation that irregular contrast staining along the stent margins, seen months to years after its implantation, might be due to the formation of multiple interstrut cavities. Moreover, the presence of the extensive cavities, in the absence of other stent-related risk factors for VLST, leads us to hypothesize that there might be a mechanistic link between the interstrut cavities and stent thrombosis. The pathophysiology responsible for the cavities is unknown, but we speculate that they might be a consequence of sirolimus-eluting stent-induced arterial inflammation or,

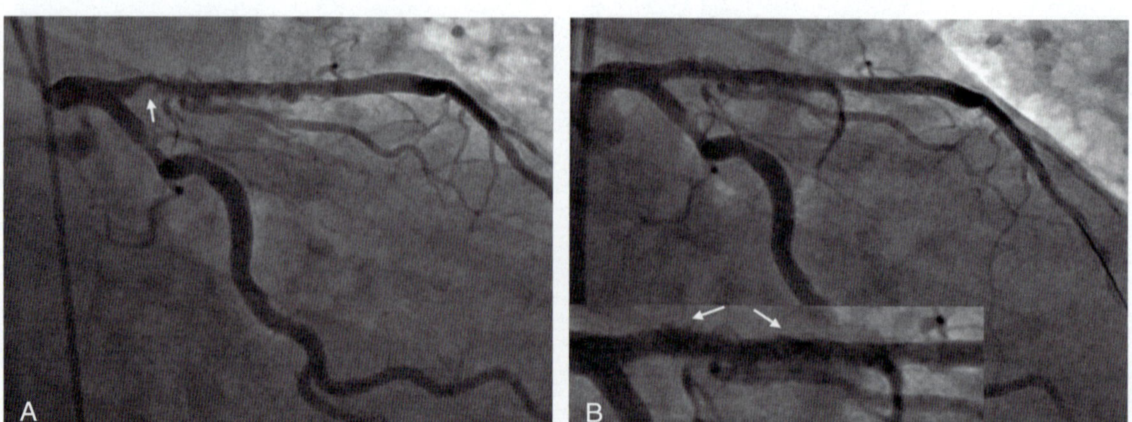

FIG. 1.122 Coronary Angiogram in a Right Anterior Oblique Projection. (A) Prethrombectomy imaging shows a filling defect (*arrow*) within the stent in the proximal left anterior descending artery. (B) Postthrombectomy imaging shows a filling defect is no longer present and contrast staining outside the stent struts (better seen in the magnified inset, *arrows*).

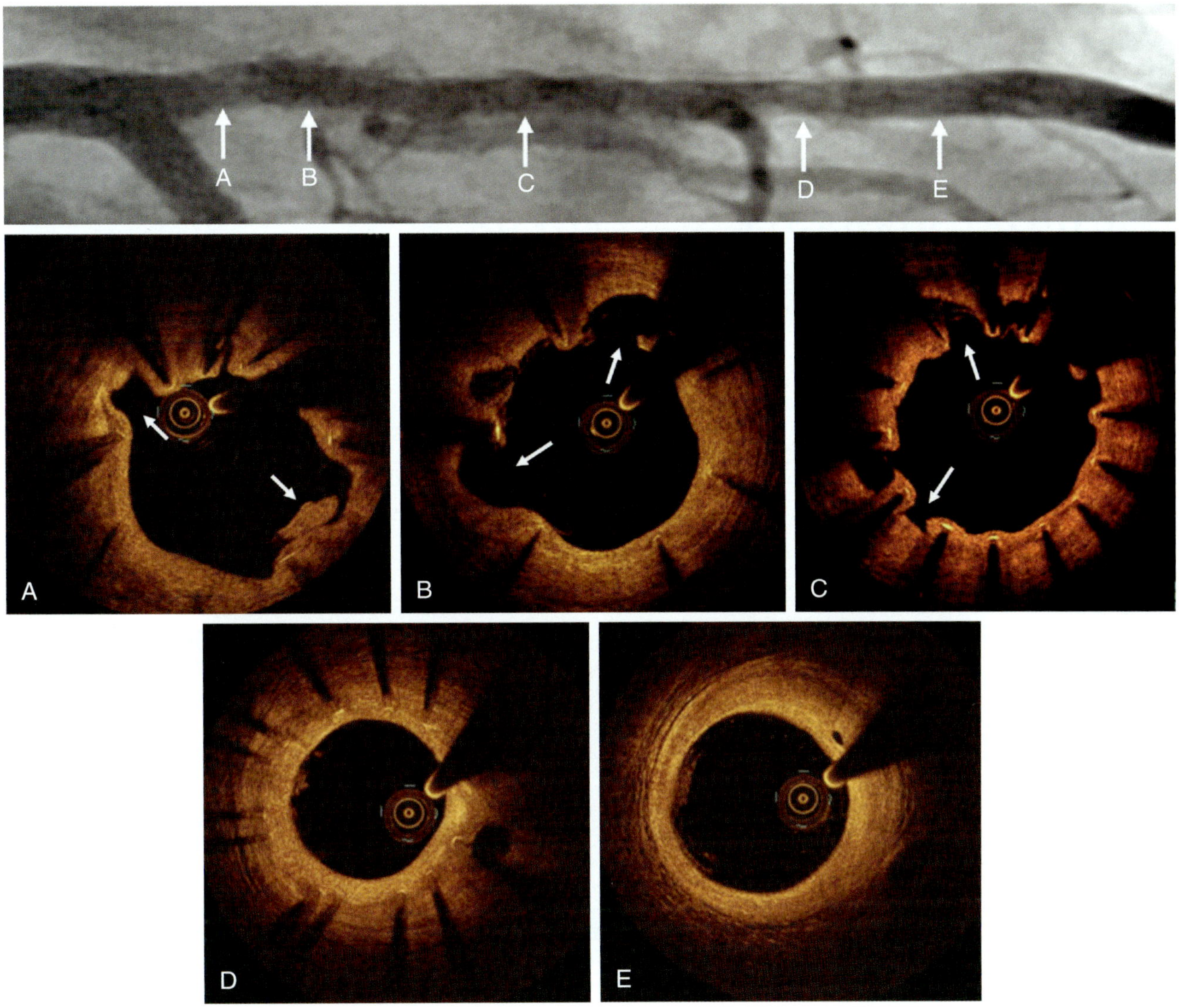

FIG. 1.123 Optical Coherence Tomography Imaging of the Stent. The images correlate to the locations identified on the coronary angiogram. (A) Thrombus is seen at the edge of an interstrut cavity. (B) Multiple interstrut cavities (*arrows*) corresponding to areas of contrast staining in the proximal segment of the stent. (C) Multiple interstrut cavities (*arrows*) corresponding to areas of contrast staining in the mid segment of the stent. (D) Distal stent showing good stent apposition with mild neointimal hyperplasia. (E) Distal reference vessel has mild atherosclerosis.

alternatively, thrombus dissolution on the abluminal edges of the stent after implantation in a patient with an acute coronary syndrome.[3] Finally, the case demonstrates the utility of optical coherence tomography for intravascular imaging owing to its high resolution.

References

1. Mauri L, Hsieh WH, Massaro JM, Ho KK, D'Agostino R, Cutlip DE. Stent thrombosis in randomized clinical trials of drug-eluting stents. *N Engl J Med.* 2007;356:1020-1029.
2. Finn AV, Joner M, Nakazawa G, et al. Pathological correlates of late drug-eluting stent thrombosis: strut coverage as a marker of endothelialization. *Circulation.* 2007;115:2435-2441.
3. Joner M, Finn AV, Farb A, et al. Pathology of drug-eluting stents in humans: delayed healing and late thrombotic risk. *J Am Coll Cardiol.* 2006;48:193-202.

New-Onset Coronary Aneurysm and Late-Acquired Incomplete Scaffold Apposition After Full Polymer Jacket of a Chronic Total Occlusion With Bioresorbable Scaffolds

Giuseppe Gargiulo, MD, Andrea Mangiameli, MD, Francesco Granata, MD, Yohei Ohno, MD, Alberto Chisari, MD, Davide Capodanno, MD, PhD, Corrado Tamburino, MD, PhD, Alessio La Manna, MD

A 60-year-old man with a chronic total occlusion of the left anterior descending coronary artery (LAD) (Fig. 1.124A) and evidence of myocardium viability was successfully treated with percutaneous coronary intervention. Four overlapping bioresorbable vascular scaffolds (BVS; Abbott Vascular, Santa Clara, California) were implanted: 2.5 × 28 mm, 3.0 × 28 mm, 3.5 × 28 mm, and 3.5 × 28 mm from distal to proximal, respectively ("full polymer jacket") (Fig. 1.124B).[1] Optical coherence tomography (OCT; Ilumien, St. Jude Medical, St. Paul, Minnesota) showed good expansion of the scaffolds and good apposition of the struts (Fig. 1.124a–g). At 8 months, elective angiographic follow-up documented a focal coronary artery aneurysm (CAA) at the mid segment of the LAD (Fig. 1.124C).[2] Optical coherence tomography revealed a CAA maximal lumen area of 16.4 mm^2 with a longitudinal length of 8.4 mm in the absence of thrombus. At the CAA site, most of the BVS struts were embedded in the aneurysmal wall and covered by neointima, whereas late-acquired incomplete scaffold apposition (ISA) was noted in some cross sections (Fig. 1.124a′–g′). To our knowledge, this is the first

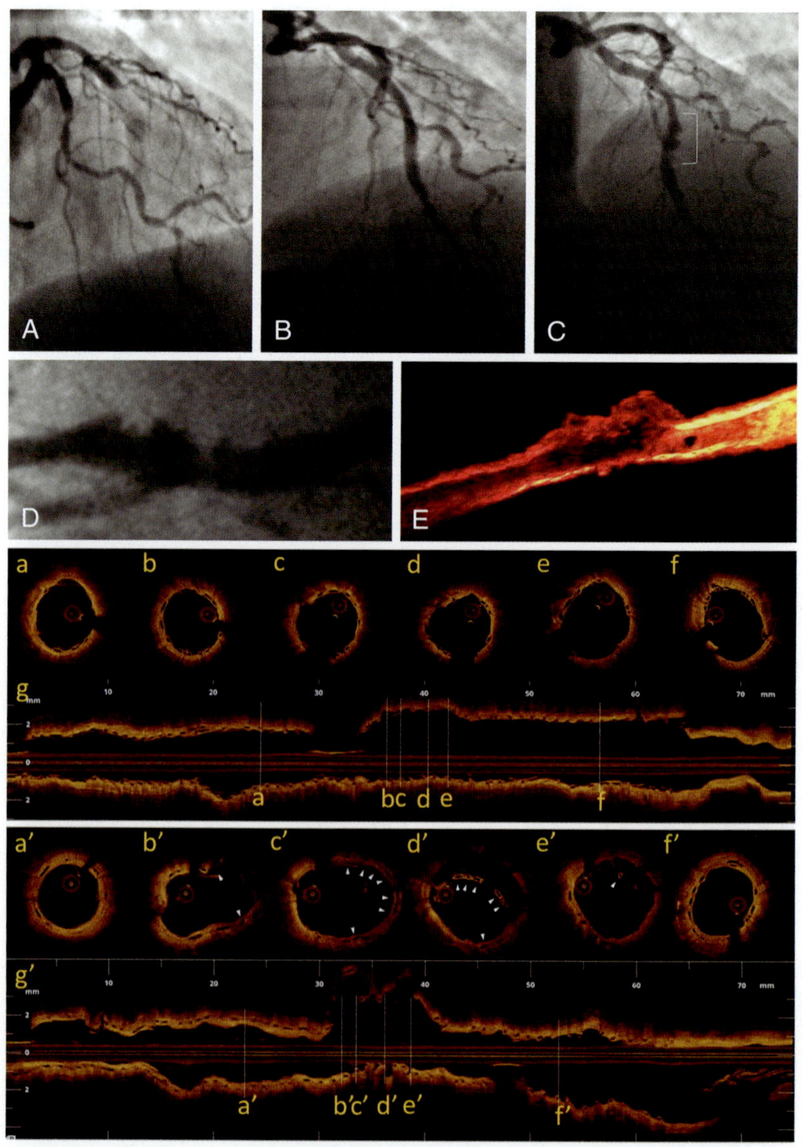

FIG. 1.124 Coronary Angiography and Optical Coherence Tomography (OCT) Findings. (A) Angiogram showing long-term total occlusion of the proximal left anterior descending coronary artery (LAD). (B) LAD angiogram after full polymer jacket with bioresorbable vascular scaffolds. (C) LAD angiogram after 8 months shows a coronary artery aneurysm (CAA) at the mid segment (*white bracket*). (D) Magnification of the CAA at angiography. (E) Magnification of the CAA with optical coherence tomography (OCD) three-dimensional reconstruction. (a–g) OCT cross sections and longitudinal view after the index procedure show good expansion and apposition of the scaffold struts. (a′–f′) Corresponding cross sections at 8-month angiographic follow-up showing normal vessel with good scaffold apposition ([a′] and [f′]) CAA with scaffold struts (*white arrowheads*) embedded in the aneurysmal vessel wall ([b′]) and [c′]) and late ISA with BVS struts (*white arrowheads*) floating in the lumen vessel ([d′]) and [e′]). The luminal surface of CAA is homogenous with no evidence of thrombus. (g′), Longitudinal view of the CAA.

described case of new-onset CAA and late-acquired ISA after BVS implantation. Potential mechanisms of late-acquired ISA after long-term total occlusion percutaneous coronary intervention include guidewire injury to the adventitial layer, creation of a false lumen, or subintimal stenting.[3] With BVS, the management is uncertain, not automatically resembling that of CAA developed after metallic stenting.[2] The potential consequences of balloon angioplasty or stent implantation inside a BVS that has lost its integrity as a result of the bioresorption process are unknown. A watchful waiting strategy with long-term dual-antiplatelet therapy and early follow-up was adopted.

References

1. La Manna A, Ohno Y, Attizzani GF, Tamburino C. Successful retrograde recanalization of chronic total coronary occlusion with multiple bioresorbable vascular scaffolds ('full polymer jacket'): initial experience and rationale. *Eur Heart J.* 2013;34:2925.
2. Aoki J, Kirtane A, Leon MB, Dangas G. Coronary artery aneurysms after drug-eluting stent implantation. *J Am Coll Cardiol Intv.* 2008;1:14-21.
3. Attizzani GF, Capodanno D, Ohno Y, Tamburino C. Mechanisms, pathophysiology, and clinical aspects of incomplete stent apposition. *J Am Coll Cardiol.* 2014;63:1355-1367.

Optical Coherence Tomography Findings in Very Late (4 Years) Paclitaxel-Eluting Stent Thrombosis

Arend F.L. Schinkel, MD, PhD, Peter Barlis, MD, Heleen M. M. van Beusekom, MD, PhD, Patrick W. Serruys, MD, PhD, FACC, Evelyn Regar, MD, PhD

The mechanisms of late coronary stent thrombosis, a complication with high morbidity and mortality,[1] are poorly understood. Late thrombosis in drug-eluting coronary stents has been associated with delayed endothelization of the stent struts or a systemic and intrastent hypersensitivity reaction.[2] We present in vivo findings in a patient with very late stent thrombosis. In 2003, a 60-year-old man with a history of stable angina and smoking had a significant stenosis of the left anterior descending artery and underwent elective placement of two overlapping paclitaxel-eluting stents (3.0 × 16 mm and 2.75 × 28 mm; Taxus stent, Boston Scientific, Natick, Massachusetts) after dilation with a noncompliant balloon. The discharge medication consisted of aspirin, clopidogrel (12 months), β-blockers, and statins. Four years after stenting the patient had an acute anterior myocardial infarction caused by late stent thrombosis while using long-term aspirin therapy (Fig. 1.125). After thrombus aspiration, intravascular ultrasonography and intravascular optical coherence tomography were performed showing incomplete coverage of 21% of the stent struts, which may reflect delayed vascular healing (Figs. 1.126 and 1.127). Pathology of the thrombotic material showed a recent multilayered thrombus (Fig. 1.128). After the procedure, the patient was treated with ReoPro (Centocor, Leiden, Netherlands) and was discharged with sustained aspirin and clopidogrel therapy.

Acknowledgments

The authors thank Anne-Marie Maugenest and Sandy van Wunnik for their assistance.

References

1. McFadden EP, Stabile E, Regar E, et al. Late thrombosis in drug-eluting coronary stents after discontinuation of antiplatelet therapy. *Lancet.* 2004;364:1519-1521.
2. Nebeker JR, Virmani R, Bennett CL, et al. Hypersensitivity cases associated with drug-eluting coronary stents: a review of available cases from the Research on Adverse Drug Events and Reports (RADAR) project. *J Am Coll Cardiol.* 2006;47:175-181.

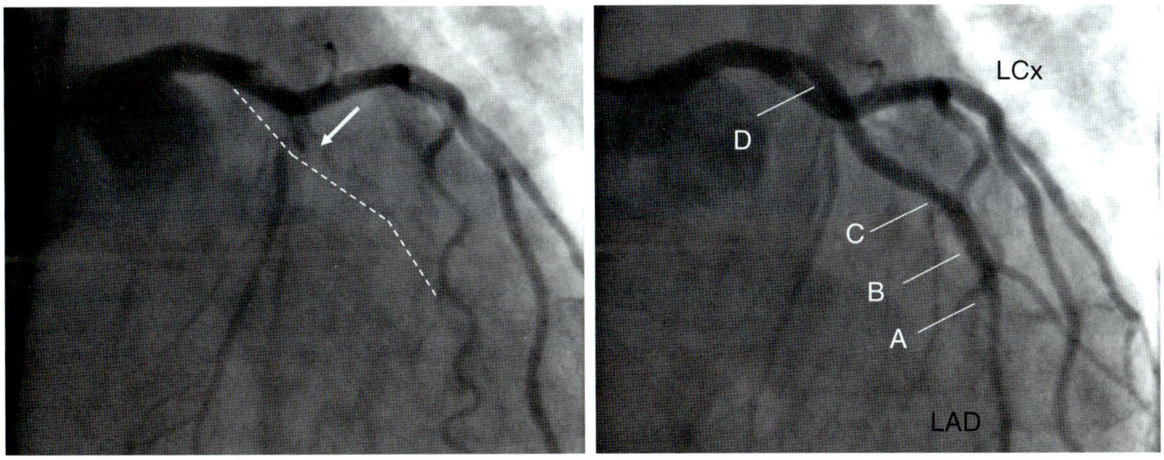

FIG. 1.125 Coronary Angiogram. The left panel shows thrombotic occlusion of the left anterior descending coronary artery; the dotted line indicates the stented segment. The right panel shows the result after thrombus aspiration (Export catheter; Medtronic, Minneapolis, Minnesota) with Thrombolysis In Myocardial Infarction grade flow 3 antegrade flow and moderate residual stenosis in the mid portion of the stented segment. Labels *A* to *D* indicate the locations of intracoronary imaging. *LAD,* left anterior descending coronary artery; *LCx,* left circumflex artery.

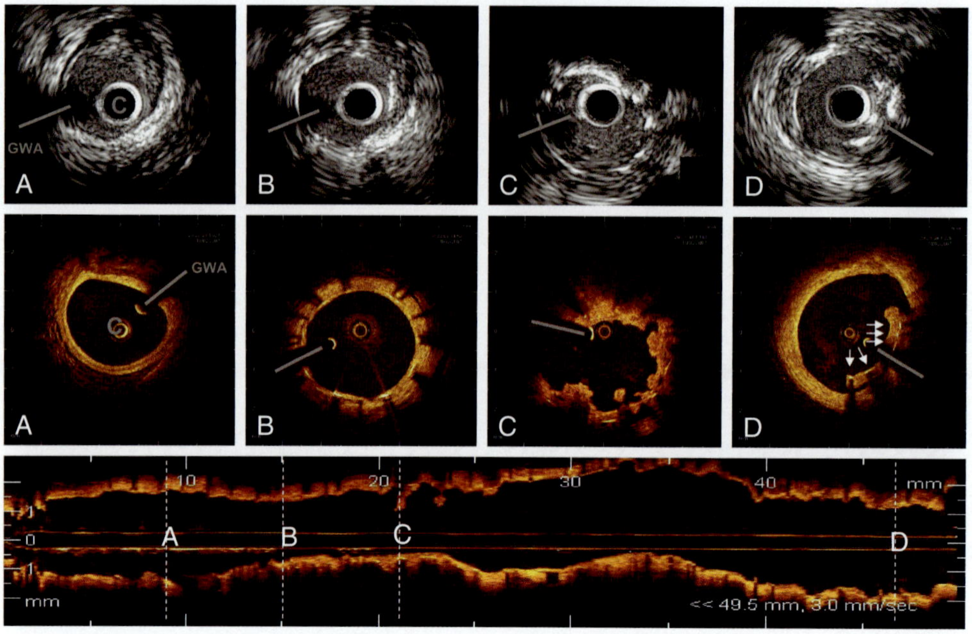

FIG. 1.126 Intracoronary Imaging After Thrombus Aspiration. The upper panel show intravascular ultrasound images (Atlantis; Boston Scientific). The lower panels show optical coherence tomography images (LightLab Imaging, Boston, Massachusetts) with cross-sectional and longitudinal views. (A) The distal reference shows eccentric plaque in 11- to 4-o'clock position. (B) The distal stent portion shows a well-expanded and apposed stent with thin tissue coverage by optical coherence tomography that is missed by intravascular ultrasound. (C) Irregular lumen borders with intraluminal remnants of the thrombus. (D) Proximal stent edge with incomplete apposition of five stent struts (*arrows*) against the vessel wall. The distance to the vessel wall is 200 f'.m. Optical coherence tomography shows tissue around the stent struts (differential diagnosis thrombus, neointima). Incomplete stent apposition may be caused by initial malaposition or acquired malaposition caused by a vascular response to the stent. *C*, catheter artifact; *GWA*, guidewire artefact.

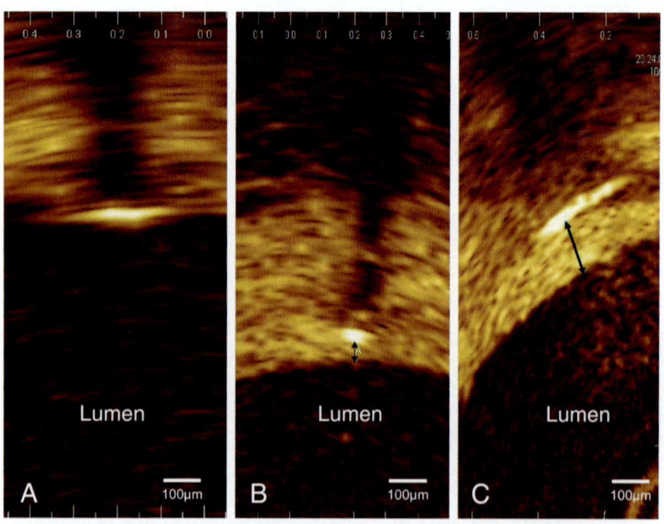

FIG. 1.127 Spectrum of Tissue Coverage as Seen by Optical Coherence Tomography (OCT) in This Stented Segment. Tissue coverage in the OCT image was not visible in 21% (n = 110) of the struts, whereas 79% (n = 411 of 521) of the struts showed tissue coverage of various thickness. (A) No visible coverage. (B) Very thin coverage (40 f'.m). (C) Maximal coverage (140 f'.m).

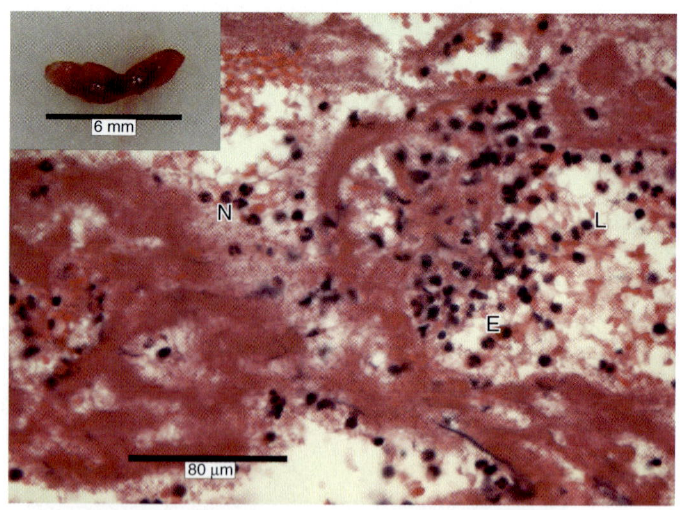

FIG. 1.128 Histology of the Aspirated Thrombus. Recent multilayered thrombus showing Zahn lines and containing abundant leukocytes consisting of eosinophils (*E*), neutrophils (*N*), and lymphocytes (*L*).

Optical Coherence Tomography Images of a Coronary Artery Aneurysm in an Infarct-Related Artery 6 Months After Bare-Metal Stent Implantation

Daiji Yoshikawa, MD, Hideki Ishii, MD, PhD, Yutaka Aoyama, MD, Hitoshi Ichimiya, MD, Yuuki Shimizu, MD, Satoshi Isobe, MD, PhD, Satoshi Shintani, MD, PhD, Yasuko Kureishi-Bando, MD, PhD, Toyoaki Murohara, MD, PhD

A 62-year-old man with hypertension and dyslipidemia underwent successful primary percutaneous coronary intervention with thrombus aspiration and bare-metal stent (3.5 × 13 mm) (Liberté, Boston Scientific, Natick, Massachusetts) implantation (12 atm) at the proximal left anterior descending coronary artery as the result of an ST-segment elevation myocardial infarction (Fig. 1.129). Optical coherence tomography (OCT) (Image Wire, LightLab Imaging, Nagoya, Japan) revealed that some stent struts were well apposed, with others embedded in intramural thrombus (Online Video 1.87, corresponds with Fig. 1.130 showing emergent procedure).

At 6-month follow-up angiography showed a coronary artery aneurysm (CAA) at the stented site without significant restenosis. The OCT imaging demonstrated that maximal luminal diameter of the CAA was 4.0 × 1.4 mm and longitudinal dimension was 4.8 mm with luminal surface described as a homogeneous, signal-rich structure absent of intramural thrombus (Fig. 1.129C–D). The intima-like structure of the CAA was continuous with vessel intima, suggesting this late-occurring CAA had a three-layer wall. This CAA was classified as small, fusiform, true, and type IV.[1] Almost all stent struts were well apposed and covered by neointimal thickening, with some stent struts malapposed with tissue coverage (Online Video 1.88, corresponds with Fig. 1.130, after 6-months images). Written informed consent was obtained before the procedure. We speculate the mechanisms for appearance of the CAA are an early fibroatheroma

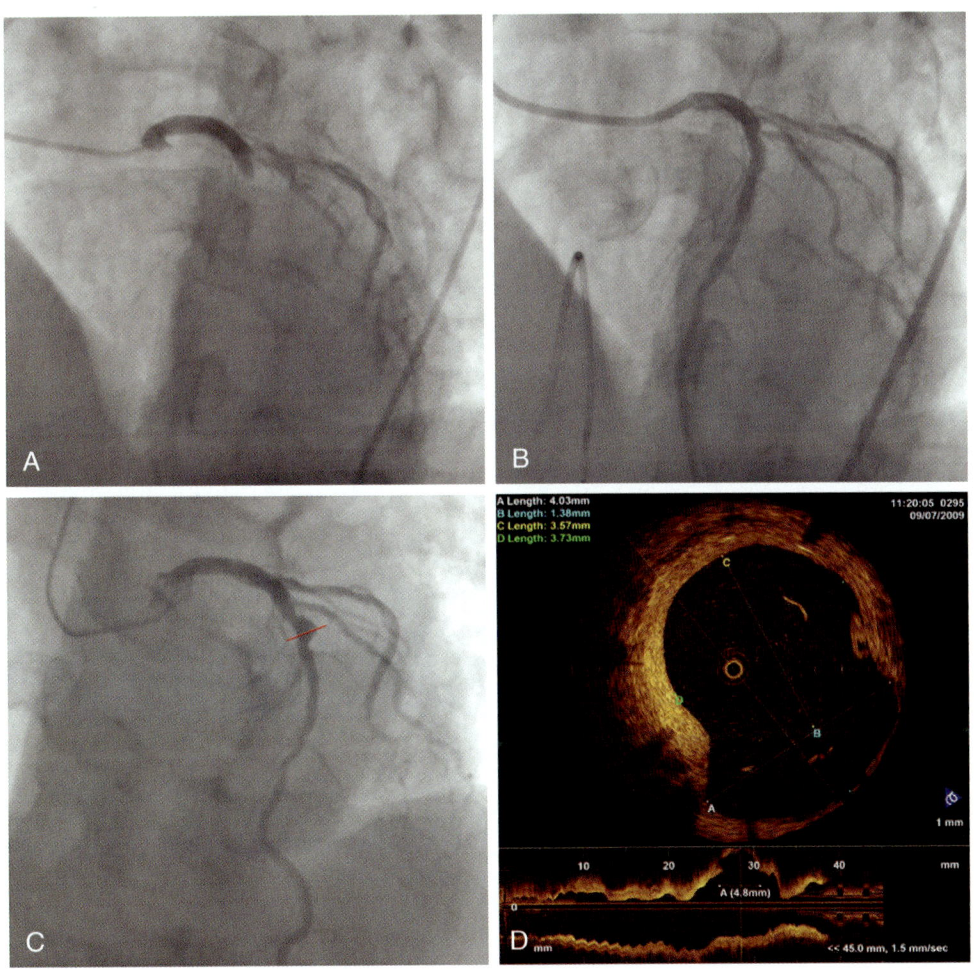

FIG. 1.129 Emergent and 6-Month Follow-Up Angiography and Optical Coherence Tomography Image of Coronary Artery Aneurysm at Maximal Luminal Diameter Site. (A) Emergent angiography reveals that the proximal left anterior descending coronary artery is totally occluded with thrombus. (B) Appearance after intervention. (C) Six-month follow-up angiography shows no restenosis with coronary artery aneurysm detected at the previously stented site. (D) Optical coherence tomography imaging of coronary artery aneurysm (*red line* in [C]) showed that the maximal luminal diameter is 4.0 × 1.4 mm and the longitudinal dimension is 4.8 mm.

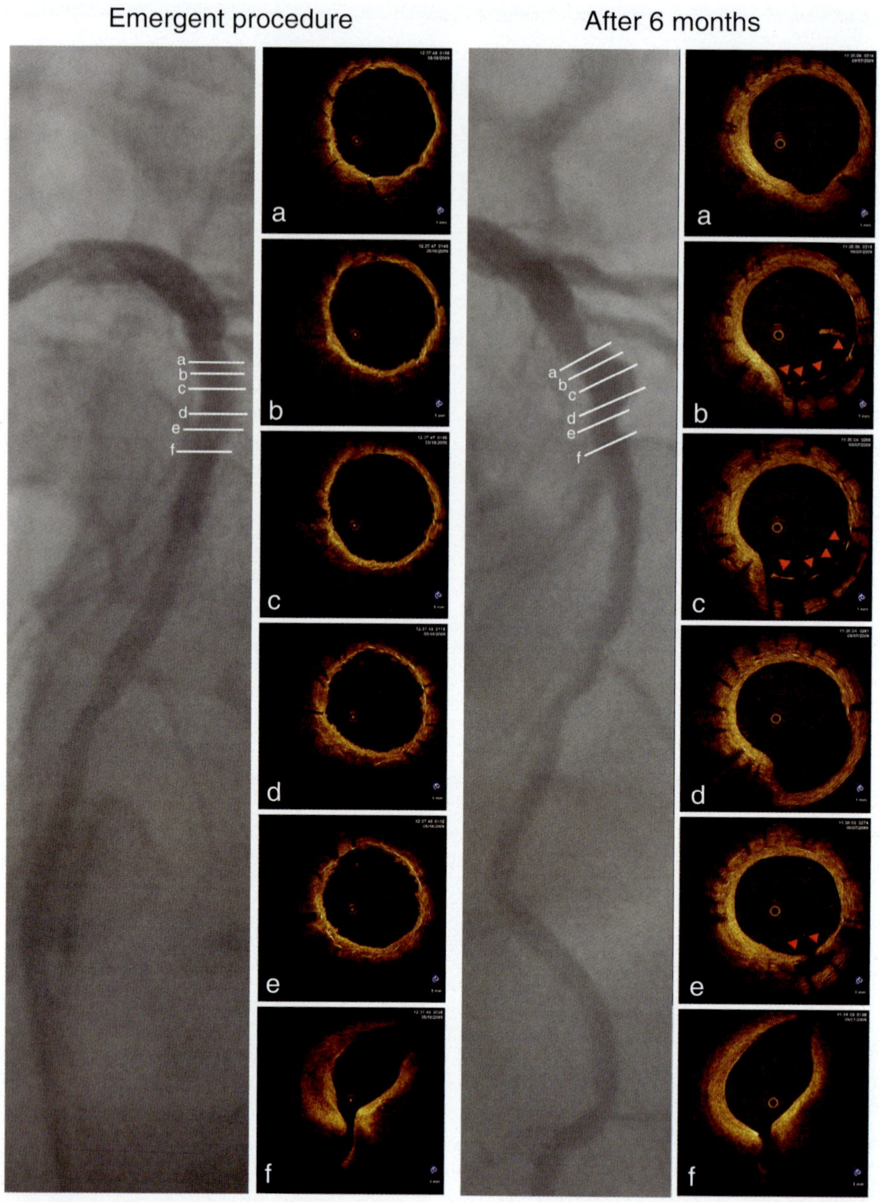

FIG. 1.130 Optical Coherence Tomography Images of the Lesion. (*Left*) Emergent procedure images (corresponding with Online Video 1.87) obtained by optical coherence tomography imaging immediately after emergent stent implantation show that some stent struts are well apposed, whereas others are embedded in intramural thrombus. (*Right*) Images obtained after 6 months (corresponding with Online Video 1.88), Each (a′) to (f′) image represents the same regions of (a) to (f) in the emergent procedure images. The luminal surface of the coronary artery aneurysm (CAA) is described as a homogeneous, signal-rich structure with no intramural thrombus in the CAA. Almost all stent struts are well apposed and covered by neointimal tissue proliferation. Some stent struts at the CAA site are malapposed with tissue coverage (*arrowheads* in [b′], [c′], and [e′]).

transformed into a vulnerable plaque with a large lipid core at the segment where excessive expansive vessel remodeling occurred.[2] Plaque rupture followed by thrombus formation caused the ST-segment elevation myocardial infarction. Thrombus accumulation might have obscured the intraplaque cavity with a ruptured fibrous cap. Antiplatelet therapy and blood flow might have dissolved the thrombus, increasing flow against the diseased cavity (vascular) wall and reducing the tolerance of the diseased cavity (vascular) wall to intraluminal pressures, causing CAA formation.[3] These mechanisms might be associated with stent malapposition or thrombosis in some cases. Long-term follow-up studies with large populations would be required to confirm the clinical significance of these findings obtained from OCT examinations.

References

1. Antonios PA, Yiannis SC, George DG. Pathogenetic mechanisms of coronary ectasia. *Int J Cardiol.* 2008;130:335-343.
2. Yiannis SC, Michael J, Ahmet UC, et al. Prediction of the localization of high-risk coronary atherosclerotic plaques on the basis of low endothelial shear stress: an intravascular ultrasound and histopathology nature history study. *Circulation.* 2008;117:993-1002.
3. Markis JE, Joffe CD, Cohn PF, Feen DJ, Herman MV, Gorlin R. Clinical significance of coronary artery ectasia. *Am J Cardiol.* 1976;37:217-222.

Recurrent Neoatherosclerosis After Bioresorbable Vascular Scaffold Treatment of In-Stent Restenosis

Teresa Bastante, MD, Fernando Rivero, MD, Amparo Benedicto, MD, Javier Cuesta, MD, Fernando Alfonso, MD, PhD

A 66-year-old man had a non–ST-segment elevation myocardial infarction 3 years after the implantation of an everolimus-eluting stent (3.5 × 12 mm) in the proximal segment of a saphenous vein graft to a marginal branch. Coronary angiography showed focal in-stent restenosis (ISR), and optical coherence tomography (OCT) confirmed severe ISR (minimal lumen area 3.1 mm^2). Notably, the tissue causing the ISR had a striking heterogeneous pattern with a very bright neointima covering large lipid pools (*plus signs,* in Fig. 1.131A and A′) that obscured the underlying stent struts, highly suggestive of neoatherosclerosis. A bioresorbable vascular scaffold (BVS) (Absorb, 3.5 × 12 mm, Abbott Vascular, Santa Clara, California) was implanted and postdilated at very high pressure (22 bar) with excellent angiographic and OCT results (minimal lumen area 8.5 mm^2) (Fig. 1.131B–B′). The classic "black box" BVS appearance (without shadowing) was readily identified fully apposed against residual tissue overlying the bright artefacts (with dorsal shadow) of the underlying metallic struts (Fig. 1.131B–B′). Seven months later, the patient had another non–ST-segment elevation myocardial infarction showing recurrent ISR on angiography. OCT showed that the obstructive tissue (minimal lumen area 3.3 mm^2) was consistent with recurrent neoatherosclerosis (Fig. 1.131C–C′). A drug-eluting stent was implanted at high pressure with excellent final result.

Treatment of patients with neoatherosclerosis remains a challenge.[1,2] Recently BVSs have been proposed as an attractive therapeutic strategy for patients with ISR to avoid the implantation of another permanent metal layer.[3] To our knowledge, this is the first report of recurrent ISR after treatment of ISR with a BVS. Our findings also suggest that recurrent neoatherosclerosis may develop after BVS implantation in this challenging scenario.

References

1. Alfonso F, Byrne RA, Rivero F, Kastrati A. Current treatment of in-stent restenosis. *J Am Coll Cardiol.* 2014;63:2659-2673.
2. Nakazawa G, Otsuka F, Nakano M, et al. The pathology of neoatherosclerosis in human coronary implants bare-metal and drug- eluting stents. *J Am Coll Cardiol.* 2011;57:1314-1322.
3. Alfonso F, Nuccio J, Cuevas C, Cárdenas A, Gonzalo N, Jimenez-Quevedo P. Treatment of coronary in-stent restenosis with bioabsorbable vascular scaffolds. *J Am Coll Cardiol.* 2014;63:2875.

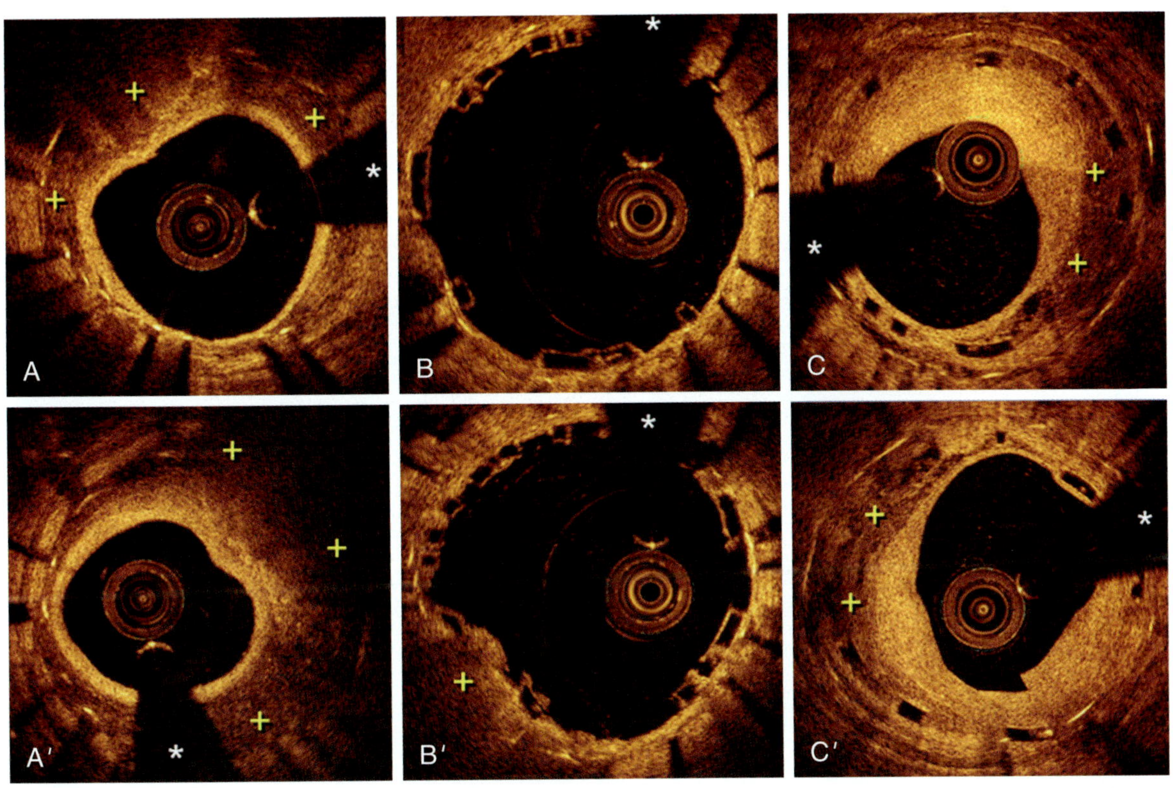

FIG. 1.131 Optical Coherence Tomography (OCT) Findings in Serial Studies. (A and A') In-stent restenosis caused by neoatherosclerosis before intervention. A glistening yellow neointima is visualized covering a heterogeneous tissue consisting mainly of large lipid areas (*plus signs*) that partially obscure the underlying metallic struts (*bright dots* with dorsal shadow). (B and B′) Results obtained immediately after bioresorbable vascular scaffold (BVS) implantation. The BVS struts appear as black boxes without shadowing. There is minor protrusion of some lipid tissue (*plus signs*). (C and C′) Recurrent neoatherosclerosis at follow-up. New lipid pools (*plus signs*) are detected within the BVS struts. The asterisk denotes the wire artifact.

Chapter 2
Complications of Coronary Intervention

Stent Thrombosis

Acute Stent Thrombosis: Technical Complication or Inadequate Antithrombotic Therapy? An Optical Coherence Tomography Study

Sammy Elmariah, MD, MPH, Ik-Kyung Jang, MD, PhD

A 68-year-old woman was admitted to the hospital with non–ST-segment elevation myocardial infarction. Coronary angiography showed a 95% mid stenosis in the left anterior descending artery (Fig. 2.1A). The lesion was treated with a 2.50 × 18 mm Xience drug-eluting stent (Abbott Vascular, Santa Clara, California) during bivalirudin infusion (Fig. 2.1B). At the end of the procedure, the patient received a 600-mg loading dose of clopidogrel and bivalirudin was discontinued. Seventy minutes later, the patient experienced chest pain with anterior ST-segment elevations. Repeat angiography demonstrated acute stent thrombosis (AST) (Fig. 2.2A). While the patient was on heparin and eptifibatide, low-pressure angioplasty was performed. Optical coherence tomography imaging showed an intravascular mass consistent with platelet-rich thrombus within the stent (Fig. 2.2B).

Technical factors or inadequate antithrombotic therapies are responsible for AST.[1,2] In this case, mechanical complications, such as dissection, underexpansion, or significant malapposition were ruled out. Review of the timing of antithrombotic therapy revealed possible gaps in therapy. Bivalirudin was discontinued simultaneous to the administration of clopidogrel. Clinical effects of bivalirudin continue for 1 hour after its discontinuation, whereas the anticipated onset of clopidogrel (600 mg) effect is 2 hours after its administration.[3] Consequently, antithrombotic therapy in our patient was insufficient for approximately 1 hour, during which the AST occurred (Fig. 2.3).

Our case highlights the usefulness of optical coherence tomography in evaluating underlying mechanisms for AST and in characterizing thrombus composition (platelets). Additionally, it emphasizes the significant increase in ischemic events with bivalirudin in subjects not pretreated with clopidogrel.[2,4] Care is needed to ensure sufficient antithrombotic therapy in these patients with the use of rapidly acting antithrombotic agents, prolongation of bivalirudin infusion, or earlier administration of the clopidogrel loading dose.

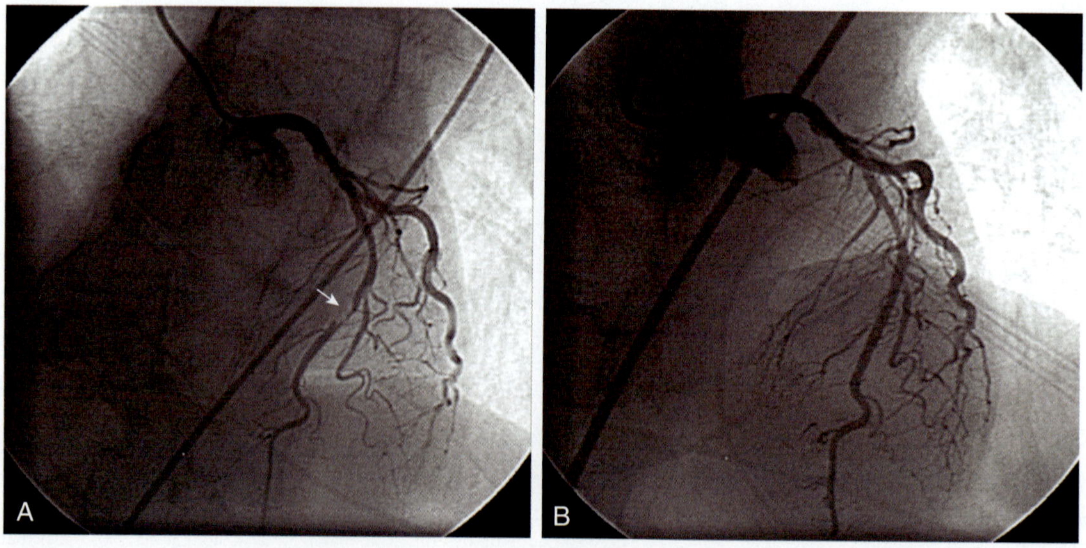

FIG. 2.1 Angiographic Frames of the Left Coronary System in the Right Anterior Oblique Cranial Projection. (A) A filling defect (*white arrow*) in the mid left anterior descending artery is present. (B) After stent deployment a good angiographic result was observed.

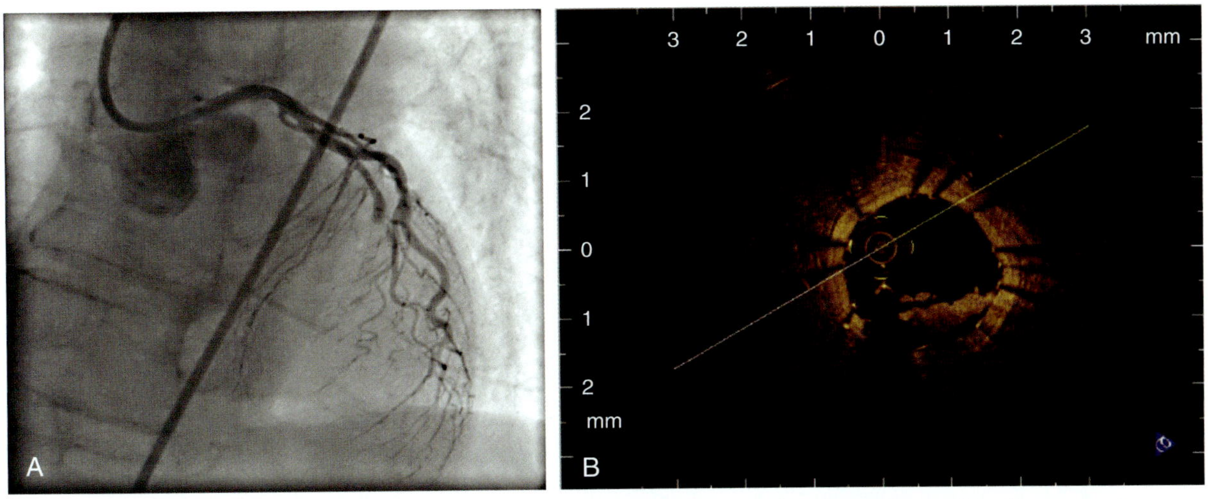

FIG. 2.2 Evaluation of Acute Stent Thrombosis. (A) Repeat coronary angiography 1 hour after the initial procedure demonstrated acute stent thrombosis. (B) After restoration of blood flow, optical coherence tomography imaging demonstrated adequate stent expansion and the absence of coronary artery dissection. Platelet-rich thrombus was noted within the stented lumen.

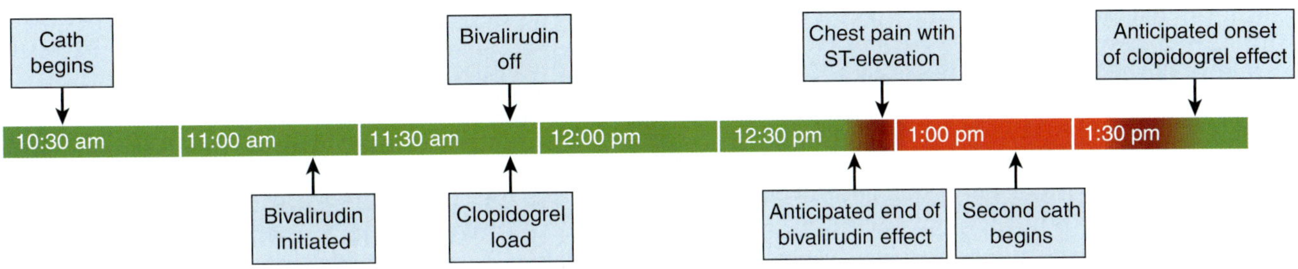

FIG. 2.3 Timeline of Antithrombatic Therapy and Stent Thrombosis. The clinical effects of bivalirudin end approximately 1 hour after its discontinuation, whereas the anticipated clinical effect of a 600-mg clopidogrel loading dose is 2 hours after its administration. Consequently, simultaneous discontinuation of bivalirudin infusion and administration of the clopidogrel load results in a 1-hour window of suboptimal antithrombotic therapy 1 hour later (*red bar*). *Cath,* catheterization.

References

1. Aoki J, Lansky AJ, Mehran R, et al. Early stent thrombosis in patients with acute coronary syndromes treated with drug-eluting and bare metal stents: the Acute Catheterization and Urgent Intervention Triage Strategy trial. *Circulation.* 2009;119:687-698.
2. Dangas GD, Caixeta A, Mehran R, et al. Frequency and predictors of stent thrombosis after percutaneous coronary intervention in acute myocardial infarction. *Circulation.* 2011;123:1745-1756.
3. Drug Information Online. Drugs.com website. Available at: http://www.drugs.com/. Accessed March 4, 2011.
4. Lincoff AM, Steinhubl SR, Manoukian SV, et al. Influence of timing of clopidogrel treatment on the efficacy and safety of bivalirudin in patients with non-ST-segment elevation acute coronary syndromes undergoing percutaneous coronary intervention: an analysis of the ACUITY (Acute Catheterization and Urgent Intervention Triage strategY) trial. *J Am Coll Cardiol Intv.* 2008;1:639-648.

An Unusual Case of Stent-in-Stent Thrombosis

Jiang Ming Fam, MBBS, W. den Dekker, MD, Paul de Graaf, BSC, Evelyn Regar, MD, PhD

A 71-year-old man was admitted for acute coronary syndrome. Six weeks earlier he had a Promus Premier 3.0 × 12 mm (Boston Scientific, Natick, Massachusetts) drug-eluting stent (DES) implanted in the obtuse marginal artery for unstable angina. On repeat coronary angiography, haziness (Fig. 2.4A, Online Video 2.1) in the ostial stented region was observed; however Thrombolysis In Myocardial Infarction grade flow was good. Optical coherence tomography (OCT) revealed a nonexpanded stent (star with struts marked with +) within and protruding out of the implanted stent. The stent appeared well expanded and apposed to the vessel wall (implanted stent with struts marked with asterisk [Fig. 2.4C–D, Online Video 2.2]). There was lumen compromise secondary to a large amount of thrombus formation seen around the unexpanded stent struts together with incomplete lesion coverage proximally. Attempts to rewire or retrieve the unexpanded stent were unsuccessful. On the basis of the OCT findings, the decision was made to crush the unexpanded stent and implant a Promus Premier 3.5 × 12-mm drug-eluting stent (Boston Scientific, Natick, Massachusetts) proximally with good results

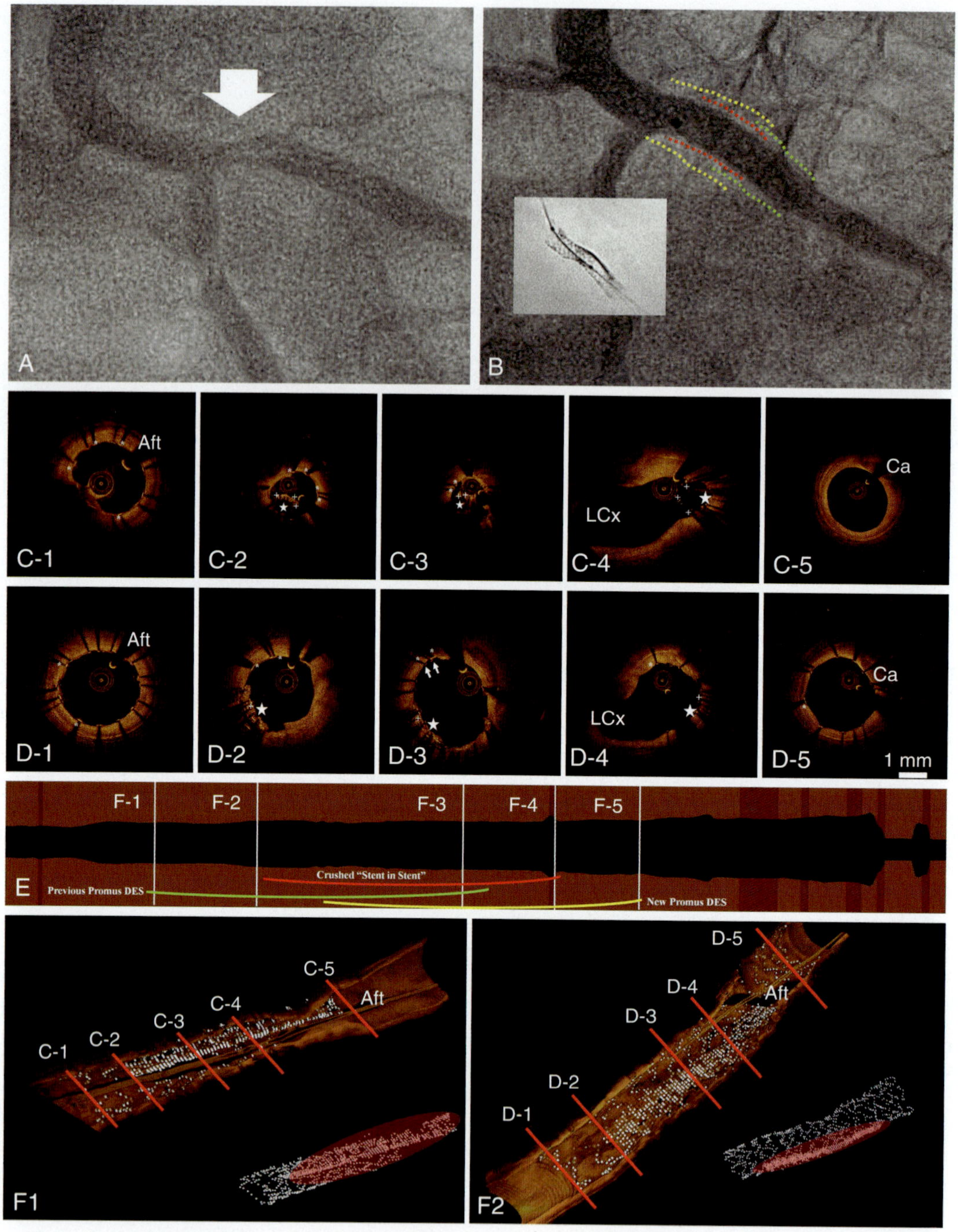

FIG. 2.4 Angiographic and Optical Coherence Tomography (OCT) Images of the Obtuse Marginal (OM) Artery With Stent-In-Stent Thrombosis. (A) Angiographic haziness (*white arrow*, Online Video 2.1) seen in the ostial segment of the OM artery that was stented (Promus Premier 3.0 × 12 mm, Boston Scientific) 6 weeks earlier. (B) Angiogram (Online Video 2.3) after implantation of a new stent (Promus Premier 3.5 × 12 mm). The inset shows a fluoroscopic image of the overlapping stents. (C) OCT of the OM/left circumflex (LCs) arteries before implantation of a Promus Premier 3.5 × 12 mm stent. The previously deployed Promus Premier 3.0 × 12-mm stent (C-1–C-3; struts are marked with *asterisks*, Online Video 2.2) appeared well expanded and apposed to the vessel wall. An unexpanded stent (C-2–C-4; star with struts marked with +) could be seen within the implanted stent. There was lumen compromise secondary to a large amount of thrombus formation seen around the unexpanded stent struts (C-3). The unexpanded stent protruded out of the deployed stent and could be seen at the bifurcation (C-4) of the OM and the LCx (C-5) arteries. (D) Corresponding OCT performed after implantation of a new Promus 3.5 × 12 mm drug-eluting stent. Multiple layers of struts (D-3, *white arrows*, Online Video 2.4) from the two overlapping unexpanded stents and the previously unexpanded stent (*star*) can be seen. (E) The lumen profile of the OM artery as seen by OCT after implantation of the Promus Premier 3.5 × 12 mm stent showing the relationship between the unexpanded and implanted stents. (F) The three-dimensional reconstruction (QAngio OCT software; Medis Specials, Leiden, Netherlands) of the vessel before (F1) and after (F2) the procedure shows the crushed stent in stent. *Aft,* artifact caused by guidewire; *Ca,* calcium; *DES,* drug-eluting stent(s); *LCx,* left circumflex artery.

(angiography shown in Fig. 2.4B, Online Video 2.3). Multiple layers of struts (OCT) (white arrows in Fig. 2.4D-3; Online Video 2.4) from the two overlapping implanted stents as well as the previously unexpanded stent can be seen in Fig. 2.4D–E. Fig. 2.4F shows the three-dimensional reconstruction (QAngio OCT software, Medis Specials, Leiden, Netherlands) of the vessel before and after procedure showing the crushed stent in stent.

We describe a rare cause of stent thrombosis, emphasizing that mechanical stent-related causes should always be ruled out, especially if stent thrombosis occurs soon after implantation. In our case, an unexpanded stent formed the nidus of thrombus formation. The unexpanded stent was likely due to loss or embolization during attempts at device delivery in a challenging procedure owing to significant calcification, severe tortuosity, and suboptimal guide catheter backup. Of note, this complication was previously undetected on angiography. This is a rare case of stent-in-stent thrombosis in which OCT demonstrates the potential to improve clinical diagnosis and procedural outcome.

ACKNOWLEDGMENT

The authors thank Dr. Shengxian Tu for providing the QAngio OCT software used for the three-dimensional rendering.

Delayed Healing of a Coronary Stent Graft

Masamichi Takano, MD, Masanori Yamamoto, MD, Toru Inami, MD, Daisuke Murakami, MD, Yoshihiko Seino, MD, Kyoichi Mizuno, MD

A polytetrafluoroethylene (PTFE)-covered stent composed of 2 metallic stents and sandwiched PTFE membrane is used especially for bailout of percutaneous intervention complicated with coronary perforation and treatment of aneurysms to prevent subsequent rupture. Detailed features within coronary stent grafts have not yet been reported in living patients. A 65-year-old man underwent implantation of a PTFE-covered stent (3.5/19 mm) to seal a giant aneurysm in the right coronary artery. Follow-up angiography at 32 months showed patency and a slightly irregular contour of the stent segment. Coronary angioscopy showed sufficient neointimal growth at the stent proximal edge. Several struts in the mid portion were regarded as exposed struts lacking neointimal coverage. Red thrombi were found in the distal portion despite continuous oral anticoagulation and dual-antiplatelet therapies (Fig. 2.5, Online Video 2.5). Optical coherence tomography confirmed the presence of uncovered struts as well as thrombus formation (Fig. 2.6). Pathologic validation using light and electron microscopy has demonstrated incomplete endothelialization and accumulation of fibrin clots within endovascular stent grafts implanted for aortic aneurysms.[1] The images for this case suggest that delayed healing and thrombogenicity of coronary stent graft persists for an extended period.

References

1. McArthur C, Teodorescu V, Eisen L, et al. Histopathologic analysis of endovascular stent grafts from patients with aortic aneurysms: does healing occur? *J Vasc Surg.* 2001;33:733-738.

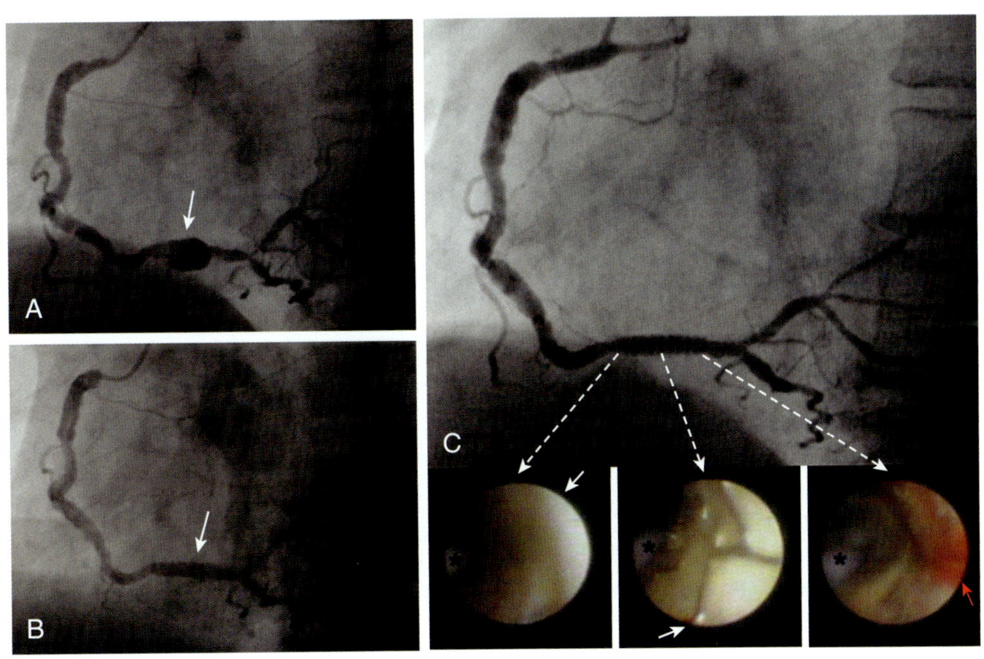

FIG. 2.5 Coronary Angiographic and Angioscopic Findings. (A) Angiography shows a giant aneurysm in the distal right coronary artery (*white arrow*). (B) The aneurysm disappears immediately after stent graft implantation (*white arrow*). (C) Angiograms 32 months later show minimum wall irregularity within the stent graft (upper panel). Angioscopic images (lower panels) exhibit bright struts of the mid portion without any surrounding tissues (*white arrow*) and red mural thrombi in the distal portion (*red arrow*). A white membranous tissue covers over struts at the proximal edge (*white arrowhead*). Asterisks indicate guidewires (Online Video 2.5).

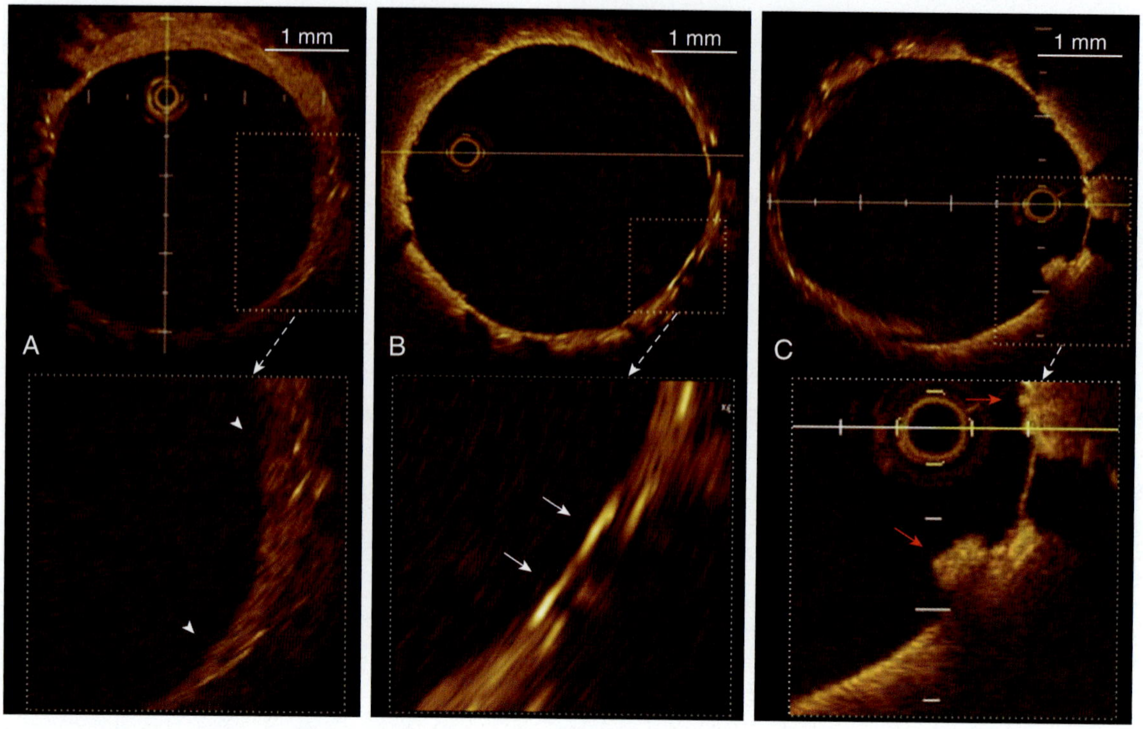

FIG. 2.6 Optical coherence tomography (OCT) Findings. OCT demonstrates relatively thick neointima at the proximal edge (*white arrowheads* in [A]), uncovered struts in the mid portion (*white arrows* in [B]), and protruding thrombi in the distal portion (*red arrows* in [C]).

Multivessel Honeycomb-Like Structure Finding in Optical Coherence Tomography

Mio Musashi, MD, Norio Tada, MD, Naoki Uemura, MD, Osamu Kawashima, MD, Tatsushi Ootomo, MD, Naoto Inoue, MD, Hideki Abe, MD, Taiichiro Meguro, MD, PhD

A 66-year-old man with a history of chronic atrial fibrillation was referred to our hospital for a preoperative cardiac evaluation for intestinal stenosis. An electrocardiogram showed negative T wave in leads II, III, aVF, and V_3 to V_5, and an echocardiogram showed moderate hypokinesis in the anteroseptal left ventricular wall. Coronary angiography revealed multiple linear filling defects with haziness in the right coronary artery and left anterior descending artery (Fig. 2.7A–B). After surgery for intestinal stenosis, we performed a staged percutaneous coronary intervention for right coronary artery and left anterior descending artery stenosis. In both lesions, optical coherence tomography revealed multiple channels of various sizes communicating with each other with smooth septa, so-called honeycomb-like structures (Fig. 2.7C–J, Online Videos 2.6 and 2.7). The septa were composed of high signal intensity and low-signal attenuation, suggesting that the structure consisted of fibrous material. We implanted Xience Prime stents (Abbott Vascular, Santa Clara, California) for both lesions, resulting in successful revascularization. Although anticoagulation therapy with warfarin in addition to dual-antiplatelet therapy was started after percutaneous coronary intervention, renal infarction occurred 3 months after percutaneous coronary intervention. Emergent angiography revealed a filling defect with thrombus in the left renal artery, and it was successfully removed with percutaneous thrombectomy. Under intensive anticoagulation therapy after the renal infarction, transesophageal echocardiography revealed no evidence of thrombus; however, spontaneous echocardiographic contrast was observed in the left atrium including an appendage.

A honeycomb-like structure finding during optical computed tomography has been reported previously.[1-3] Authors of the studies reported a honeycomb-like structure that represented recanalization of an organized thrombus. However, its etiology is still controversial. To our knowledge, there has been no report of a honeycomb-like structure at multiple vessels. The patient had received no anticoagulation therapy on the first visit. From the history of atrial fibrillation and renal thromboembolic infarction, we speculated that, in our case, the honeycomb-like structure represented recanalization of cardiogenic embolism.

References

1. Kang SJ, Nakano M, Virmani R, et al. OCT findings in patients with recanalization of organized thrombi in coronary arteries. *J Am Coll Cardiol Img.* 2012;5:725-732.
2. Toutouzas K, Karanasos A, Stathogiannis K, et al. A honeycomb-like structure in the left anterior descending coronary artery. *J Am Coll Cardiol Intv.* 2012;5:688-689.
3. Cho JM, Raffel OC, Stone JR, Kim CJ, Jang IK. Spontaneous recanalization of a coronary artery after thrombotic occlusion: in vivo demonstration with optical coherence tomography. *J Am Coll Cardiol.* 2010;55:1274.

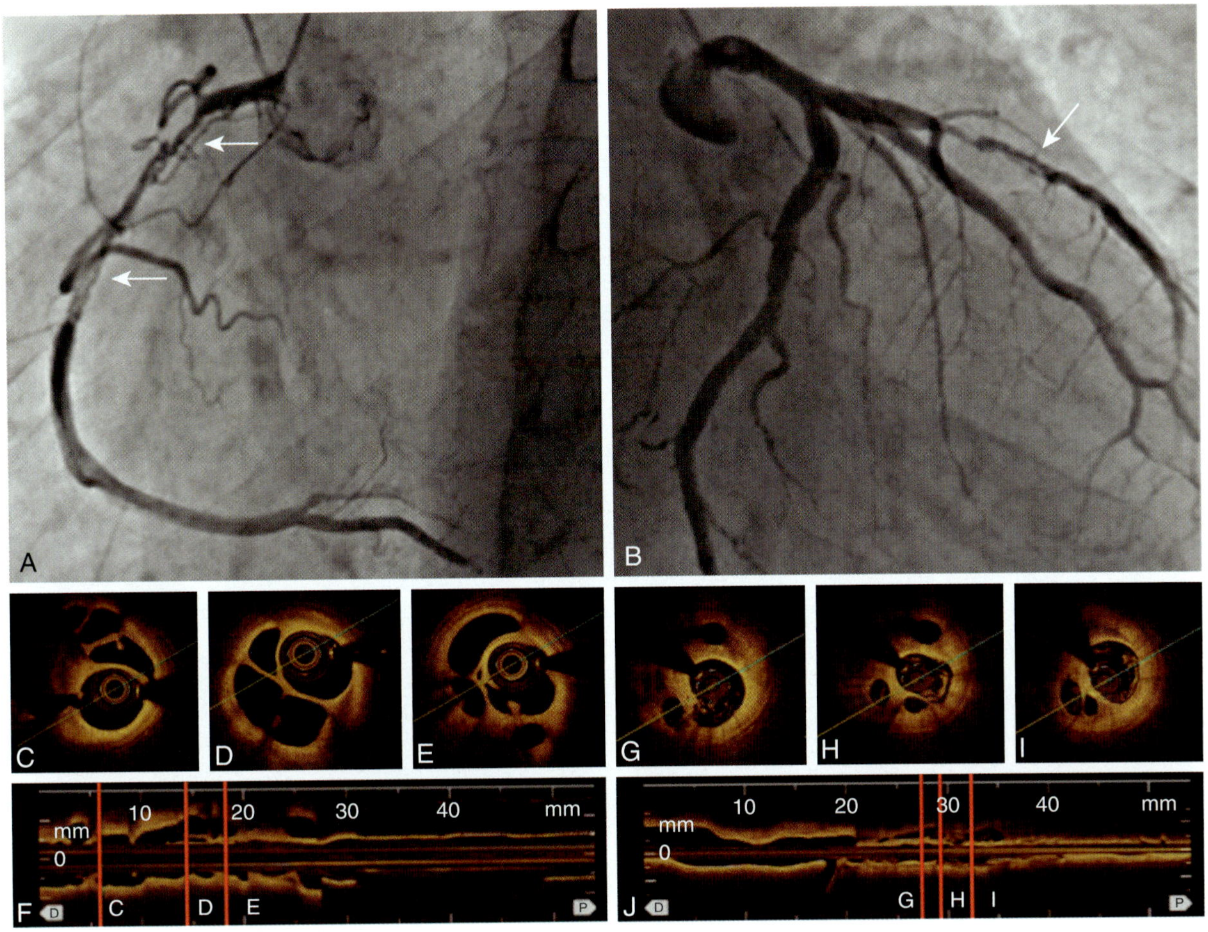

FIG. 2.7 Angiographic and Optical Coherence Tomography Findings of Right and Left Coronary Arteries. Angiography revealed multiple linear filling defects (*white arrows*) and haziness in the proximal to middle portion of right coronary artery (RCA) (A) and in the middle of the left anterior descending artery (LAD) (B). Optical coherence tomography findings of cross-sectional images (C–E in RCA, G–I in LAD) and longitudinal images (F in RCA, J in LAD) revealed multiple channels of various sizes communicating with each other with smooth septa. The septa were composed of high-signal intensity and low-signal attenuation (Online Videos 2.6 and 2.7).

Optical Coherence Tomography Assessment of Late Intrascaffold Dissection: A New Challenge of Bioresorbable Scaffolds

Yohei Ohno, MD, Andrea Mangiameli, MD, Guilherme F. Attizzani, MD, Davide Capodanno, MD, PhD, Corrado Tamburino, MD, PhD

A 48-year-old man was admitted because of a non–ST-segment elevation myocardial infarction. Fifteen months earlier, a 3.0 × 28 mm bioresorbable vascular scaffold (BVS) (Absorb, Abbott Vascular, Santa Clara, California) was implanted in the mid left anterior descending coronary artery for stable angina. Coronary angiography showed a focal in-scaffold restenosis (Fig. 2.8A). Optical coherence tomography (Ilumien, St. Jude Medical, St. Paul, Minnesota) revealed a heterogeneous pattern consisting of neointimal hyperplasia (Fig. 2.8C), mural white thrombus (Fig. 2.8C), and lipidic plaque with attenuation (Fig. 2.8D). Optical coherence tomography after predilation with a 2.0 × 15 mm semicompliant balloon showed outer migration of scaffold struts (Fig. 2.8E, G, and H) visible in several frames leading to intrascaffold dissection (Fig. 2.8E–H) extending behind the disrupted scaffolds. Good angiographic result was obtained after a 3.0 × 15 mm noncompliant balloon was dilated and administration of an abciximab infusion (Fig. 2.8B); no further intervention was performed.

Although a BVS promotes acute vessel scaffolding similar to metallic stents, it carries a unique feature of complete resorption approximately 3 years after implantation.[1] It is known that 6 months after the implantation, a BVS loses radial strength and structural continuity; therefore it no longer functions as a scaffold,[2] which was

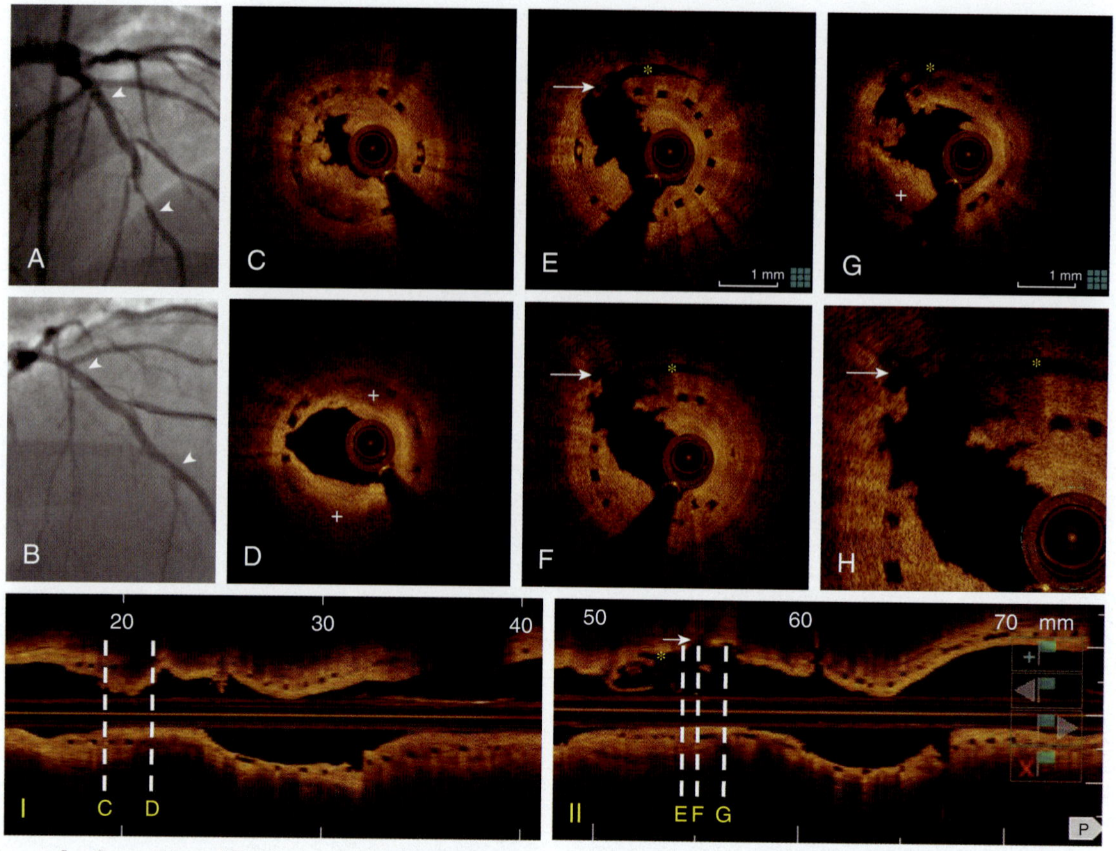

FIG. 2.8 Coronary Angiography and Optical Coherence Tomography Cross-Sectional Images With Longitudinal Views. Coronary angiography (A and B) and optical coherence tomography cross-sectional images (C–H) with longitudinal views (I, II) are demonstrated. (A) Coronary angiography demonstrates focal in-scaffold restenosis. The *white arrowheads* indicate the position of the platinum markers of the BVS. (B) A good angiographic result after balloon dilation and abciximab infusion is shown. (C–G), The *white dashed lines* in the longitudinal views correspond to the cross sections, respectively, before intervention (I) and after intervention (II). Neointimal hyperplasia (12- to 4-o'clock position) and mural white thrombus (*white asterisks*) are revealed in (C), whereas lipidic plaque with attenuation (*white plus signs*) is visualized in (D). Outer migration of scaffold struts (*white arrow*) and intrascaffold dissection (*yellow asterisk*) are visualized in (E) to (H). The magnification of (G) is shown in (H).

likely the potential mechanism that favored in-scaffold dissection after balloon dilation in our case. Although clinicians should be aware that in-scaffold dissections might occur after performing in-BVS balloon dilation for late BVS failure (i.e., theoretically after 6 months), as herewith presented, the best management of BVS restenosis (i.e., implanting another BVS in BVS or balloon dilation only) remains to be determined.

References

1. Serruys PW, Onuma Y, Garcia-Garcia HM, et al. Dynamics of vessel wall changes following the implantation of the absorb everolimus-eluting bioresorbable vascular scaffold: a multi-imaging modality study at 6, 12, 24 and 36 months. *EuroIntervention*. 2014;9:1271-1284.
2. Oberhauser JP, Hossainy S, Rapoza RJ. Design principles and performance of bioresorbable polymeric vascular scaffolds. *EuroIntervention*. 2009;5 Suppl F:F15-F22.

Phantom Stent Thrombosis Intracoronary Imaging Insights

Fernando Rivero, MD, Javier Cuesta, MD, Amparo Benedicto, MD, Teresa Bastante, MD, Daniel Rodriguez-Alcudia, MD, M. Cruz Aguilera, MD, Fernando Alfonso, MD

A 72-old-year-man was admitted for an inferior ST-segment elevation acute myocardial infarction. Seven years earlier, a 2.75 × 15 mm bare-metal stent was successfully implanted in the posterolateral branch of the right coronary artery at another institution. Emergent coronary angiography showed a thrombotic occlusion at the mid segment of the right coronary artery (Fig. 2.9). After multiple unsuccessful attempts to cross the occlusion, eventually a hydrophilic guidewire was advanced across the occluded segment. Thromboaspiration was unsuccessful despite the use of two different aspiration devices that were unable to cross the lesion. Optical coherence tomography (OCT) was performed to clarify the underlying substrate. A large intracoronary red thrombus with intense posterior

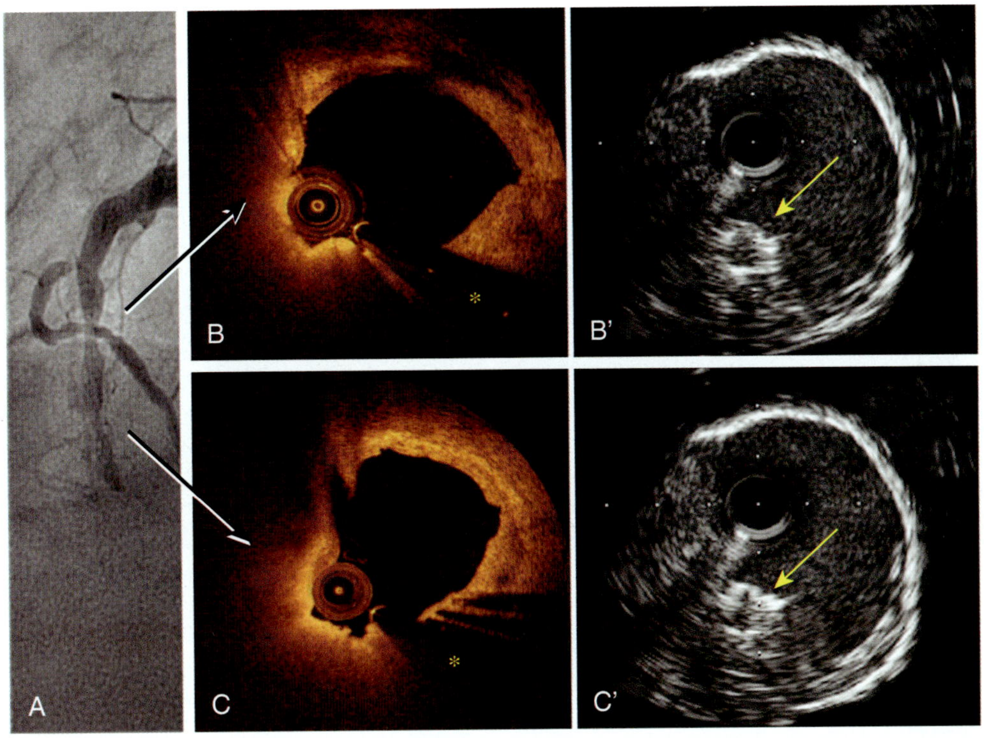

FIG. 2.9 Optical Coherence Tomography and Intravascular Ultrasound Findings. (A) Angiogram of the right coronary artery. (B and C) Optical coherence tomography images show a red intracoronary thrombus with major posterior shadowing, preventing visualization of the arterial wall at this segment. (B′ and C′) Intravascular ultrasound images show a large thrombus containing a clear circular image of metal density related to a previously (7 years ago) lost and underexpanded stent in the coronary artery. The *asterisks* indicate wire artifacts.

shadowing that prevented an adequate visualization of the underlying vessel wall was revealed with OCT. At this point, the use of intravascular ultrasonography (IVUS) was considered to further clarify the anatomy of this challenging lesion. IVUS revealed the presence of a metal structure embedded within the thrombus, highly suggestive of the presence of an "abandoned," underexpanded intracoronary stent at this coronary segment. The abandoned stent was eventually crushed to the arterial wall with a new bare-metal stent. Subsequent hospitalization was uneventful.

Intracoronary loss of unexpanded stents is an infrequent but potentially serious complication that may occur unnoticed during the procedure.[1,2] Despite its unique axial resolution, OCT may have major problems in identifying the culprit "phantom" underlying stent in the setting of a large thrombus burden. In this scenario, IVUS, despite its lower spatial resolution, readily visualizes structures behind thrombus content and fully delineates the complete vessel wall and the outer vessel contour, even without any coronary flow. Our findings demonstrate that IVUS may be especially useful for revealing the presence and disclosing the characteristics of an underlying phantom stent, even in the presence of a large thrombus burden.[3]

References

1. Brilakis ES, Best PJ, Elesber AA, et al. Incidence, retrieval methods, and outcomes of stent loss during percutaneous coronary intervention: a large single-center experience. *Catheter Cardiovasc Interv.* 2005;66:333-340.
2. Alomar ME, Michael TT, Patel VG, et al. Stent loss and retrieval during percutaneous coronary interventions: a systematic review and meta-analysis. *J Invasive Cardiol.* 2013;25:637-641.
3. Alfonso F, Dutary J, Paulo M, et al. Combined use of optical coherence tomography and intravascular ultrasound imaging in patients undergoing coronary interventions for stent thrombosis. *Heart.* 2012;98:1213-1220.

Two Cases of Coronary Stent Thrombosis Very Late After Bare-Metal Stenting

Masamichi Takano, MD, Masanori Yamamoto, MD, Kyoichi Mizuno, MD

The medical literature has recently focused on very late stent thrombosis (VLST) after drug-eluting stent implantation, while its mechanistic issue was not fully explored in the bare-metal stent (BMS) era. The first case is that of a 59-year-old man with inferior non–ST-segment elevation myocardial infarction 4 years after BMS implantation (NIR 3.5/18 mm, Boston Scientific, Galway, Ireland) for a long-term total occlusion lesion in the proximal right coronary artery. Coronary angiograms showed Thrombolysis In Myocardial Infarction (TIMI) grade flow 1 and filling defects in the BMS previously implanted, and massive red thrombi attaching to uncovered stent struts were found by angioscope (Fig. 2.10, Online Video 2.8). Thrombectomy and adjunctive balloon angioplasty

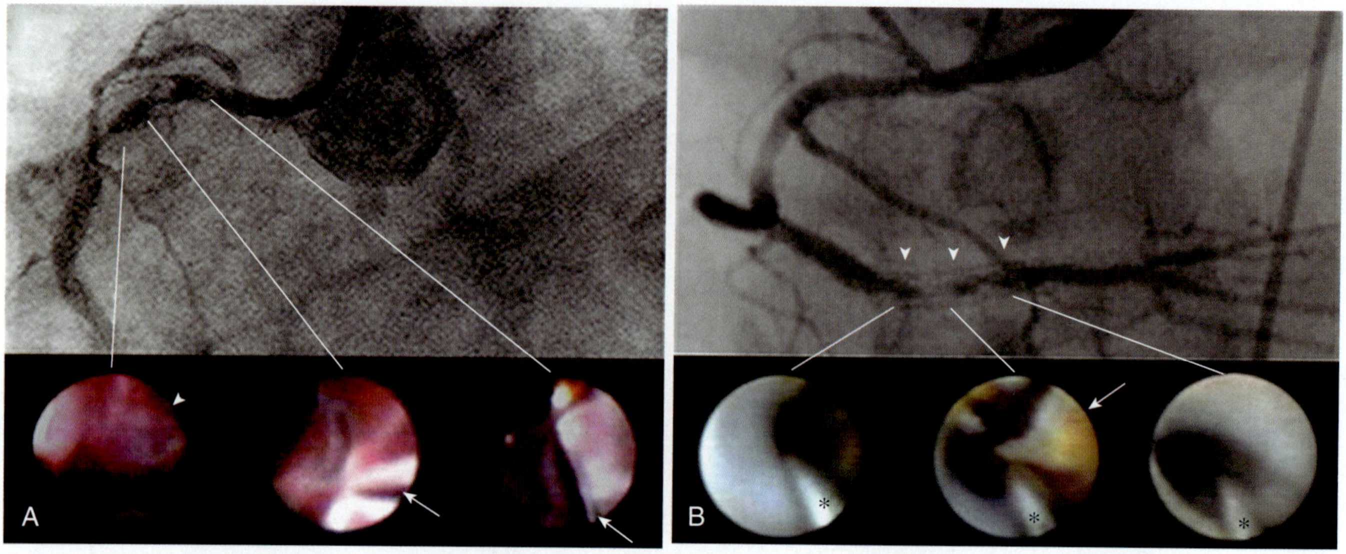

FIG. 2.10 Findings of Coronary Angiography and Angioscopy. (A) Coronary angiograms show thrombolysis in myocardial infarction (TIMI) grade flow I with filling defects of the stent segment. In this segment, occlusive red thrombi (*arrows*) and uncovered stent struts (*arrowhead*) are identified by angioscopy. (B) Angiograms show TIMI plaque (*arrow*) and thrombi are found by angioscopy. Any stent struts are not visible in this angioscopic view. The *asterisk* indicates a guidewire.

were performed based on the angioscopic findings, and TIMI grade flow 3 was obtained.

The second case is that of a 71-year-old man who was admitted for a diagnosis of inferior non–ST-segment elevation myocardial infarction 10 years after a treatment with BMS (gfx 3.0/18 mm, Applied Vascular Engineering, Santa Rosa, California) for the culprit lesion of stable angina pectoris in the distal right coronary artery. Angiographic haziness in the BMS segment was seen despite TIMI grade flow 3. Any progressive lesions on angiography were not seen in other segments. Angioscopic observation for the stent segment demonstrated absence of the uncovered struts. Remarkably, ruptured yellow plaque accompanied by thrombi occupied the lumen (Fig. 2.10, Online Video 2.9). Direct stenting was consequently performed for sealing the ruptured plaque. Although both cases were definite VLST standardized by the Academic Research Consortium,[1] the lumen appearance of direct visualization by angioscope was quite different. Previous autopsy studies showed that plaque disruption outside the BMS with extensive prolapse could lead to thrombosis.[2] For the first time, angioscopic findings in the second case propose strong evidence that atherosclerotic plaque disruption inside the BMS may be one potential trigger of thrombosis. However, persistent uncovered struts in the first case may lead to VLST, as well as those of the drug-eluting stent.[3] The images presented cannot generalize VLST to all cases. However, contrastive angioscopic images suggest that various pathogeneses may contribute to the occurrence of definite VLST after BMS implantation, and different interventional strategies for VLST may be chosen.

References

1. Cutlip DE, Windecker S, Mehran R, et al., Academic Research Consortium. Clinical end points in coronary stent trials: a case for standardized definitions. *Circulation.* 2007;115:2344-2351.
2. Farb A, Burke AP, Kolodgie FD, Virmani R. Pathological mechanisms of fatal late coronary stent thrombosis in humans. *Circulation.* 2003;108:1701-1706.
3. Takano M, Mizuno K. Late coronary thrombosis in a sirolimus-eluting stent due to the lack of neointimal coverage. *Eur Heart J.* 2006;27:1133.

Very Late Stent Thrombosis 5 Years After Implantation of a Sirolimus-Eluting Stent Observed by Angioscopy and Optical Coherence Tomography

Takayuki Ishihara, MD, Masaki Awata, MD, PhD, Masashi Fujita, MD, PhD, Tetsuya Watanabe, MD, PhD, Osamu Iida, MD, Yoshio Ishida, MD, PhD, Shinsuke Nanto, MD, PhD, Masaaki Uematsu, MD, PhD

Drug-eluting stents have dramatically reduced the rate of in-stent restenosis.[1] However, very late stent thrombosis (VLST) is one of the clinical issues with regard to the safety of drug-eluting stents.[2,3] To date there are no articles that report VLST evaluated by both angioscopy and optical coherence tomography (OCT). A 50-year-old man came to the emergency department with chest pain. Five years earlier a 3.0 × 13 mm sirolimus-eluting stent (SES) was implanted in the left anterior descending artery. Coronary angiography revealed severe stenosis with a contrast filling defect at the SES site (Fig. 2.11A) that was attributed to VLST. The OCT demonstrated the presence of a

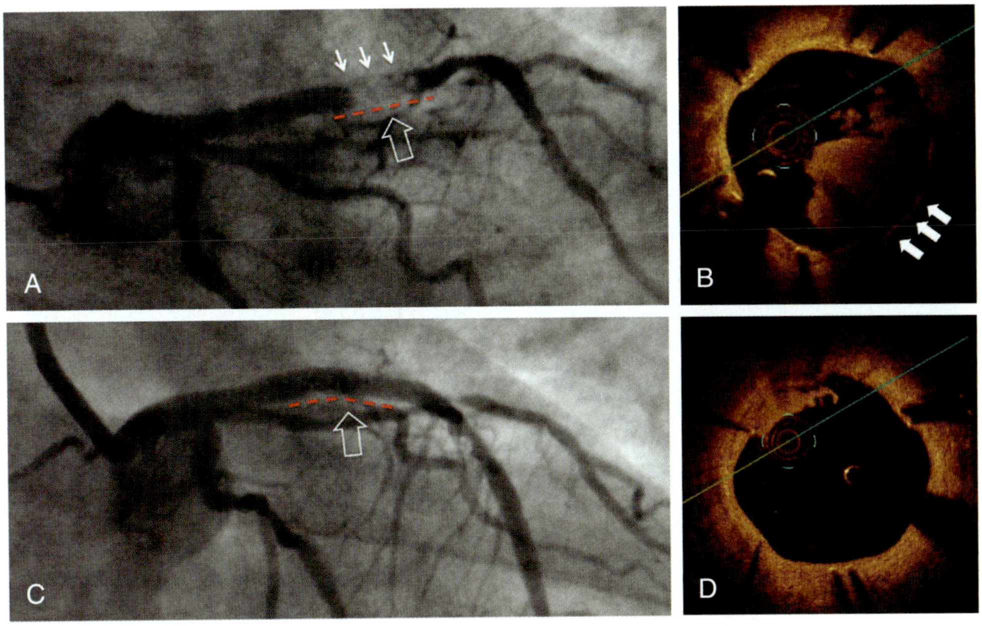

FIG. 2.11 Images of Coronary Angiography and Optical Coherence Tomography (OCT) of Pre– and Post–Percutaneous Coronary Intervention. (A) Initial coronary angiography demonstrated severe stenosis with a contrast filling defect in the sirolimus-eluting stent (SES) implantation site of the left anterior descending artery (*small arrows*). The *dashed red line* shows the SES implantation site. (B) OCT revealed massive thrombus in the SES (*solid arrows*) at the site of the open arrow. (C) Vessel patency was restored after an aspiration procedure. The *dashed red line* shows the SES implantation site. (D) The OCT image demonstrated restored vessel patency at the site of the *open arrow* (as shown in A and C).

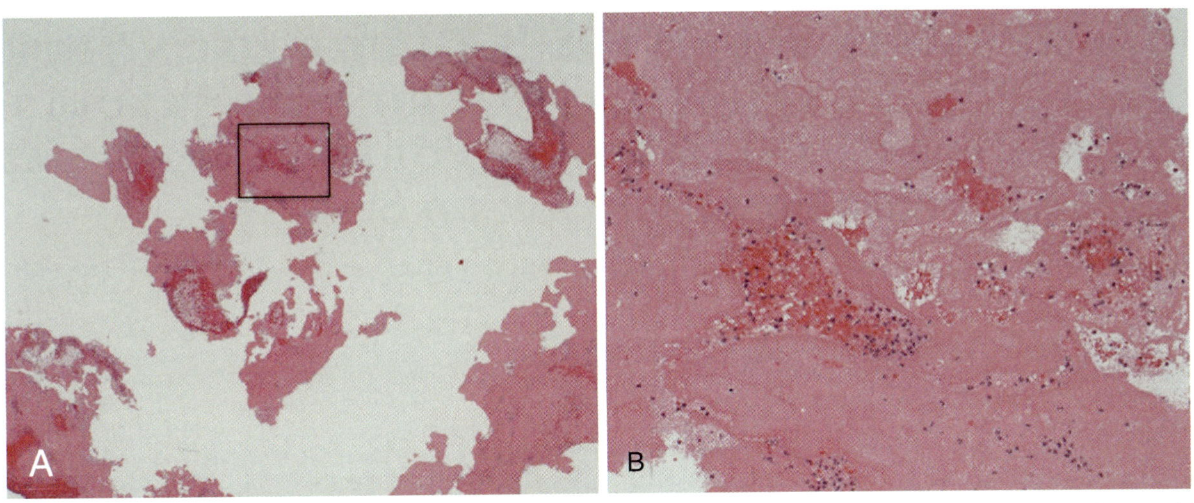

FIG. 2.12 Histopathology of Aspirated Materials. Aspirated materials contained fresh red and white thrombus. Plaque debris and eosinophils were not present. Hematoxylin and eosin stain; original magnification (A) ×20; (B) ×100.

massive thrombus (Fig. 2.11B). Thrombus aspiration resulted in disappearance of the filling defect (Fig. 2.11C). The OCT demonstrated dramatic reduction of the thrombus (Fig. 2.11D). On pathologic evaluation the aspirated contents contained thrombi but no plaque or eosinophil (Fig. 2.12). Coronary angiography 12 days after the procedure showed patency of the SES without peri-stent contrast staining (Fig. 2.13A). Angioscopic observation showed presence of fully visible struts with red thrombus (Fig. 2.13B, Online Video 2.10). The OCT also revealed uncovered struts (Fig. 2.13C). It has been reported that the main cause of early stent thrombosis is usually a procedure-related issue, whereas the cause of late stent thrombosis is delayed arterial healing, and the cause of VLST is an abnormal vascular response.[4] However, an abnormal vascular response was thought to be less relevant as a cause of VLST in this case because strut malapposition was not severe, and the material aspirated from the strut did not contain eosinophils. In contrast, judging from the fully visible struts observed by angioscopy without neointima formation and the presence of uncovered struts observed by OCT, delayed arterial healing was thought to be the main cause of VLST in this case.

References

1. Moses JW, Leon MB, Popma JJ, et al. Sirolimus-eluting stents versus standard stents in patients with stenosis in a native coronary artery. *N Engl J Med*. 2003;349:1315-1323.
2. Kastrati A, Mehilli J, Pache J, et al. Analysis of 14 trials comparing sirolimus-eluting stents with bare-metal stents. *N Engl J Med*. 2007;3056:1030-1039.
3. Kon H, Sakai H, Otsubo M, et al. Contrast staining outside the sirolimus-eluting stent leading to coronary aneurysm formation: a case of very late stent thrombosis associated with hypersensitivity reaction. *Circ Cardiovasc Interv*. 2011;4:e1-e3.
4. Kimura T, Morimoto T, Kozuma K, et al. Comparisons of baseline demographics, clinical presentation, and long-term outcome among patients with early, late, and very late stent thrombosis of sirolimus-eluting stents: observations from the Registry of Stent Thrombosis for Review and Reevaluation (RESTART). *Circulation*. 2010;122:52-61.

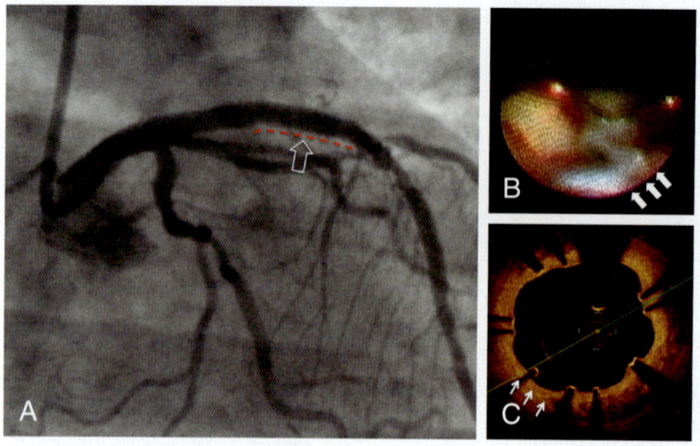

FIG. 2.13 Images of Coronary Angiography, Angioscopy, and Optical Coherence Tomography 12 Days After Initial Procedure. (A) Follow-up coronary angiography revealed patency without peri-stent contrast staining or the presence of a thrombotic filling defect. The *dashed red line* shows the sirolimus-eluting stent. (B) Angioscopic evaluation demonstrated fully visible struts with red thrombus and yellow plaques at the site of the *open arrow* in (A) (*large arrows*). (C) Optical coherence tomographic evaluation demonstrated uncovered struts and malapposition at the site of the *open arrow* in (A). The maximum interval between the stent strut and the vessel was 240 μm (*small arrows*) (Online Video 2.10).

Cross-Sectional and Longitudinal Positive Remodeling After Subintimal Drug-Eluting Stent Implantation: Multiple Late Coronary Aneurysms, Stent Fractures, and a Newly Formed Stent Gap Between Previously Overlapped Stents

Kenichi Tsujita, MD, PhD, Akiko Maehara, MD, Gary S. Mintz, MD, Michael Poon, MD, Giuseppe Maiolino, MD, PhD, Teppei Sugaya, MD, Keiichi Igarashi, MD, PhD, Masahiko Ochiai, MD, PhD

A 50-year-old man with a history of smoking and hyperlipidemia, but no chest pain, was admitted because of an abnormal electrocardiogram and regional wall motion abnormality on echocardiography (mild inferior hypokinesis). Coronary angiography revealed two chronic total occlusions (CTOs): ostial right coronary artery (RCA) and mid left circumflex artery. The long RCA CTO lesion was treated by intentional retrograde creation of a subintimal lumen with a "knuckled" Fielder XT wire (Asahi Intecc, Nagoya, Japan) (Fig. 2.14) followed by deliberate implantation of four overlapping paclitaxel-eluting stents into the subintimal space. Complete stent—vessel wall apposition and overlapping of adjacent stents was confirmed by post-procedural intravascular ultrasonography (Figs. 2.15 and 2.16). The 8-month follow-up coronary angiogram showed multiple aneurysms in the RCA, but not in the mid left circumflex artery, that had been treated using a conventional antegrade CTO approach and single-stent implantation into the true lumen. At the sites of the RCA aneurysms, intravascular ultrasonography showed large areas of late acquired stent malapposition (LSM) as the result of vessel remodeling (an increase in cross-sectional and longitudinal vessel dimensions), changes that were most marked at the sites of subintimal stent implantation (Fig. 2.15). These areas of LSM were accompanied by stent fractures and a newly formed gap between the (previously overlapped) most distal stent and the proximal adjacent partial stent segment (Fig. 2.16). Serial intravascular ultrasound quantitative analysis revealed positive remodeling (increase in mean vessel area from 15.0 to 20.8 mm^2). The newly formed gap between the previously overlapped stents suggested that positive vessel remodeling occurred in the longitudinal direction and cross-sectionally.

Drug-eluting stents reduce restenosis even after treatment of CTO lesions. However, the frequency of LSM appears to be greater after the implantation of drug-eluting stents versus bare-metal stents, especially in the setting of treatment of CTO lesions. Hong et al.[1] reported that predictors of LSM were total stent length, primary stenting in acute myocardial infarction, and stenting of CTO lesions. Hong et al.[1,2] found that LSM may be associated with less neointimal hyperplasia, but it has also been implicated in patients with very late stent thrombosis.[3] In our case, large areas of LSM were observed at the sites of angiographic aneurysms that were detected 8 months after treatment of an RCA CTO. The complex procedure included deliberate subintimal passage of the guidewire and implantation of drug-eluting stent into the subintimal space. This technique might have exaggerated injury to the medial and adventitial layers, or the adventitial location of the drug and polymer may have induced a local hypersensitivity to cause cross-sectional and longitudinal vessel remodeling, LSM, and aneurysm formation. Of note, there were no areas of aneurysm formation or LSM 16 months after treatment of the left circumflex artery CTO using a conventional antegrade approach with sirolimus-eluting stent implantation into the true lumen.

References

1. Hong MK, Mintz GS, Lee CW, et al. Late stent malapposition after drug-eluting stent implantation: an intravascular ultrasound analysis with long-term follow-up. *Circulation*. 2006;113:414-419.
2. Hong MK, Mintz GS, Lee CW, et al. Incidence, mechanism, predictors, and long-term prognosis of late stent malapposition after bare-metal stent implantation. *Circulation*. 2004;109:881-886.
3. Cook S, Wenaweser P, Togni M, et al. Incomplete stent apposition and very late stent thrombosis after drug-eluting stent implantation. *Circulation*. 2007;115:2426-2434.

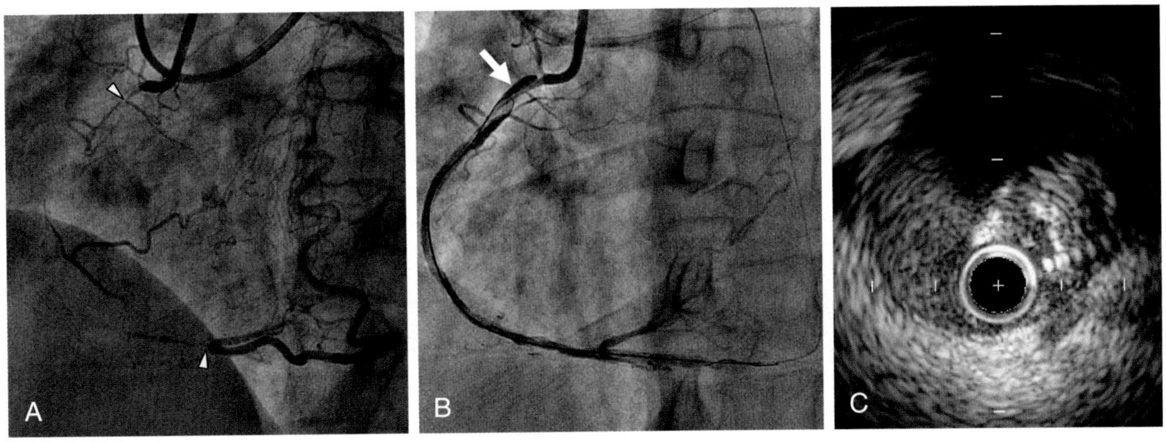

FIG. 2.14 Baseline Coronary Angiogram and Subintimal Wiring. (A) An extremely long chronic total occlusion (CTO) from the ostium of the right coronary artery (RCA) to the distal bifurcation (*arrowheads*) was seen in the preintervention angiogram. The contralateral injection showed an epicardial collateral from left anterior descending coronary artery to the RCA. (B) The CTO was successfully crossed using a retrograde approach via this epicardial collateral combined with the intentional creation of subintimal lumen using a stiff guidewire. Coronary angiography showed a large coronary dissection in the proximal RCA. (C) The intravascular ultrasound catheter (*white arrow* in [B]) was placed in the subintimal space, and the true lumen was collapsed at the 2-o'clock position.

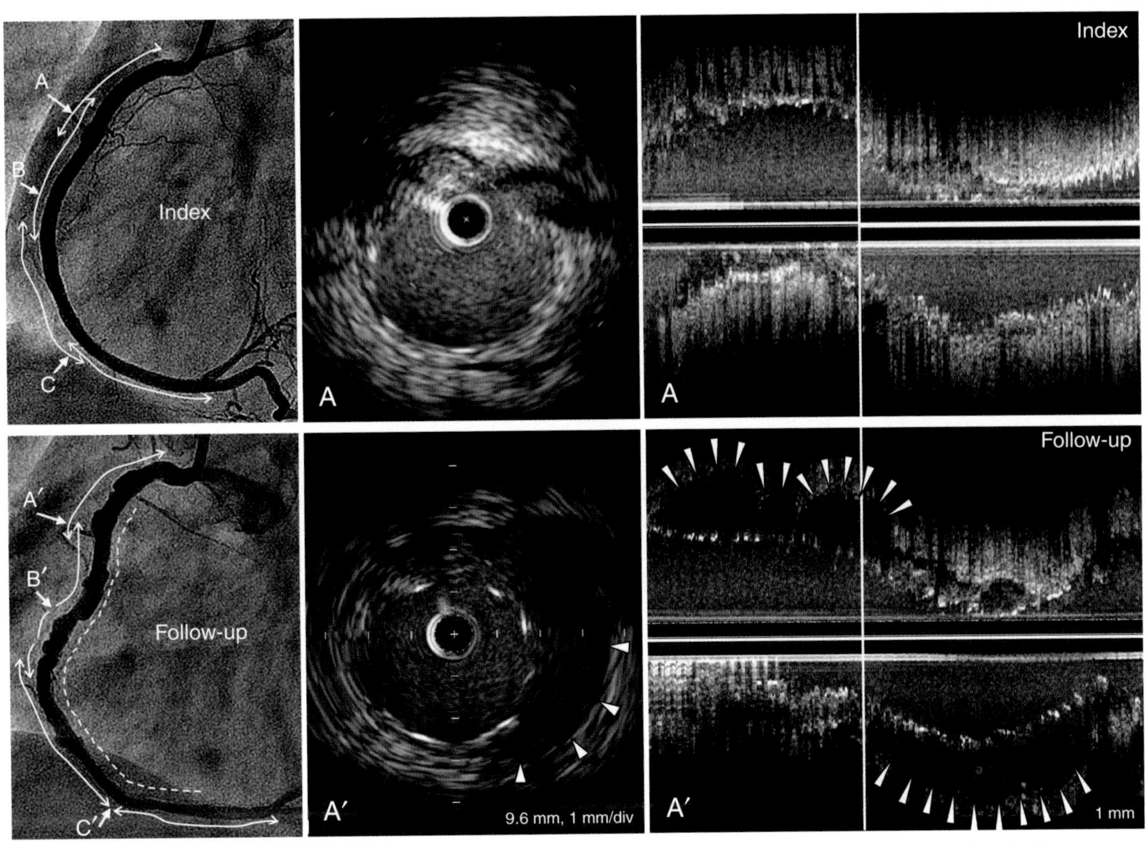

FIG. 2.15 Cross-Sectional Positive Remodeling. The index and follow-up angiograms (*left*) after four overlapping paclitaxel-eluting stents (2.75 × 32 mm, 3.0 × 32 mm, 3.0 × 32 mm, and 3.5 × 28 mm) were implanted from the distal bifurcation to the orifice of the right coronary artery (RCA) to treat a long chronic total occlusion (CTO) lesion. The dashed line indicates the subintimal stents; the four double-headed white arrows indicate the location of each of the four stents. The follow-up angiogram demonstrated multiple aneurysms, especially in the proximal segment where a large dissection was observed at the index procedure. Cross-sectional and longitudinal intravascular ultrasonography (IVUS) panels (A) correspond to A on the baseline angiogram; cross-sectional and longitudinal IVUS panels (A′) correspond to A′ on the follow-up angiogram. The baseline and follow-up cross-sectional IVUS images are from the same anatomic location(s) in the RCA; note the small right ventricular branch at the 1- to 2-o'clock position on the baseline and follow-up images that correspond to the same small right ventricular branch on the angiograms. At baseline, both the cross-sectional and longitudinal IVUS images (A) showed well-apposed and well-expanded stents. At follow-up (A′), there were large areas of late acquired stent malapposition as the result of positive vessel remodeling (*white arrowheads*) on both the cross-sectional and longitudinal IVUS images.

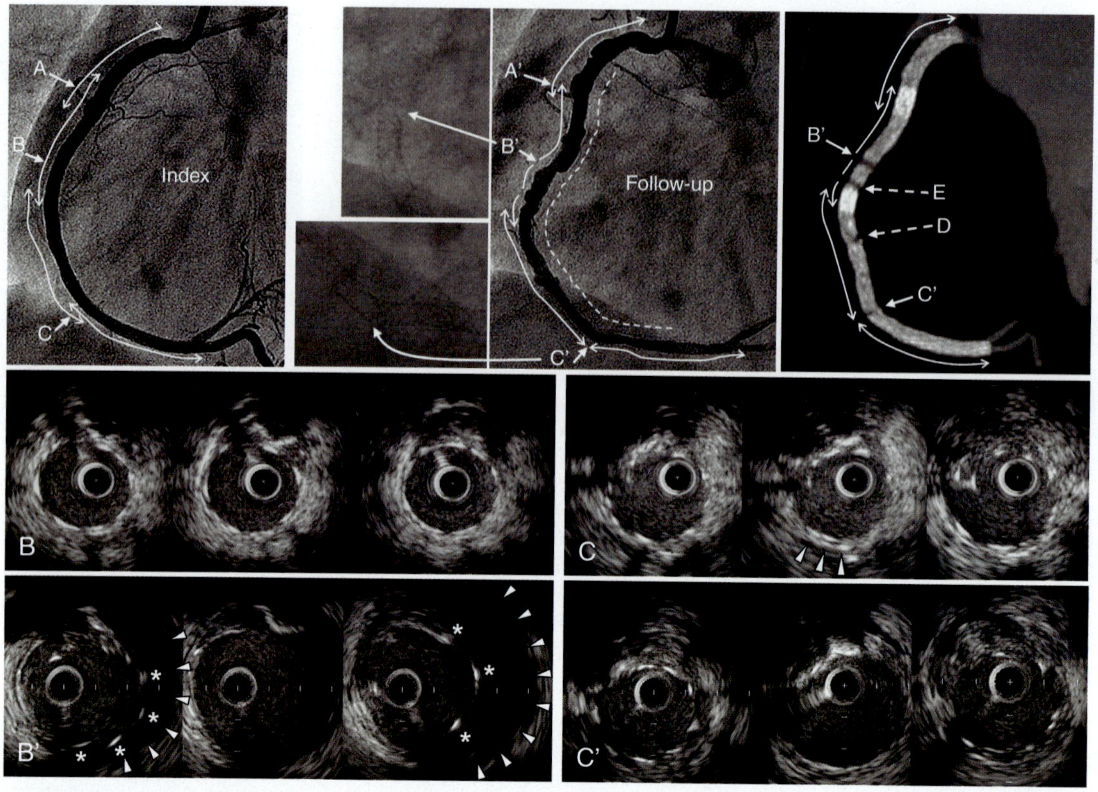

FIG. 2.16 Longitudinal Positive Remodeling. The index and follow-up angiograms (*top, left, and center*) after four paclitaxel-eluting stents (2.75 × 32 mm, 3.0 × 32 mm, 3.0 × 32 mm, and 3.5 × 28 mm) were implanted from the distal bifurcation to orifice of the right coronary artery (RCA) to treat a long chronic total occlusion lesion. Unlike the focus in Fig. 2.15, here we focus on segments B and B′ and C and C′; note that at follow-up, both locations contain fluoroscopic evidence of absence of stent struts indicating either fracture (B′) or separation of overlapped stents (C′). The intravascular ultrasonographic (IVUS) sequences B and B′ are from the same anatomic location in the RCA and correspond to B on the baseline and follow-up angiograms; IVUS sequences C and C′ are from the same anatomic location in the RCA and correspond to C on the baseline and follow-up angiograms. In IVUS sequences B and B′ from baseline to follow-up, there has been positive remodeling (*white arrowheads*), development of LSM (*asterisks*), and stent fracture (absence of stent struts in the middle IVUS image). In IVUS sequences C and C′ from baseline to follow-up, an absence of stent struts was seen at the site of previously overlapping stents (*small white arrows*, double stent layers at baseline, but no struts at follow-up in the middle IVUS image). The follow-up 64-slice multidetector computed tomography (MDCT) of the RCA confirmed the IVUS findings of complete (B′) stent fracture and separation of the previously overlapped stents (C′). The MDCT image showed two additional areas of incomplete (D) and complete (E) stent fracture; these were also seen on the IVUS studies but are not included here for the sake of simplicity.

In-Stent Protrusion After Implantation of a Drug-Eluting Stent in a Honeycomb-Like Coronary Artery Structure: Complete Resolution Over 6 Months and the Role of Optical Coherence Tomography Imaging in the Diagnosis and Follow-Up

Kohei Koyama, MD, Kihei Yoneyama, MD, PhD, Takanobu Mitarai, MD, Shingo Kuwata, MD, Yuki Ishibashi, MD, PhD, Ken Kongoji, MD, PhD, Yoshihiro J. Akashi, MD, PhD

A 61-year-old woman had chest pain while walking. The patient had positive electrocardiographic findings for ischemia and a slightly elevated troponin level I (0.271 ng/mL), suggesting acute coronary syndrome. Optical coherence tomography (OCT) confirmed a honeycomb-like structure with multiple signal-free channels (Fig. 2.17). A drug-eluting stent (DES) (everolimus-eluting stent 2.5 × 15 mm) was then implanted because of atherosclerosis at the distal culprit lesion. OCT after stent implantation showed thrombi protrusion and the complete resolution over 6 months (Fig. 2.18).

A spontaneous recanalization of thrombi, forming a honeycomb-like structure, is rare in patients undergoing coronary angiography.[1] The primary concerns are stent thrombosis

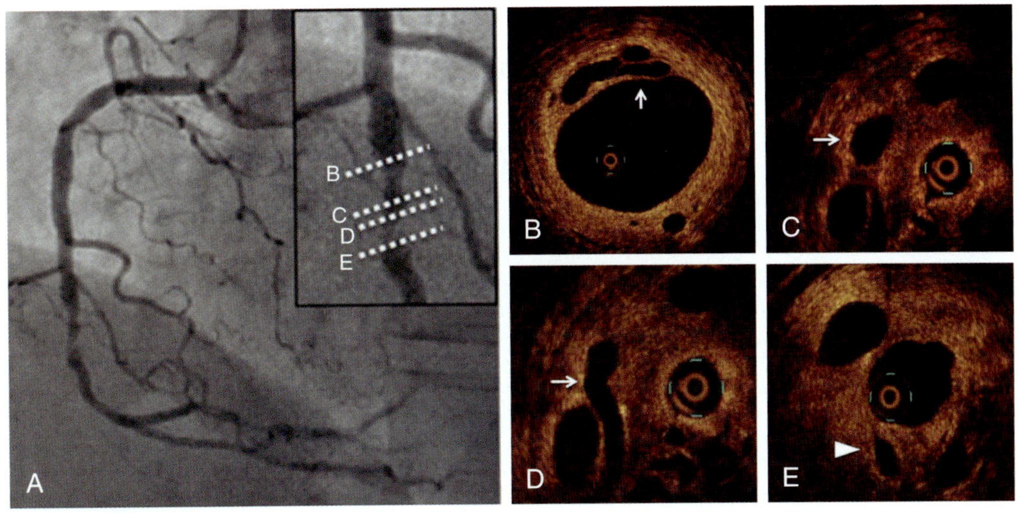

FIG. 2.17 A Honeycomb-Like Structure. (A) Coronary angiography at the acute phase. (B–E) Optical coherence tomography shows that the channels communicated with one another (*arrows*), and some of those converged toward the large central lumen (*arrowhead*).

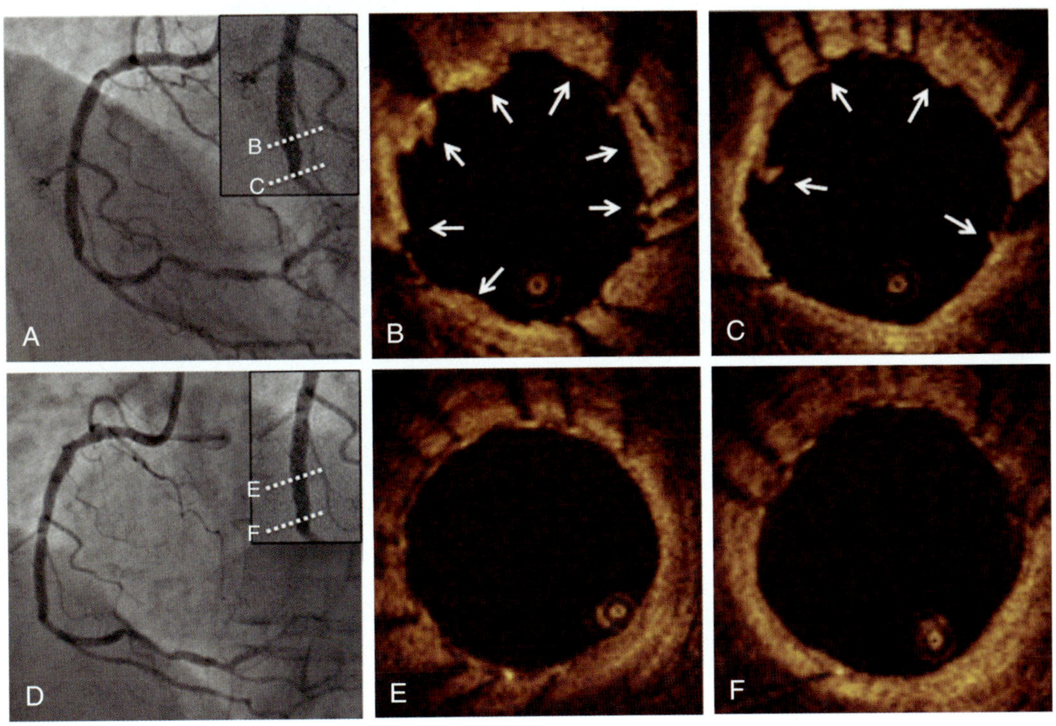

FIG. 2.18 Drug-Eluting Stent (DES) Implantation and Follow-Up Findings. (A) The final coronary angiogram result was satisfactory. (B and C) Optical coherence tomography (OCT) after DES implantation showed well-apposed stent struts with thrombi protrusion in the spontaneously recanalized thrombus (*arrows*). (D) The coronary angiogram at 6 months after DES implantation showed no stenosis in the stent. (E and F) The OCT images at 6 months showed the complete absence of the thrombus protrusion and stent struts that were well apposed to the vessel wall.

because of malposition after DES stenting on the thrombi lesion, and in-stent restenosis of the atherosclerotic plaque with bare-metal stent implantation. Follow-up OCT at 6 months confirmed the successful DES deployment and its efficacy in acute coronary syndrome.

Reference

1. Toutouzas K, Karanasos A, Stathogiannis K, et al. A honeycomb-like structure in the left anterior descending coronary artery: demonstration of recanalized thrombus by optical coherence tomography. *J Am Coll Cardiol Intv.* 2012;5:688-689.

Coronary Dissections and Hematomas

INTRAMURAL HEMATOMA APPEARING AS A NEW LESION AFTER CORONARY STENTING

Jennifer A. Tremmel, MD, SM, Tomomi Koizumi, MD, PhD, Aiden O'Loughlin, MBBS, BSc, MB, Alan C. Yeung, MD

A 51-year-old man with hypertension and hyperlipidemia had exertional chest pain and underwent a stress echocardiogram that showed anterior and lateral ischemia. Coronary angiography revealed a 70% stenosis of the mid left circumflex artery and an 80% stenosis of the proximal left anterior descending artery (Fig. 2.19A). The left circumflex artery was directly stented with a 2.5 × 12 mm drug-eluting stent (DES). The left anterior descending artery stenosis was predilated with a 3.0 × 9 mm balloon and a 3.5 × 16 mm DES was placed, with a maximal inflation pressure of 16 atm. After stent placement there appeared to be a new lesion at the distal end of the stent (Fig. 2.19B). The angiographic abnormality was not relieved by intracoronary nitroglycerin or verapamil. The patient remained hemodynamically stable without electrocardiographic changes or chest pain.

Intravascular ultrasonography was used to determine the etiology of this new lesion and showed an intramural hematoma originating at the distal end of the stent (Fig. 2.20). There was no identifiable entry point. The intramural hematoma was treated with an overlapping 3.0 × 20 mm DES implanted at a maximal pressure of 12 atm. The stent length was chosen to cover beyond the distal extent of the intramural hematoma. Final intravascular ultrasonography showed resolution of the intramural hematoma, and angiography demonstrated no residual stenosis and Thrombolysis In Myocardial Infarction grade flow 3. The creatinine kinase-myocardial band the next morning was normal.

Intramural hematomas after percutaneous coronary intervention are defined as an accumulation of blood within the media that displaces the internal elastic membrane inward and the external elastic membrane outward, with or without identifiable entry and exit points.[1] They have been demonstrated in up to 7% of all percutaneous coronary interventions and are most common in patients with diabetes and those with less-diseased coronary arteries. The angiographic appearance of an intramural hematoma is generally a dissection (60% of cases), but in 11% it appears as spasm or a new lesion, and in 29% there is no significant angiographic abnormality.

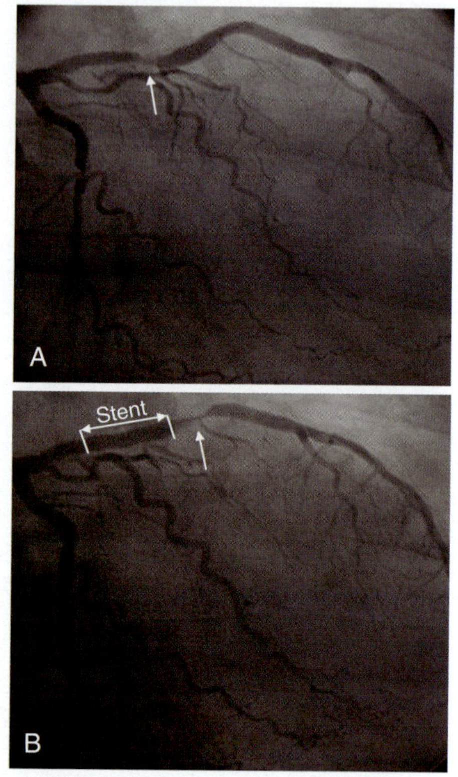

FIG. 2.19 Left Coronary Artery Angiogram Before and After Stenting. (A) Angiography of the left coronary artery showing the original stenosis in the proximal left anterior descending artery (*arrow*). (B) Angiography of the left anterior descending artery after stent implantation showing a new luminal narrowing just distal to the stent (*arrow*).

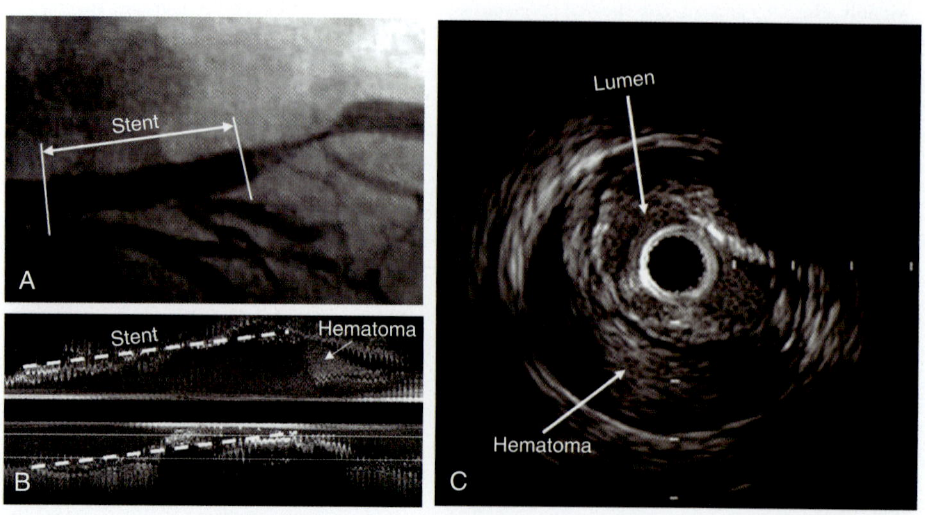

FIG. 2.20 Intravascular Ultrasound of New Lesion Appearing at Distal End of Stent. (A) Angiography of the left anterior descending artery showing a new luminal narrowing just distal to the stent. (B) Longitudinal intravascular ultrasound image of the artery segment seen in (A). The *white dotted line* outlines the stent, and the *white arrow* indicates the hematoma, which occupied much of the lumen of the distal reference segment. (C) Intramural hematoma seen in the cross-sectional intravascular ultrasound image at the site of luminal narrowing in (A).

Intramural hematomas can occur at both the distal (55%) and proximal stent edges (45%). Up to 26% are complicated by a non–Q-wave myocardial infarction. The proper management of intramural hematomas remains poorly defined.[2]

References

1. Mintz GS, Nissen SE, Anderson WD, et al. American College of Cardiology clinical expert consensus document on standards for acquisition, measurement, and reporting of intravascular ultrasound studies (IVUS): a report of the American College of Cardiology task force on clinical expert consensus documents. *J Am Coll Cardiol.* 2001;37:1478-1492.
2. Maehara A, Mintz GS, Bui AB, et al. Incidence, morphology, angiographic findings, and outcomes of intramural hematomas after percutaneous coronary interventions: an intravascular ultrasound study. *Circulation.* 2002;105:2037-2042.

Ruptured Neoatherosclerosis Presenting as a Large Intrastent Neointimal Dissection

Fernando Rivero, MD, Javier Cuesta, MD, Amparo Benedicto, MD, Teresa Bastante, MD, Fernando Alfonso, MD

A 77-year-old man was admitted for a prolonged chest pain. Nine years earlier he required implantation of a bare-metal stent in the proximal left anterior descending coronary artery for stable angina. In the emergency department, the electrocardiogram showed dynamic ST-segment depression on the anterior leads. A significant increase in cardiac biomarkers was subsequently confirmed. Coronary angiography showed no significant coronary stenosis, although a faint, linear haziness was visualized within the stent (Fig. 2.21A). Optical coherence tomography revealed a typical pattern of nonocclusive intrastent neoatherosclerosis (NA) (Fig. 2.21B). However, at the mid segment of the stent, a clear rupture of a bright, glistening neointima was readily demonstrated (Fig. 2.21C). Interestingly, this tear induced a relatively large intrastent dissection (up to 5 mm in length) and a striking double-lumen morphology (Fig. 2.21D–F). The mean dissection thickness was 340 mm. The minimal lumen area of the true lumen was 1.7 mm^2, and the maximal area of the false lumen was 3.6 mm^2. No residual intracoronary thrombi were recognized. An excellent result was obtained with the implantation of an everolimus-eluting stent.

NA is a well-defined cause of very late in-stent restenosis and stent thrombosis.[1] Because of its unsurpassed resolution, optical coherence tomography provides a unique tool in the diagnosis of

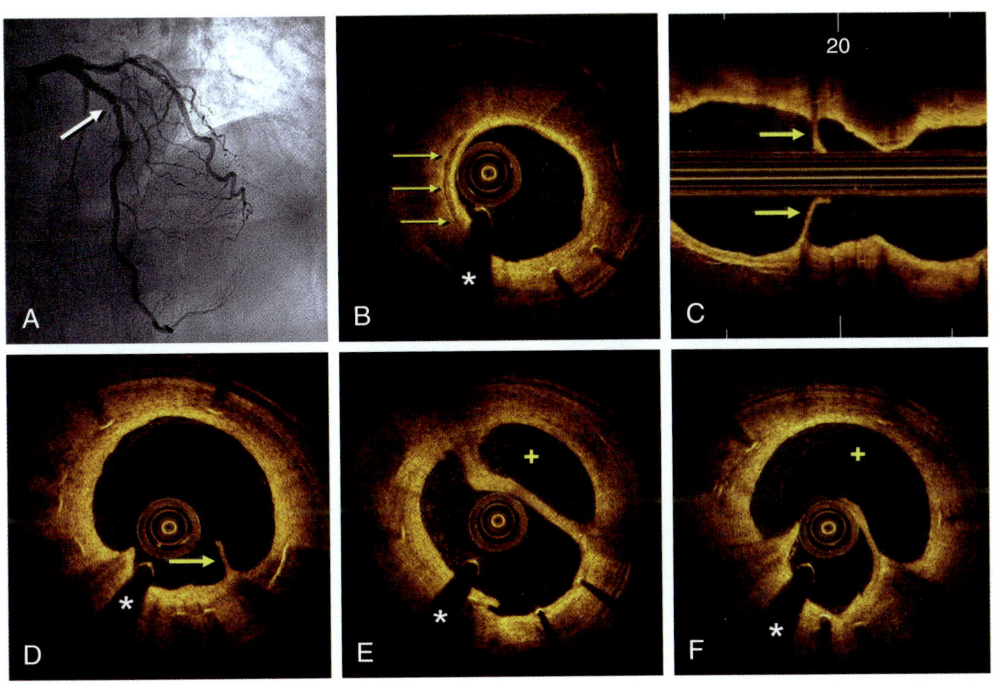

FIG. 2.21 Intracoronary Insights of the Intrastent Neointimal Dissection. (A) Coronary angiography showing a linear haziness within the stent (*arrow*). (B) Optical coherence tomography (OCT) disclosing neoatherosclerosis with large lipid pools and a layered area (*arrows*) suggestive of in-stent calcified tissue. (C) OCT imaging showing a neointimal dissection (*arrows*). (D–F) From proximal to distal segments, a large intrastent dissection with double-lumen morphology was observed. The *arrow* in (D) indicates neointimal dissection. A plus sign indicates the false lumen. An *asterisk* denotes a wire artifact.

NA.[2] Characteristic findings include infiltrated neointima, lipid pools, thin-cap fibroatheroma, calcification, and even macrophage accumulation.[2,3] Complicated NA is characterized by relatively confined neointimal ruptures with associated intracoronary thrombus.[2,3] However, our unique findings suggest that complicated NA may also present as a relatively large, angiographically silent, intrastent coronary dissection.

References

1. Nakazawa G, Otsuka F, Nakano M, et al. The pathology of neoatherosclerosis in human coronary implants bare-metal and drug-eluting stents. *J Am Coll Cardiol.* 2011;57:1314-1322.
2. Alfonso F, Dutary J, Paulo M, et al. Combined use of optical coherence tomography and intravascular ultrasound imaging in patients undergoing coronary interventions for stent thrombosis. *Heart.* 2012;98:1213-1220.
3. Kang SJ, Mintz GS, Akasaka T, et al. Optical coherence tomographic analysis of in-stent neoatherosclerosis after drug-eluting stent implantation. *Circulation.* 2011;123:2954-2963.

Acute Closure Caused by Extramedial Hematoma 3 Hours After Stenting

Shinji Inaba, MD, Gary S. Mintz, MD, Michael B. Collins, MD, Khady N. Fall, MD, Jeffrey W. Moses, MD, Akiko Maehara, MD

A 53-year-old woman was admitted for unstable angina pectoris. Coronary angiography revealed a stenosis in the right coronary artery (Fig. 2.22A). A 2.75 × 18 mm zotarolimus-eluting stent was implanted at 16 atm. Intravascular ultrasonography showed a distal edge dissection (Fig. 2.22C), which appeared to extend beyond the media with a lumen of 5.8 mm^2 and TIMI (Thrombolysis In Myocardial Infarction) grade flow 3 (Fig. 2.22B).

Sustained chest pain occurred 3 hours after the procedure. Emergent angiography revealed flow-limiting obstruction at the distal stent edge (Fig. 2.23). Optical coherence tomography showed a hematoma (hyporeflective-backscattering with attenuation) that was clearly located outside the media but inside the adventitia (Fig. 2.24). Intravascular ultrasonography also showed the development of an extramedial hematoma. The mechanism is shown in Fig. 2.25.

We report a progression from dissection to extramedial hematoma. Optical coherence tomography can localize a poststent hematoma as intramedial or extramedial.

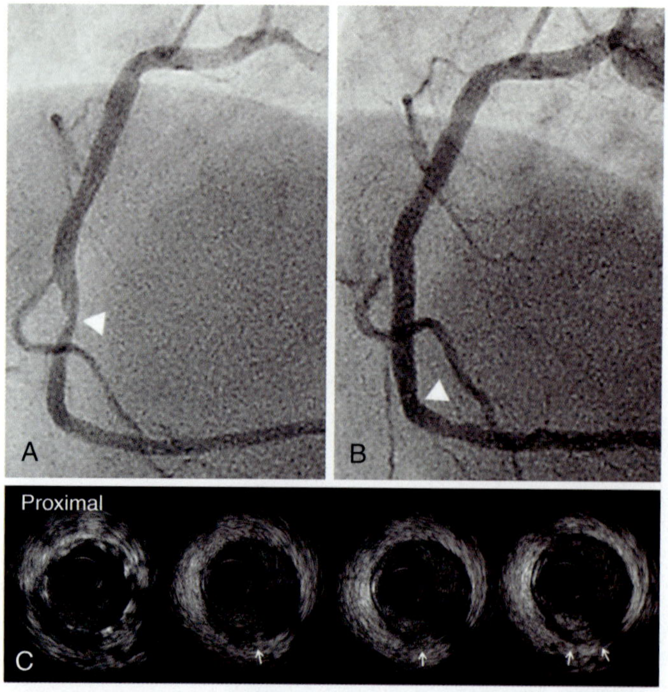

FIG. 2.22 Baseline Angiography and Intravascular Ultrasonography. (A) Angiography showing focal stenosis (*arrowhead*). (B) Postprocedure angiography showing the distal stent edge (*arrowhead*). (C) Postprocedure intravascular ultrasonography showing the edge dissection extending to the outside of the media (*arrows*).

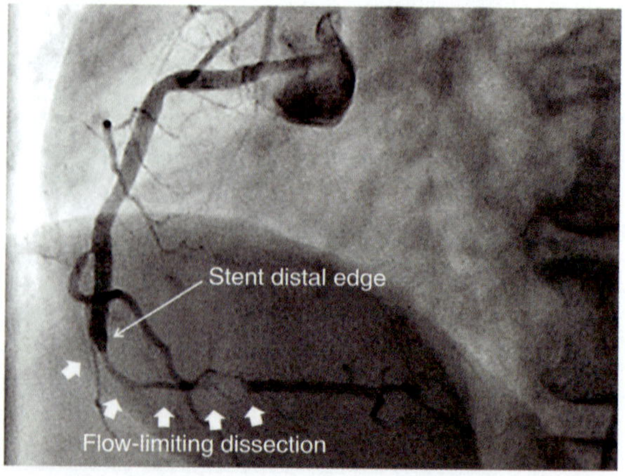

FIG. 2.23 Angiography 3 Hours Later. Angriography 3 hours later shows a flow-limiting obstruction (*large white arrows*) observed from the stent distal edge.

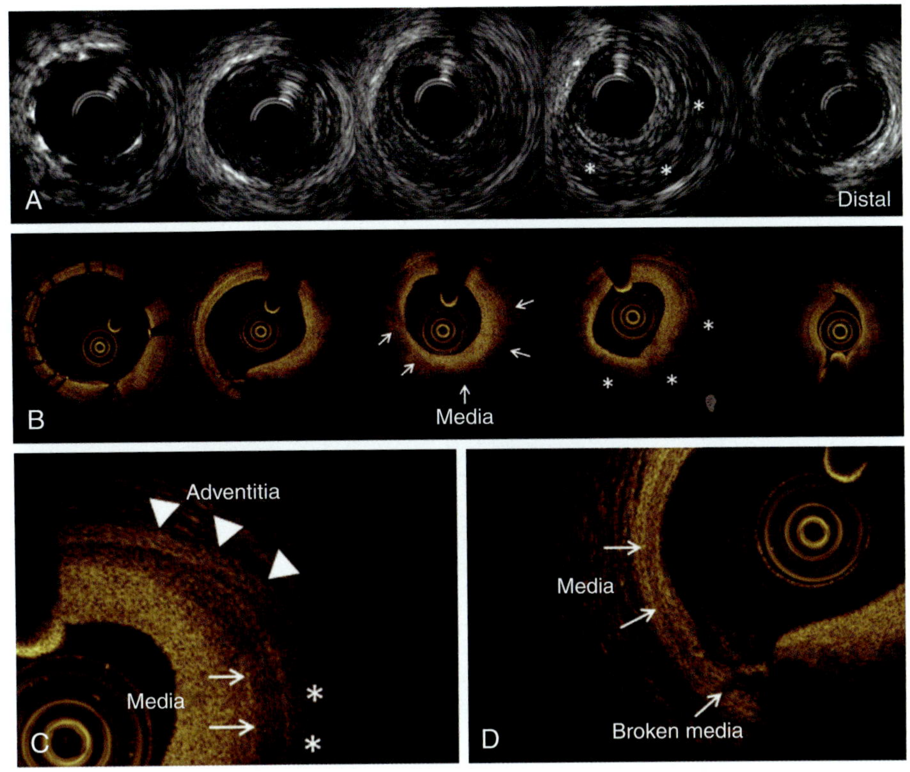

FIG. 2.24 Intravascular Ultrasonography and Optical Coherence Tomography Images. (A) Intravascular ultrasonography showing a hematoma (*asterisk*) that appeared outside the media (*arrows*) but inside the adventitia (*triangle*) by optical coherence tomography (B–D).

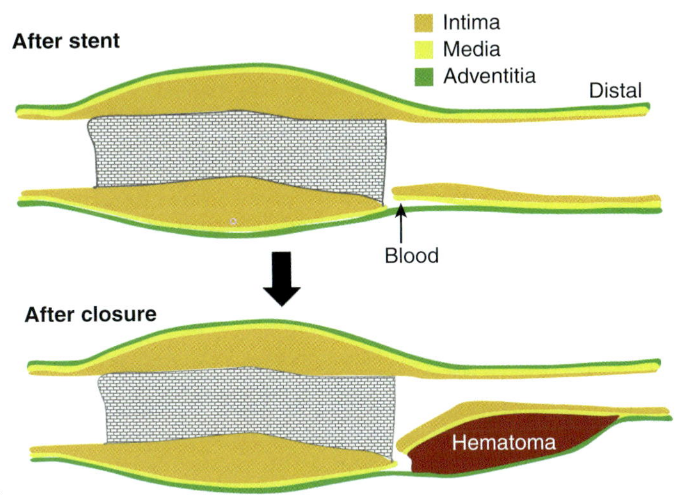

FIG. 2.25 Mechanism of extramedial hematoma.

Aortocoronary Dissection With Extension to the Suprarenal Abdominal Aorta: A Rare Complication After Percutaneous Coronary Intervention

Min-Tsun Liao, MD, Shih-Chi Liu, MD, Jen-Kuang Lee, MD, Fu-Tien Chiang, MD, PhD, Cho-Kai Wu, MD

A 53-year-old man was seen with chest tightness and a positive treadmill test result. A percutaneous coronary intervention (PCI) was performed on the distal total occlusion of the right coronary artery (RCA) with a 6F Amplatz Left 1 guiding catheter (Amplatz, Abbott, Plymouth, Minnesota) and a Runthrough floppy wire (Terumo Europe, Leuven, Belgium). However, a proximal RCA dissection along with an aortic dissection was found during wiring (Fig. 2.26A). A Driver 3.5 × 24 mm stent (Medtronic, Minneapolis,

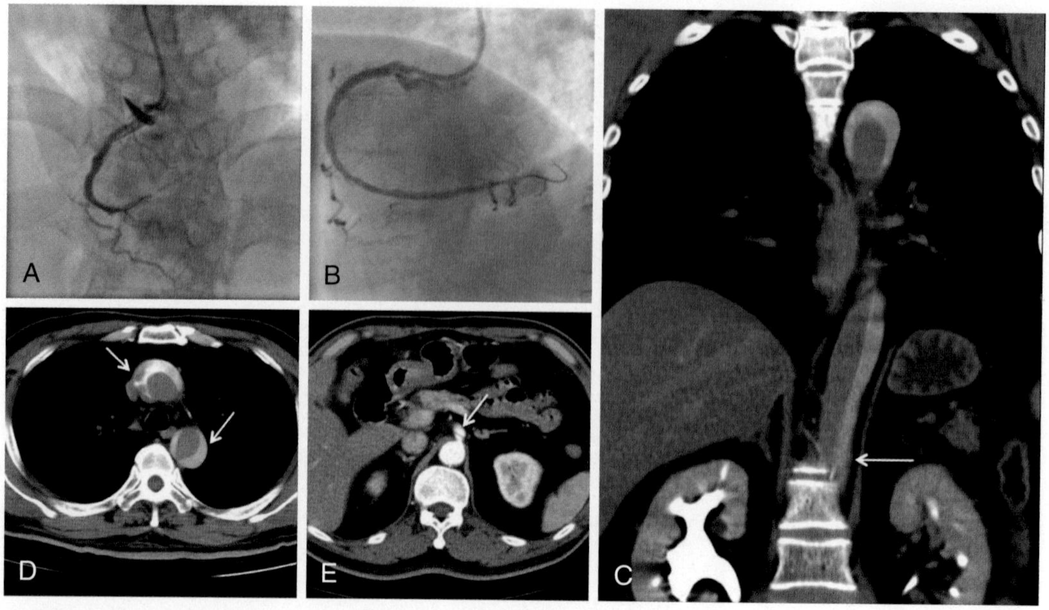

FIG. 2.26 Angiography and Computed Tomography. (A) Angiography demonstrating the proximal long segment dissection of the right coronary artery, extending to sinus of Valsalva. (B) After stenting (Driver 3.5 × 24 mm [Medtronic, Minneapolis, Minnesota]), the final angiogram revealed limited dissection to the sinus of Valsalva. (C and D) Computed tomography imaging demonstrated a type A aortic dissection *(arrows)* extending from ascending aorta to the suprarenal abdominal level with involvement of the aortic arch and celiac trunk *(arrow)* (E).

Minnesota) was implanted in the proximal RCA. Next, a guidewire was placed across the distal total occlusion, and a 2.5 × 30 mm Endeavor Resolute stent (Medtronic) was implanted. The final angiogram showed limited aortic dissection (Fig. 2.26B). The patient's state of consciousness changed 30 minutes after the PCI while he was in the intensive care unit. An emergent computed tomography scan (within 15 minutes) revealed a type A aortic dissection extending from the ascending aorta to the suprarenal abdominal level (Fig. 2.26C–D) with involvement of the aortic arch and celiac trunk (Fig. 2.26E). An emergent ascending aortic graft and venous bypass graft were performed. The patient was discharged 16 days later in stable condition. To the best of our knowledge, this case is the first report of an extensive aortic dissection after PCI to the level of the suprarenal abdominal aorta.

Aortic dissection after PCI is a rare and life-threatening complication with an incidence of approximately 0.02%.[1] Most reported iatrogenic aortic dissections have been related to procedures in the RCA.[2] The extent of dissection might be underestimated by angiography, especially if the entry point has been sealed by stenting. Management of aortic dissection after PCI remains controversial. Dunning et al.[3] summarized the results from 9 patients and suggested that patients might be managed by coronary artery stenting if the dissection extends less than 40 mm from the coronary ostium and that surgical intervention might be required if the dissection extends beyond 40 mm from the ostium.

References

1. Pérez-Castellano N, García-Fernández MA, García EJ, Delcán JL. Dissection of the aortic sinus of Valsalva complicating coronary catheterization: cause, mechanism, evolution, and management. *Cathet Cardiovasc Diagn.* 1998;43:273-279.
2. Yip HK, Wu CJ, Yeh KH, et al. Unusual complication of retrograde dissection to the coronary sinus of Valsalva during percutaneous revascularization: a single-center experience and literature review. *Chest.* 2001;119:493-501.
3. Dunning DW, Kahn JK, Hawkins ET, O'Neill WW. Iatrogenic coronary artery dissections extending into and involving the aortic root. *Catheter Cardiovasc Interv.* 2000;51:387-393.

Catheter-Induced Stent Occlusion: An Uncommon Complication During Diagnostic Angiography

Shinichi Furuichi, MD, Yoshifumi Sasamori, CE, Takeichi Yamaji, RT, Toshiya Satoh, MD

A 76-year-old man with cardiac risk factors of hypertension and smoking was referred to our hospital for elective follow-up angiography because he was due to undergo carotid artery stenting. Sirolimus-eluting stents had been implanted in the mid to proximal portion of the right coronary artery 3 years previously. Control angiography showed minimal neointimal proliferation inside the stents (Fig. 2.27A). Immediately after the first injection, the catheter pressure fell and the patient reported chest pain. Further angiography demonstrated an occlusion of the stent with a radiolucent dissection flap inside the stent (Fig. 2.27B); consequently, we performed bailout emergency angioplasty. After guidewire placement, Thrombolysis In Myocardial Infarction grade flow 3 was restored

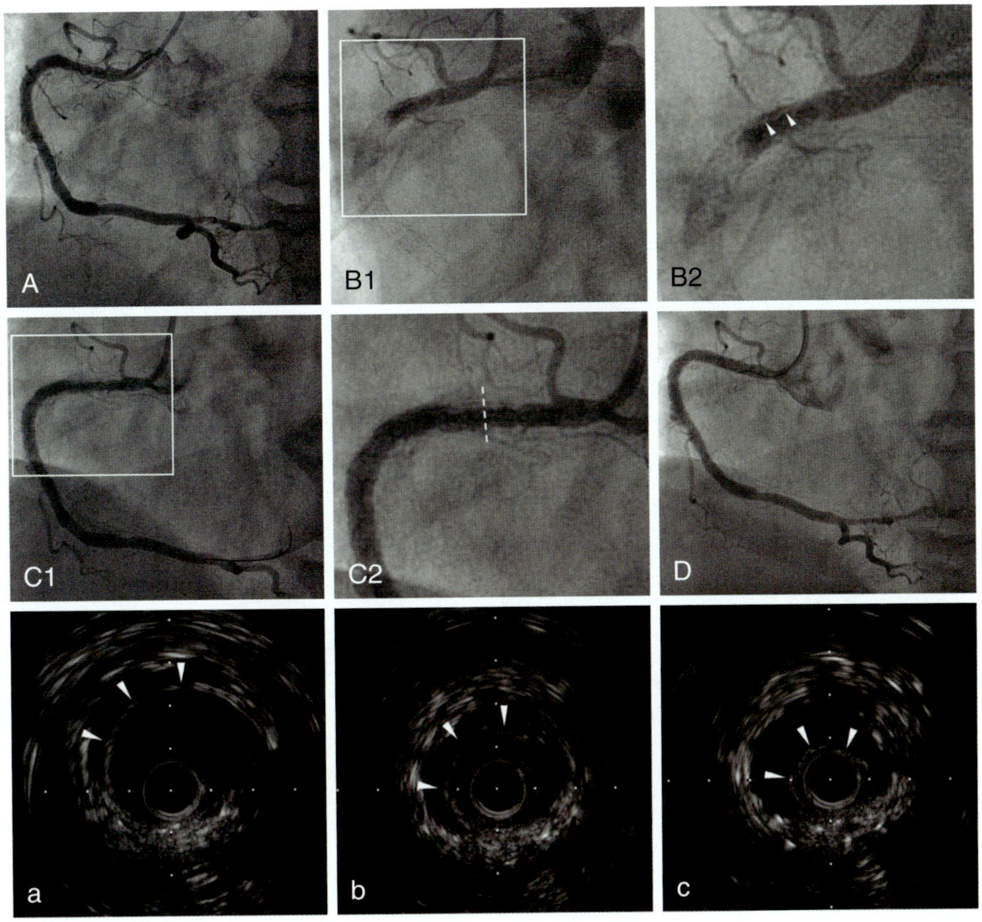

FIG. 2.27 Angiography and Intravascular Ultrasonography. (A) Baseline angiography. (B1 and B2) Angiography showing acute stent occlusion. (C1 and C2) Angiography after guidewire placement. (D) Final angiography. Intravascular ultrasonography showing neointimal dissection flap (a–c, *arrowheads*) inside the stent with a transiently compromised true lumen by the dissection flap (c) (Online Video 2.11).

(Fig. 2.27C). To evaluate the cause of the occlusion, intravascular ultrasound was performed. Intravascular ultrasound with saline solution injection through the guiding catheter revealed a neointimal dissection flap inside the stent with a transiently compromised true lumen by the dissection flap (Fig. 2.27a–c and Online Video 2.11). The dissection flat originated only from within the stent and started from the proximal edge of the stent where the catheter tip had been positioned during the first injection. Another sirolimus-eluting stent was implanted to seal the entire dissection plane, and final angiography showed a good result (Fig. 2.27D).

Extraordinary Subintimal Bleeding After Coronary Stenting

Sei Komatsu, MD, Tomoki Ohara, MD, Satoru Takahashi, MD, Mitsuhiko Takewa, MD, Chikao Yutani, MD, Kazuhisa Kodama, MD

A 76-year-old man underwent coronary angiography to treat unstable angina with rest angina for a week. Imaging showed a severe stenosis in the middle of left circumflex artery (Fig. 2.28A, *arrow*). Percutaneous coronary intervention was performed using a 3.0 × 15 mm Xience V stent (Abbott Vascular, Santa Clara, California), with subsequent predilation using a 3.0 × 15 mm Trek balloon (Abbott Vascular) (Fig. 2.28B). Coronary angiography did not show aneurysmal formation or dissection proximal to the stented site (Fig. 2.28B, *arrow*). Nonobstructive angioscopy revealed yellow intima at the proximal edge of the stent (Fig. 2.28C).

The yellow surface then suddenly changed to wide subintimal bloody staining with some branches like flames (Fig. 2.28C–D, Online Video 2.12) and pulsated flows (Fig. 2.28E–F, *arrows*). They did not communicate with the coronary blood flow. The irregular subintimal arterial bleeding might be related to injury of plaque smaller than the detection limit of intravascular ultrasound images because they did not reveal a slit or dissection (Fig. 2.28G–H).

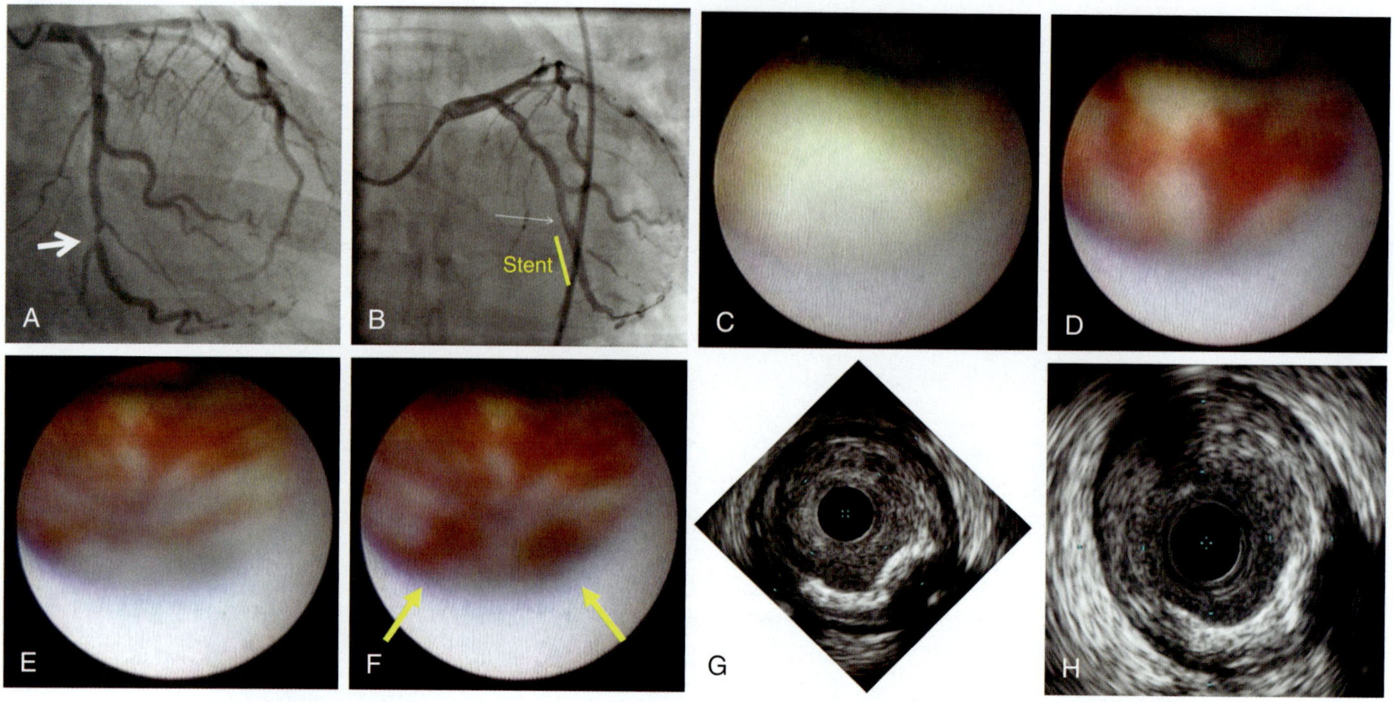

FIG. 2.28 Coronary Angiography Imaging. Coronary angiography images before (A) and after (B) percutaneous coronary intervention. Angioscopic image just proximal of the stent without (C) and with (D) wide subintimal bleeding (Online Video 2.12), and without (E) and with (F) pulsated flow. Intravascular ultrasound images of corresponded site for bleeding before (G) and after (H) intervention.

Index and Follow-Up Optical Coherence Tomography Imaging Demonstrating Resolution of Poststent Intramural Hematoma Managed Conservatively

Ashish Shah, MD, Anirban Choudhury, MD, Richard A. Anderson, MBBS BSC, MD

A 46-year-old man presented with non−ST-segment elevation myocardial infarction. Electrocardiography showed new T-wave inversion in the inferior leads. Coronary angiography demonstrated a severe lesion in the proximal right coronary artery (RCA) (Fig. 2.29A–B).

Immediately after implantation of 4.5 × 16 mm bare-metal stent, there was no flow down the RCA (Fig. 2.29C). The vessel just beyond the stent was dilated, and another 4.5 × 12 mm bare-metal stent was implanted. Flow was reestablished, but there was a residual long segment of moderate luminal narrowing with smooth edges. Angiographic suggestion of a possible intramural hematoma (IH) (Fig. 2.29D–F) was confirmed by intracoronary optical coherence tomography (Fig. 2.30A–B). The patient was treated conservatively and underwent check angiography 5 weeks later, which demonstrated angiographic resolution (Fig. 2.31A) confirmed by optical coherence tomography (Fig. 2.31B).

IH is defined as blood collection within the media, displacing the internal and external elastic membranes, with or without identifiable entry or exit points.[1] IH occurs more often in patients with diabetes and those with less advanced coronary disease, in de novo eccentric lesions, and in the RCA. There are no existing treatment guidelines, but in a follow-up study of patients with IH, there were more non−ST-segment elevation myocardial infarctions and revascularizations within 1 month in those managed conservatively, whereas more revascularization and deaths from 1 to 12 months occurred in those treated with stenting.[2] This case illustrates the course of IH with conservative treatment.

References

1. Mintz GS, Nissen SE, Anderson WD, et al. American College of Cardiology clinical expert consensus document on standards for acquisition, measurement and reporting of intravascular ultrasound studies (IVUS). A report of the American College of Cardiology Task Force on Clinical Expert Consensus Documents. *J Am Coll Cardiol.* 2001;37:1478-1492.
2. Maehara A, Mintz GS, Bui AB, et al. Incidence, morphology, angiographic findings, and outcomes of intramural hematomas after percutaneous coronary interventions: an intravascular ultrasound study. *Circulation.* 2002;105:2037-2042.

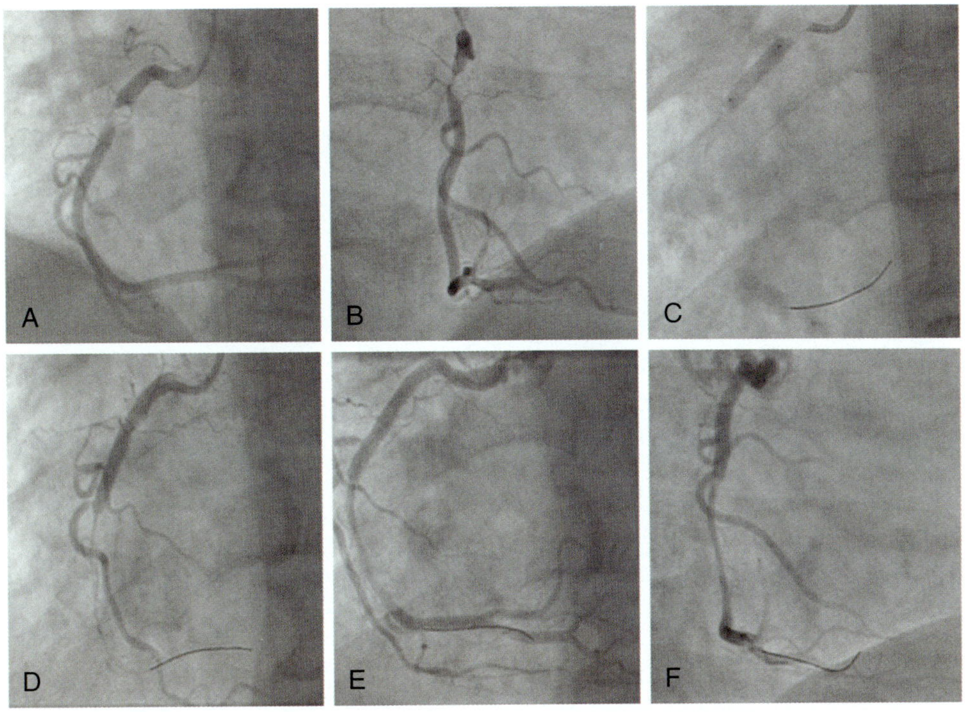

FIG. 2.29 Index Procedure. Angiography images before stenting (A and B), during stenting (C), immediately after stenting (D), and by the end of the procedure (E and F) showing a newer long segment of luminal narrowing with smooth edges, which improved with time.

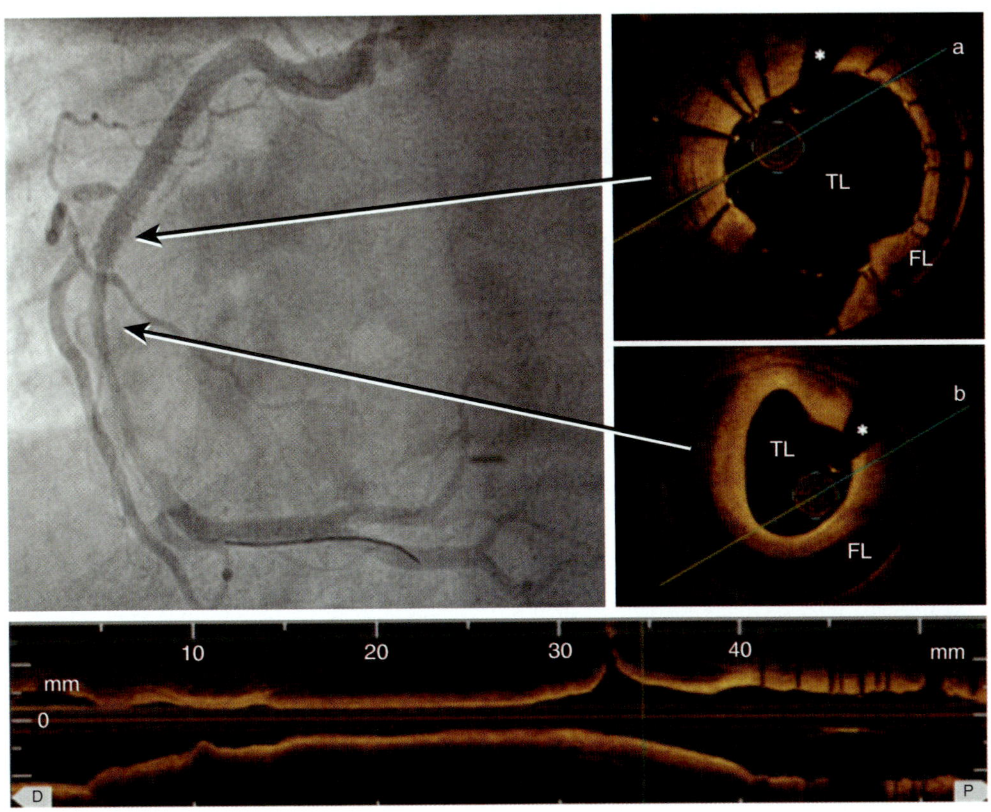

FIG. 2.30 Optical Coherence Tomography Demonstrating the Lesion Pathology. Optical coherence tomography showing intima media separation from the adventia by an intramural hematoma. The *asterisks* indicate wire artifacts. *FL*, false lumen; *TL*, true lumen.

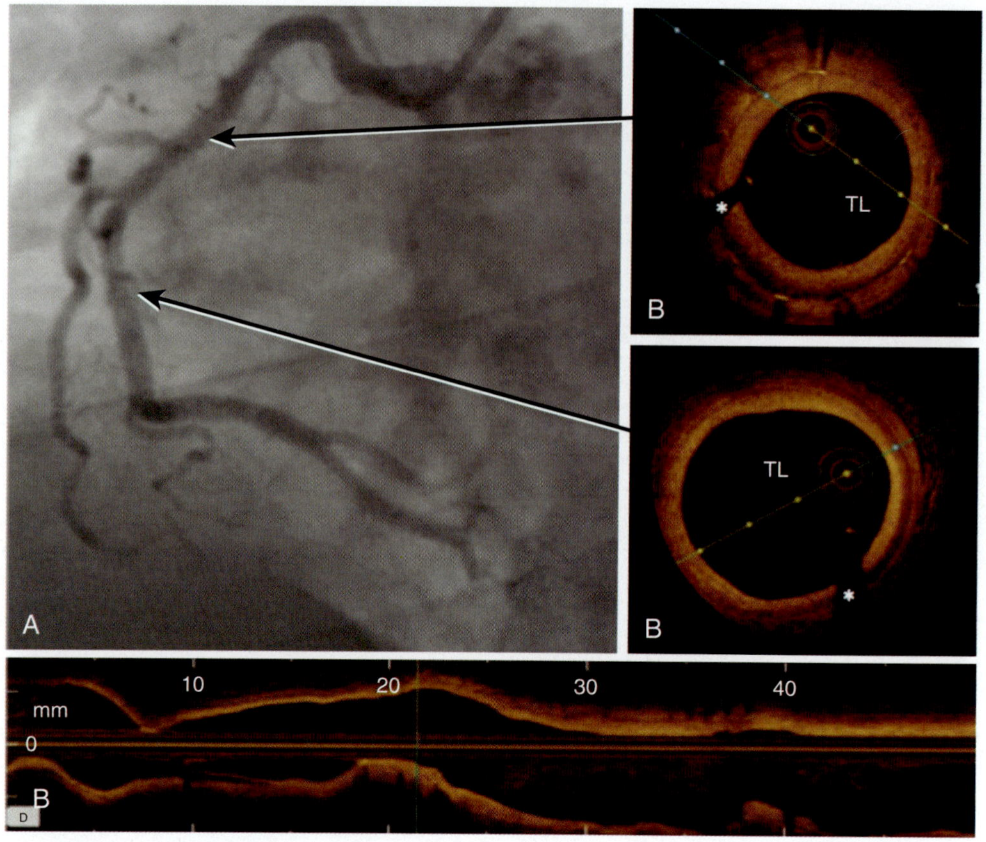

FIG. 2.31 5 Weeks Post-Index Procedure. Angiography (A) and optical coherence tomography (B) demonstrated hematoma resorption and well-apposed stent struts. The *asterisks* indicate wire artifacts. *TL*, true lumen.

In-Stent Dissection Causes No Flow During Percutaneous Coronary Intervention

Fumiaki Yashima, MD, Shinsuke Yuasa, MD, PhD, Yuichiro Maekawa, MD, PhD, Mai Kimura, MD, PhD, Keitaro Akita, MD, Ryo Yanagisawa, MD, Makoto Tanaka, MD, Kentaro Hayashida, MD, PhD, Takashi Kawakami, MD, Hideaki Kanazawa, MD, PhD, Jun Fujita, MD, PhD, Keiichi Fukuda, MD, PhD

A 71-year-old woman with chest pain consulted us 1 week after an emergent operation for a small intestine perforation. She had previously undergone percutaneous coronary intervention (PCI) twice for the left anterior descending artery. The first was performed with a bare-metal stent 5 years earlier, and the second was performed for in-stent restenosis (ISR) treated with a biolimus A9–eluting stent. Angiography revealed 99% restenosis at the same location as that of the previous in-stent restenosis (Fig. 2.32A, Online Video 2.13); therefore PCI was performed. Immediately after initial dilation using a semicompliant 2.0-mm balloon, the coronary flow abruptly disappeared (Fig. 2.32B, Online Video 2.14). The slow-flow/no-reflow phenomenon is associated with myocardial injury, less favorable clinical outcomes, and generally with microthromboemboli. Despite standard treatments such as manual thrombus aspiration and intracoronary vasodilator administration, we could not reestablish coronary flow. To determine the mechanism underlying the no flow, we performed intravascular ultrasound testing, which did not reveal the cause of the no flow (Fig. 2.32D–E, Online Video 2.15). We then performed optical coherence tomography, which clearly showed a dissection within the previous stent (Fig. 2.32F–H, Online Video 2.16). Subsequent dilation by a cutting balloon reestablished coronary flow (Fig. 2.32I, Online Video 2.17). We speculated that neoatherosclerosis within the stent caused the restenosis, and the initial dilation induced a dissection that caused occlusion and resulted in no flow. This report is the first to show that in-stent dissection can cause no flow during PCI and that optical coherence tomography would uncover the mechanism.

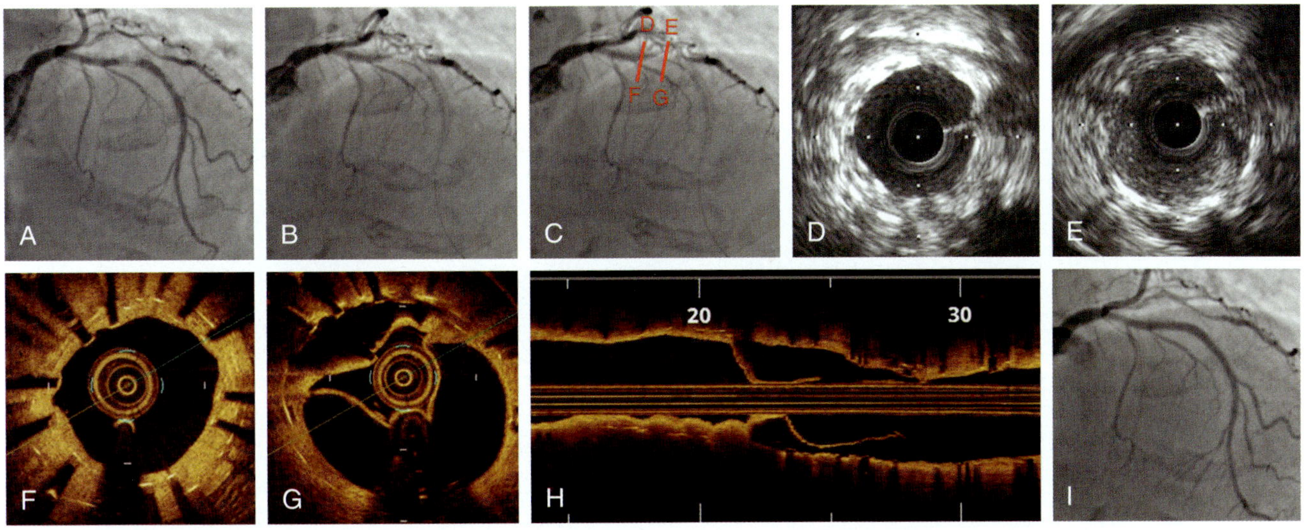

FIG. 2.32 Angiography, Intravascular Ultrasound (IVUS), and Optical Coherence Tomography (OCT) Images. (A) Angiography before percutaneous coronary intervention (Online Video 2.13). (B) No flow after initial dilation (Online Video 2.14). (C) The locations of IVUS/OCT images. (D and E) IVUS images showing the locations in (C) (Online Video 2.15). (F and G) OCT cross-sectional images showing the locations in (C) (Online Video 2.16). (H) OCT longitudinal image. (I) Final angiography (Online Video 2.17).

Intimomedial Abrasion Complicating Coronary Thrombus Aspiration

Milosz Jaguszewski, MD, PhD, Brunilda Alushi, MD, PhD, Leif-Christopher Engel, MD, Juan Luis Gutiérrez-Chico, MD, PhD

A 73-year-old man referred for primary percutaneous coronary intervention had complete occlusion of the proximal left anterior descending artery (LAD) (Online Video 2.18). Aspiration thrombectomy was performed with an Export AP catheter (forward-facing tip, 1.09-mm inner lumen diameter, 1.73-mm outer diameter; Medtronic Cardiovascular, Santa Rosa, California), thus removing a red thrombus (Fig. 2.33) and restoring distal Thrombolysis In Myocardial Infarction flow grade 3. Milking (i.e., muscular bridge) was then observed in the mid-LAD (Online Video 2.19). After stent implantation in the proximal LAD, the ST-segment leveled out and chest pain remitted. However, 5 minutes later and before sheath removal, chest pain relapsed with transient recurrent ST-segment reelevations. Repeat angiography found only a slightly hazy region around the milking segment (Online Video 2.20). Optical coherence tomography (OCT) revealed an intracoronary structure proximal to the milking segment, with high optical backscattering and low attenuation, attached to the vessel wall by a filiform proximal pedicle (Fig. 2.34A–B) in direct continuity with a proximal intimomedial abrasion (Fig. 2.35). These OCT findings suggested the intracoronary mass to be a pediculated intimomedial flap versus a white thrombus as the differential diagnosis; therefore a second careful aspiration was performed and the mass was successfully removed (Fig. 2.33). A final OCT scan confirmed removal and absence of new iatrogenic lesions (Fig. 2.35C). Milking shows a regular oval shape of the 3 vascular layers in the first pullback (obtained in systole) (Fig. 2.36A), absent in the corresponding matched cross sections in the second pullback (obtained in diastole) (Fig. 2.36B).

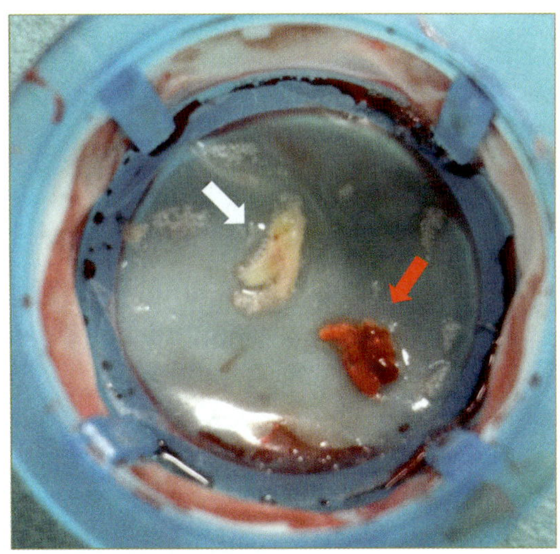

FIG. 2.33 Macroscopic Appearance of the Specimens Harvested in the Aspiration Thrombectomy. Red thrombus aspirated during primary percutaneous coronary intervention of a proximal left anterior descending artery (LAD) (*red arrow*); intimomedial flap aspirated from the mid-LAD after abrasion during thrombectomy (*white arrow*) (Online Video 2.18).

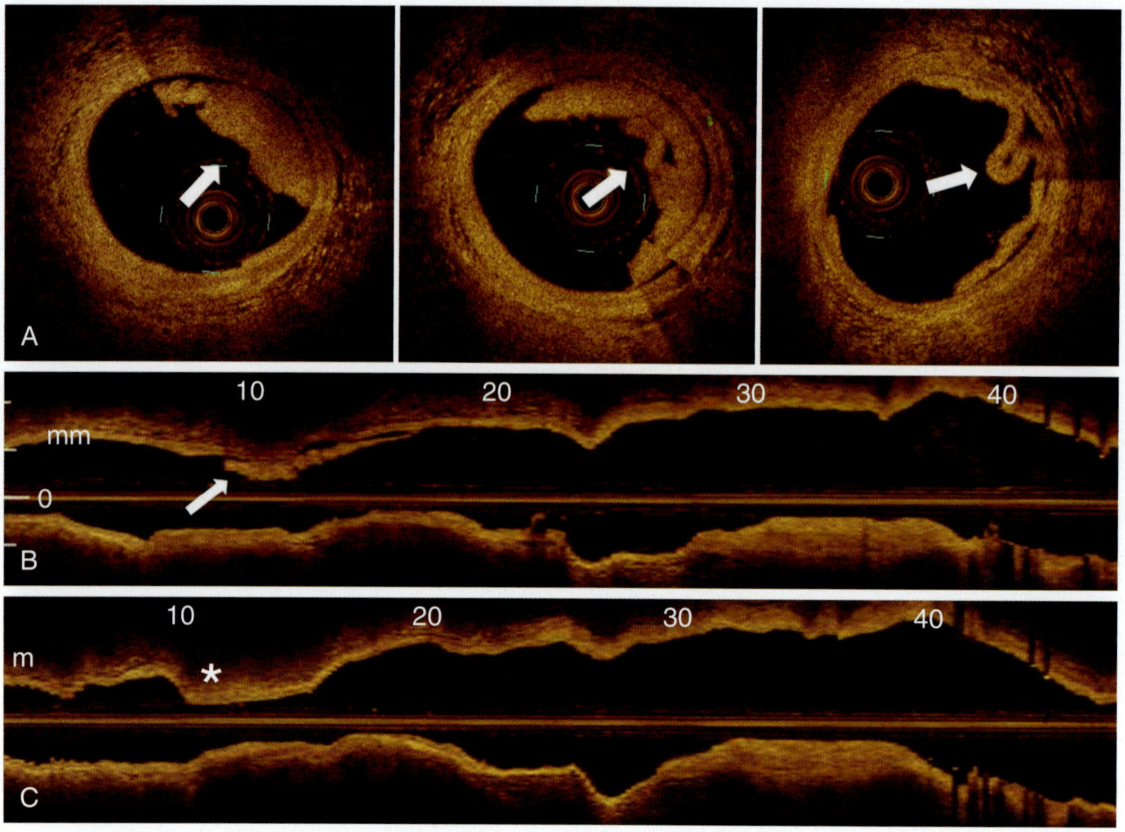

FIG. 2.34 Intimomedial Flap Detected in the Optical Coherence Tomography (OCT) Pullback. Intimomedial flap on OCT ([A], [B], *white arrow*). (C) OCT image of the same coronary segment after removal of the flap; notice the milking phenomenon in systole (*asterisk*). *m*, media.

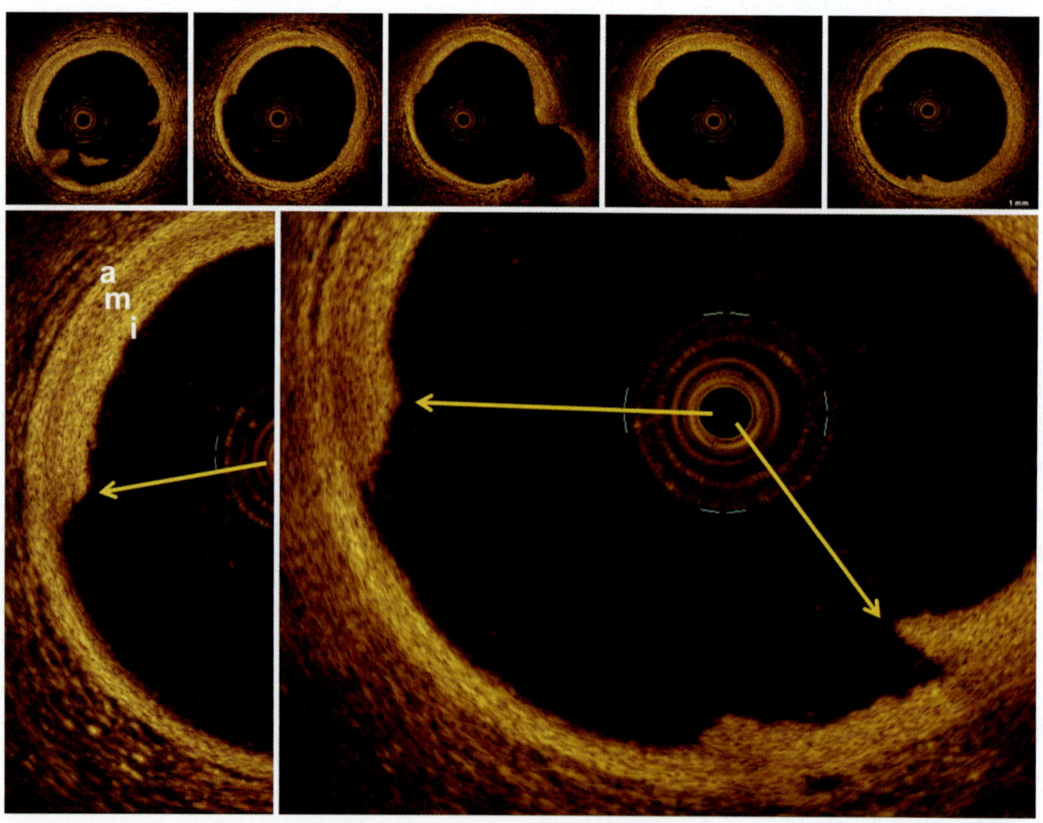

FIG. 2.35 Intimomedial Abrasion in a Coronary Sector After Aspiration Thrombectomy. Note the 3 vascular layers in the noninjured sector: intima (*i*), media (*m*), and adventitia (*a*), whereas in the injured sector, only 1 medioadventitial layer is seen (Online Video 2.19).

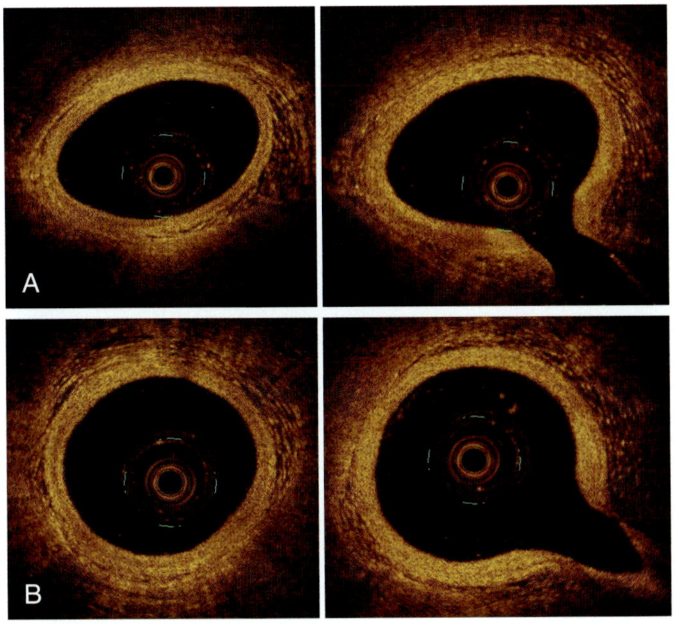

FIG. 2.36 Milking Phenomenon (i.e., Muscular Bridge) as Observed in Optical Coherence Tomography. Matched cross sections of a coronary segment with the milking phenomenon imaged during systole (A) and diastole (B) (Online Video 2.20). *a,* adventitia; *i,* intima; *m,* media.

The optical properties of the intraluminal mass and the clinical course strongly suggest an intimomedial flap abraded during thrombectomy, attached to the wall by a distal filiform endothelial pedicle, and everted distally into the lumen. This flap might cause recurrent transient ischemia via a valvular mechanism. A white thrombus might have a similar macroscopic appearance and optical properties,[1,2] but the relatively regular contour and the thickness gradient (thicker distally than proximally) do not support this differential diagnosis. Milking might have increased the risk of intimomedial abrasion as the result of the dynamic reduction of the vessel caliber (Fig. 2.34B–C).

References

1. Kume T, Akasaka T, Kawamoto T, et al. Assessment of coronary arterial thrombus by optical coherence tomography. *Am J Cardiol.* 2006;97:1713-1717.
2. Tearney GJ, Regar E, Akasaka T, et al. Consensus standards for acquisition, measurement, and reporting of intravascular optical coherence tomography studies: a report from the International Working Group for Intravascular Optical Coherence Tomography Standardization and Validation. *J Am Coll Cardiol.* 2012;59:1058-1072.

Rapid Growth of Giant Coronary Artery Aneurysm After Treatment of Stent Edge Dissection

Reiko Shiomura, MD, Nobuaki Kobayashi, MD, PhD, Noritake Hata, MD, PhD, Wataru Shimizu, MD, PhD

A 73-year-old man with diabetes mellitus, hypertension, chronic renal failure, and prior myocardial infarction was admitted with acute non–ST-segment elevation myocardial infarction. Coronary angiography (CAG) showed severe stenosis at the ostial left main trunk and the proximal left circumflex artery (Fig. 2.37A, Online Video 2.21). We decided to perform percutaneous coronary intervention using a T-stent technique. Intravascular ultrasound imaging after stenting (Xience Xpedition 3.5 × 18 mm [Abbott Vascular, Santa Clara, California]) for the proximal left anterior descending coronary artery to the left main trunk and Xience Xpedition 3.0 × 18 mm for the proximal left circumflex coronary artery) revealed a coronary dissection and intramural hematoma at the distal edge of the left anterior descending coronary artery stent (Fig. 2.37B, Online Video 2.22). After additional stenting (Xience Xpedition 2.5 × 23 mm) from the distal edge of the left anterior descending coronary artery stent, final CAG revealed optimal luminal dilation without flow limitation (Fig. 2.37C, Online Video 2.23). Final intravascular ultrasound imaging showed that the dissection was fully covered by the additional stent, without any gaps (Fig. 2.37D, Online Video 2.24).

Ten days after the procedure, the patient reported severe chest pain. Repeated CAG showed a giant coronary artery aneurysm (12.7 × 14.6 mm; calculated by quantitative CAG) causing a flow limitation at the site of the treated dissection (Fig. 2.37E, Online Video 2.25). Computed tomography (Fig. 2.37F) revealed a stent gap at the site of the aneurysm. As a result, the patient underwent coronary artery bypass grafting and aneurysm repair (aneurysmorrhaphy). The possible mechanism responsible for the rapid growth of this giant coronary artery aneurysm was the treated stent edge dissection, and the aneurysm may have caused the early stent fracture.

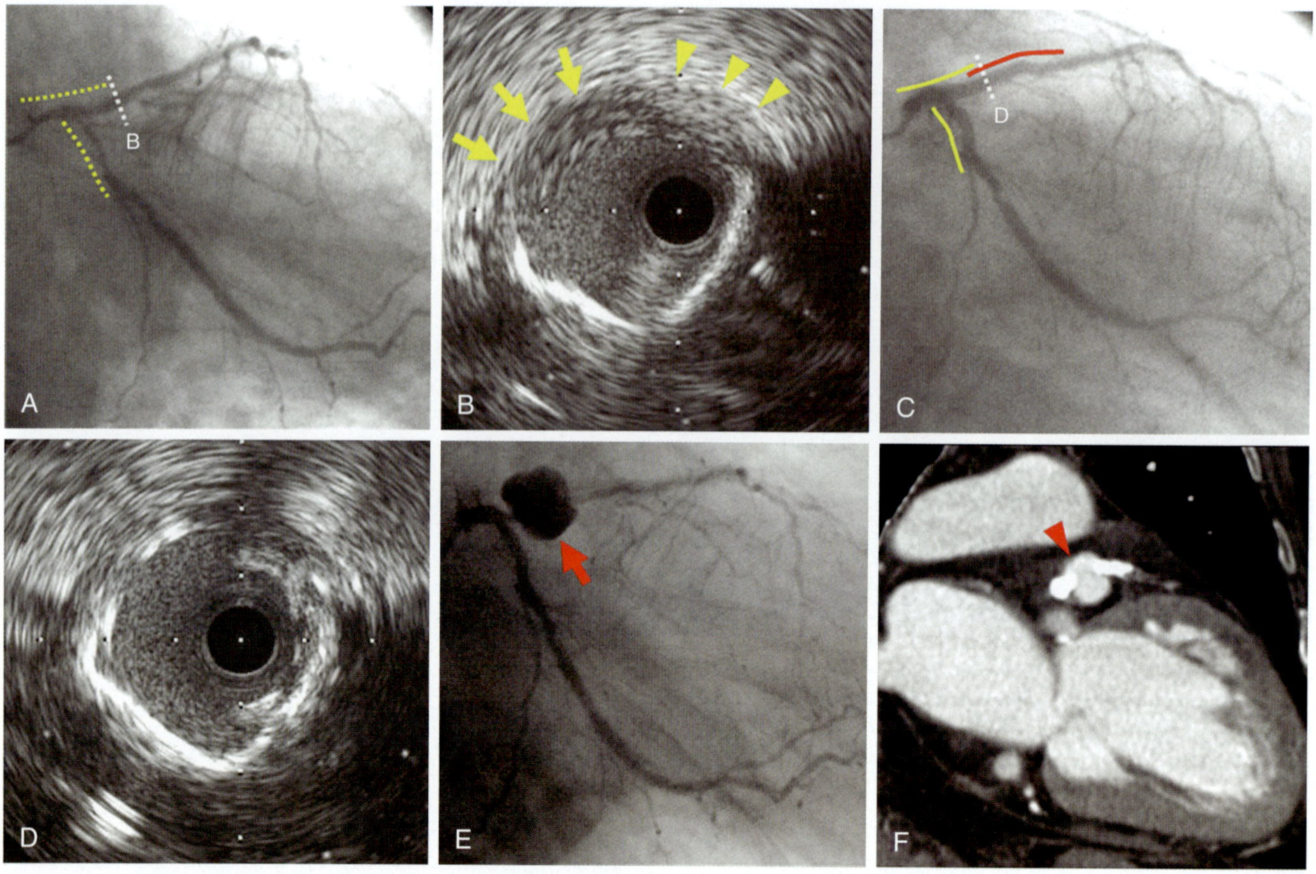

FIG. 2.37 Multiple Imaging Modalities for the Left Anterior Descending Coronary Artery. (A) Initial coronary angiography (CAG) showing severe stenosis at the ostial left main trunk and the proximal left circumflex coronary artery. The *yellow dotted lines* indicate the initial stenting strategy (see Online Video 2.21). (B) Intravascular ultrasound (IVUS) image of the left anterior descending coronary artery (LAD) after stenting, showing the distal edge dissection reaching the media (*yellow arrows*) and intramural hematoma (*yellow arrowheads*) (see Online Video 2.22). (C) Final CAG showing optimal luminal dilation. The *solid lines* represent the implanted stents (see Online Video 2.23). (D) Final IVUS image showing the stent edge dissection fully covered by an additional stent (see Online Video 2.24). (E) Repeat CAG 10 days after the procedure, showing rapid growth of coronary aneurysm (*red arrow*) at the site of the dissection that was treated with additional stenting (see Online Video 2.25). (F) Computed tomography showing a stent gap at the site of the aneurysm (*red arrowhead*).

Coronary Perforations

Respect the Septal Perforator: Septal Artery Perforation During CTO PCI Resulting in Massive Interventricular Septal Hematoma and Biventricular Cardiac Obstructive Shock

Tiberio M. Frisoli, MD, Majed Afana, MD, Sagger Mawri, MD, Mazen Hadid, MD, Luay Sayed, MD, William W. O'Neill, MD, Dee Dee Wang, MD, Sachin Parikh, MD, Akshay Khandelwal, MD, Khaldoon Alaswad, MD

A 70-year-old man with debilitating refractory angina underwent percutaneous coronary intervention of a right coronary artery chronic total occlusion. Previous echocardiogram showed normal biventricular function with an interventricular septum (IVS) diameter of 1.0 cm. Through a microcatheter several hydrophobic and hydrophilic wires were used in the left anterior descending septal perforator coronary arteries to attempt passage, unsuccessfully, into the right coronary artery. Angiography showed septal perforation (Online Video 2.26). An echocardiogram after the procedure showed massive IVS thickening (4.1 cm) (Fig. 2.38).

The patient was transferred to our institution in cardiogenic shock. Right heart catheterization revealed left heart failure (pulmonary capillary wedge pressure 24 mm Hg, cardiac index 1.3 L/min per meter squared) and right heart failure (pulmonary artery pulsatility index 1.13, right atrial pressure/pulmonary capillary wedge pressure ratio 0.75).

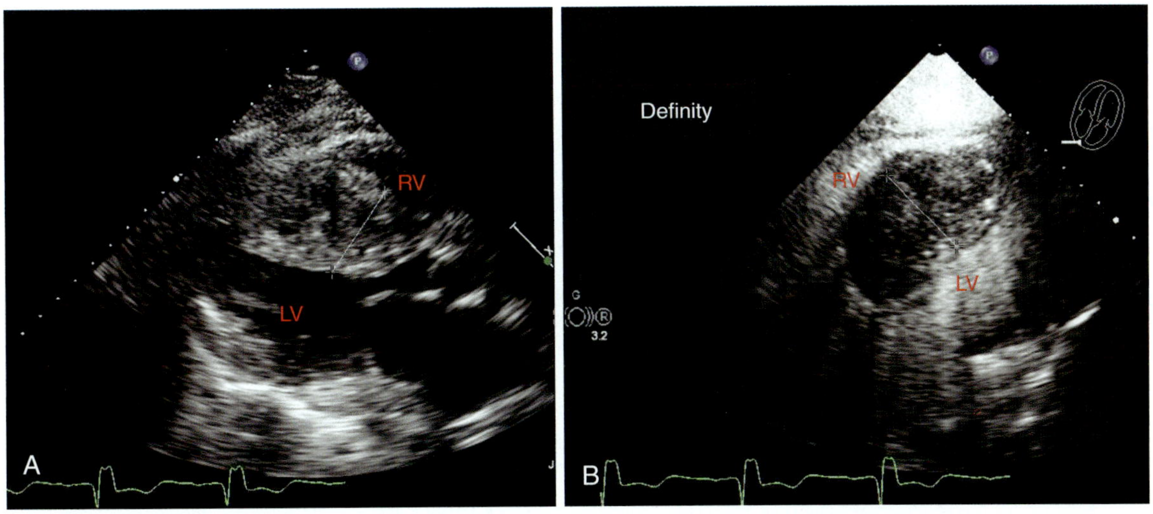

FIG. 2.38 Interventricular Septum (IVS) Hematoma. (A) Parasternal long-axis views shows IVS hematoma. (B) Apical four-chamber view with contrast for endocardial border delineation shows IVS hematoma roughly 4 cm in width. *LV*, left ventricle; *RV*, right ventricle. See Online Videos 2.26 and 2.27.

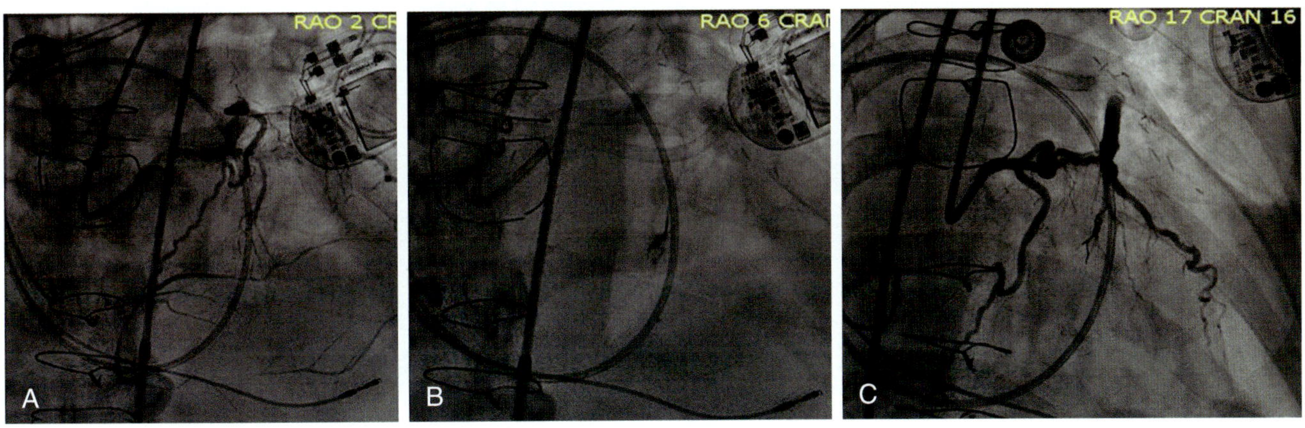

FIG. 2.39 Septal Coiling Intervention. (A) Initial angiogram during septal coiling intervention. (B) Angiogram through microcatheter in culprit septal perforator. (C) Coiling of septal perforator with four VortX-18 coils (Boston Scientific, Natick, Massachusetts).

Coil embolization of the culprit septal artery was performed (Fig. 2.39). Despite right-sided tandem heart implantation, the patient remained in cardiogenic shock (cardiac index 1.4, left ventricular end-diastolic pressure 30 mm Hg); therefore a left-sided Impella device (Abiomed, Danvers, Massachusetts) was placed. Frequent Impella suction alarm events and progressive cardiogenic shock prompted escalation to venoarterial extracorporeal membrane oxygenation, which allowed off-titration of high-dose vasopressor medications. The patient died 10 days later of multiorgan failure. Transesophageal echocardiography on extracorporeal membrane oxygenation before the patient's death illustrates the sheer size of the IVS hematoma—its heterogeneous core, likely to represent blood and necrotic tissue; the compressive effect on the right ventricle and left ventricle sufficient to greatly impair filling; and the IVS dyskinesis and its contribution to low output (Online Video 2.27).

IVS hematoma is associated with morbidity after coronary artery bypass grafting,[1] chest trauma,[2] surgical ventricular septal defect closure,[3] and myocardial infarction.[4] Although septal wire perforations can often be treated conservatively,[5] device perforations, as with a microcatheter, likely deserve closer surveillance and lower threshold for early intervention. Septal perforation yielding IVS hematoma sufficient to cause biventricular obstructive shock has not been reported.

Percutaneous coronary intervention procedures for chronic total occlusion are becoming more prevalent; complications such as this may increase and should be brought to awareness.

References

1. Ettles DF, Firth N, Nair RU, Williams GJ. Fatal acute left ventricular outflow obstruction due to interventricular septal haematoma–diagnosis by transoesophageal echocardiography. *Eur Heart J.* 1989;10:479-481.
2. Tejada Artigas A, Laperal Mur JR, Calvo Cebollero I, Fernández González B, González Manzanares JL, Placer Peralta L. Contusion and post-traumatic hematoma of the interventricular septum. *Rev Esp Cardiol.* 1992;45:663-664.
3. Jensen R, Burg P, Anderson C, et al. Post-operative ventricular septal hematoma: natural history of two pediatric cases. *J Thorac Cardiovasc Surg.* 2007;133:1651-1652.
4. Pliam MB, Sternlieb JJ. Intramyocardial dissecting hematoma: an unusual form of subacute cardiac rupture. *J Card Surg.* 1993;8:628-637.
5. Fairley SL, Donnelly PM, Hanratty CG, Walsh SJ. Images in cardiovascular medicine. Interventricular septal hematoma and ventricular septal defect after retrograde intervention for a chronic total occlusion of a left anterior descending coronary artery. *Circulation.* 2010;122:e518-e521.

Right Ventricular Free Wall Hematoma: Contemporary Multimodal Imaging

M. Fuad Jan, MBBS, MD, Suhail Allaqaband, MD, Khawaja Afzal Ammar, MD, Sara Fetke, APNP, A. Jamil Tajik, MD

Successful percutaneous coronary intervention (PCI) was performed on a 75-year-old woman for an inferior ST-segment elevation myocardial infarction (Fig. 2.40A–B, Online Videos 2.28 and 2.29). Persistent staining of contrast material (Fig 2.40C, Online Videos 2.30 and 2.31) after PCI prompted emergent transthoracic echocardiography (TTE) in the catheterization laboratory to rule out pericardial effusion. TTE revealed a small intramural base-to-mid right ventricular free wall hematoma (RVFWH). The latter progressively increased in size (maximal size, 4 × 2.4 cm) over the next few days to become bilobed, but with no communication with the RV cavity (Fig. 2.40D–G, Online Videos 2.32–2.36). Multimodality imaging with computed tomography (Fig. 2.40H) and magnetic

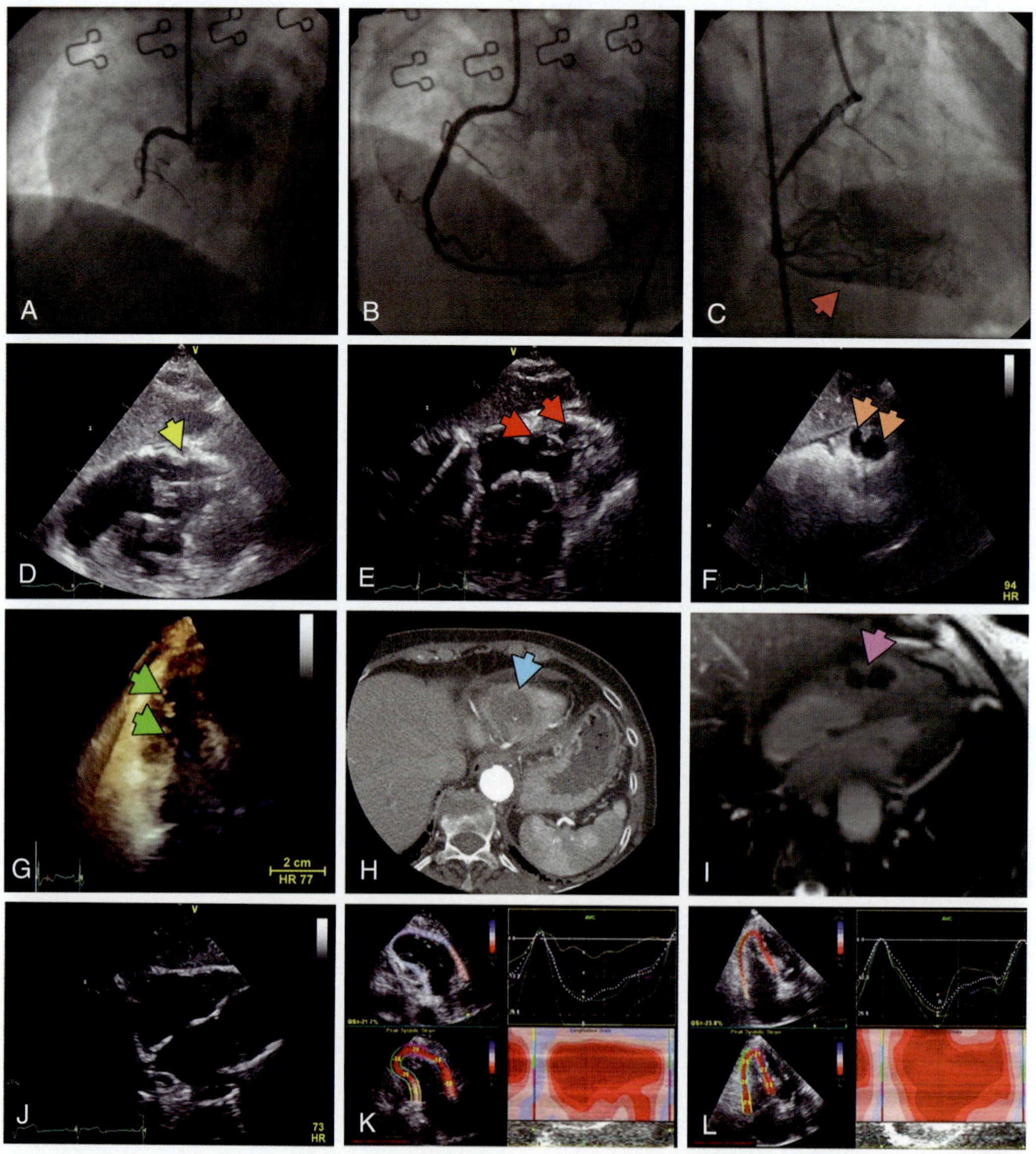

FIG. 2.40 Multimodal Imaging of a Right Ventricular Free Wall Hematoma After Percutaneous Coronary Intervention (PCI) for an Acute Myocardial Infarction. (A) Complete occlusion Thrombolysis In Myocardial Infarction (TIMI grade flow 0) of the right coronary artery followed by restoration of the TIMI grade flow 3 (B, Online Videos 2.28 and 2.29). (C) Persistent staining (*arrowhead*) (Online Videos 2.30 and 2.31) led to emergent transthoracic echocardiography that demonstrated an area of hemorrhagic transformation in the RV free wall (*arrowhead*) (D) that progressively increased in size (*arrowheads*) (E–G, Online Videos 2.32–2.36). (H–I) Computed tomography and magnetic resonance imaging of the heart performed on days 3 and 5 after PCI (Online Video 2.37) confirmed the hemorrhagic transformation in the RV free wall. (J) Nearly complete resolution of the RV hematoma at 8 weeks (Online Video 2.38); note also the reduced peak systolic strain of the right ventricle on day 3 after PCI (−5%) (K) and its resurgence 8 weeks after development of the hematoma (−25%) (L, Online Video 2.32). *PCI*, percutaneous coronary intervention; *RV*, right ventricular.

resonance imaging (Fig. 2.40I, Online Video 2.37) confirmed the diagnosis of RVFWH. Repeat TTE 2 months later showed nearly complete resolution of the RVFWH (Fig. 2.40J, Online Video 2.38) with excellent recovery of peak systolic strain of the right ventricle (from −5% to −25%) (Fig. 2.40K–L, Online Video 2.32).

Postinfarction intramyocardial hemorrhage/hematoma (involving either the right or left ventricle) after PCI for ST-segment elevation myocardial infarction is a singular event. The incidence and natural history after PCI in the contemporary era are unknown. Reperfusion post-PCI in the distressed endothelium is likely followed by a complex cascade of events culminating in increased matrix metalloproteinase concentrations, providing a ripe bed for the development of intramyocardial hemorrhage. No comparative studies exist on the best imaging modality to optimize identification of a postinfarction intramyocardial hematoma. Multimodality cardiac imaging as delineated can be useful for both diagnosis and risk stratification.

Severe Intramyocardial Hematoma as a Complication of Retrograde Approach in Chronic Total Occlusion

Rebeca Lorca, MD, Isaac Pascual, MD, PhD, Alfonso Suarez-Cuervo, MD, María Martín, MD, PhD, Juan Calvo, MD, PhD, Cecilia Corros, MD, Helena Cigarrán, MD, Pablo Avanzas, MD, PhD, Daniel Hernández-Vaquero, MD, PhD, César Morís, MD, PhD

Interventricular septal hematoma is a rare but potentially dangerous complication of retrograde chronic total occlusion (CTO) percutaneous coronary interventions (PCI).[1,2]

A 58-year-old man was referred for right coronary artery CTO-PCI performed by a retrograde approach via the collateral septal artery (Fig. 2.41A–B). The procedure was successful, although a little contrast "stain" was visualized surrounding the collateral septal (Fig. 2.41C, Online Video 2.39). Two hours later, he had chest pain with ST-segment elevation, hypotension, and tachycardia. Emergent coronary angiography ruled out both stent occlusion and progression of the contrast stain.

An impressive interventricular septal hematoma (5 × 3.9 cm) was found on echocardiogram (Fig. 2.41D, Online Video 2.40), with a mass effect producing left ventricular outflow tract obstruction. This could explain both the symptoms and hemodynamic situation. To complete the study computed tomography angiography and cardiac magnetic resonance imaging (Fig. 2.41E–H) were performed later.

Three days after monitoring and strictly controlled medical treatment in the coronary unit, the clinical situation improved, the hematoma diminished, and left ventricular outflow tract obstruction disappeared.

This severe intramyocardial hematoma as the result of a retrograde CTO-PCI complication, with functional repercussions, was successfully managed with a conservative approach.

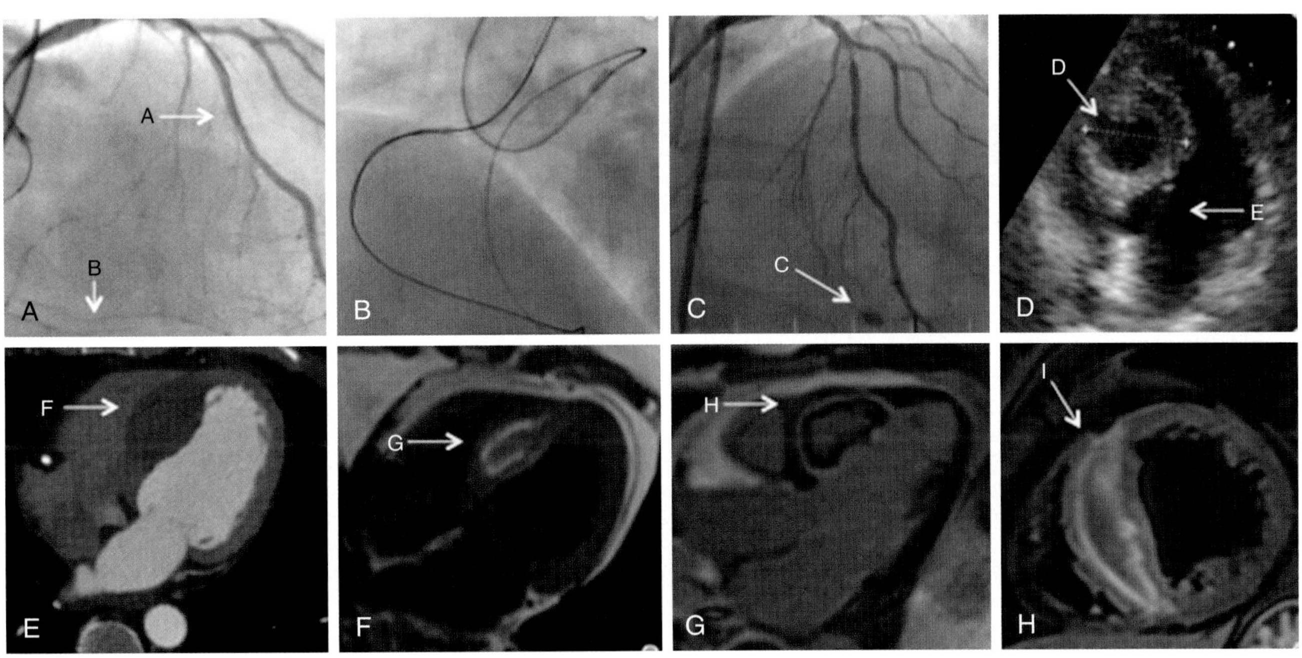

FIG. 2.41 Cardiac Imaging Techniques. (A) Left anterior descending artery (*arrow A*) supplying septal collaterals (*arrow B*) to the right coronary artery, with a chronic total occlusion. (B) Successful retrograde wire crossing. (C) Septal collateral perforation (*arrow C*) visualized with right coronary angiography (Online Video 2.39). (D) Interventricular septal hematoma (*arrow D*) visualized in echocardiogram (Online Video 2.40), producing a mass effect that interferes with the flow in the left ventricular outflow tract (*arrow E*). (E) Interventricular septal hematoma shown on cardiac computed tomography (*arrow F*). (F–H) Interventricular septal hematoma shown by T1 cardiac magnetic resonance (*arrow G*), late gadolinium enhancement (*arrow H*), and T2 fat saturation (*arrow I*).

References

1. Fairley SL, Donnelly PM, Hanratty CG, Walsh SJ. Images in cardiovascular medicine. Interventricular septal hematoma and ventricular septal defect after retrograde intervention for a chronic total occlusion of a left anterior descending coronary artery. *Circulation.* 2010;122:e518-e521.
2. Lin TH, Wu DK, Su HM, et al. Septum hematoma: a complication of retrograde wiring in chronic total occlusion. *Int J Cardiol.* 2006;113:e64-e66.

When Collateral Damage Does Matter: Iatrogenic Ventricular Septal Rupture After Percutaneous Coronary Intervention of the Left Anterior Descending Artery

Vincent Michiels, MD, Martin J. Swaans, MD, Bastiaan J. Sorgdrager, MD, Rolf F. Veldkamp, MD, PhD, Robin H. Heijmen, MD, PhD, Jurrien M. ten Berg, MD, PhD

An 83-year-old woman with no cardiac history was admitted because of a non–ST-segment elevation myocardial infarction for which she underwent a diagnostic coronary angiography. The culprit lesion was considered to be a 70% stenosis in the mid left anterior descending coronary artery just after the origin of a large septal branch (Fig. 2.42A). Percutaneous coronary intervention (PCI) was performed with implantation of a drug-eluting stent (3.0 × 12 mm Promus Element, Boston Scientific, Natick, Massachusetts). After stent implantation, there was an occlusion of the septal branch, presumably caused by plaque shift. Despite several attempts, the branch could not be rewired, so the occlusion was accepted (Fig. 2.42B). The patient was discharged in good clinical condition 2 days after the procedure (maximum creatine kinase level 1760 U/L).

However, 8 days later, the patient was readmitted because of acute pulmonary edema. Transthoracic echocardiography showed a ventricular septal rupture with a large interventricular septal defect,

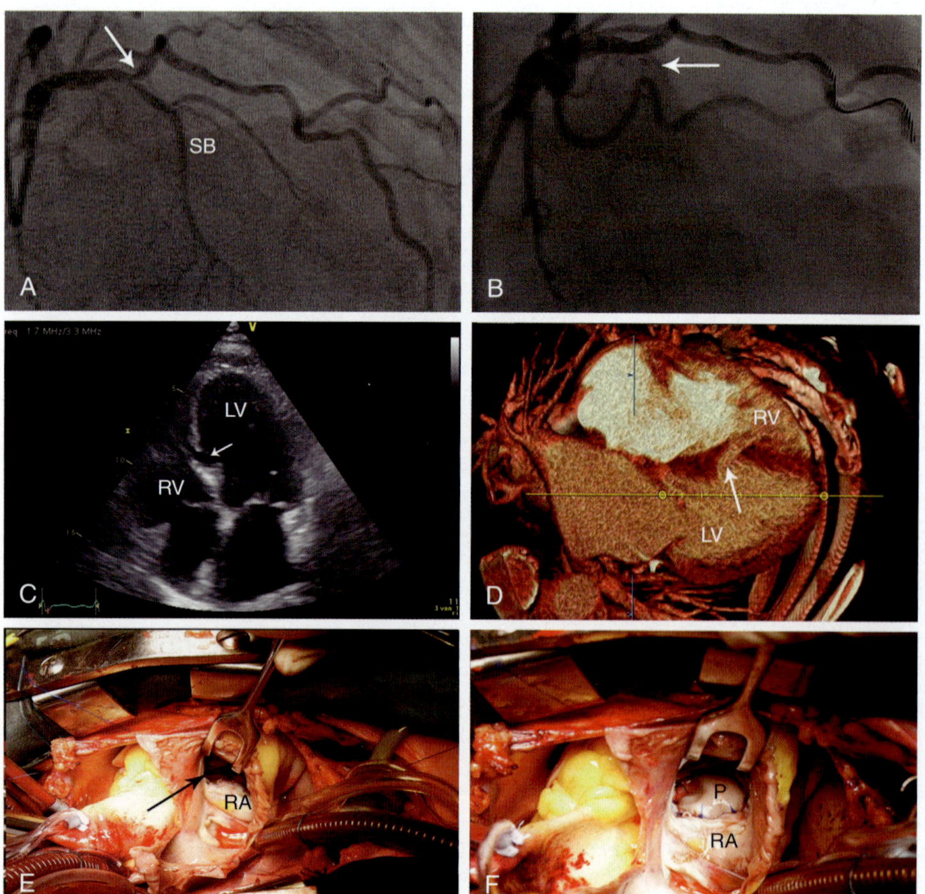

FIG. 2.42 Different Stages and Imaging Modalities of the Ventricular Septal Rupture (VSR) After Percutaneous Coronary Intervention (PCI). (A) Angiography before PCI. The *arrow* indicates stenosis. (B) Angiography after PCI. The *arrow* indicates the occluded septal branch. (C) Transthoracic echocardiogram, four-chamber view. The *arrow* indicates the septal defect. (D) Volume-rendered cardiac computed tomography image, four-chamber view. The *arrow* indicates the septal defect. (E) Perioperative photograph before closure of the VSR. The *arrow* indicates the septal defect. (F) Perioperative photograph after closure of the VSR. *LV,* left ventricle; *P,* patch; *RA,* right atrium; *RV,* right ventricle; *SB,* septal branch.

as confirmed on cardiac computed tomography (Fig. 2.42C–D). Initially, the patient's condition was stabilized and recompensated with the use of intravenous diuretics and an intraaortic balloon pump. The defect was closed surgically with a bovine pericardial patch (Fig. 2.42E–F). The patient had an uneventful postoperative recovery.

This case shows the post-PCI complication of an iatrogenic occlusion of a septal branch that caused extensive infarction of the interventricular septum leading to ischemic rupture. It reminds us that leaving a septal branch occluded after PCI for the LAD is not without risk, and every attempt should be made to restore flow.

Complications of Diagnostic Catheterization

Intracoronary Bubbles Iatrogenic Air Embolism Assessed With Optical Coherence Tomography

Ramón Maruri-Sánchez, MD, Fernando Rivero, MD, Teresa Bastante, MD, Javier Cuesta, MD, Marcos García-Guimaraes, MD, Fernando Alfonso, MD, PhD

An 82-year-old man with hypertension, diabetes mellitus type 2, and chronic renal failure treated with hemodialysis was admitted with rest angina. Coronary angiography showed two-vessel coronary artery disease, with significant stenosis in the first and second diagonal branches that were small vessels, and a severe heavily calcified focal stenosis in the proximal segment of the posterolateral branch. This lesion was treated with percutaneous coronary intervention (PCI) using sequential high-pressure balloon dilations (diameter 1.5, 2.0, and 3.0 mm) followed by the implantation of a 3 mm × 12 mm drug-eluting stent. Immediate angiography after stent implantation showed good result of the stent, but also revealed a localized slow-flow phenomenon subsequently accompanied by chest pain and inferior ST-segment elevation. A filling defect in the ectatic proximal segment of the posterolateral branch was also recognized (Fig. 2.43A, Online Video 2.41). The differential diagnosis of the repletion contrast defect included thrombus and air embolism, and therefore optical coherence tomography (OCT) was indicated. No image of thrombus was detected by OCT. Instead, two circumferential, low-refringence lines (without brightness inside) occupied the entire vessel lumen, confirming the suspicion diagnosis of air embolism (Fig. 2.43B). The air leakage was probably produced during the balloon dilation secondary to a pinhole balloon rupture because a mild pressure drop was observed during the inflation of the device.

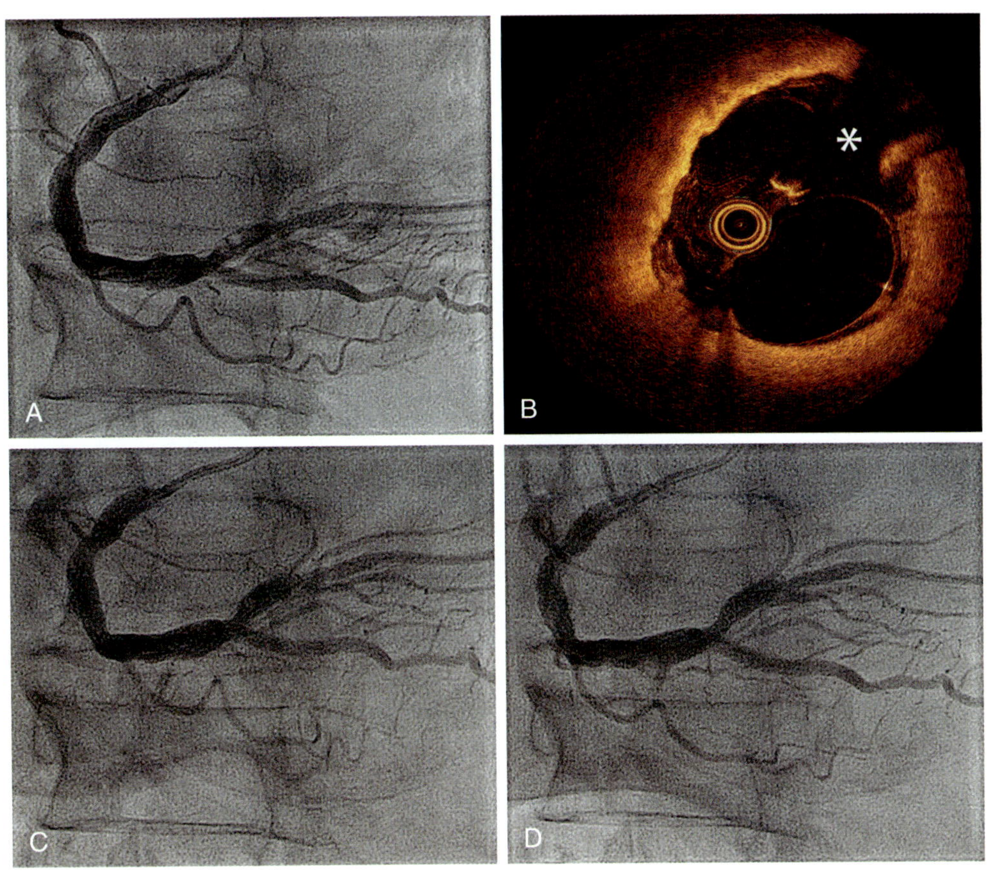

FIG. 2.43 Imaging of Diagnosis, Treatment, and Resolution of Air Embolism. (A) Coronary angiography showing a filling defect in the proximal segment of the posterolateral branch (Online Video 2.41). (B) Optical coherence tomography depicting two circumferential, low-refringence lines without any brightness inside the vessel lumen. The *asterisk* indicates the guidewire artifact. (C) Repletion defect decrease on coronary angiography during aspiration with 6F Export catheter (Medtronic, Minneapolis, Minnesota) (Online Video 2.42). (D) After full air aspiration, coronary angiography shows no residual repletion defects. Normal coronary flow and a good result of percutaneous coronary intervention were eventually achieved.

Air aspiration was performed using a 6F Export aspiration catheter (Medtronic, Minneapolis, Minnesota) with several passages. After this maneuver, the angiographic repletion defect eventually disappeared (Fig. 2.43C–D, Online Video 2.42), and coronary flow and ST-segment changes normalized. The patient's hospital course was uneventful.

Coronary air embolism is a rare complication during PCI that may be asymptomatic or cause chest pain, ST-segment elevation, or systemic hypotension.[1,2] Massive air embolism may cause hemodynamic derangement, severe life-threatening arrhythmias, and even death.[1,2] The diagnosis of air embolism is readily suspected in cases with the typical "moving round bubbles" that are easily detected on angiography and are often associated with slow coronary flow. However, sometimes, particularly during complex PCI procedures in ectatic vessels, the bubbles may remain still, and therefore the haziness or repletion defect may be difficult to differentiate from intracoronary thrombus formation. To the best of our knowledge, this is the first report in the literature describing the value of OCT to help in the differential diagnosis of coronary air embolism. Our findings suggest that OCT readily allows the differentiation of this condition from intracoronary thrombus and therefore may be helpful in selected cases to guide subsequent management. Air embolism treatment options include 100% oxygen administration as well as atropine and epinephrine injections.[1] Air aspiration has been previously described as an alternative treatment.[3] This case nicely illustrates that bubble aspiration using an Export catheter is useful in removing the air from the coronary artery, avoiding the potential damage of distal microvasculature owing to distal air embolization.

References

1. Khan M, Schmidt DH, Bajwa T, Shalev Y. Coronary air embolism: incidence, severity, and suggested approaches to treatment. *Cathet Cardiovasc Diagn.* 1995;36:313-318.
2. Dib J, Boyle AJ, Chan M, Resar JR. Coronary air embolism: a case report and review of the literature. *Catheter Cardiovasc Interv.* 2006;68:897-900.
3. Solodky A, Birnbaum Y, Assali A, Ben Gal T, Strasberg B, Herz I. Coronary air embolism treated by bubble aspiration. *Catheter Cardiovasc Interv.* 2000;49:452-454.

Aortic Regurgitation After Cardiac Catheterization

Benjamin Safar, MD, Olivier Milleron, MD, Patrick Mesnildrey, MD, Simon Cattan, MD

A case of iatrogenic aortic regurgitation caused by laceration of a cusp fenestration of the aortic valve during diagnostic coronary angiography is presented. This complication was finally cured by aortic valve replacement. Images of transthoracic, 64-slice multidetector computed tomography and macroscopic surgery pictures illustrate this case.

A 66-year-old man was admitted to our department for coronary disease. Physical examination results were normal, without any heart murmur, and transthoracic echocardiography did not show evidence of valvular disease. Coronary angiography revealed triple-vessel disease with moderate left ventricular dysfunction and medical treatment was decided.

After the procedure a grade 3/6 diastolic murmur appeared. Transthoracic echocardiography revealed a severe aortic regurgitation caused by posterior cusp prolapse (Fig. 2.44A) confirmed by transesophageal echocardiography.

At 6 months, the patient developed severe dyspnea and surgery was planned. Cardiac 64-slice multidetector computed tomography reassessed coronary stenosis and showed the noncoronary cusp prolapse (Fig. 2.44B–C). Intraoperative findings were a rupture of posterior cusp fenestration, which was responsible for an 8-mm tear (Fig. 2.44D), and intact congenital fenestrations were also present on the right and left coronary cusps (Fig. 2.44E). Mechanical valve replacement combined with coronary artery bypass grafting was performed. The patient's postoperative course was uneventful.

Aortic cusp fenestrations are frequent findings during aortic valve surgery for dystrophic aortic insufficiency.[1-4] These congenital fenestrations are located in the paracommissural area, in the coaptation zone, and do not directly result in regurgitation when they are intact. Fenestrations consist of thin fibrous strands connecting the central part of the cusp to the commissure. In this case report, guidewires may have passed through the noncoronary cusp fenestration, leading to its rupture resulting in cusp prolapse and regurgitation. If the remaining cusps are macroscopically normal, valve repair might be performed as an alternative to prosthetic replacement.

References

1. Fundarò P, Di Mattia DG, Cialfi A, Santoli C. Repair of aortic cusp traumatic laceration caused by cardiac catheterization. *J Heart Dis.* 1996;5:281-282.
2. Blaszyk H, Witkiewicz AJ, Edwards WD. Acute aortic regurgitation due to spontaneous rupture of a fenestrated cusp: report in a 65-year-old man and review of seven additional cases. *Cardiovasc Pathol.* 1999;8:213-216.
3. Mora´n SV, Casanegra P, Maturana G, Dubernet J. Spontaneous rupture of a fenestrated aortic valve. Surgical treatment. *J Thorac Cardiovasc Surg.* 1977;73:716-718.
4. Akiyama K, Hirota J, Taniyasu N, Maisawa K, Kobayashi Y, Tsuda M. Pathogenetic significance of myxomatous degeneration in fenestration-related massive aortic regurgitation. *Circ J.* 2004;68:439-443.

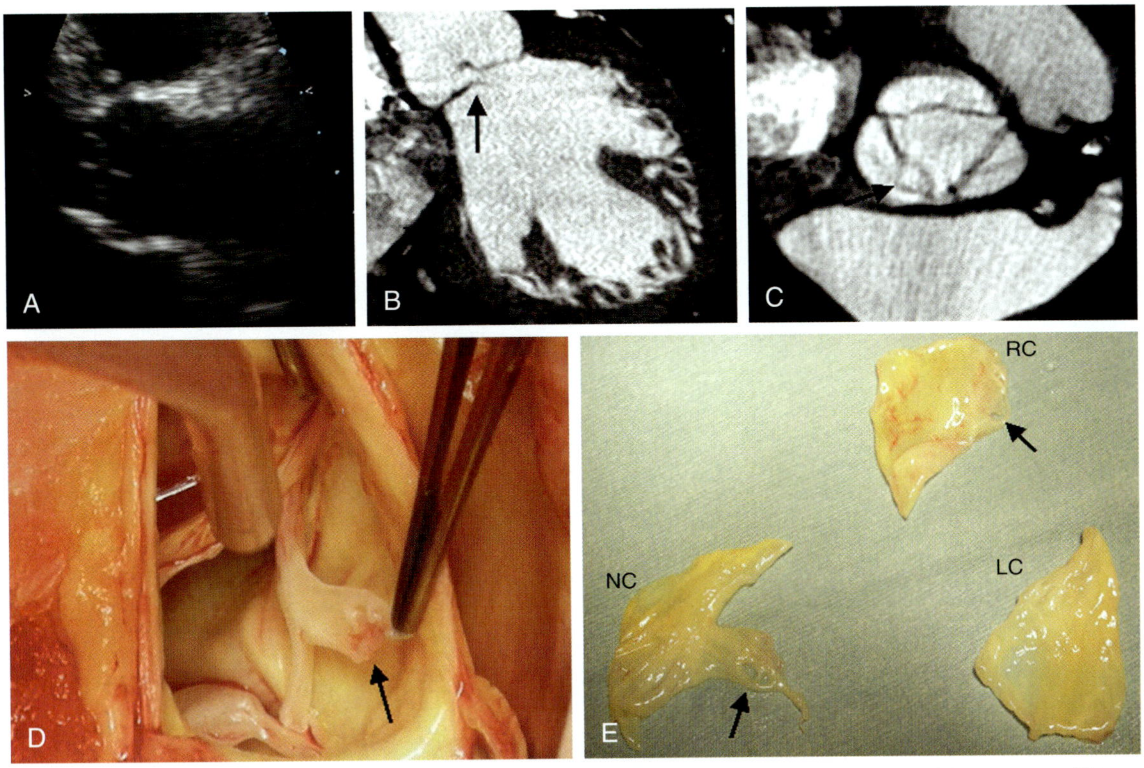

FIG. 2.44 Iatrogenic Aortic Regurgitation Repair Images. (A) Transthoracic echocardiography image: parasternal long-axis view. This end-diastole image shows an aortic posterior cusp prolapse (*arrow*) with complete coaptation defect, responsible for an important aortic regurgitation. (B and C) Cardiac 64-slice multidetector computed tomography images: left ventricle long-axis view (B) and transverse section of the aortic valve (C). The posterior cusp prolapse (*arrows*) visible on echocardiography is confirmed by cardiac computed tomography realized to reassess coronary stenosis. (D) Intraoperative findings during aortic valve replacement and coronary artery bypass grafting. This intraoperative image shows the laceration of the aortic posterior cusp with an 8-mm tear where the cusp fenestrations (*arrow*) are found. (E) Operative piece of the aortic valve replaced. Millimetric fenestrations are visible on the posterior but also on the right coronary cusp (*RC*) (*arrows*). This image also shows clearly the posterior cusp tear responsible for the important aortic regurgitation. *LC*, left coronary cusp; *NC*, noncoronary or posterior cusp.

Equipment Dislodgement and Fracture

A Potential Procedural Complication 2 Years After Percutaneous Coronary Intervention to Treat Left Anterior Descending Artery Lesions With the T-Stenting and the Small Protrusion Technique

Kenichi Karube, MD, Yusuke Fujino, MD, Toru Naganuma, MD, Satoko Tahara, MD, Shotaro Nakamura, MD, Sunao Nakamura, MD, Antonio Colombo, MD

A 72-year-old man had exertional angina 22 months after percutaneous coronary intervention in the proximal segment of left anterior descending artery (LAD) and first diagonal branch (D1) with the provisional T-stenting and small protrusion (TAP) technique (Xience Prime 2.5 × 23 mm stent on D1, Abbott Vascular, Santa Clara, California). Coronary angiography demonstrated significant in-stent restenosis of the mid LAD (Fig. 2.45A).

A floppy guidewire was passed through the lesion. Then a balloon (Lacrosse nonslip element, 2.5 × 13 mm, Goodman, Nagoya, Japan) was advanced and inflated. After deflation we removed the balloon with some difficulty and observed a deformed stent attached to it (Fig. 2.45F). Coronary angiography confirmed removal of the D1 stent and showed focal stenosis with probable dissection in the D1 (Fig. 2.45C–D). Frequency-domain optical coherence tomography revealed intimal tears (Fig. 2.46Ba–Bc) and trails of the extracted

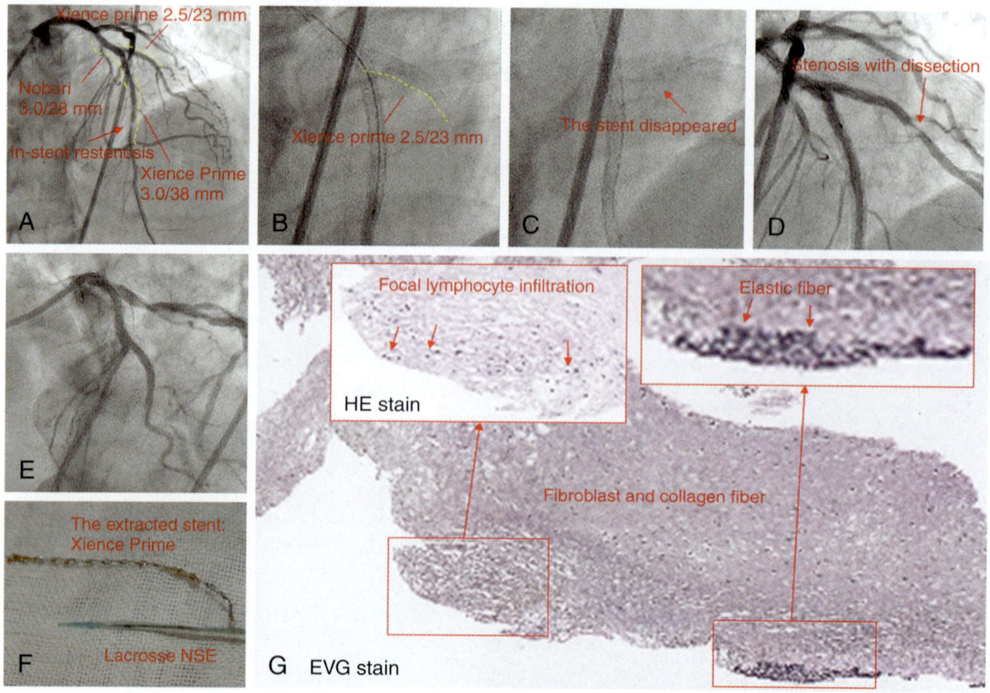

FIG. 2.45 Images of the Left Coronary Artery Angiogram During Percutaneous Coronary Intervention, the Extracted Stent, and Histology of Tissue Attached to the Removed Stent. (A and B) A 2.5 × 13 mm Lacrosse nonslip element (*NSE*) balloon (Goodman, Nagoya, Japan) was introduced into the mid left anterior descending artery in-stent restenosis and inflated. (C) A drug-eluting stent (DES) (Xience Prime, Abbott Vascular, Santa Clara, California), previously inserted in the first diagonal branch (D1), had disappeared. (D) Coronary angiography showed stenosis with probable dissection at the previously stented site in D1. (E) Final coronary angiography showed an excellent result after implantation of a new DES. (F) The extracted D1 stent was attached to the balloon. (G) Histologic study of the tissue adhering to the extracted stent showed fibrous thickening of the intima and part of media and focal inflammatory infiltration (lymphocytes). *EVG*, Elastica van Gieson; *HE*, hematoxylin and eosin.

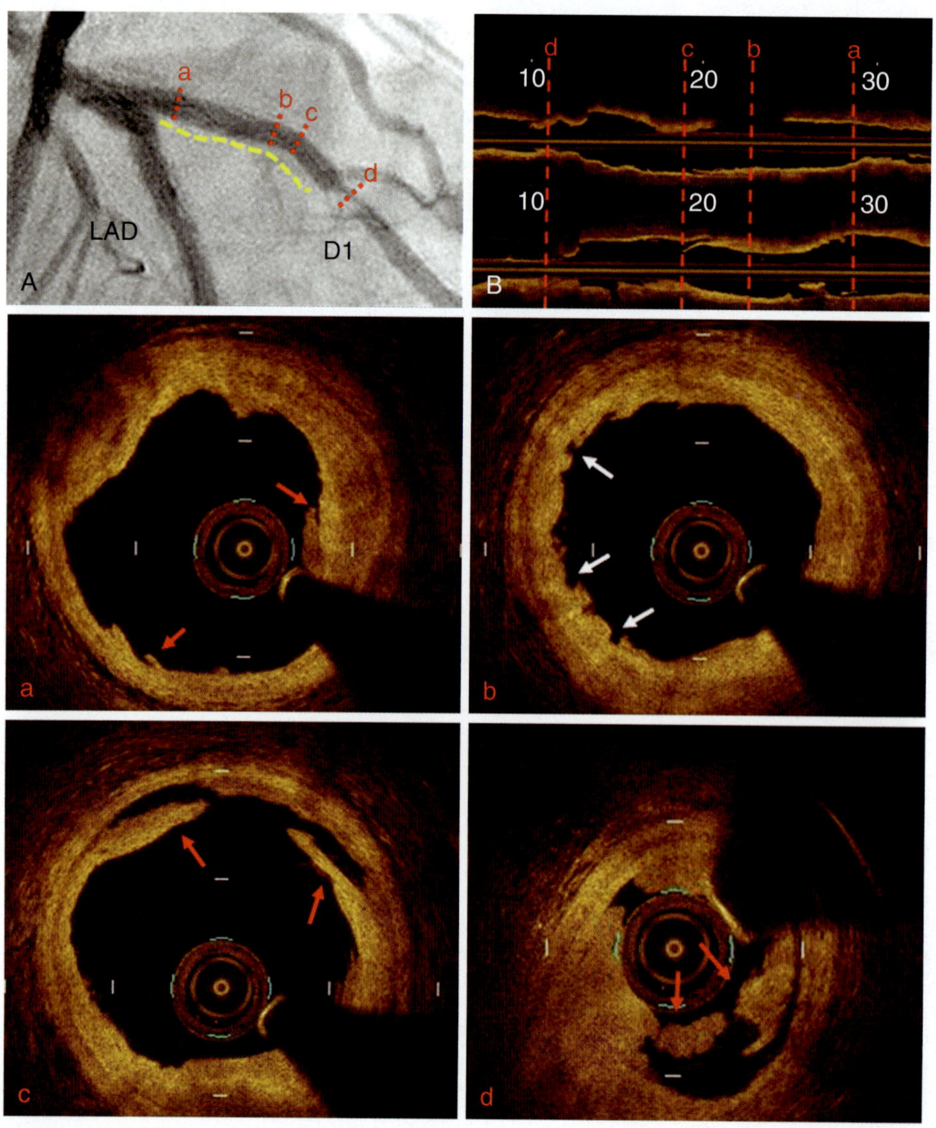

FIG. 2.46 Frequency-Domain Optical Coherence Tomography Images and Coronary Angiography of the First Diagonal Branch (D1). (A) Coronary angiography after extraction of the stent showed stenosis with probable dissection in the DI. (B) Frequency-domain optical coherence tomography showed intimal tears (*red arrows* in a, c, and d) and trails of the extracted stent struts (*white arrows* in b) (Online Video 2.43). There was neither significant stenosis nor coronary dissection at the previously stented site in D1. Letters indicate the proximal (a), middle (b, c), and distal (d) segment of the previously stented site in D1. *LAD,* left anterior descending artery.

stent struts (Fig. 2.46Bb, Online Video 2.43). A drug-eluting stent was successfully inserted into the D1 (Fig. 2.45E).

To our knowledge, this is the first report of the extraction of a previously implanted side-branch stent after the T-stenting and small protrusion (TAP) technique. This rare complication appeared to be due to the entrapment of the deflated balloon in the struts of the D1 stent protruding into the LAD, secondary to the guidewire passing through the struts. Histologic study of the tissue adhered to the extracted stent identified fibrous thickening of the intima and part of the media and focal inflammation. The connection between the vessel wall and the stent might have been loosened as the result of the suppression of neointimal proliferation by everolimus and/or chronic inflammation. The TAP technique is associated with favorable clinical outcomes.[1] However, this report suggests that care is needed when a guidewire is passed through a lesion distal to the bifurcation previously treated with the TAP technique, and a J-type wire should be considered.

Reference

1. Naganuma T, Latib A, Basavarajaiah S, et al. The long-term clinical outcome of T-stenting and small protrusion technique for coronary bifurcation lesions. *J Am Coll Cardiol Intv.* 2013;6:554-561.

Accidental Extraction of a Stent Implanted 3 Years Earlier by a Dislodged Stent: A Rare Complication of Percutaneous Coronary Intervention

Qing Qin, MD, Jianying Ma, MD, Chenguang Li, MD, Lei Ge, MD, Juying Qian, MD, Junbo Ge, MD

A 60-year-old man had angina 3 years after implantation of a 3.0 × 36 mm sirolimus-eluting stent (SES) (Excel, JW Medical Systems, Weihai, China) crossing over from the distal left main coronary artery (LM) to the mid left anterior descending coronary artery (LAD). He had an acute inferior myocardial infarction 4.5 years earlier, and four SESs were implanted to revascularize an occluded right coronary artery. An implantable cardioverter-defibrillator was later implanted for ventricular tachycardia. Current coronary angiography (CAG) showed a 70% stenosis in the left circumflex coronary artery (LCx), but no in-stent restenosis was observed in the previously placed stent (Fig. 2.47A).

After predilation with a 2.0 × 15 mm balloon, multiple attempts to deliver a 2.5 × 38 mm SES (Helios, Kimley Medical, Shenzhen, China) through the previous LM stent to the left circumflex coronary artery lesion were made but failed. While retrieving the stent, it caught on the LM stent and partly detached from the balloon (Fig. 2.47B). A 2.5 × 15 mm balloon was inflated in the guide catheter to squeeze the stent before it was pulled out with difficulty with another deformed stent (Fig. 2.47D) attached with intima. CAG showed the disappearance of the LM-LAD stent (Fig. 2.47C) and a mid-LAD occlusion (Fig. 2.47E–F). After dilation with a 2.0 × 15 mm balloon, intravenous ultrasound demonstrated dissection at the mid-LAD and intimal injury at the proximal LAD (Fig. 2.47F–I). Finally, a 2.5 ×18-mm SES (Firebird 2, MicroPort Medical, Shanghai, China) was implanted at the mid LAD with good CAG results (Fig. 2.47J). The patient was symptom free at 6-month follow-up.

To our knowledge, this is the fourth reported case of stent extraction by a dislodged stent[1-3]; however, the extracted stent was in place for 3 years, the longest endothelialization period. Fortunately, only intimal injury was observed at the distal LM and proximal LAD, and 1 stent implanted at the dissection site perfectly achieved revascularization. This report suggests that caution is needed when passing a stent through old stent struts as the previous stent could still be extracted after long-term endothelialization.

References

1. Cheema JK, Shroff AR, Vidovich MI. Unintentional extraction of an endothelialized bare metal stent. *Cardiovasc Revasc Med.* 2013;14:187-190.
2. Hsu PC, Lin TH, Lee WH, Sheu SH. Inadvertent extraction of a deployed stent after using twisted wire technique. *Kaohsiung J Med Sci.* 2014;30:55-56.
3. Kim JW, Kim W. Unintentional extraction of a coronary stent deployed two months prior during a dislodged left main stent retrieval. *Int J Cardiol.* 2012;156:e45-e48.

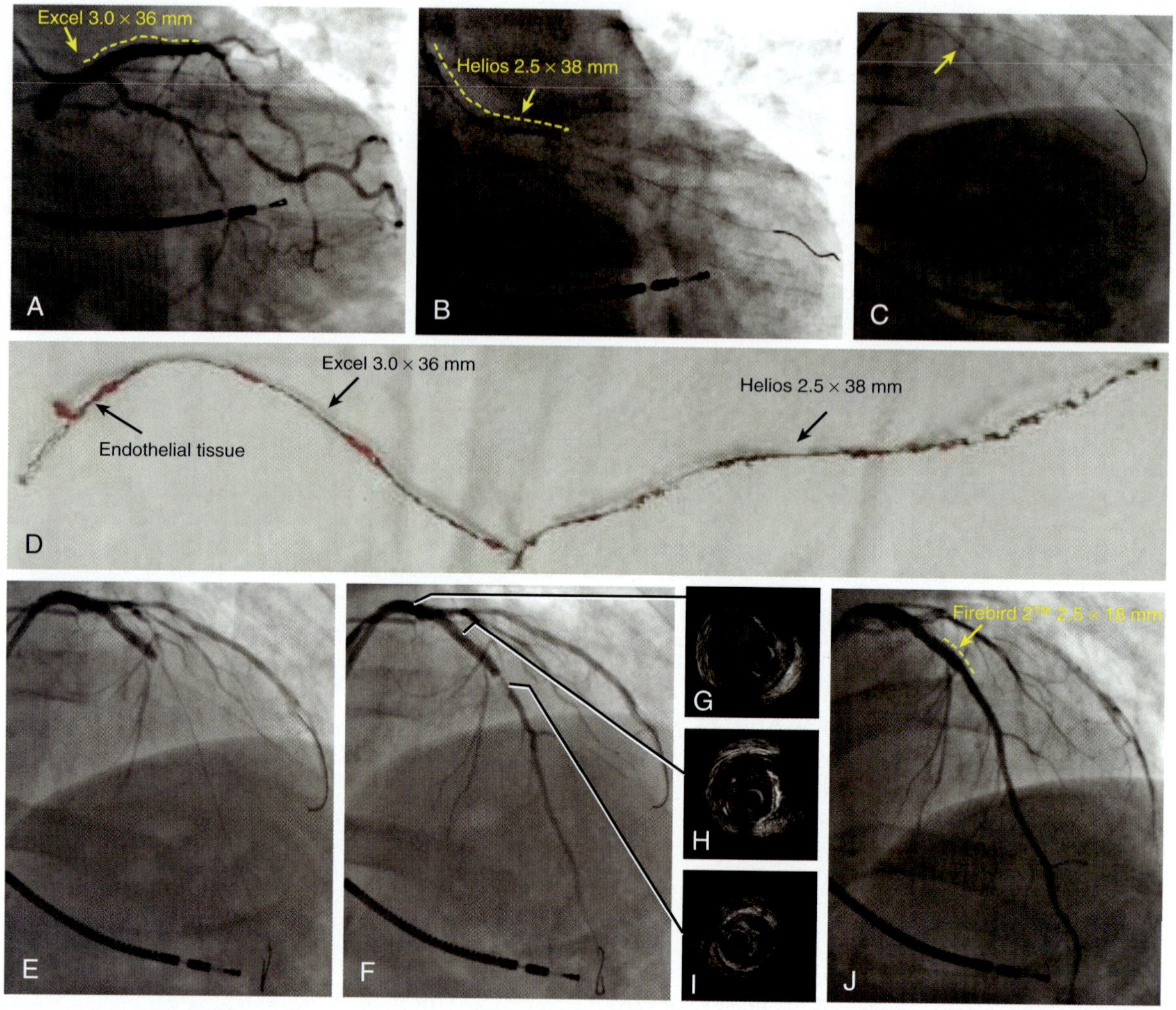

FIG. 2.47 Images of the Left Coronary Angiogram During a Percutaneous Coronary Intervention, the Extracted Stent, and Intravascular Ultrasound of the Left Anterior Descending Coronary Artery (LAD) After Stent Extraction. (A) Coronary angiography (CAG) demonstrated no in-stent restenosis in the left main coronary artery (LM) to mid LAD stent (*arrow*), but diffuse stenosis at the left circumflex artery. (B) The stent is dislodged at the ostium of the LM (*arrow*). (C) The LM-LAD stent is invisible after the dislodged stent is pulled out (*arrow*). (D) Morphologies of the distorted stent and dislodged stent (*Helios*, Kimley Medical, Shenzhen, China) caught in the proximal part of a scattered-shaped previously implanted LM-LAD stent (*Excel*, JW Medical Systems, Weihai, China) with endothelial tissue attached to it. (E) CAG indicated LAD occlusion immediately after the stent as extracted. (F) Residual stenosis and dissection remained (*arrow*) after dilation. (G–I) Intravascular ultrasound demonstrated intimal injury at the proximal LAD (G and H) dissection at the mid LAD (I), as indicated. (J) Final CAG results after implantation of a stent at the mid LAD.

Frequency-Domain Optical Coherence Tomography Assessment of Stent Constriction 9 Months After Sirolimus-Eluting Stent Implantation in a Highly Calcified Plaque

Yusuke Fujino, MD, Guilherme F. Attizzani, MD, Sunao Nakamura, MD, Marco A. Costa, MD, PhD, Hiram G. Bezerra, MD, PhD

A 60-year-old man with a history of chronic renal failure in hemodialysis was admitted because of angina symptoms. Coronary angiography showed an eccentric lesion of the distal unprotected left main coronary artery involving the ostium of the left anterior descending artery (Fig. 2.48A). Frequency-domain optical coherence tomography (FD-OCT) revealed a calcified plaque protruding to the lumen (Fig. 2.48Aa). Rotational atherectomy with a 2.0-mm burr (Fig. 2.48Ab) was conducted before the implantation of a 3.5 × 18 mm sirolimus-eluting stent at 12 atm, which was followed by intrastent postdilation with a noncompliant 4.0 × 12 mm balloon at

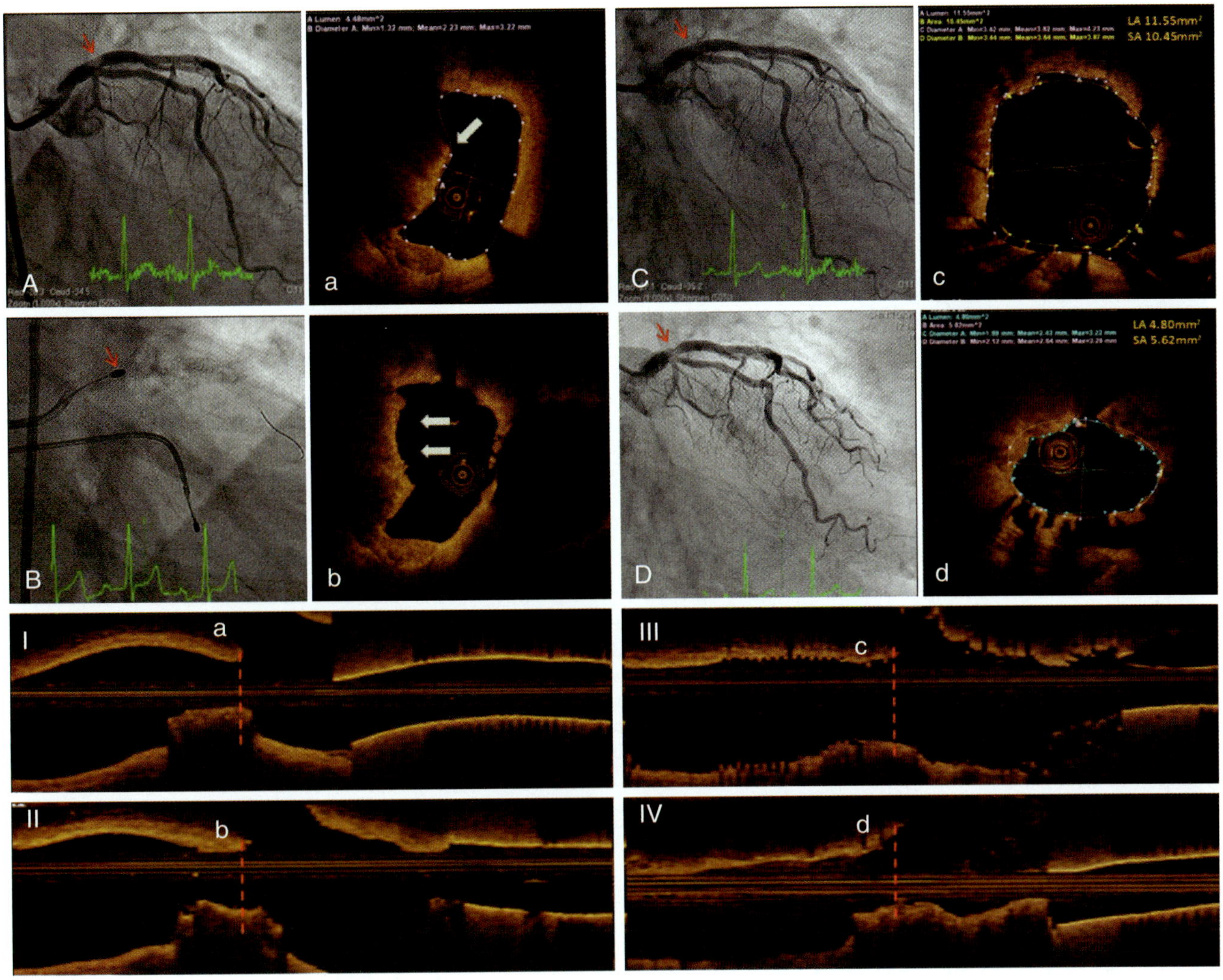

FIG. 2.48 Stent Constriction Document by Frequency-Domain Optical Coherence Tomography (FD-OCT). Angiography shows a narrowing in the distal unprotected left main coronary artery/origin of left anterior descending artery (A, *red arrow*). FD-OCT reveals a protruding calcified plaque (I and a, *white arrow*) that was intervened with rotational atherectomy (B, *red arrow*) (II and b, *white arrows*). A good result is demonstrated after stent implantation (C, *red arrow*) by angiography, and by FD-OCT (stent area 10.45 mm^2; III and c). At follow-up, although angiography reveals a late luminal loss (D, *red arrow*), FD-OCT demonstrates minimal neointimal hyperplasia and important stent constriction (stent area 5.62 mm^2) (IV and d). *LA*, lumen area.

18 atm (Fig. 2.48Cc). The patient underwent 9-month follow-up coronary angiography that showed luminal loss (Fig. 2.48D). The FD-OCT imaging exhibited a constricted sirolimus-eluting stent (Fig. 2.348d). Three-dimensional FD-OCT images revealed a well-expanded stent at baseline, whereas stent constriction was depicted in a highly calcified region at follow-up (Fig. 2.49).

Although it is a rare phenomenon, stent constriction might be responsible for target lesion failure.[1] In our case, FD-OCT images helped to clarify the mechanisms that led to late luminal loss, demonstrating the longitudinal distribution of stent constriction, as well as its relationship with a highly calcified plaque, therefore playing an important role in treatment proposal.

Reference

1. Hong MK, Park SW, Lee CW, et al. Intravascular ultrasound comparison of chronic recoil among different stent designs. *Am J Cardiol.* 1999;84: 1247-1250.

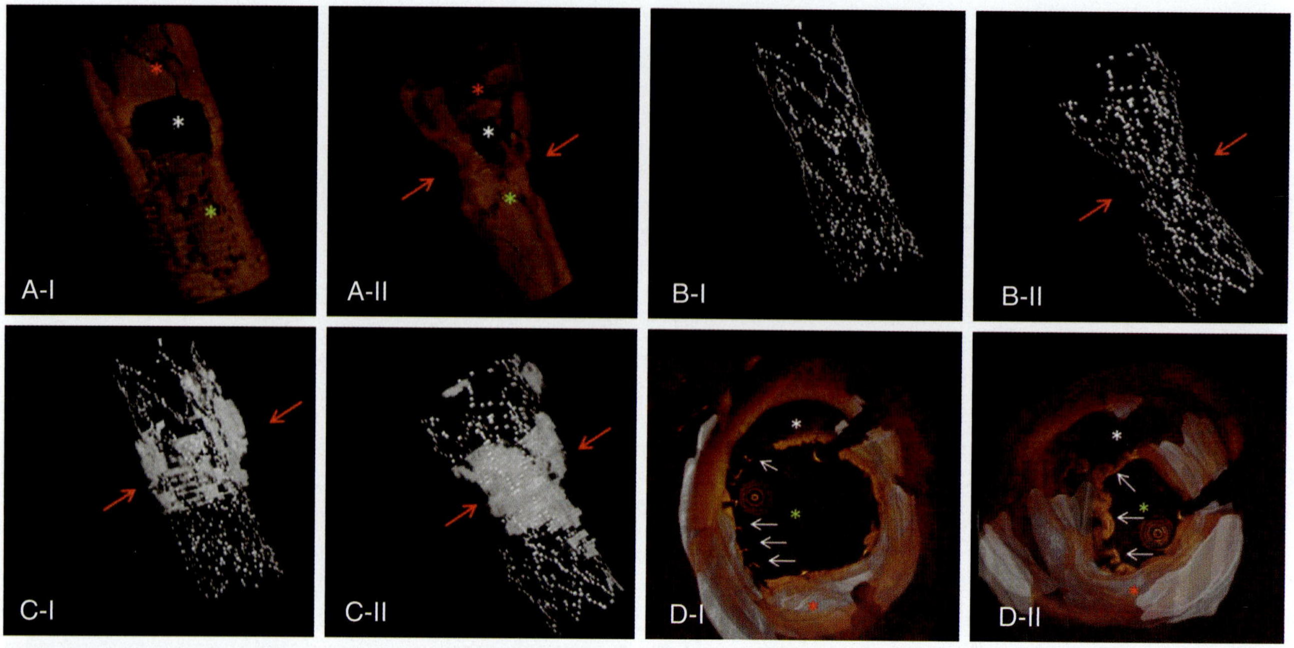

FIG. 2.49 Three-dimensional (3D) Frequency-Domain Optical Coherence Tomography (FD-OCT) Assessment of Stent Constriction. (A-I) A 3D FD-OCT reconstruction of the left coronary artery after stent implantation. Longitudinal assessment of stent expansion is shown in image (B-I), whereas (C-I) shows the stent relationship with calcium (highlighted in *light gray, red arrows*). At follow-up, 3D reconstruction shows late luminal loss (A-II, *red arrows*). Stent 3D rendering shows marked constriction (B-II, *red arrows*) and its relationship with calcium (C-II, *red arrows*). In (D-I) and (D-II), respectively, baseline and follow-up 3D views of the region of interest show stent struts (*white arrows*) and their relationship with calcium (highlighted in *light gray*). The *red, white,* and *green asterisks* represent the unprotected left main coronary artery, left circumflex ostium, and left anterior descending artery, respectively.

First Experience With Successful Percutaneous Retrieval of Retained Fractured Impella Device

Qusai A. Saleh, MD, Michael Foster, MD, Nidal Abi Rafeh, MD

A 50-year-old man underwent successful high-risk percutaneous coronary intervention in the setting of non–ST-segment elevation myocardial infarction and cardiogenic shock. An Impella CP device (Abiomed Inc., Danvers, Massachusetts) was implanted via the right femoral artery. Soon after the intervention was finished, the patient became agitated and was moving forcefully on the catheter laboratory table, causing the Impella alarm to be set off, indicating that it had moved out of the left ventricle.

Multiple attempts to advance the Impella device back into the left ventricle were unsuccessful. During one such attempt, the Impella device buckled at the angle between the inlet and outflow areas. The decision was then made to remove the Impella device and exchange it for a new one. As the Impella device was being pulled out through the repositioning sheath (a tapered sheath from 15F to 9F), the tip was fractured at the junction of the cannula and the inlet area and retained in the right common femoral artery. The retained fragment subsequently embolized into the proximal right deep femoral artery (Fig. 2.50A–B).

In an attempt to percutaneously retrieve the fractured Impella tip, the left common femoral artery was accessed. A 6F 45-cm Destination sheath (Terumo Interventional Systems, Somerset, New Jersey) was advanced over a wire and positioned in the right common iliac artery. The repositioning sheath in the right common femoral artery was then exchanged for a 14F Impella sheath. A 12 to 20 EN Snare device (Merit Medical Systems, Inc., South Jordan, Utah) was advanced through the 6F Destination sheath and used to snare the Impella tip up to the right common iliac artery (Fig. 2.50C, Online Video 2.44). A 27 to 45 EN Snare system was then advanced through the 14F sheath into the right common iliac artery. After multiple attempts, we were able to successfully snare the Impella tip and externalize it through the 14F sheath (Fig. 2.50D–E, Online Video 2.45). A new Impella CP device was then successfully placed through the right common femoral artery.

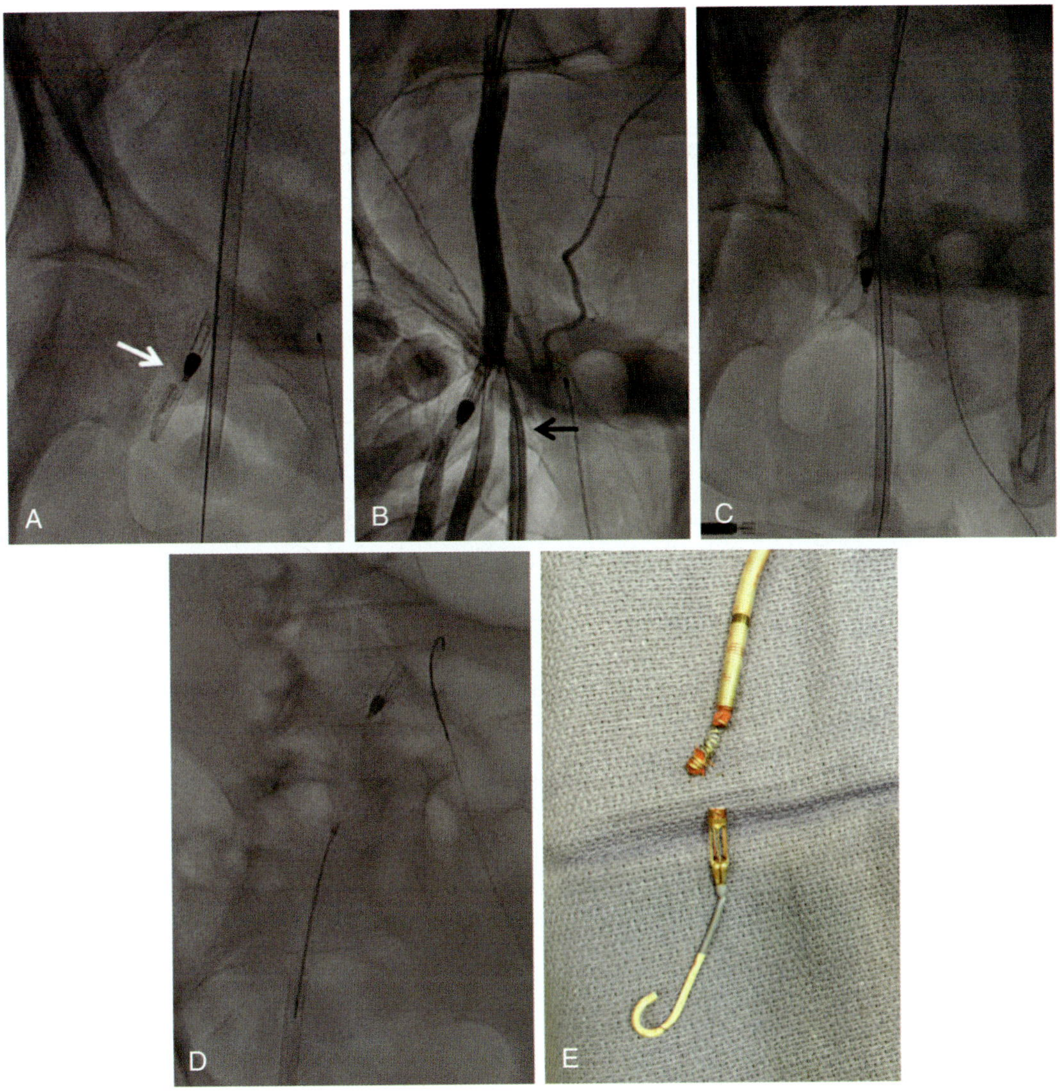

FIG. 2.50 Percutaneous Retrieval of Retained Fractured Impella Device. (A) Fluoroscopy showing the retained fractured tip (*white arrow*) in the right deep femoral artery. (B) Angiography through contralateral access with the 14F sheath (*black arrow*) withdrawn and manual compression at the access site. (C) Snaring of the fractured tip through contralateral access (Online Video 2.44). (D) Successful capture and snaring of the fractured tip in the right common iliac artery (Online Video 2.45). (E) Fractured Impella (Abiomed, Danvers, Massachusetts) device after retrieval.

Guidewire Self-Extrusion After Entrapment of Distal Protection Device During Saphenous Vein Graft Angioplasty

Rodrigo Vugman Wainstein, MD, MSc, ScD, Felipe Homem Valle, MD, Fernando Pivatto Júnior, MD, Ivan Morzoletto Pedrollo, MD, Luiz Carlos Corsetti Bergoli, MD, MSc, Marco Vugman Wainstein, MD, McC, ScD

A 66-year-old man with previous coronary artery bypass graft surgery was referred to cardiac catheterization because of a non–ST-segment elevation acute myocardial infarction. On arrival he was hemodynamically stable and reported mild chest discomfort. Coronary angiography showed a patent saphenous vein graft (SVG) to the distal right coronary artery with severe stenosis in the proximal and mid segment (Fig. 2.51A). The choice for percutaneous coronary intervention was made. The SVG was cannulated with a JR4 6F guiding catheter (Launcher, Medtronic, Santa Rosa, California) and a distal protection device (SpyderFX 5.0, Covidien, Mansfield, Massachusetts) was positioned. Three (3.5 mm × 23 mm, 3.5 mm × 38 mm, and 4.0 mm × 28 mm) everolimus drug-eluting stents (Xience,

Abbott Vascular, Santa Clara, California) were implanted from the distal to the proximal segment of the vessel, respectively (Fig. 2.51B). Stents were post dilated with a 4.0 mm × 15 mm noncompliant balloon at 18 atm. Subsequent angiography showed satisfactory result. At filter recovery, entrapment of distal protection device into struts of the more distal stent occurred (Fig. 2.51C). After several unsuccessful attempts to retrieve the filter, an unusual strategy was taken: the device's 0.014-inch guidewire was cut at its entry site in the right femoral artery. At the end of the procedure, SVG to the distal right coronary artery was occluded proximally. No extravasation of dye was observed in final angiograms. The patient left the laboratory with severe chest pain and 3-mm ST-segment elevation in inferior leads. He was admitted to the coronary care unit and after an uneventful recovery was discharged home 5 days later.

One month after discharge, the patient came to the emergency department with abdominal discomfort. Surprisingly, an extrusion of the previously retained guidewire through abdominal wall was noted (Figs. 2.52–2.54, Online Video 2.46). No signs of infection were observed. Spontaneous and progressive self-extrusion of the guidewire occurred during the hospital stay until its complete exit. The patient was finally discharged home 3 days after admission.

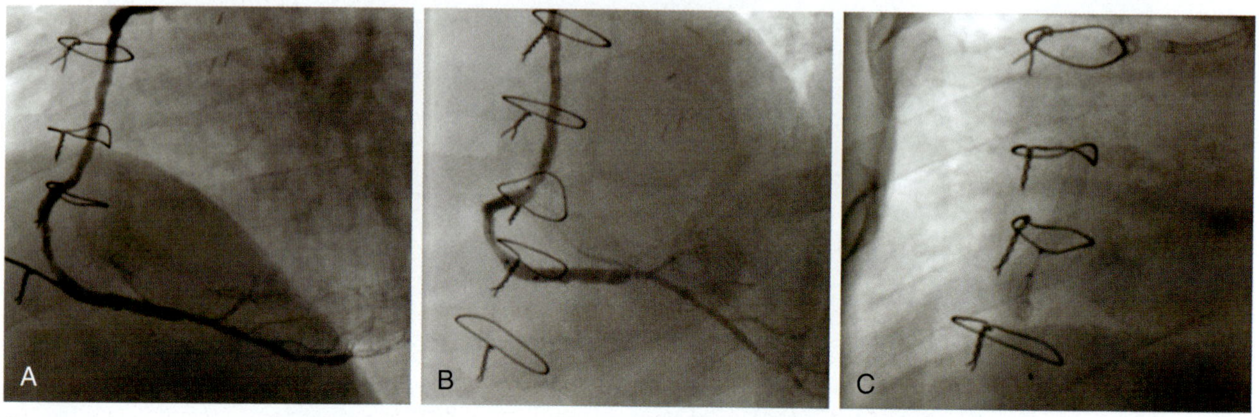

FIG. 2.51 Selective Angiography of Saphenous Vein Graft to Distal Right Coronary. (A) Coronary angiography showing a patent saphenous vein graft to the distal right coronary artery with severe stenosis in the proximal and mid segment. (B) Distal protection device (SpyderFX 5.0, Covidien, Mansfield, Massachusetts). (C) Entrapment of the distal protection device into the struts of the more distal stent.

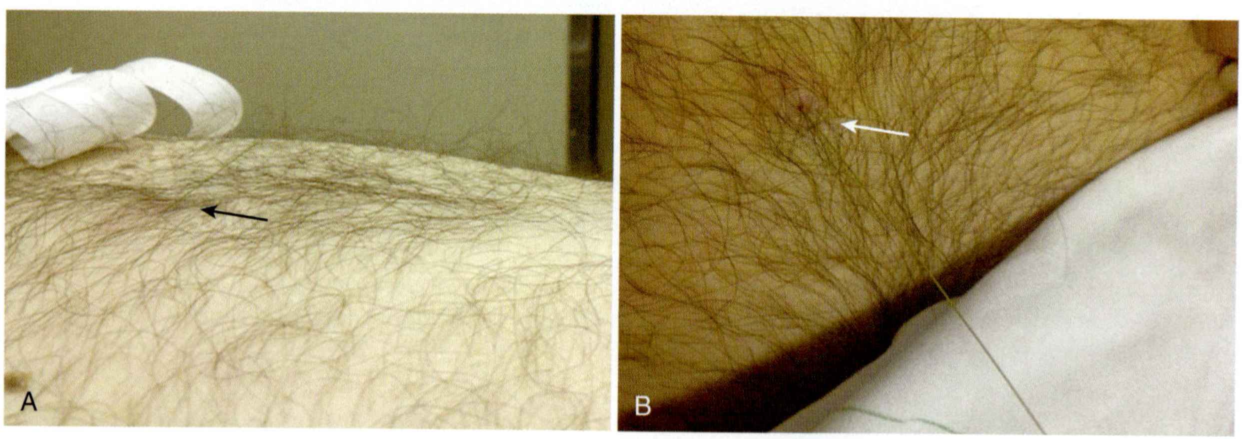

FIG. 2.52 Guidewire Self-Extrusion. (A and B) Distal protection device guidewire exit through the abdominal wall.

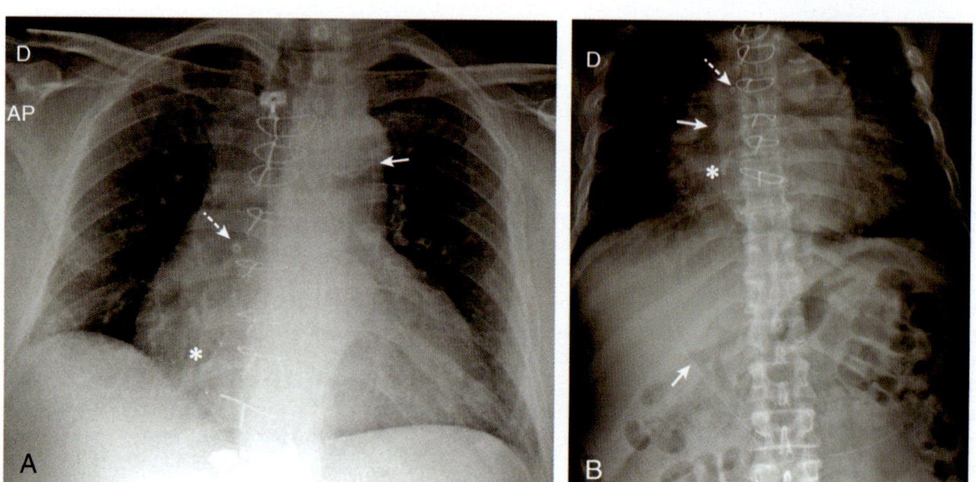

FIG. 2.53 Guidewire Migration on Frontal Radiographs. (A) Frontal anteroposterior (*AP*) chest radiograph image after the procedure showing the guidewire's path inside the aorta (*solid arrow*) and its proximal extremity within the saphenous vein graft. (B) Frontal AP chest and superior abdomen radiograph image 1 month later showing the guidewire's distal migration (*solid arrows*) and path through the abdomen. The distal protection device (*asterisk*) and saphenous vein graft ostial stent (*dashed arrow*) can be observed in both images.

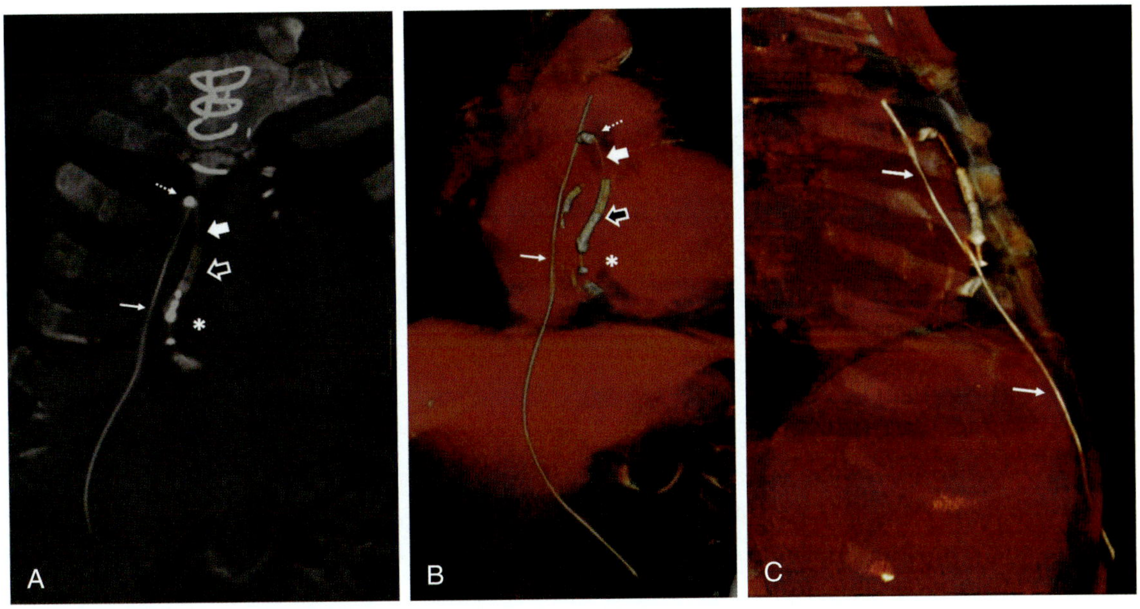

FIG. 2.54 Guidewire Extrusion on Tomography Reformations. (A) Maximum intensity projection reformatting of coronal computed tomography (CT) and (B) coronal three-dimensional reformatted CT showing guidewire (*thin solid arrow*) attached proximally to the saphenous vein graft ostium stent (*dashed arrow*) with a pathway through the superior abdomen, fractured guidewire (*thick solid arrow*), saphenous vein graft distal stent (*thick open arrow*), and distal protection device (*asterisk*). (C) Sagittal three-dimensional reformatted CT showing the guidewire (*arrows*) along the anterior mediastinum, crossing the right hemidiaphragm and the intraperitoneal fat anteriorly to the liver, externalizing distally in the mesogastrium region. The pathway is also demonstrated in an axial CT video (Online Video 2.46).

Identification of Fragmented Balloon Materials in Coronary Arteries by Optical Coherence Tomography

Naveed A. Adoni, MD, Grace W. Huang, DO, Umamahesh C. Rangasetty, MD, Syed Gilani, MD, Ken Fujise, MD

A critical calcific mid left anterior descending stenosis of a 54-year-old man with unstable angina was treated with a drug-eluting stent. Except for the rupture of a noncompliant balloon during postdilation, the procedure was uneventful (Fig. 2.55A). Shortly before the procedure ended, however, the patient became hypotensive with his typical angina pain. Repeat angiography now showed a hazy opacity in the left main coronary artery (LMCA) with no flow to the left circumflex (Fig. 2.55B). Dissection and thrombus formation of the LMCA was suspected. Further hemodynamic deterioration required emergent endotracheal intubation and inotropes. The intravenous infusion of a glycoprotein IIb/IIIa receptor blocker was started. The left anterior descending and 2 obtuse marginal (OM) branches were promptly wired. The small first OM branch was not wired. Multiple balloon inflations established the TIMI (Thrombolysis In Myocardial Infarction) grade flow 2 to the arteries (Fig. 2.55C). An intravascular ultrasound catheter was advanced to the distal LMCA (Fig. 2.55C-1) and the segment was interrogated with and without ChromaFlo imaging (Volcano, San Diego, California) (Fig. 2.55E–D, respectively) (size bar = 1 mm) yielding no definitive findings. At that time, an optical coherence tomography (OCT) catheter was advanced and a pullback image was obtained from the mid portion of the second OM branch into the LMCA. Strikingly, a small circular material (Fig. 2.55G, corresponding to image 2.55C-3) and a thin membranous material (Fig. 2.551F–G, corresponding to images 2.55C-1–C-2, respectively) were now evident, most likely representing a portion of the ruptured balloon trapped in the proximal second OM branch and the LMCA. Three 0.014-inch wires were also visualized by OCT in the LMCA (Fig. 2.55F, corresponding to image 2.55C-1) (size bar = 1 mm). After unsuccessful attempts to retrieve the foreign body, the patient successfully underwent emergent coronary artery bypass graft surgery.

This is the first case report to demonstrate the ability of OCT to image a balloon fragment trapped in the coronary arteries to a resolution sufficiently high for clinicians to accurately identify the object. In this case, the accurate characterization and identification of the object allowed the cardiologists not to proceed with the stenting of the LMCA, which would have had a suboptimal outcome because of the uncompressible (Fig. 2.55H) and highly thrombogenic (Fig. 2.55F–G) materials.

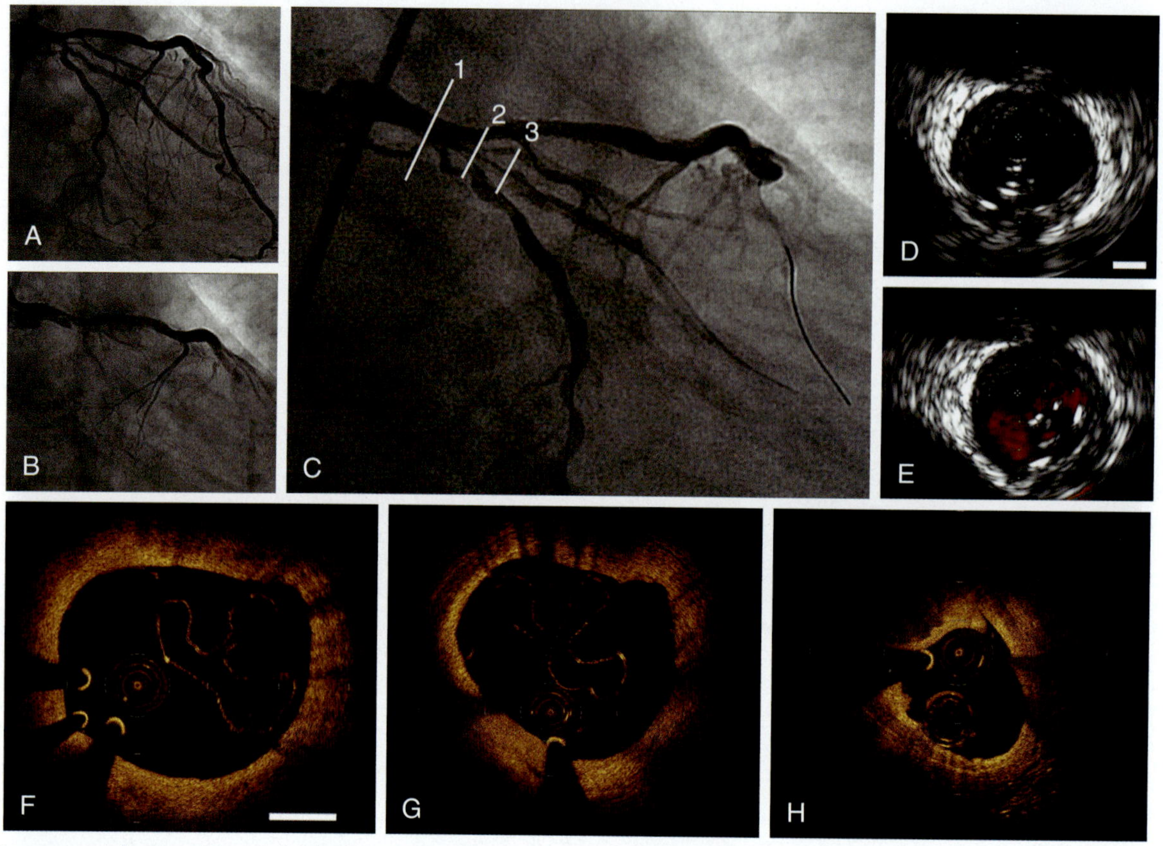

FIG. 2.55 Fragmented Balloon Materials Manifesting Themselves in the Translucency in the Coronary Arteries. (A) Coronary angiogram after successful stenting of the left anterior descending artery. (B) Repeat coronary angiogram obtained when the patient became hypotensive with his typical chest pain. (C) Coronary angiogram obtained at the time of optical coherence tomography (OCT) image acquisition. Multiple balloon inflation and the administration of a GPIIb/IIIa receptor blocker had restored the coronary flow. The OCT catheter was placed in the second obtuse marginal branch (OM2). The OM2 and the left main coronary artery (LMCA) were visualized. (D and E) Intravascular ultrasound (IVUS) images of the LMCA at the level of C-1 with (E) and without (D) ChromaFlo enhancement (Volcano, San Diego, California). (F, G, and H) OCT images of the LMCA (F), the ostial OM2 (G), and the proximal OM2 (H) at the levels of C-1, C-2, and C-3, respectively. A round noncompressible material (H) and thin membranous structure (F and G) were evident by OCT, but not by IVUS. Three (F) and one (G and H) 0.014-inch guidewires were visualized by OCT at the levels of C-1 and C-2/C-3, respectively. Size bar = 1 mm.

Impella 5.0 Device Fracture and Transcatheter Retrieval

Castigliano M. Bhamidipati, DO, PhD, MSC, Moses Mathur, MD, MS, Ravi S. Hira, MD, James M. McCabe, MD, Jay D. Pal, MD, PhD

A 35-year-old man with a history of Kawasaki disease was seen in cardiogenic shock after an ST-segment elevation myocardial infarction. He underwent percutaneous intervention of the culprit vessel. He subsequently had a cardiac arrest, during which time an Impella 5.0 device (Abiomed, Danvers, Massachusetts) was placed percutaneously via the right common femoral artery. The patient continued to experience ventricular tachyarrhythmias, and venoarterial extracorporeal life support was initiated. The Impella device was left in the left ventricle to aid in decompression.

Over the next 5 days, biventricular function improved enough to consider weaning mechanical support. The Impella device driveshaft was manually pulled back, but intraoperative transesophageal echocardiography did not show a corresponding change in pump body position. Attempts to readvance the Impella device were similarly unsuccessful. The Impella device motor current was then noted to be flat, which is worrisome for pump failure. When surveyed under fluoroscopy, we noted a fracture at the distal edge of the 21F pump motor (now located in the right iliac artery near the repositioning sheath). The pigtail and inlet were still in the left ventricle (Fig. 2.56).

The common femoral artery was exposed and controlled. To maintain wire access to the vessel lumen, the repositioning sheath was cut and removed. The Impella device driveshaft was used as a rail to insert a 10F sheath into the common femoral artery. A 0.035-inch J wire was then placed adjacent to the driveshaft into the descending thoracic aorta. With luminal wire access secured, the 10F sheath was removed, followed by the 21F Impella motor. A 26F Gore DrySeal sheath (W. L. Gore & Associates, Flagstaff, Arizona) was advanced over the J wire. A 6F multipurpose guide catheter was inserted in

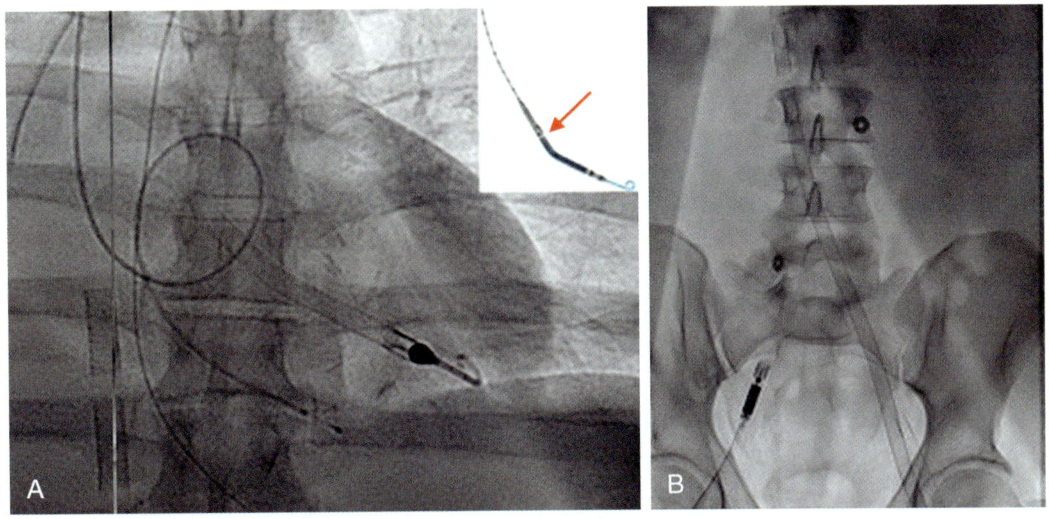

FIG. 2.56 Impella Fracture. Baseline fluoroscopic views showing the fractured Impella 5.0 device (Abiomed, Danvers, Massachusetts). (A) The distal ("pigtail") segment is positioned in the left ventricle. The proximal segment of the plastic tubing is positioned in the left ventricular outflow tract (just below the aortic valve). The inset diagram shows the site of fracture (*arrow*). (B) The outlet area of the Impella device is seen withdrawn to the level of the right common iliac artery.

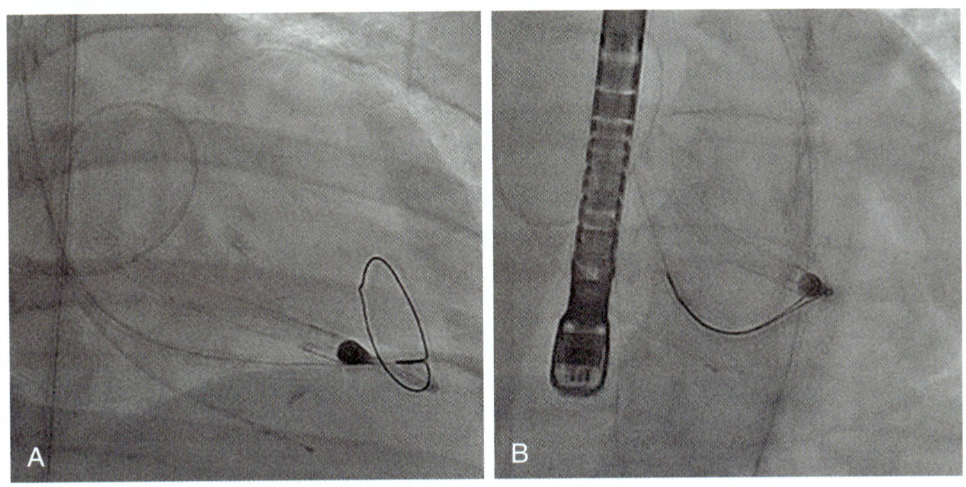

FIG. 2.57 Snare Retrieval. (A) An 8F multipurpose guide catheter is seen inserted into the left ventricle to assist delivery of a 36-mm Gooseneck snare (ev3, Endovascular, Plymouth, Minnesota) toward the distal tip of the Impella 5.0 device. (B) The 36-mm Gooseneck snare is seen capturing the pigtail portion of the Impella 5.0 device.

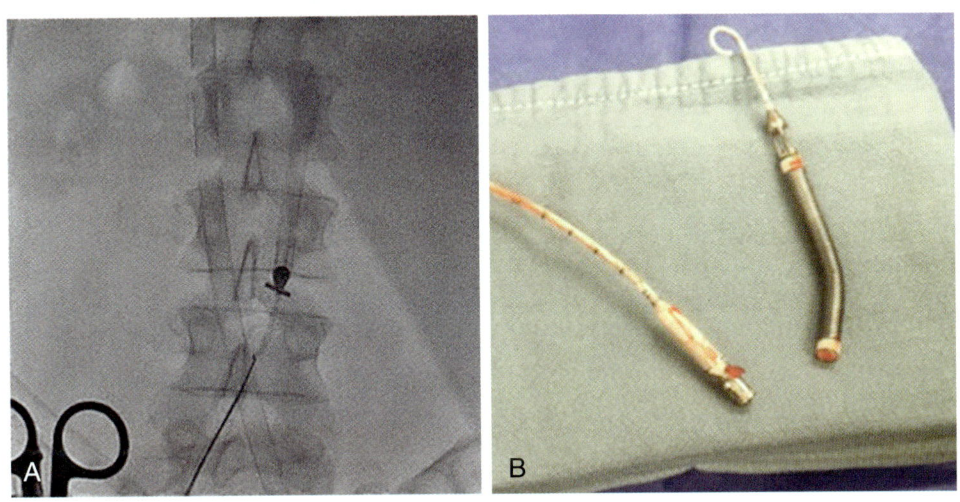

FIG. 2.58 Retrieval Impella. (A) The Impella 5.0 device is retrieved into the 26F Gore DrySeal sheath (W. L. Gore & Associates, Flagstaff, Arizona), with the distal end in first. (B) Ex vivo image of the fractured segments.

the left ventricle, and a 36-mm Gooseneck snare (ev3, Endovascular, Plymouth, Minnesota) was directed to the left ventricular apex. The pigtail was then snared and removed through the femoral sheath (Figs. 2.57 and 2.58).

Neither a fracture of an Impella device nor its successful transcatheter retrieval has been previously described.[1,2] We highlight this case to demonstrate the importance of multidisciplinary collaboration and creative hybrid solutions for favorable patient outcomes.

References

1. Eftekhari A, Eiskjaer H, Terkelsen CJ, et al. Perforation of the anterior mitral leaflet after Impella LP 5.0 therapy in cardiogenic shock. *Am J Cardiol.* 2016;117:1539-1541.
2. Eleid MF, Melduni RM, Joyce DL. Snare-facilitated retrieval of entangled Impella device. *J Interv Cardiol.* 2016;29:332-333.

Late Complication: Xience V Stent Fractures With Restenosis

Jason R. Foerst, MD, Timothy C. Ball, MD, PhD, Masataka Nakano, MD, Renu Virmani, MD, Aaron V. Kaplan, MD

A 70-year-old morbidly obese woman with severe emphysema was seen with unstable angina. Coronary angiography revealed high-grade, calcified, ostial left circumflex (LCx) and distal right coronary artery (RCA) lesions. The patient was deemed a high-risk surgical candidate and underwent stenting of the left main coronary artery into the LCx with a 3.5 × 18 mm Xience V stent (Abbott Vascular, Santa Clara, California). A second 3.5 × 18 mm Xience V stent was overlapped distally to cover a mid LCx lesion, and both stents were postdilated to 16 atm with a 3.5-mm noncompliant balloon. The RCA lesion was stented with a 3.0 × 12 mm Xience V and postdilated to 16 atm with a 3.0-mm noncompliant balloon (Fig. 2.59). The patient did well for 6 months until she returned with unstable angina. Angiography revealed restenosis at the ostium of the stented LCx and within the distal RCA stent (Fig. 2.59). During repeat intervention, wiring of the LCx resulted in abrupt closure. Refractory ventricular fibrillation developed and the patient died.

A postmortem examination was performed in which the coronary arteries were pressure flushed, formalin fixed, and perfused with a lead-based contrast agent (Microfil MV-120, FlowTech, Carver, Massachusetts), and the stented segments were resected under fluoroscopic guidance. The explanted arterial segments were then scanned using a GE eXplore SP MicroCT scanner (GE Healthcare, London, Ontario, Canada).[1] Three-dimensional reconstructions at 23-μ resolution demonstrated heavy calcification and stent fracture at the sites of maximal restenosis. Both Xience V stents fractured in the middle of the hairpin bend in the connecting element and along the crown at the base of the connecting element. Histologic study of both stents revealed underlying heavy fibrocalcific plaque and extensive neointimal hyperplasia at the fracture site without thrombus (Figs. 2.60 and 2.61). The histology of the RCA stent shows inflammation and fibrin accumulation, possibly related to sloughed polymer at the site of fracture (Fig. 2.62). Autopsy studies have suggested a correlation between severe first-generation stent fracture and restenosis.[2] In this case of clinical everolimus drug-eluting stent restenosis at 6 months, it is unclear whether stent fracture–induced restenosis or vessel pathoanatomic characteristics, such as calcium, tortuosity, torsion, and local plaque composition, led to restenosis with coincidental stent fracture.

References

1. Vorpahl M, Foerst JR, Kelm M, Kaplan AV, Virmani R, Ball T. The complementary role of microct and histopathology in characterizing the natural history of stented arteries. *Expert Rev Cardiolvasc Ther.* 2011;9:939-948.
2. Nakazawa G, Finn AV, Vorpahl M, et al. Incidence and predictors of drug-eluting stent fracture in human coronary artery a pathologic analysis. *J Am Coll Cardiol.* 2009;54:1924-1931.

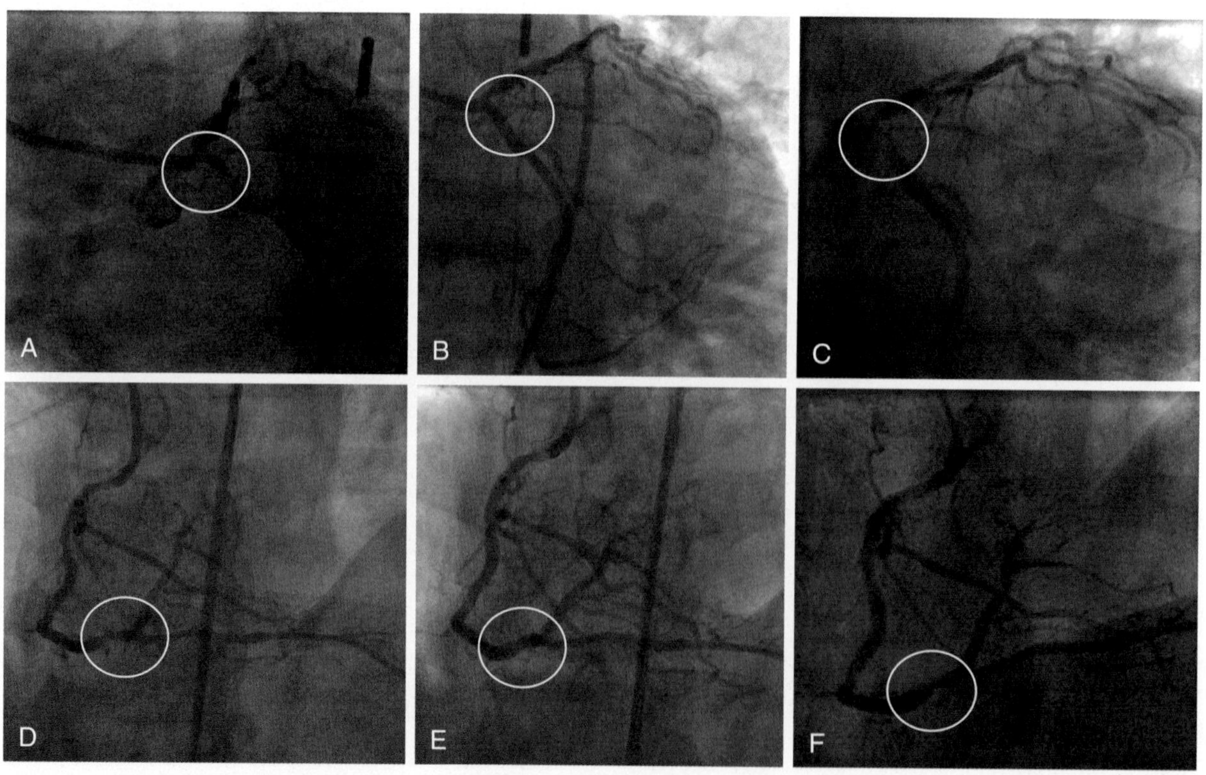

FIG. 2.59 Coronary Angiographic Findings at Index Procedure and Follow-Up. Angiography of the left coronary system at the index procedure showing high-grade ostial and proximal circumflex coronary artery lesions (A), after intervention (B), and 6 months later, revealing severe in-stent restenosis (C). Angiography of the right coronary artery demonstrating a distal stenosis (D), after intervention (E), and 6 months later with in-stent restenosis (F).

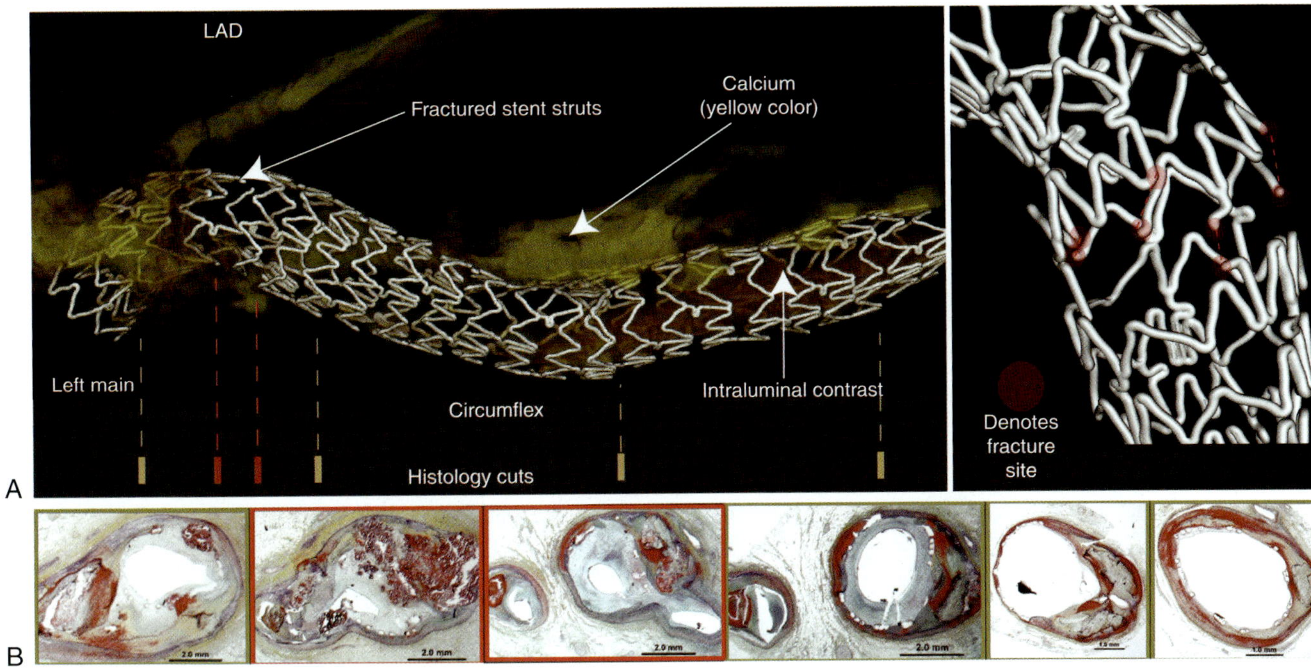

FIG. 2.60 Micro-Computed Tomography (MicroCT) and Histology Findings in the Left Main (LM) and Left Circumflex (LCx). (A) MicroCT three-dimensional reconstruction of the LM and LCx coronary artery stents with a magnified image of the fractured segment to the right. The *red dots* highlight fracture points, with the *dotted lines* indicating the original connection. The calcified plaque is colored *yellow*, and residual intraluminal contrast is *red*. (B) Corresponding histologic cross sections of the LM/LCx stents demonstrating focal restenosis at the area of fracture. *LAD*, left anterior descending coronary artery.

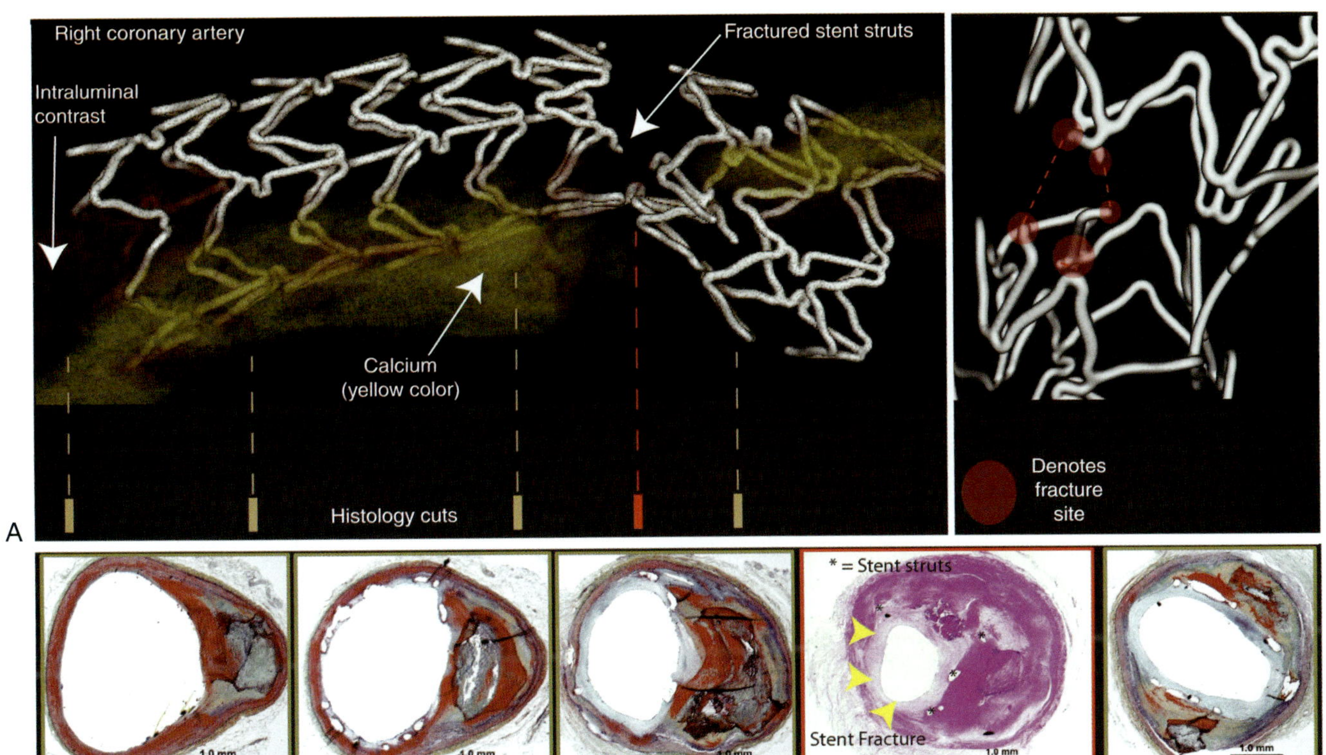

FIG. 2.61 Micro-Computed Tomography (MicroCT) and Histology Findings in the Right Coronary Artery (RCA). (A) MicroCT three-dimensional reconstruction of the RCA stent with a magnified image of the fractured segment to the right. The *red dots* highlight fracture points, with the *dotted line* indicating the original connection. The calcified plaque is colored *yellow*, and residual intraluminal contrast is *red*. (B) Corresponding histologic cross sections of the RCA stent showing focal restenosis at the area of fracture, with inflammation and fibrin accumulation at areas of polymer displacement.

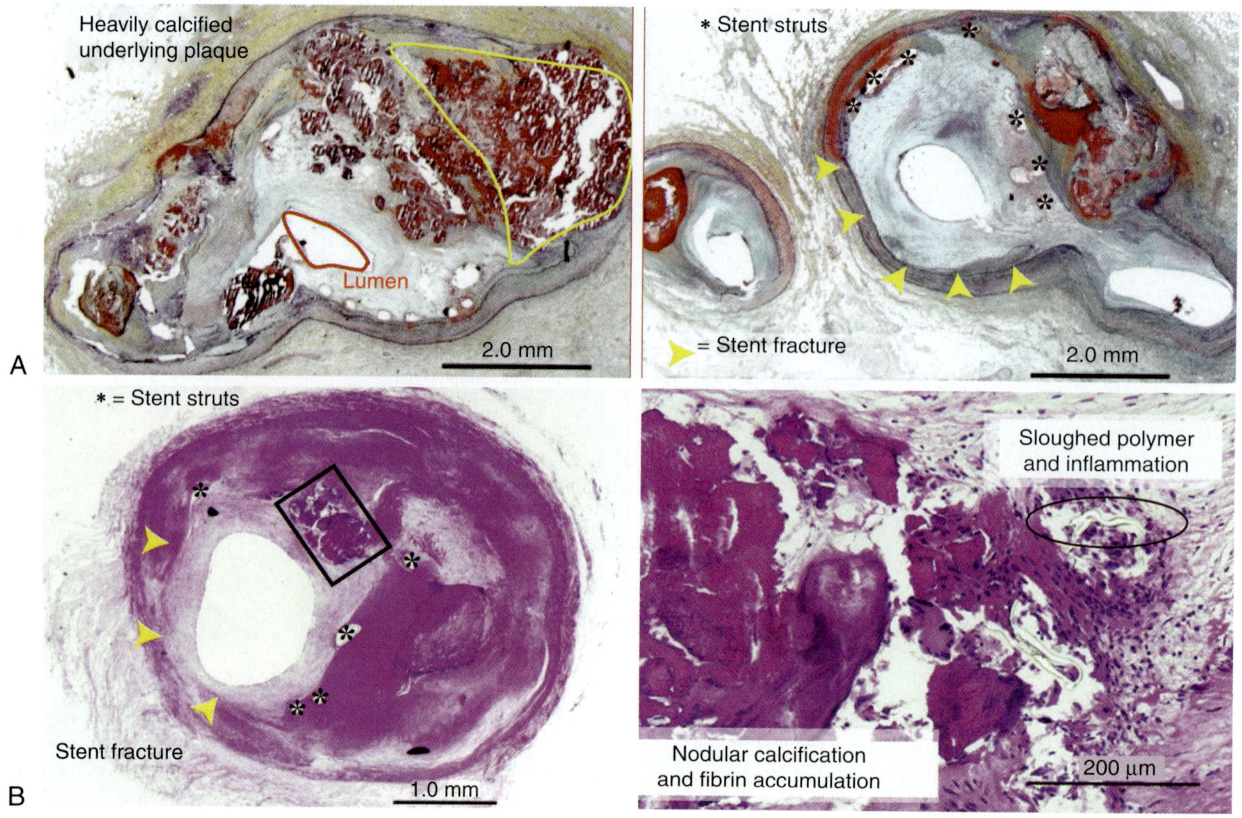

FIG. 2.62 Fracture Site Histology. (A) Histologic cross sections at the left circumflex artery stent fracture site showing heavy underlying fibrocalcific plaque (bordered by *yellow*) and extensive neointimal hyperplasia (Movat stain, original magnification ×12.5). (B) Right coronary artery stent fracture site on the left demonstrating underlying fibrocalcific plaque (hematoxylin and eosin stain, original magnification ×20). The right image is a higher magnification of an area of sloughed drug-eluting stent polymer with surrounding inflammation (original magnification ×200).

Simple Solution for an Undeflatable Stent Balloon in the Left Main Stem

Jonathan Watt, MB CHB, MD, Ayush Khurana, MB CHB, Javed M. Ahmed, MBBS, Ian F. Purcell, MB CHB, MD

A 52-year-old woman with uncontrolled angina underwent coronary angiography, which showed stenosis of the left anterior descending artery and first diagonal bifurcation (Fig. 2.63A). Culotte stenting was performed using a 2.5 mm × 18 mm Xience ProX drug-eluting stent (Abbott Vascular, Abbott Park, Illinois) in the diagonal, followed by a 3.5 mm × 18 mm Xience Prime drug-eluting stent (Abbott Vascular) in the left anterior descending artery. However, it was impossible to deflate the stent balloon using the indeflator. The undeflatable stent balloon completely obstructed the distal left main stem (Fig. 2.63B). No defect was visible in the stent assembly. Severe chest pain and hypotension developed, and the patient was treated for ventricular fibrillation. We could not burst the balloon using a Confianza Pro 12 guidewire (Asahi Intecc, Aichi, Japan) or by overinflating to 28 atm. The stuck balloon was unresponsive to significant pulling. Finally, we cut the hypotube using sterile scissors (Fig. 2.63C), optimizing the patency of the lumen using the stiff end of a coronary guidewire. The balloon passively deflated and was removed. The total inflation time was 21 minutes. Kissing balloon dilation was performed, and a good final result was achieved. The peak troponin T level was 80 ng/L (normal range 0 to 14 ng/L). Echocardiographic results were normal. We believe an undeflatable angioplasty balloon is most likely caused by an invisible kink in the metallic hypotube near the plastic attachment, which allows positive pressure inflation but not negative pressure deflation. Therefore our simple solution, hitherto unpublished, should be strongly considered to avert a potentially fatal outcome.

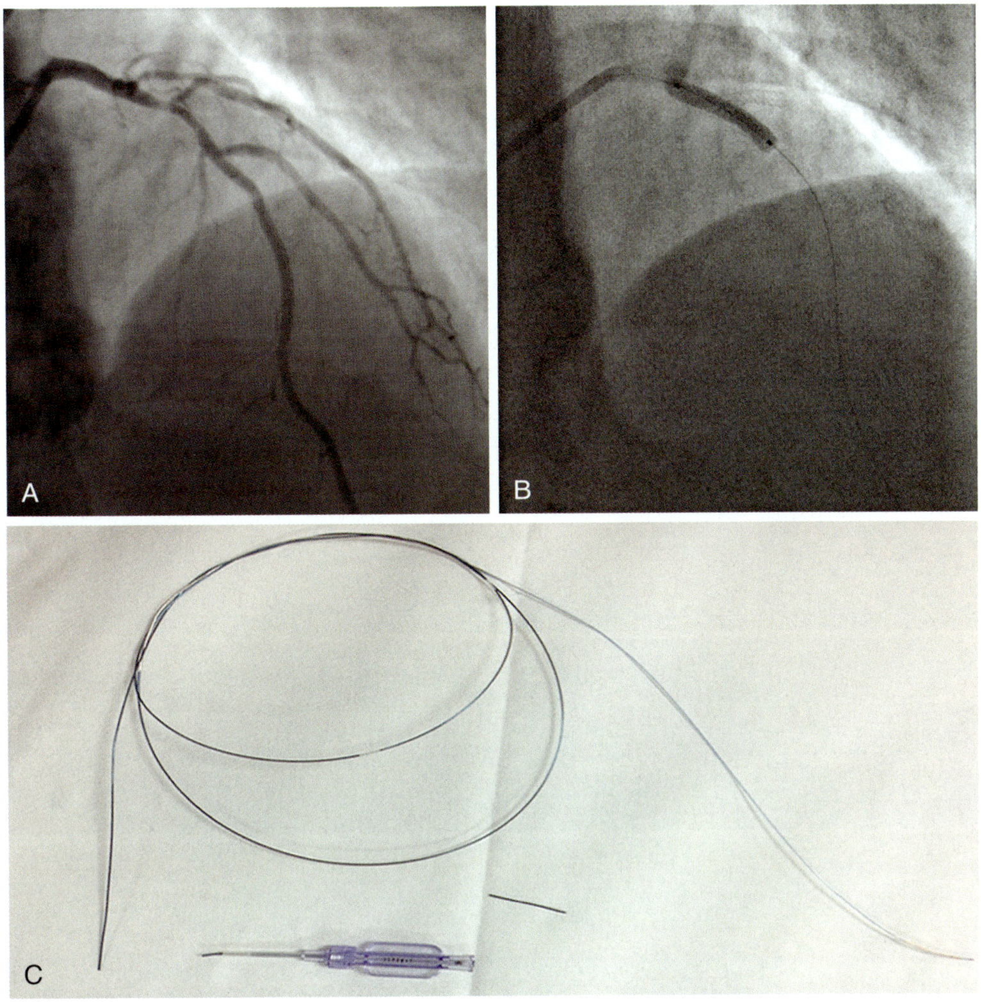

FIG. 2.63 Coronary Angiographic Findings and Final Solution. (A) Left coronary angiography demonstrating left anterior descending/first diagonal bifurcation stenosis. (B) Undeflatable stent balloon obstructing the left main stem after culotte stenting. (C) Photograph of the stent hypotube after cutting with sharp sterile scissors to facilitate passive balloon deflation.

Successful Retrieval of Entrapped Balloon With Optical Coherence Tomography Guidance

Yoshiyasu Minami, MD, PhD, Kentaro Meguro, MD, PhD, Takao Shimohama, MD, PhD, Tomoyoshi Yanagisawa, MD, PhD, Ryota Kakizaki, MD, Taiki Tojo, MD, PhD, Junya Ako, MD, PhD

A 75-year-old woman underwent percutaneous coronary intervention (PCI) for her tight calcified lesion at proximal left anterior descending artery (Fig. 2.64A). After debulking the thick calcified lesion using rotational coronary atherectomy, further dilation using a noncompliant balloon was attempted. However, the lesion was too rigid to expand, resulting in balloon rupture. When retracting the balloon, the ruptured balloon fractured in the middle. The distal portion of the balloon was left behind, trapped between the lesion and the tip of the guiding catheter. Angiography and intravascular ultrasound images of the left main artery (Fig. 2.64B) failed to identify the location of remaining balloon; therefore we performed optical coherence tomography (OCT). The structure of remaining balloon was clearly visualized by OCT (Fig. 2.64C–F). Because a part of the balloon was already inside the guiding catheter, we captured it by dilating another balloon inside the catheter. The ruptured balloon was successfully retrieved by withdrawing the entire system, including the guiding catheter and the coronary wires (Fig. 2.64G).

We report successful retrieval of an entrapped ruptured balloon under OCT guidance. Device entrapment during PCI is a rare but a serious complication[1] that may lead to adverse events, including intracoronary thrombus formation and emergent coronary artery bypass grafting.[2] It is of utmost importance to accurately locate the

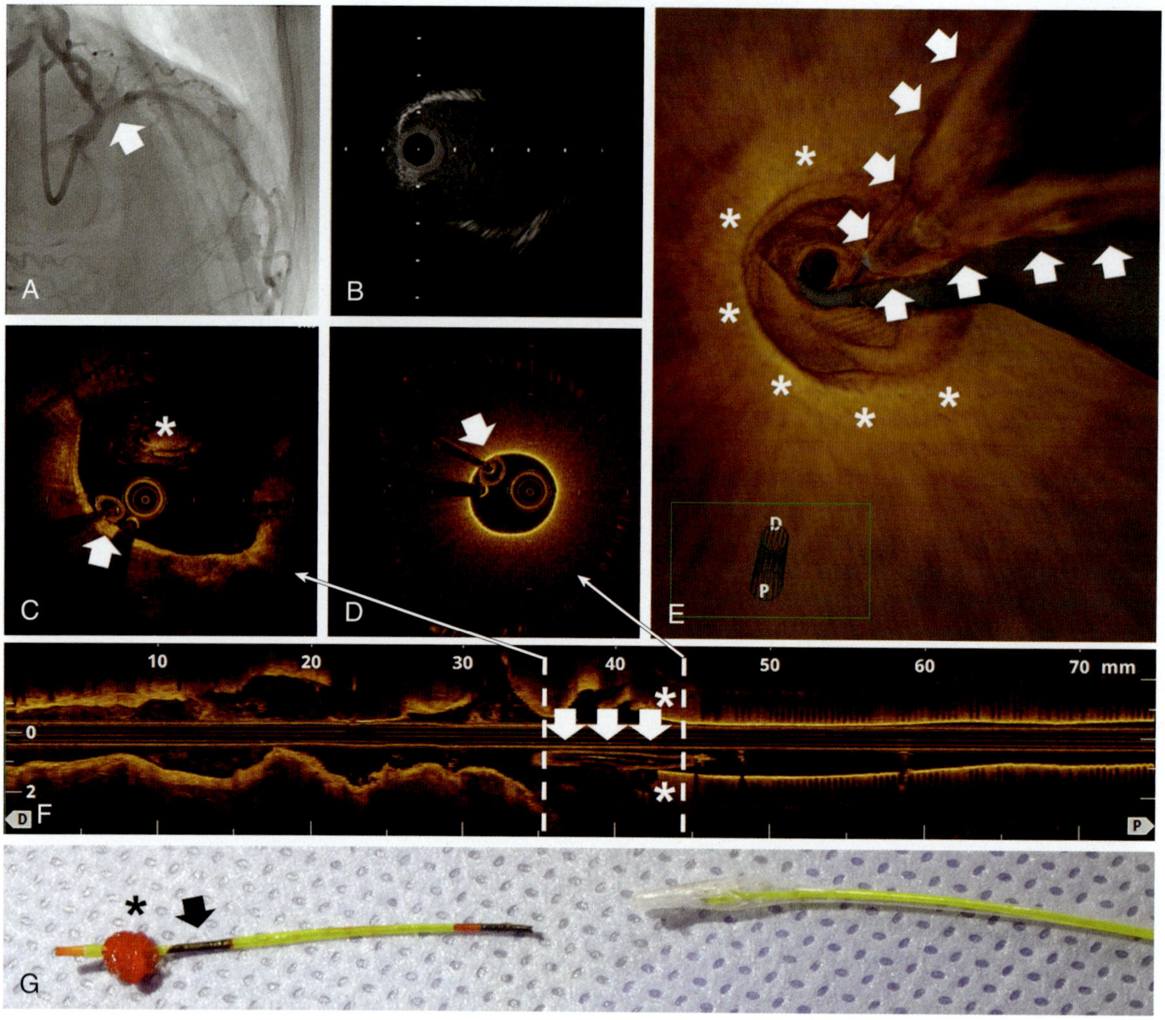

FIG. 2.64 Images of Entrapped Balloon on Angiography, Intravascular Ultrasound, and Optical Coherence Tomography (OCT). (A) Angiography revealed a tight lesion (*arrow*) at the proximal left anterior descending artery. (B) The remaining balloon was not visualized by intravascular ultrasonography. (C and D) OCT clearly imaged the remaining balloon (*arrow*) within the left main artery and guiding catheter. The *asterisk* represents residual red blood cells. (E and F) Three-dimensional and longitudinal reconstructed OCT images showed an abnormal ductal mass (*arrow*) over the tip of guiding catheter (*asterisk*). *Dotted lines* represent the location of cross-sectional OCT images in (C) and (D). (G) The removed balloon, which shrunk during the retrieval (*asterisk*). The x-ray marker was stretched (*arrow*) and nearly invisible on angiography.

intracoronary foreign body for safe retrieval.[3] In our case, it was impossible to detect the remaining balloon on angiography because the x-ray marker was stretched and nearly invisible. In addition, the remaining balloon was not imaged by intravascular ultrasonography, whereas the entire structure of the remaining balloon was clearly imaged by OCT because of its superior spatial resolution. OCT is a powerful option to accomplish safe bailout in device entrapment during PCI.

References

1. Brilakis ES, Best PJ, Elesber AA, et al. Incidence, retrieval methods, and outcomes of stent loss during percutaneous coronary intervention: a large single-center experience. *Catheter Cardiovasc Interv.* 2005;66:333-340.
2. Alexiou K, Kappert U, Knaut M, Matschke K, Tugtekin SM. Entrapped coronary catheter remnants and stents: must they be surgically removed? *Tex Heart Inst J.* 2006;33:139-142.
3. Madronero JL, Hein F, Bergbauer M. Removal of a ruptured, detached, and entrapped angioplasty balloon after coronary stenting. *J Invasive Cardiol.* 2000;12:102-104.

Usefulness of Rotational Atherectomy in Preventing Polymer Damage of Everolimus-Eluting Stent in Calcified Coronary Artery

Nehiro Kuriyama, MD, Yoshio Kobayashi, MD, Masashi Yamaguchi, PhD, Yoshisato Shibata, MD

A 78-year-old woman with an 80% stenosis with moderate calcification in the mid left circumflex artery (Fig. 2.65A–B) was referred for coronary angioplasty. Delivery of a 28-mm everolimus-eluting stent (EES) was initially attempted. However, it would not advance to the lesion (Fig. 2.65C). Rotational atherectomy was performed (Fig. 2.65D). Another 28-mm EES was delivered to the lesion without significant resistance (Fig. 2.65E). The EES was withdrawn to examine damage to its polymer. Another 28-mm EES was implanted. The final angiogram showed a good result (Fig. 2.65F). Scanning electron microscopy demonstrated damage to the polymer of the EES that would not advance to the lesion (Fig. 2.66A–D). By contrast, there was no damage to the polymer of the EES that was implanted without significant resistance after rotational atherectomy (Fig. 2.66E).

Even with EES, damage to its polymer may occur when it is delivered through a calcified coronary artery. In this situation, rotational atherectomy may be useful to prevent damage to its polymer.

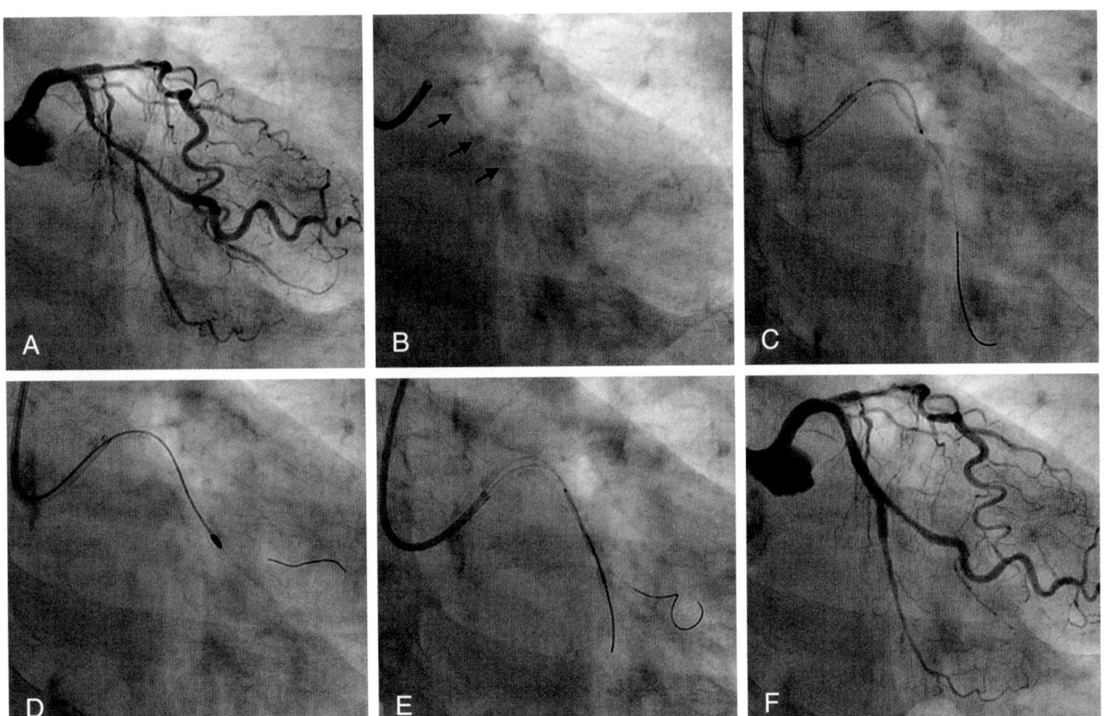

FIG. 2.65 Everolimus-Eluting Stent Implantation in a Calcified Coronary Artery. (A) Coronary angiography showing an 80% stenosis in the mid left circumflex artery. (B) Fluoroscopy shows moderate calcification (*arrows*) in the proximal and mid left circumflex artery. (C) An everolimus-eluting stent is not able to be advanced to the lesion. (D) Rotational atherectomy is performed. (E) Another everolimus-eluting stent is advanced to the lesion without significant resistance. (F) The final angiogram shows a good result.

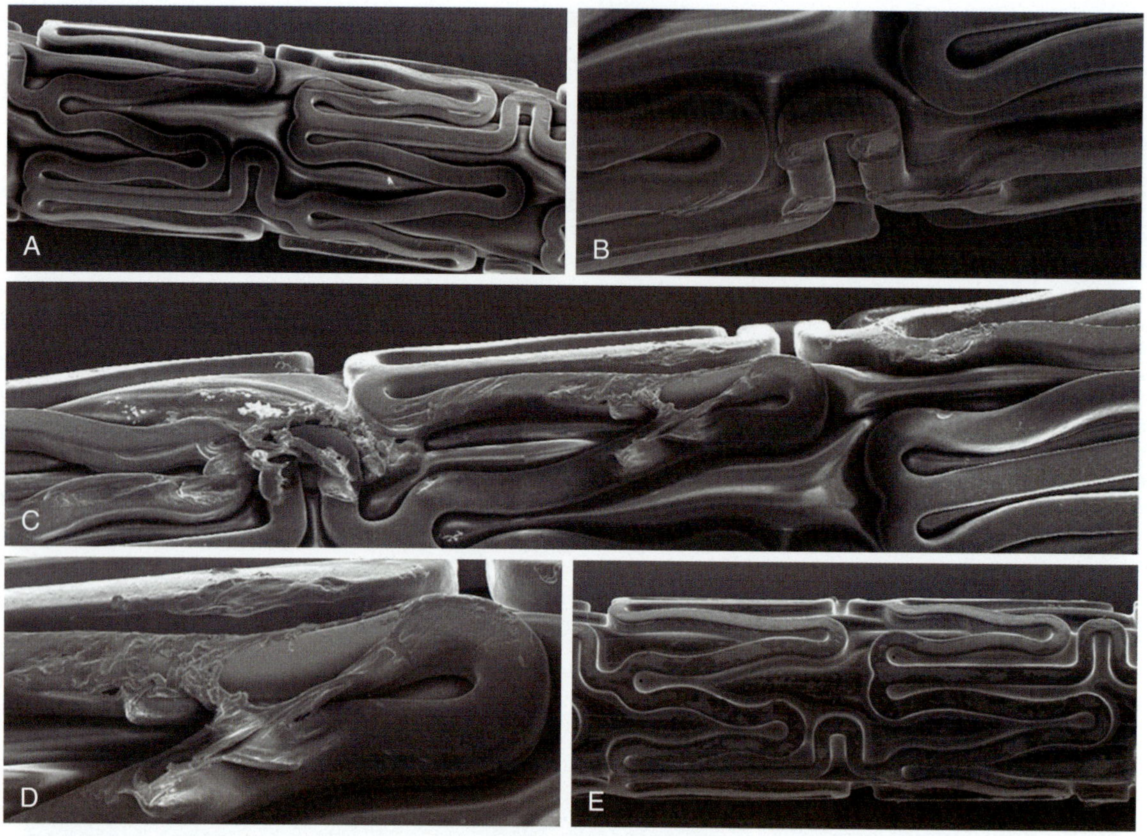

FIG. 2.66 Scanning Electron Microscopy Showing Damage and No Damage to Polymer. (A–D) Scanning electron microscopy shows damage to the polymer of the everolimus-eluting stent that would not advance to the lesion. (E) By contrast, there is no damage to the polymer of the everolimus-eluting stent that was delivered without significant resistance after rotational atherectomy.

Access Site Complications

Aberrant Right Subclavian Artery Hematoma Following Radial Catheterization

George Kassimis, MD, MSc, Nikant Sabharwal, BM BCh, BSc, Niket Patel, MBBS, BSc, Adrian Banning, MBBS, MD

A 66-year-old man with previous stenting to the left anterior descending coronary artery and the right coronary artery performed from the femoral approach was seen with chest pain. Elective coronary angiography was performed from the right radial artery. Accessing the ascending aorta required extensive manipulation, but both right and left arteries were visualized using Judkins diagnostic catheters and were shown to have no evidence of obstruction. Four hours later the patient experienced severe chest pain without ischemic electrocardiographic changes. Examination revealed a difference in blood pressure between the right (80/50 mm Hg) and left (140/95 mm Hg) arms. Multidetector computed tomography was performed to exclude aortic dissection, and an iatrogenic intramural hematoma of an aberrant right subclavian artery (ARSA) was diagnosed. Pain relief was administered and the pain settled with medical therapy, allowing discharge within 72 hours. The patient was asymptomatic at clinical follow-up.

ARSA arising from the descending thoracic aorta is an uncommon congenital variant that occurs in about 0.2% to 1.7% of the population.[1] In such cases, the tortuous course of the ARSA creates difficulty in passing a guidewire to the ascending aorta during right transradial catheterization. The catheter has to follow a zigzag course through the RSA to the descending aorta, and then to the ascending aorta (Fig. 2.67A–B).[2] In this case, catheter manipulation caused an intramural hematoma (Fig. 2.67C–D), diagnosed by multidetector computed tomography. Management of this condition is conservative with pain relief and blood pressure control. It can be suspected by angiographic visualization, in the anteroposterior view, of the angle of the catheter when it engages the ascending aorta, or by manual angiography at the ostium of the right subclavian artery.[2] Clinicians should be vigilant for this anatomic anomaly during right transradial coronary angiography, and although technically difficult, it is feasible to continue the procedure without switching to the femoral artery approach.[3]

References

1. Valsecchi O, Vassileva A, Musumeci G, et al. Failure of transradial approach during coronary interventions: anatomic considerations. *Catheter Cardiovasc Interv.* 2006;67:870-878.
2. Abhaichand RK, Louvard Y, Gobeil JF, et al. The problem of arteria lusoria in right transradial coronary angiography and angioplasty. *Catheter Cardiovasc Interv.* 2001;54:196-201.
3. Yiu KH, Chan WS, Jim MH, Chow WH. Arteria lusoria diagnosed by transradial coronary catheterization. *J Am Coll Cardiol Intv.* 2010;3: 880-881.

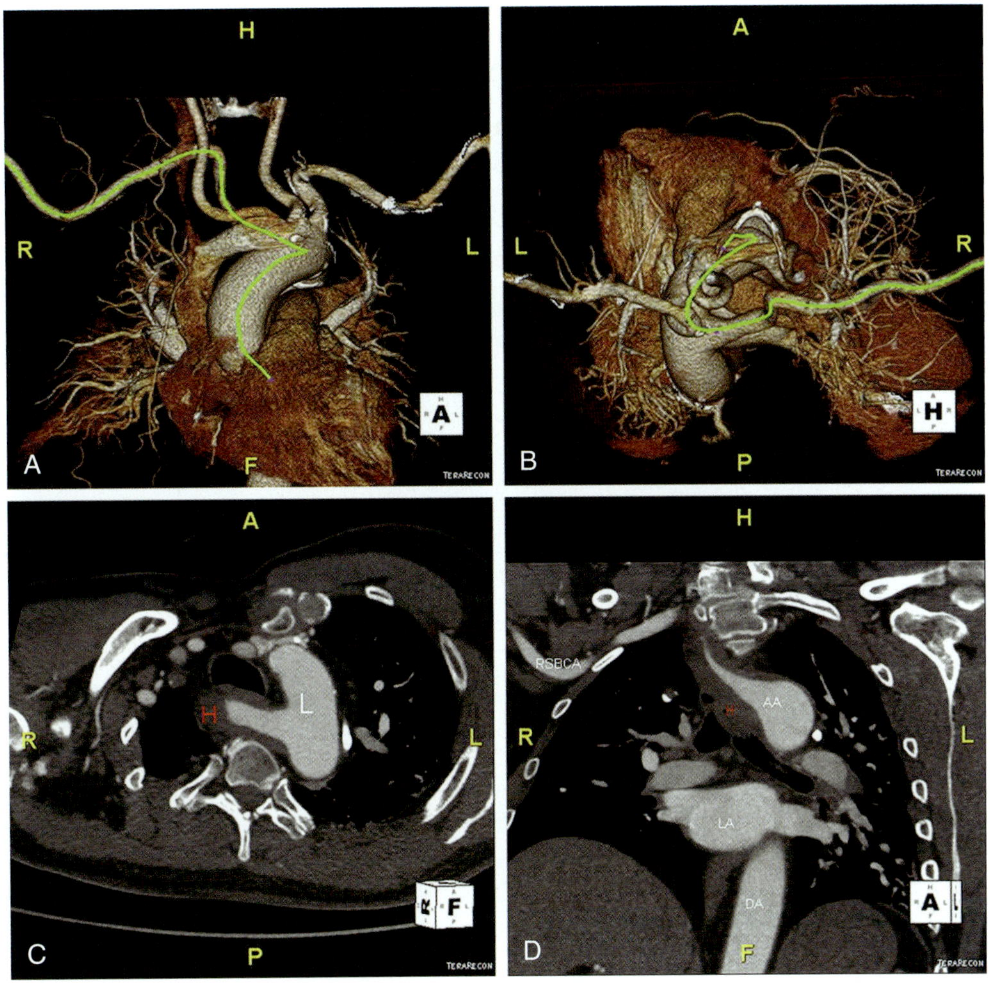

FIG. 2.67 Aberrant Right Subclavian Artery Hematoma Following Radial Catheterization. Multidetector computed tomography three-dimensional volume-rendered reconstruction of the great vessels. The course of the catheter from the right subclavian artery to the aortic root is highlighted in *green* in the anteroposterior projection (A) and the inferior view from the head (B). (C) Oblique projection in the axis of the insertion of the right subclavian artery to the aortic arch. The hematoma (*H* in *red*) and lumen (*L* in *white*) are marked accordingly. (D) Rotated coronal projection of the right subclavian artery and its insertion to the aortic arch. *AA*, aortic arch; *DA*, descending aorta; *H*, hematoma of the right subclavian artery; *L*, lumen; *LA*, left atrium; *RSBCA*, right subclavian artery.

Arteriovenous Radial Fistula: A Rare and Delayed Complication of Coronary Angiography

Isaac Pascual, MD, PhD, Rebeca Lorca, MD, Pablo Avanzas, MD, PhD, Daniel Hernández-Vaquero, MD, PhD, César Morís, MD, PhD

A 76-year-old man underwent revascularization with implantation of two drug-eluting stents in the middle right coronary artery because of an inferior infarct 11 years previously, through right radial access. Posterior clinical evolution was good with preserved systolic function. He was referred to our center for coronary angiography for the development of angina in the past 3 months. On examination of vascular access before the procedure, a large venous system development was detected in the medial region of the right forearm (Fig. 2.68A) with a large radial pulse with a manifest thrill.

Coronary angiography was performed through right femoral access with good results from the previous stents and a severe circumflex coronary artery lesion that was treated with implantation of two drug-eluting stents. Afterward, selective angiography was performed in the right humeral artery, which showed a well-developed fistula between the radial artery and the ipsilateral ulnar vein (Fig. 2.68B, Online Video 2.47). The study was completed with vascular ultrasonography, which confirmed the existence of an arteriovenous fistula (Fig. 2.68C, Online Video 2.48). A hyperflux in the venous system and a large diastolic component in the Doppler wave of the radial artery, typical of arteriovenous continuity, which disappeared upon compression of the fistula, were found. In the vascular surgery department, a conservative treatment approach was chosen.

We illustrate a highly developed arteriovenous fistula, which is a rare and delayed documented complication of coronary angiography through radial access.

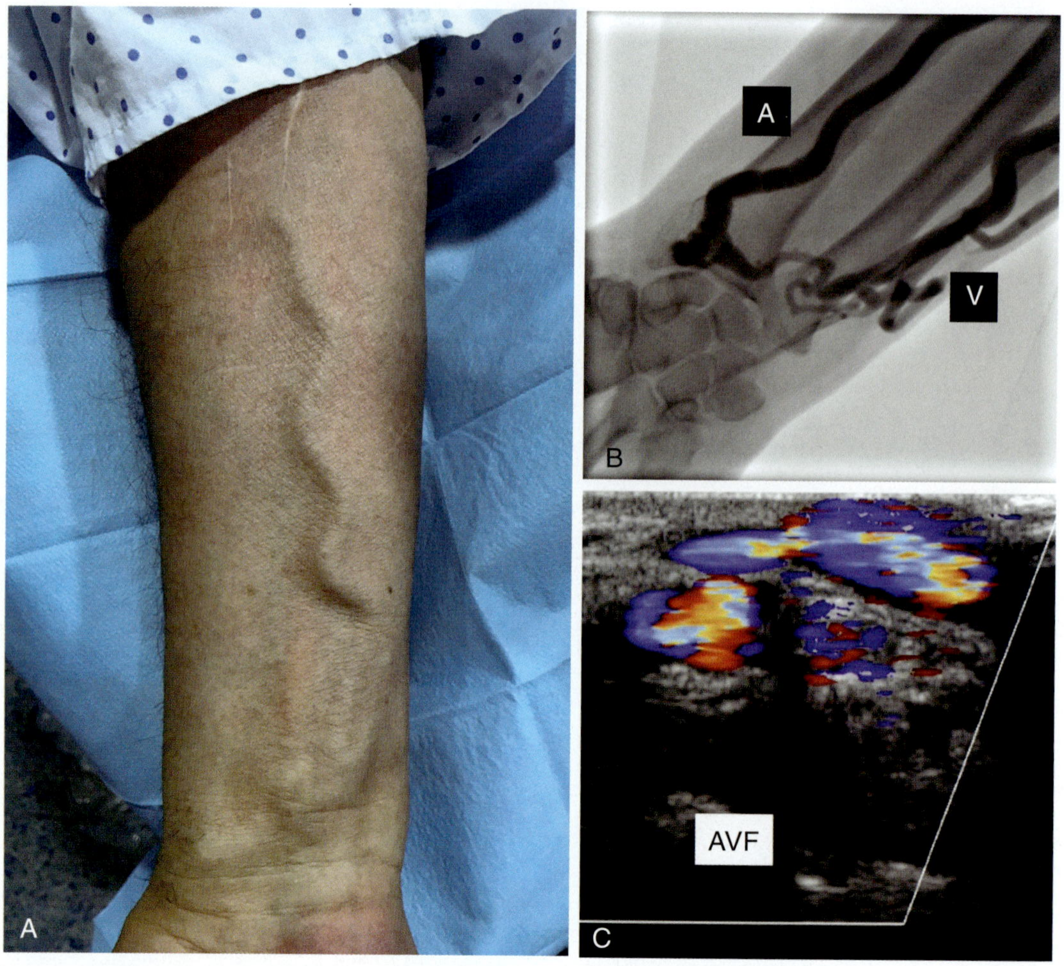

FIG. 2.68 Arteriovenous Radial Fistula. (A) Visual venous system development in the right forearm. (B) Angiography showing the fistula between the radial artery (*A*) and the ipsilateral ulnar vein (*V*). See Online Video 2.47. (C) Color Doppler vascular ultrasonography of the arteriovenous fistula (*AVF*) showing hyperflux in the venous system. See Online Video 2.48.

Digital Gangrene After Transradial Coronary Angiogram

Kuljit Singh, MD, PhD, Joseph Abunassar, MD, Derek Y.F. So, MD

A 60-year-old woman who received thrombolytic treatment for an inferoposterior myocardial infarction in a peripheral hospital was referred for rescue angioplasty for ongoing chest pain. Her relevant history included active smoking, diabetes, and reversible cerebral vasoconstrictive syndrome. At the time of myocardial infarction, she was being evaluated for symptoms suggestive of possible Raynaud phenomenon. Because of administration of thrombolytic medication, a right radial artery (RA) approach for coronary angiography was chosen to avoid femoral artery–related bleeding complications. An Allen test result was positive (normal), and before the procedure 2.5 mg of verapamil and 200 mg of glyceryl trinitrate were administered in the RA. During the procedure, the severe spasm of the RA developed, and the procedure was completed using 5F guide catheters. We administered further intraradial glyceryl trinitrate and verapamil along with intravenous midazolam and fentanyl to relieve the spasm. Acute lesions were noticed in both the right and left circumflex coronary arteries, which were treated with drug-eluting stents. Within the first 24 hours after coronary angiography, pain, numbness, and pallor of the distal right ring finger developed. The ischemic changes gradually transformed to dry gangrene of the distal phalanx of the ring finger (Figs. 2.69 and 2.70). After urgent vascular surgery consultation unfractionated heparin therapy was started. Transthoracic echocardiography and bilateral carotid ultrasonography were used to rule out any obvious cause of embolization. Contrast computed tomography demonstrated occlusion of the distal right radial and proximal second proper palmar digital arteries (Fig. 2.71). It was decided to manage the patient's condition conservatively with anticoagulation as any further intervention in the radial artery during the acute period could lead to further embolization. The digital ischemia was thought to be secondary to microembolization during right radial instrumentation that was exacerbated by severe radial artery spasm. Management of the dry gangrene required partial amputation of the distal phalanx.

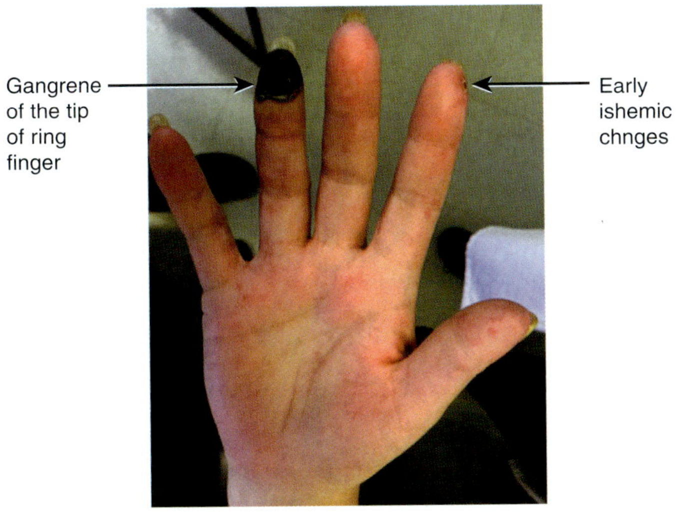

FIG. 2.69 Palmar Aspect of the Right Hand. Digital gangrene of the right ring finger. Early ischemic changes secondary to embolism can be seen on the other fingers.

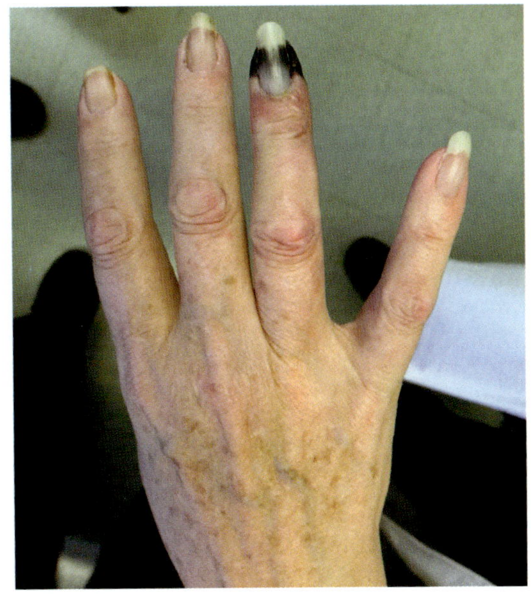

FIG. 2.70 Dorsal Aspect of the Right Hand. Right ring finger digital gangrene.

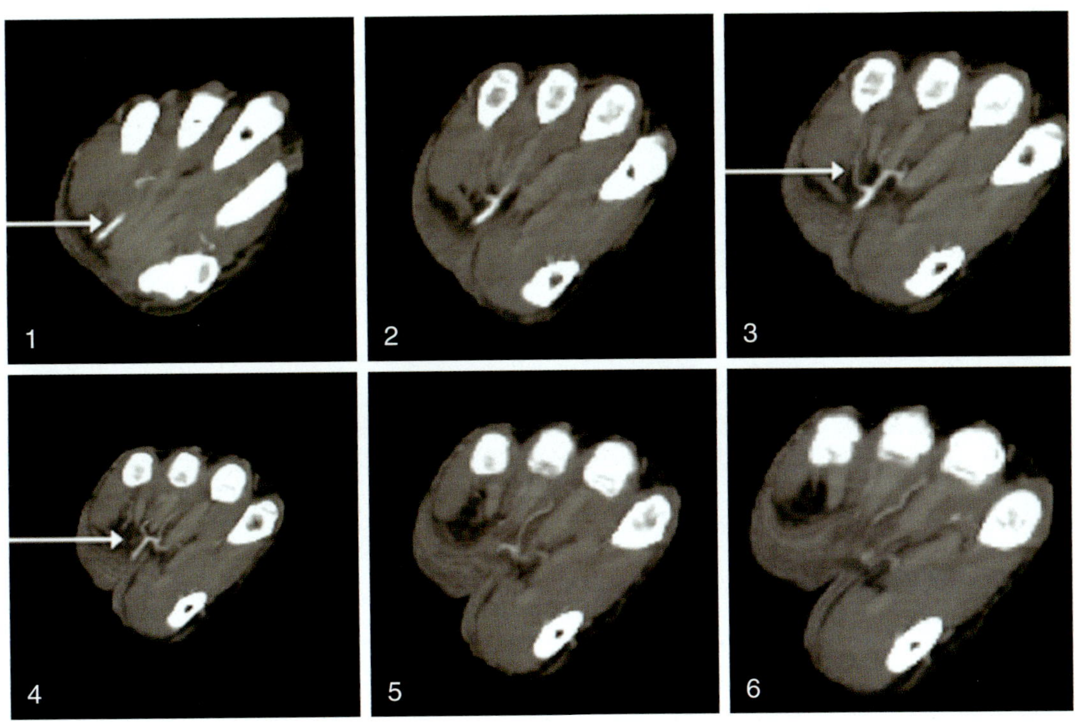

FIG. 2.71 Computed tomography (CT) Vascular Run of the Right Upper Limb. CT scan images showing the ulnar artery, common palmar digital arteries, and proper palmar digital arteries (shown by *arrows*). The radial artery cannot be seen because of occlusion. On CT scan, there was occlusion of the proximal second proper palmar digital artery with collateral flow noted distally in the artery.

From Radial Artery to Embolus: A Rare Complication of Transradial Angiography

Catherine Jaworski, MD, Adam J. Brown, MD, Stephen P. Hoole, MD, Martin Goddard, MD, Nick E.J. West, MD

A 77-year-old woman with effort angina returned for intervention to her proximal circumflex and second obtuse marginal (OM2) artery. Angiography was undertaken transradially. Mild radial intraarterial spasm was treated with intraarterial glyceryl trinitrate, and a hydrophilic-coated guidewire flex artery was passed to the aortic root. The circumflex artery was selectively engaged owing to a short left main stem, with maintenance of a normal arterial pressure trace. The first acquisition showed a new hazy filling defect (arrow) in the first obtuse marginal branch (OM1) artery (Fig. 2.72A, Online Video 2.49). The patient remained stable and pain free. Subsequent acquisitions demonstrated an occluded OM1 (*arrow* in Fig. 2.72B, Online Video 2.50). Because the patient's condition was stable, the uninvolved OM2 stenosis was treated with a drug-eluting stent. With some difficulty, a Sion wire (Asahi Intecc, Nagoya, Japan) was successfully passed beyond the OM1 occlusion. Several passes of manual thrombectomy were performed without yield and with an unchanged angiographic appearance. A third pass did not deliver any debris into the syringe; however, on exiting the guide catheter, a long, 25-mm object was expelled (Fig. 2.72C). The angiographic appearance completely resolved (Thrombolysis In Myocardial Infarction grade flow III), and the procedure was completed with stent implantation in the proximal circumflex (Fig. 2.72D, Online Video 2.51). Histopathology confirmed radial artery embolus (Fig. 2.72E–F). The patient's forearm remained unchanged. Radial artery embolization is a very rare complication of transradial intervention, not previously documented in the literature, fortuitously with a good ending on this occasion. Aggressive treatment of arterial spasm is prudent before guide insertion to prevent intraarterial stripping.

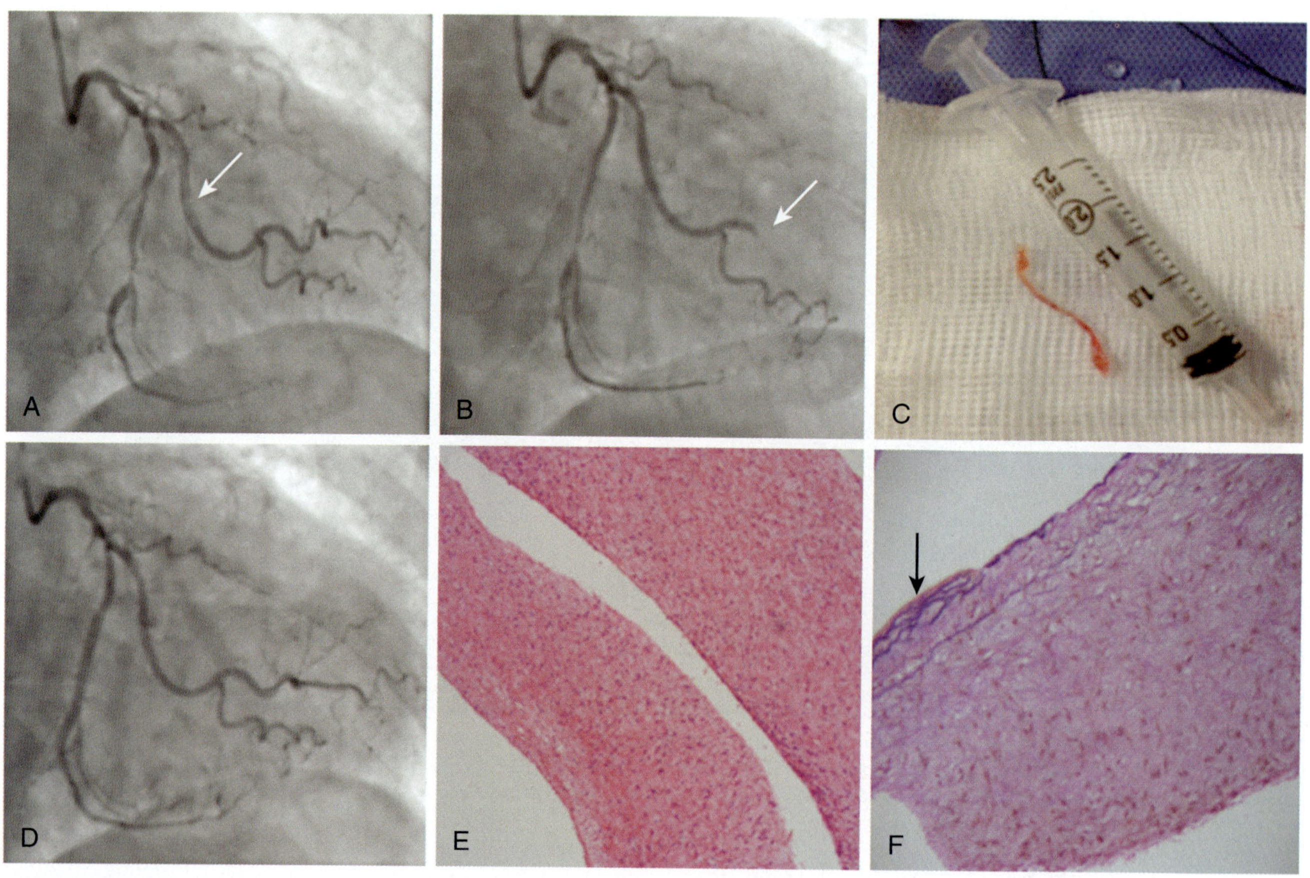

FIG. 2.72 Coronary Intervention Complicated by Radial Artery Embolus. Angiography demonstrating a hazy filling defect (*arrow*, [A], Online Video 2.49) and complete occlusion in the first obtuse marginal branch (OM1) (*arrow*, [B], Online Video 2.50). (C) Macroscopic appearance of radial artery embolus. (D) Complete resolution in the first obtuse marginal artery (Online Video 2.51). (E) Hematoxylin and eosin stain showing loose fibrous tissue and smooth muscle cells. Elastic Van Gieson stain showing nonatherosclerotic intimal thickening of the internal elastic lamina in keeping with radial endarterectomy (*arrow*, [F]).

Iatrogenic Subclavian Artery Pseudoaneurysm Complicating a Transradial Percutaneous Coronary Intervention

Iñaki Villanueva-Benito, MD, Itziar Solla-Ruiz, MD, Raquel Rodriguez-Calveiro, MD, Jose Luis Maciñeiras-Montero, MD, Carlos Manuel Rodriguez-Paz, MD, Alberto Ortiz-Saez, MD

A transradial approach has gained progressive acceptance because it has been shown to have fewer hemorrhagic and vascular-related complications than the femoral approach for diagnostic and therapeutic percutaneous coronary artery procedures. However, transradial access is not free of complications.[1] A 43-year-old man was admitted with a non–ST-segment elevation acute coronary syndrome. A transradial coronary angiography was performed, followed by a drug-eluting stent implantation in the proximal descendent artery. Twenty-four hours after the procedure, the patient experienced an intense, continuous chest pain in his right upper hemithorax that irradiated to the right forearm, without electrocardiographic changes or elevated marker levels of myocardial damage, and required a high dose of analgesia. A computed tomogram was performed, showing a subclavian artery pseudoaneurysm that compressed the brachial plexus (Fig. 2.73A–D). A few days later, an endovascular covered self-expanding stent was successfully placed, excluding the pseudoaneurysm (Fig. 2.73E–H). Chest pain disappeared and the patient was discharged uneventfully.

Subclavian artery pseudoaneurysm is a well-described complication as an inadvertent arterial puncture after central venous catheterization.[2] There are a few reported cases of subclavian artery dissection complicating mammary artery graft catheterization performed via the transfemoral approach,[3] but to our knowledge, this is the first description of a subclavian pseudoaneurysm complicating a transradial artery cardiac catheterization.

References

1. Kanei Y, Kwan T, Nakra NC, et al. Transradial cardiac catheterization: a review of access site complications. *Catheter Cardiovasc Interv.* 2011;78:840-846.
2. Najafi A, Moharari RS, Khajavi MR, Salimi J, Khashayar P. A giant subclavian pseudoaneurysm following central venous catheterization. *J Anesth.* 2009;23:628-629.
3. Collins NJ, Beecroft JR, Horlick EM. Complex right subclavian artery dissection during diagnostic cardiac catheterization. *J Invasive Cardiol.* 2008;20:E61-E63.

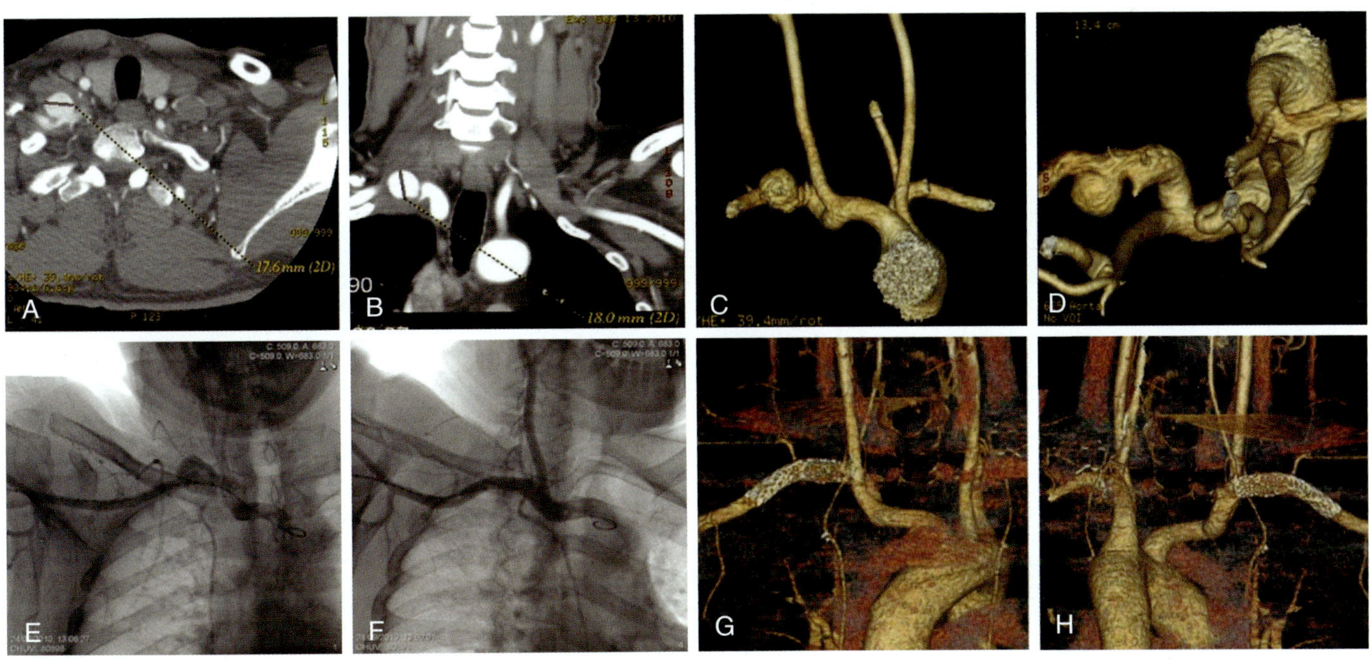

FIG. 2.73 Computed Tomography and Angiographic Images of Pseudoaneurysm. (A and B) Computed tomography two-dimensional images and three-dimensional reconstruction (C and D) showing the subclavian pseudoaneurysm. Angiographic images of the pseudoaneurysm before (E) and after (F) deployment of a covered self-expanding stent. (G and H) Computed tomography three-dimensional reconstruction showing the complete exclusion of the pseudoaneurysm.

Recurrent Vasospastic Myocardial Infarctions and Hand Necrosis

Florian Rey, MD, Marco Roffi, MD, Cindy Bouvet, MD, Romain Bréguet, MD, Peter Jandus, MD, Fabio Rigamonti, MD

A 30-year-old male smoker came to the emergency department with anterior ST-segment elevation myocardial infarction. Primary percutaneous coronary intervention performed via the right radial artery showed an ostial thrombotic subocclusion of the left anterior descending artery (Fig. 2.74A, *black arrow*) successfully treated with two drug-eluting stents under abciximab perfusion.

Two days later the patient had an inferior ST-segment elevation myocardial infarction, and repeat percutaneous coronary intervention via the same vascular access showed a subocclusion of the previously normal mid right coronary artery (Fig, 2.74B, *black arrow*). Intravascular optical coherence tomography confirmed the angiographic suspicion of focal vasospasm (Fig. 2.74C), showing a concentric narrowing without atherosclerosis, dissection, or thrombus. After an ineffective injection of intracoronary nitroglycerin and verapamil, balloon angioplasty without stenting achieved resolution of the spasm and alleviation of symptoms. Although drug test results were negative, the patient admitted occasional consumption of cocaine and methylamphetamine. He was discharged taking oral calcium channel blocker and dual-antiplatelet therapy and the cardiac rehabilitation was uneventful.

Three months later severe right hand ischemia developed as the result of extensive spastic and thrombotic occlusions of the forearm and finger arteries (Fig. 2.74D, *black arrows*) refractory to vasodilators, fibrinolytic agents, and endovascular revascularization. Despite fasciotomy (Fig. 2.74E), transradial amputation was required for extensive necrosis. The vascular histologic studies showed an intimal mononuclear infiltration. Cocaine-associated thromboangiitis obliterans was retained as the final diagnosis.

As shown in our case, the cocaine-derived cardiovascular risks are present not only in the consumption period but could occur weeks or months later and should be considered as risk factors for dramatic outcomes.

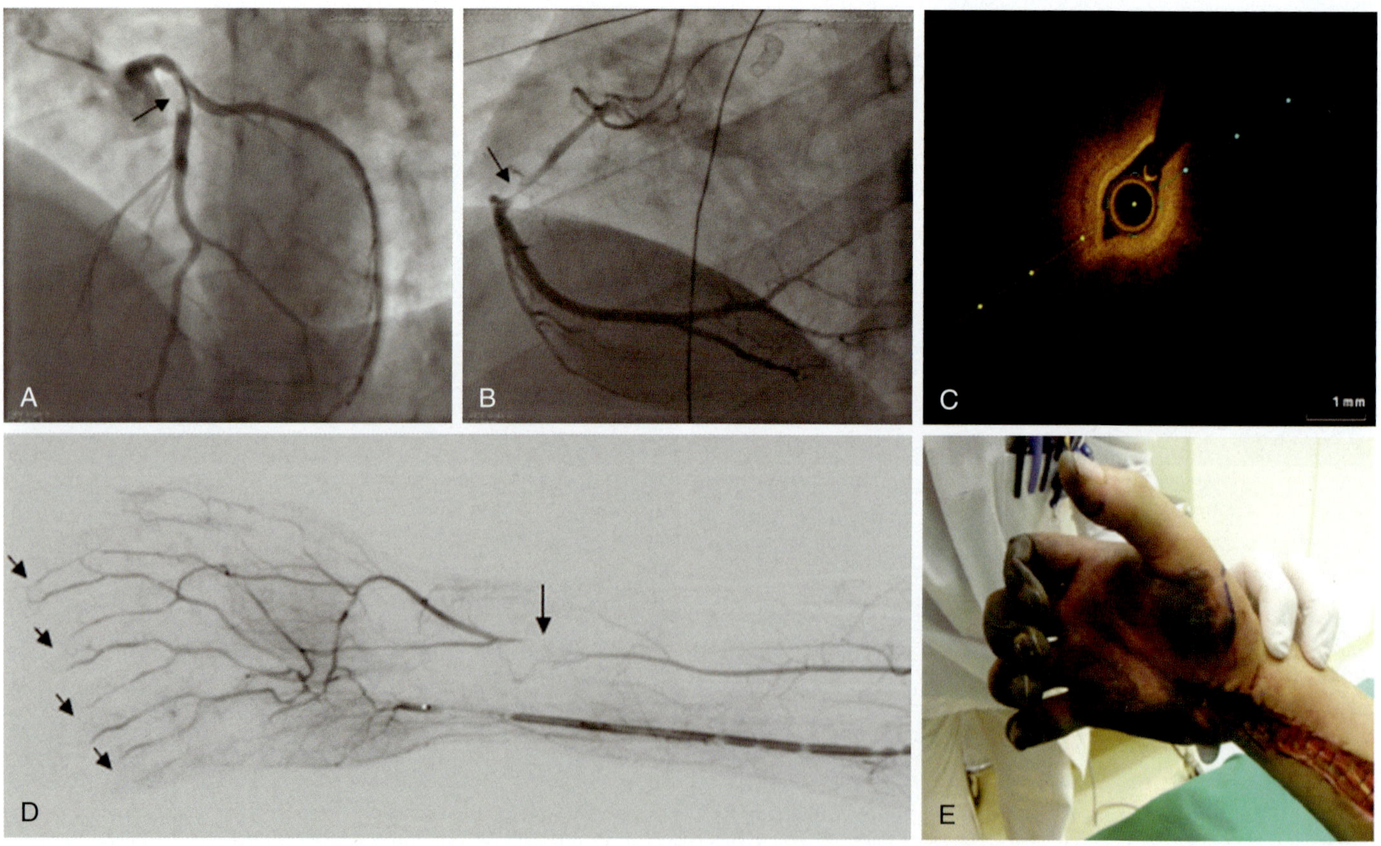

FIG. 2.74 Images. (A) Ostial thrombotic subocclusion of the left anterior descending artery (*black arrow*). (B) Subocclusion of the previously normal mid right coronary artery (*black arrow*). (C) Intravascular optical coherence tomography confirmed the angiographic suspicion of focal vasospasm. (D) Extensive spastic and thrombotic occlusions of the forearm and finger arteries (*black arrows*). (E) Fasciotomy of the forearm.

Chapter 3
Coronary Interventional Techniques

Coronary Aneurysms

A Giant Coronary Artery Aneurysm Treated With Multiple Overlapping Covered Stents

Alberto F. Cereda, MD, Gianluca Tiberti, MD, Isidoro G. Pera, MD, Edoardo Cantù, MD, Luca A. Ferri, MD, Stefano Savonitto, MD, Luigi Piatti, MD

A 62-year-old man with known coronary artery ectasias was referred to our center in 2001 for ischemic symptoms and mild inferior hypokinesis on echocardiography. Coronary angiography showed diffused coronary artery ectasias with an aneurysmatic appearance of the proximal and mid left circumflex coronary artery without stenotic lesions (Fig. 3.1A); a conservative medical approach with aspirin and warfarin was advised. The patient did well with medical therapy thereafter until December 2016, when he was admitted with an inferolateral ST-segment elevation myocardial infarction. Emergency angiography showed the evolution of the mid left circumflex coronary artery lesion into a giant aneurysm with distal thrombotic embolization causing occlusion of the vessel (Fig. 3.1B–C, Online Video 3.1). Because of the large amount of thrombus, rheolytic coronary mechanical thrombectomy was chosen to remove the occluding clot, with ST-segment resolution (Fig. 3.1D–E). One week later, despite triple therapy with aspirin, clopidogrel, and warfarin, recurrent coronary thrombosis occurred, and balloon angioplasty was needed to bridge the patient to the next definitive coronary intervention. The procedure was performed via right radial access, using a 6F extra backup 3.5 catheter. An intravascular ultrasound preevaluation of the distal and proximal landing zones of the giant aneurysm was undertaken, and 4 PK Papyrus stents (Biotronik, Berlin, Germany) were implanted in sequence from the distal to the proximal edge, with 4 to 5 mm of overlap (Fig. 3.1F1–F2, G1–G2). The proximal and distal landing zones were postdilated with noncompliant balloons with good angiographic results (Fig. 3.1H, Online Video 3.2). Intravascular ultrasound grayscale and ChromaFlo (Philips, Volcano, San Diego, California) imaging (Online Video 3.3) highlighted the successful apposition of the covered stents and the complete sealing of the aneurysm, also visible on echocardiography (Fig. 3.1I, Online Video 3.4). At 4 months, the patient is doing well with aspirin and clopidogrel therapy. We succeeded in sealing a giant coronary artery aneurysm, with good angiographic and clinical outcomes, by means of a novel transradial intravascular ultrasound–guided percutaneous technique.

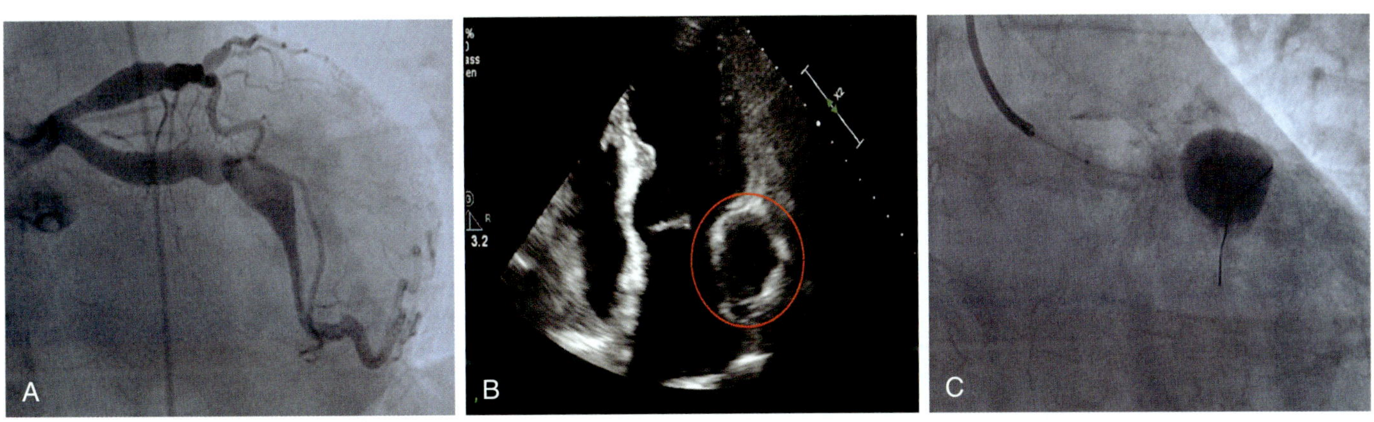

FIG. 3.1 Stove Pipe Technique. (A) Diffused coronary artery ectasia, more significant in the proximal left circumflex coronary artery (15 × 30 mm) 3 years before the acute coronary syndrome. (B) Giant left coronary artery aneurysm visible on echocardiography in the intensive care unit after clinical stabilization of the patient's condition with mild left ventricular function reduction (four-chamber view); the giant aneurysm *encircled in red.* (C) Attempted wiring of the thrombotic occluded left circumflex coronary artery with contrast opacification of the aneurysm.

Continued

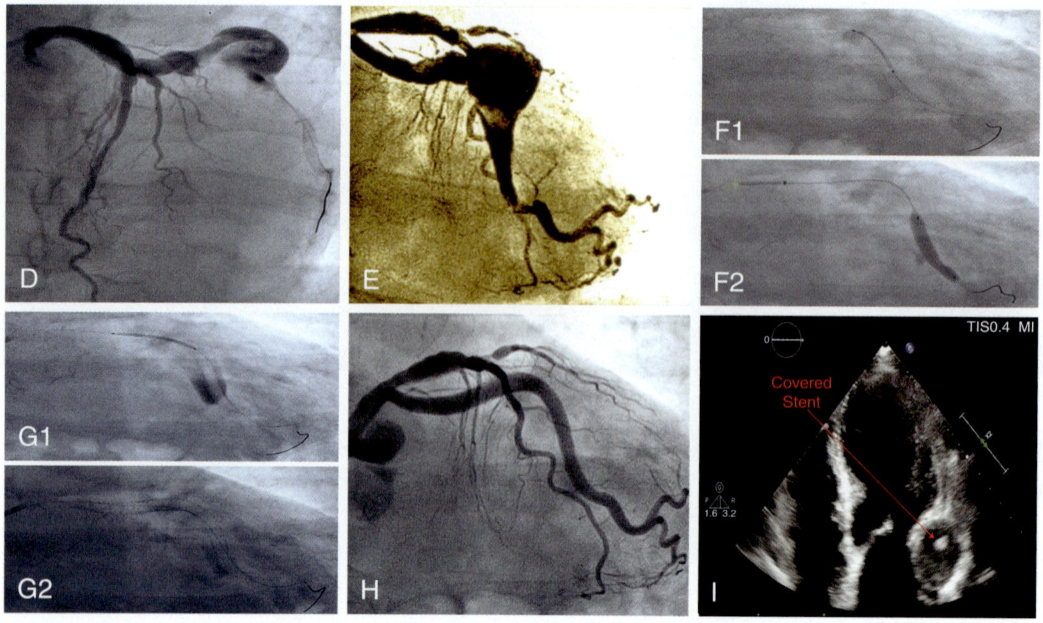

FIG. 3.1, cont'd (D) Distal flow after rheolytic thrombectomy. Note the flow vortex inside the aneurysm (Online Video 3.1). (E) Angiography of the giant aneurysm (30 × 50 mm) before covered stenting. (F1) Apposition of the distal PK Papyrus stent (Biotronik, Berlin, Germany) (4.0 × 26 mm). (F2) Apposition in overlapping of the second Papyrus stent (4.0 × 26 mm). (G1) Apposition of the third Papyrus stent (4.5 × 26 mm) overlapping the second stent. (G2) Apposition of the last proximal Papyrus stent (4.0 × 26 mm) and complete sealing of the aneurysm. (H) Final angiographic result. Distal staining of contrast is due to the previous injection before sealing off the aneurysm. Intravascular ultrasonography and ChromaFlo confirmed the results (see Online Video 3.2). (I) Image of the covered stents on echocardiography (four-chamber view). The red *arrow* indicates the covered stent (see Online Videos 3.3 and 3.4).

Endovascular Coil Embolization of Behçet Disease–Related Giant Aneurysm of the Right Coronary Artery After Failure of Surgical Suture

Patrick T. Siegrist, MD, Satoru Sumitsuji, MD, Keigo Osuga, MD, PhD, Taichi Sakaguchi, MD, PhD, Kouichi Tachibana, MD, PhD, Shinsuke Nanto, MD, PhD

A 69-year-old man with Behçet disease was referred for treatment of a rapidly growing giant aneurysm (38 × 31 mm) of the right coronary artery (RCA), as detected by computed tomography (Fig. 3.2A). The patient initially underwent surgery for single coronary artery bypass grafting and RCA ligature. However, because of a heavily calcified vessel wall (Fig. 3.2B), probably related to chronic inflammation, the RCA remained patent (Fig. 3.2C). Consequently, percutaneous placement of a covered stent graft (CSG) followed by coil embolization (CE) was planned to seal the aneurysm orifice and avoid occlusion of the arterial bypass graft. Considering the orifice length of 32 mm, a long bare-metal stent (BMS) was implanted first to prevent migration of the CSG (our maximal length for CSG is 19 mm). However, the following CSG delivery failed owing to friction in a mild, but calcified, stenosis (Fig. 3.2C) and resistance at the proximal edge of the previously implanted BMS. Ultimately, CE within the BMS was performed. The final angiogram showed only mild leakage through the coil and stent struts (Fig. 3.2D). Alternative percutaneous strategies involve additional stenting of the proximal stenosis to facilitate CSG placement or multiple-layer BMS along with CE to further enhance sealing of the aneurysm ostium. However, the remaining mild leakage is expected to be self-limiting as a result of thrombus formation.

Because data on coronary involvement of Behçet disease are scarce, treatment of coronary aneurysm is controversial. Reports of rupture and thromboembolization-related myocardial infarction suggest prophylactic invasive treatment. Conversely, vascular complications after interventional treatment have been reported.[1] Thus invasive treatment should be considered in case of aneurysm growth, massive size, and recurrent ischemia. For conservative treatment, close monitoring and suppression of underlying vasculitis should be warranted. Additionally, antiplatelet or anticoagulant therapy has been suggested to prevent thromboembolic complications.[2]

References

1. Yildiz A, Arslan C, Erol C. Cardiac tamponade due to rupture of a right coronary artery aneurysm in a patient with Behcet's disease: a case report. *J Cardiovasc Med (Hagerstown)*. 2012;13:243-245.
2. Li D, Wu Q, Sun L, et al. Surgical treatment of giant coronary artery aneurysm. *J Thorac Cardiovasc Surg*. 2005;130:817-821.

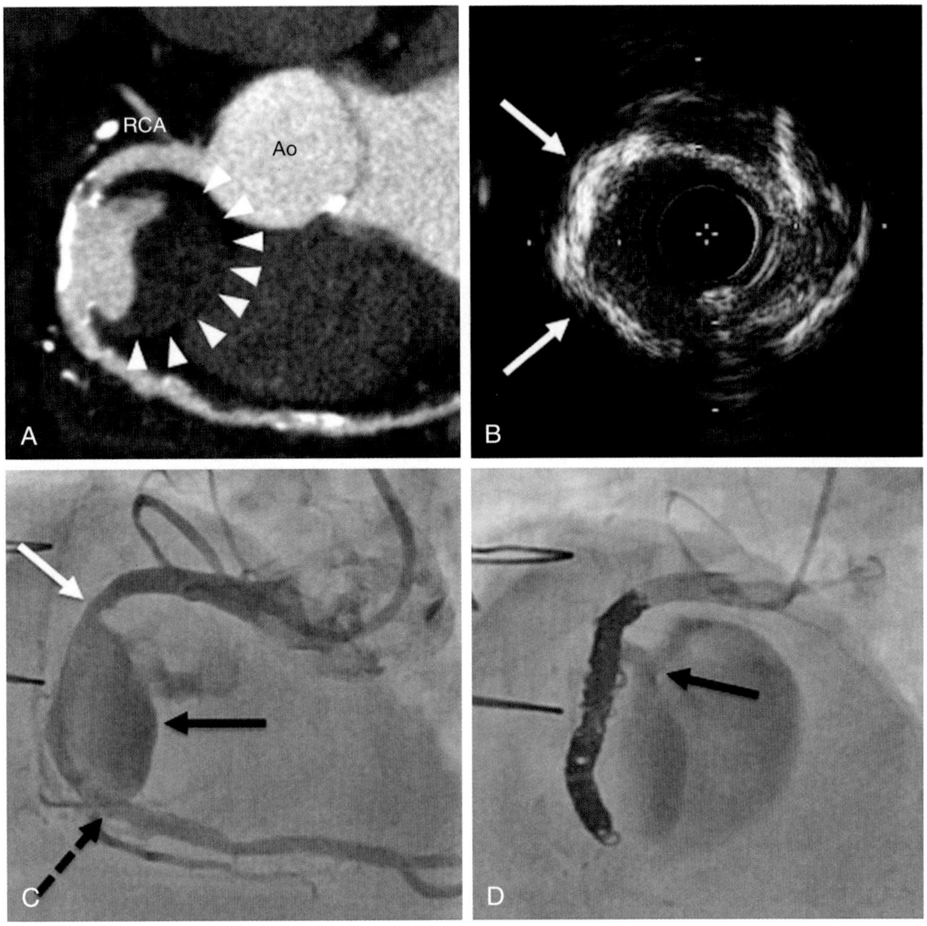

FIG. 3.2 Endovascular Coiling of Behçet Disease–Related Giant Coronary Aneurysm After Successful Bypass Grafting But Failure of Ligature. (A) Computed tomography showing a giant aneurysm of the right coronary artery (*RCA*) (*arrowheads*). (B) Intravascular ultrasound (IVUS) shows a heavily calcified vessel wall (*arrows*), rendering proximal and distal surgical sutures inefficient. (C) On follow-up angiography, remaining flow into the aneurysm (*black arrow*), level of previous IVUS image (*dashed arrow*), and a mild, but calcified, stenosis (*white arrow*) are shown. (D) The final angiogram shows only mild leakage through the coil and stent struts (*arrow*). *Ao*, aorta.

Occlusion of a Large Expanding Saphenous Vein Bypass Graft Aneurysm With Percutaneously Injected Ethylene–Vinyl Alcohol Copolymer

Brian Sonnenberg, MD, Jennifer Rutledge, MD, Robert C. Welsh, MD

A 63-year-old man with prior coronary artery bypass graft surgery (9 years earlier) had an incidental diagnosis of a saphenous vein graft (SVG) aneurysm during investigation of an abdominal aortic aneurysm. Computed tomographic scan showed expansion of the SVG aneurysm from 2.3 to 4.5 cm maximal diameter over 2 years (Fig. 3.3A). The patient had multiple comorbidities, including peripheral vascular disease, renal failure with a failed prior renal transplant, a hereditary C4 deficiency, and lupus-like syndrome, and was not considered a candidate for repeat open heart surgery. Given the uncertain rupture risk of the expanding SVG aneurysm, he was taken to the cardiac catheterization laboratory for planned coil occlusion. At time of angiography the anatomy was considered incompatible with standard coil occlusion, owing to expansion of the aneurysm with gentle contrast injections and the extensive size (Fig. 3.3B–C). Subsequently, a 7F guide catheter was used to engage the SVG with a Marathon microcatheter (EV3 Neurovascular, Irvine, California) advanced over a guidewire into the aneurysm neck. Percutaneously injected ethylene–vinyl alcohol copolymer was used to seal the ostium of the graft aneurysm with successful occlusion of the aneurysm and no residual flow into the aneurysm; a tiny residual tag of the copolymer was left protruding into the ascending aorta (Fig. 3.3D). On transesophageal echocardiography 5 weeks later, the ostial vein graft plug was seen, and the patient remains clinically stable. This is the first reported case of percutaneous injection of ethylene–vinyl alcohol copolymer in this situation.

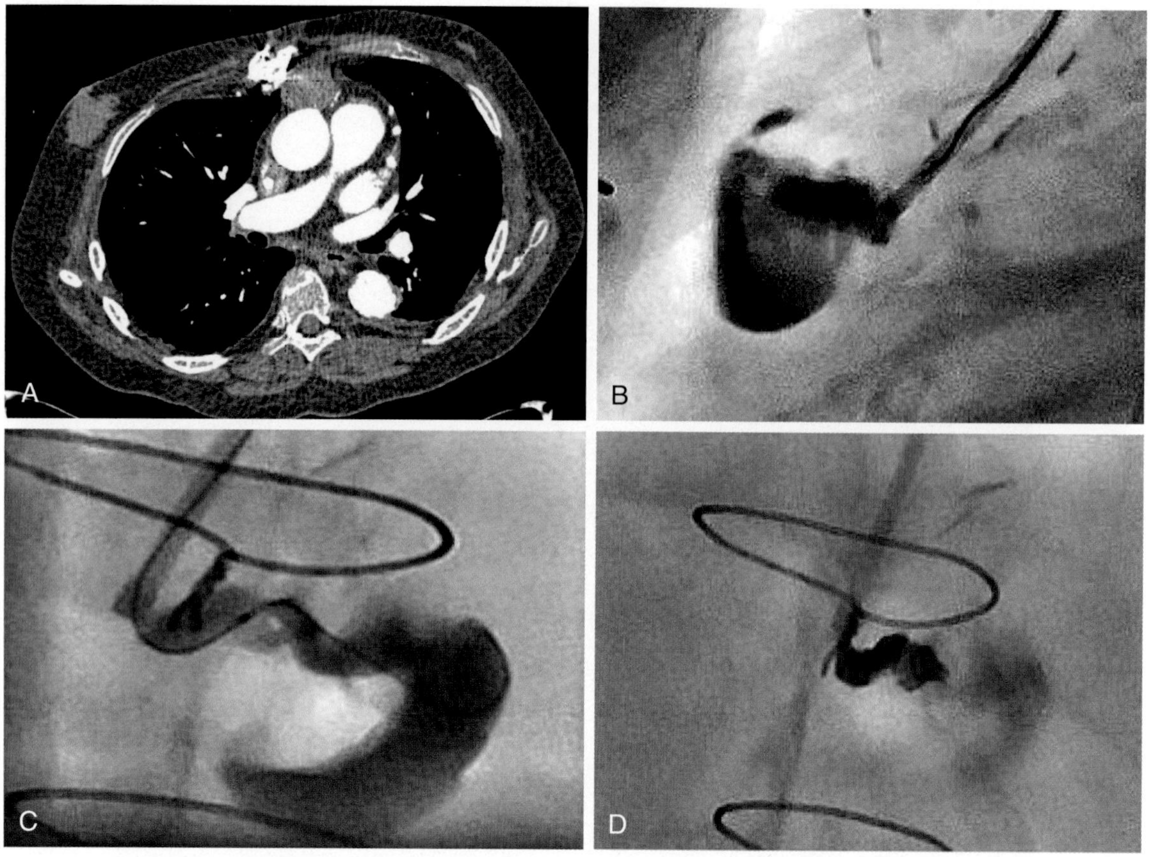

FIG. 3.3 Percutaneous Occlusion of a Saphenous Vein Graft Aneurysm With Ethylene Vinyl Alcohol Copolymer. (A) An expanding saphenous vein graft aneurysm was discovered in a patient with multiple comorbidities. Percutaneous coil occlusion was planned, given the uncertain rupture risk and high risk of reoperation, but this was not possible because of expansion of the aneurysm with contrast injections and the extensive size (B and C). Subsequently, a guide catheter with a Marathon microcatheter (EV3 Neurovascular, Irvine, California) was advanced into the aneurysm neck. Percutaneously injected ethylene–vinyl alcohol copolymer was used to seal the ostium of the graft aneurysm with successful occlusion and no residual flow into the aneurysm (D).

Overlapping Stent Intervention Treatment of a Giant Right Coronary Artery Pseudoaneurysm

Hai-Long Dai, MD, PhD, Xue-Feng Guang, MD, Li-Hong Jiang, MD, PhD, Qiang Xue, MD, Wei-Hua Zhang, MD

A 69-year-old woman was seen with chest heaviness. She had no remarkable medical history and no history of Kawasaki disease or other inflammatory disease. Echocardiography showed a large paracardiac mass in the lateral free wall of the right atrium. Dual-source 64-slice cardiac computed tomography angiography showed a giant right coronary artery (RCA) pseudoaneurysm (4.4 × 4.5 cm) (Fig. 3.4A). Coronary angiography revealed a large pseudoaneurysm in the RCA with 90% stenosis (Fig. 3.5A, Online Video 3.5).

This coronary pseudoaneurysm may have been spontaneous. Treatment options included resection with bypass grafting, coil embolization, and covered stents.[1] However, aneurysms with collateral branches cannot be treated with covered stents, delayed endothelialization, or thrombosis after covered stent implantation.[2,3] Some authors reported that treatment of carotid pseudoaneurysms using overlapping stents produced good results.[4]

We decided to perform a percutaneous coronary intervention. After balloon dilation of the stenotic lesion of the RCA, a percutaneous procedure using 3 overlapping stents (Lepu drug-eluting stents, 4.0 × 36 mm, 4.0 × 24 mm, and 4.0 × 18 mm, Lepu Medical, Beijing, China) was performed (The jet of contrast decreased somewhat after the first stent was implanted. A second stent was implanted with reduction in the leak, and we then inserted a third stent.). Although small leaks remained, an overlapping stent intervention induced a slow-velocity flow field in the pseudoaneurysmal sac (Fig. 3.5B, Online Video 3.6). After the procedure, the patient took aspirin and clopidogrel. One month after the procedure, the patient reported no discomfort. The coronary angiogram revealed that the

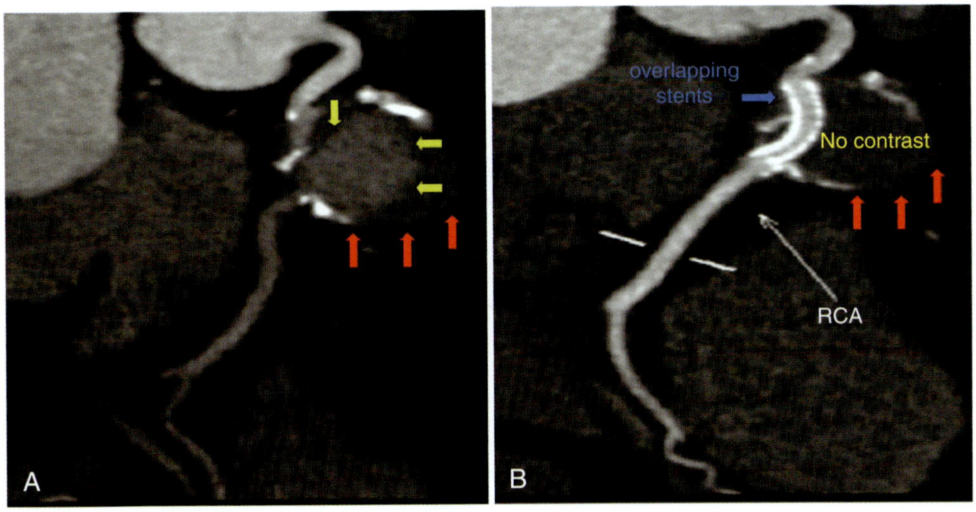

FIG. 3.4. Dual-Source 64-Slice Cardiac Computed Tomography Angiography. (A) A giant right coronary artery pseudoaneurysm (*red arrows*) containing contrast (*yellow arrows*). The vessel distal to the pseudoaneurysm shows impaired contrast filling. (B) Nine months after placement of three overlapping stents, total exclusion of the pseudoaneurysm is accomplished and normal distal contrast filling is obtained. *RCA,* right coronary artery.

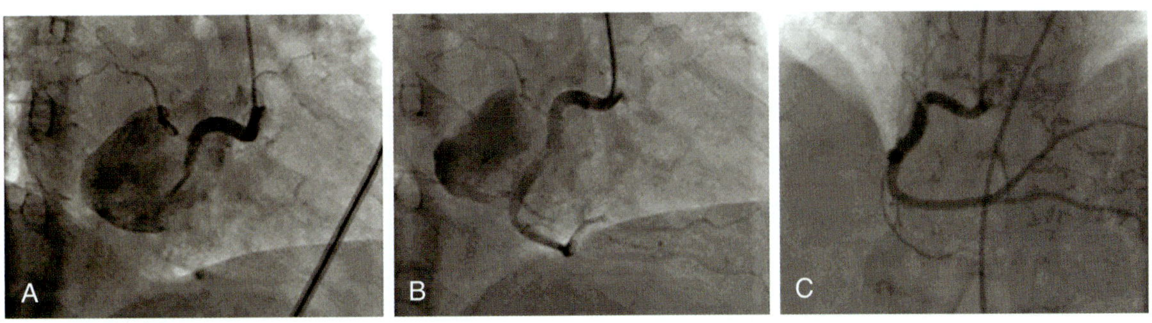

FIG. 3.5. Coronary Angiography. (A) A large pseudoaneurysm in the right coronary artery with 90% stenosis (Online Video 3.5). (B) Three overlapping stents were placed, after which only small leaks remained, with an aneurysmal flow reduction (Online Video 3.6). (C) One month after the procedure, the pseudoaneurysm was successfully occluded (Online Video 3.7).

pseudoaneurysm was completely sealed off, and the branch of the RCA was not affected (Figure 3.5C, Online Video 3.7). At 9 month follow-up, the patient was symptom free. Cardiac computed tomography angiography demonstrated stent patency and complete coverage of the neck with total exclusion of the pseudoaneurysm (Fig. 3.4B). The patient remains asymptomatic at 20-month clinical follow-up.

To the best of our knowledge, this is the first reported percutaneous treatment of a coronary pseudoaneurysm with multiple overlapping stents.

References

1. Aqel RA, Zoghbi GJ, Iskandrian A. Spontaneous coronary artery dissection, aneurysms, and pseudoaneurysms: a review. *Echocardiography.* 2004; 21:175-182.
2. Takano M, Yamamoto M, Inami S, et al. Delayed endothelialization after polytetrafluoroethylene- covered stent implantation for coronary aneurysm. *Circulation.* 2009;73:190-193.
3. Alston EA, Brott BC, Misra VK, Athanasuleas CL, Anderson PG, Litovsky SH. Histologic analysis of a covered stent implanted for pseudoaneurysm in a coronary artery. *Cardiovasc Pathol.* 2013;22:e19-e21.
4. Amistà P, Barbisan D, Beghetto M, Cavasin N, Zucchetta P, Frego M. Three-stent placement for treatment of carotid artery pseudoaneurysm. A case report. *Interv Neuroradiol.* 2006;12:339-343.

Percutaneous Closure of a Saphenous Vein Graft Aneurysm Causing Left Internal Mammary Artery Compression and Left Ventricular Systolic Dysfunction

Razi Khan, MD, Nirmal Kakani, MD, Pantelis Diamantouros, MD

A 58-year-old man was admitted for aortobifemoral bypass with a diagnosis of bilateral iliac occlusions. He had coronary artery bypass graft surgery 15 years earlier, which included left internal mammary artery (LIMA) grafting to the left anterior descending artery and saphenous vein grafting (SVG) to the second obtuse marginal artery. Preoperative chest x-ray films showed a potential mediastinal mass. Assessment with computed tomography demonstrated a patent 5.1 cm (sagittal) × 7.6 cm (anteroposterior) × 6.3 cm (transverse) SVG aneurysm, with associated compression of the LIMA graft (Fig. 3.6A–B).

Angiography confirmed a patent SVG aneurysm (Fig. 3.6C) with reduced contrast density within the LIMA distal to its aneurysmal contact point (Fig. 3.6D), suggesting diminished blood flow through the graft. Left ventriculography showed severe anterior wall hypokinesis (Online Video 3.8). Because of its size and associated compression of the LIMA, aneurysmal closure using a percutaneous Amplatzer vascular plug (AGA Medical, Golden Valley, Minnesota) was decided. Risk of LIMA injury with surgical reentry was considered high given its proximity to the sternum.

Given the patient's bilateral iliac occlusions, vascular access was obtained via the left brachial artery. The SVG graft was engaged using a 6F VL 3.5 guide catheter (Boston Scientific, Natick, Massachusetts) manipulated to the aneurysm neck. The SVG diameter at the site of intended device implantation was 10 mm based on computed tomography/fluoroscopic imaging. A 12-mm Amplatzer vascular plug I was then introduced successfully proximal to the aneurysm. Fluoroscopic and computed tomography imaging confirmed appropriate occluder positioning (Fig. 3.6E) with minimal contrast flowing through the device.

Two months after the procedure, angiography demonstrated complete aneurysmal thrombosis, with no flow distal to the vascular plug. Additionally, dense contrast passage was visualized through the LIMA graft with marked improvement of left ventricular function and anterior wall motion (Fig. 3.1F, Online Video 3.9).

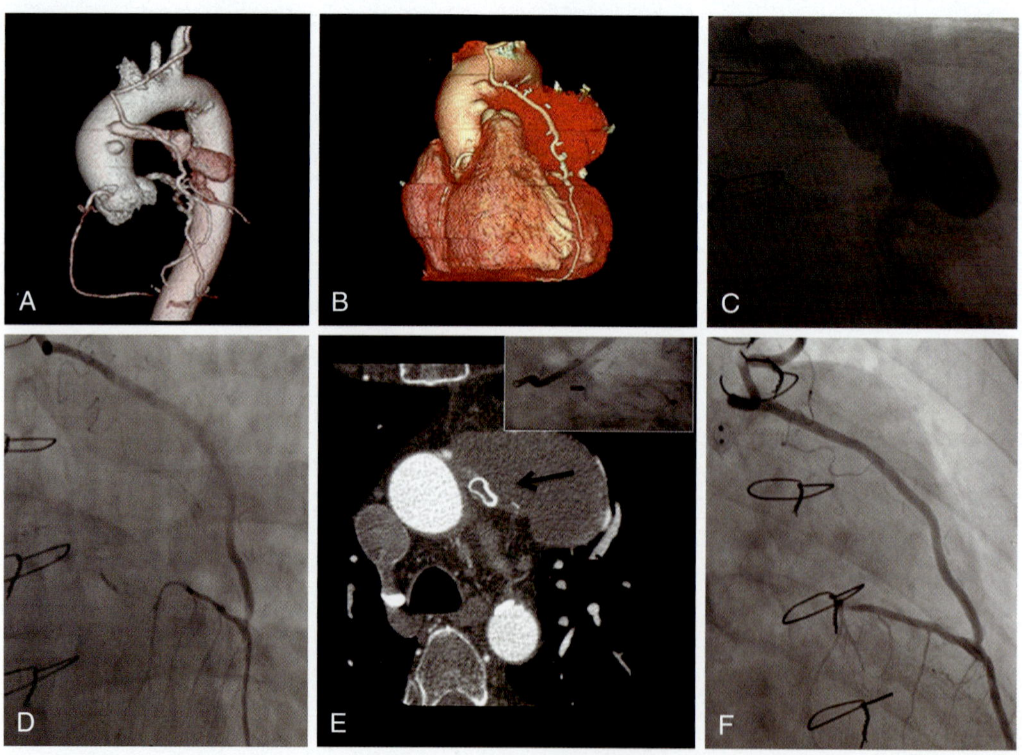

FIG. 3.6 Assessment of Saphenous Vein Graft Aneurysm Before and After Percutaneous Closure. (A) Computed tomography (CT) (three-dimensional reconstruction) showing luminal flow in the saphenous vein graft (SVG) aneurysm (the thrombosed portion of the aneurysm is not visualized). (B) CT (three-dimensional reconstruction) showing the SVG aneurysm with compression of the left internal mammary artery (LIMA). Angiographic imaging showing a patent SVG aneurysm (C) and attenuation of contrast through the LIMA graft distal to aneurysmal point of contact (D). (E) CT (two-dimensional) and angiographic (inset) imaging of successful implantation of the Amplatzer vascular plug I (AGA Medical, Golden Valley, Minnesota) (*black arrow*). (F) Angiographic imaging showing restoration of dense contrast passage through the LIMA (see Online Videos 3.8 and 3.9).

SVG aneurysms are rare complications of coronary artery bypass graft surgery.[1] The natural history of these aneurysms is not well known; however, complications include thrombus embolization, rupture, and erosion into neighboring structures.[2] To our knowledge, this is the first case of SVG aneurysm–associated LIMA compression with resultant left ventricular dysfunction. Although treatment has traditionally involved surgical ligation or excision, percutaneous closure is being increasingly performed, particularly in high-risk surgical patients, such as the patient described in our case.[3,4]

ACKNOWLEDGMENT

The authors thank Hamid Neshat for his help with figure modifications.

References

1. Williams ML, Rampersaud E, Wolfe WG. A man with saphenous vein graft aneurysms after bypass surgery. *Ann Thorac Surg.* 2004;77:1815-1817.
2. Gupta S, Khan T, Stephenson LW, Cooley D, Schnader J. Clinical conference on management dilemmas: a growing vascular mass in the chest. *Chest.* 2000;118:1769-1775.
3. Cruden NL, Turnbull C, Starkey IR. Saphenous vein graft aneurysm. *Eur Heart J.* 2007;28:1071.
4. Sura AC, Douglas JS Jr. Percutaneous closure of giant saphenous vein graft aneurysm. *J Am Coll Cardiol Intv.* 2010;3:784-785.

Percutaneous Closure of Giant Saphenous Vein Graft Aneurysm

Amish C. Sura, MD, John S. Douglas Jr., MD

A 78-year-old man was referred to our institution for treatment of an unusual expanding aneurysm. He had earlier coronary artery bypass surgery in 1999. Subsequently, exertional dyspnea developed, and chest x-ray films showed a right chest mass that was increasing in size. Multislice computed tomography revealed a partially thrombosed 16.5 × 6.5 cm aneurysm arising from the site of the saphenous vein conduit to the right coronary artery and extending in the distribution of this graft, suggesting a true saphenous vein graft aneurysm (Fig. 3.7A–B). This aneurysm impinged on the diaphragm, compressed the liver inferiorly, and did not communicate with the distal right coronary artery.

Closure was recommended because of the expanding aneurysm and potential for rupture. A surgical approach was judged possible but required repeat sternotomy and use of cardiopulmonary bypass. Percutaneous closure was judged to be feasible and much less invasive and was elected by the patient.

From a femoral approach, a 7F JR4 guide catheter (Medtronic, Minneapolis, Minnesota) was used to engage the neck of the aneurysm. Angiography was performed (Fig. 3.8A) and a 5 × 20 mm balloon was used to "size" the neck at approximately 3 mm in diameter (Fig. 3.8B). A stiff guidewire was introduced (Fig. 3.8C) over which a 9F Amplatzer delivery sheath was cannulated into the neck of the aneurysm. A 4-mm Amplatzer Septal occluder device (AGA Medical, Golden Valley, Minnesota) was implanted (Fig. 3.8D), occluding the aneurysm neck. Aortic angiography and transesophageal echocardiography confirmed the absence of flow into or out of the aneurismal cavity (Fig. 3.8E).

The patient was discharged the next day taking aspirin and clopidogrel (75 mg). At 3 months after the procedure, the patient was asymptomatic and fully active.

Aortocoronary saphenous vein graft aneurysms are a rare complication of coronary artery bypass graft surgery. The incidence

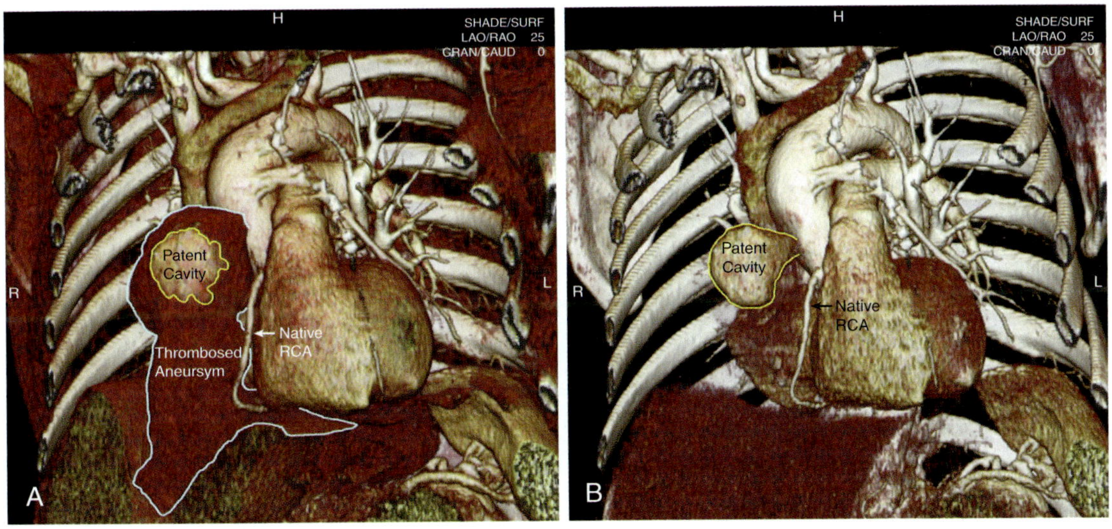

FIG. 3.7 Multislice Computed Tomography. (A) Shallow left anterior oblique view with multislice computed tomography showing a large aneurysm filled with thrombus with a smaller patent cavity that communicates with the aorta. (B) Image reconstruction showing the relationship of the aneurysm cavity to the aorta. *RCA*, right coronary artery.

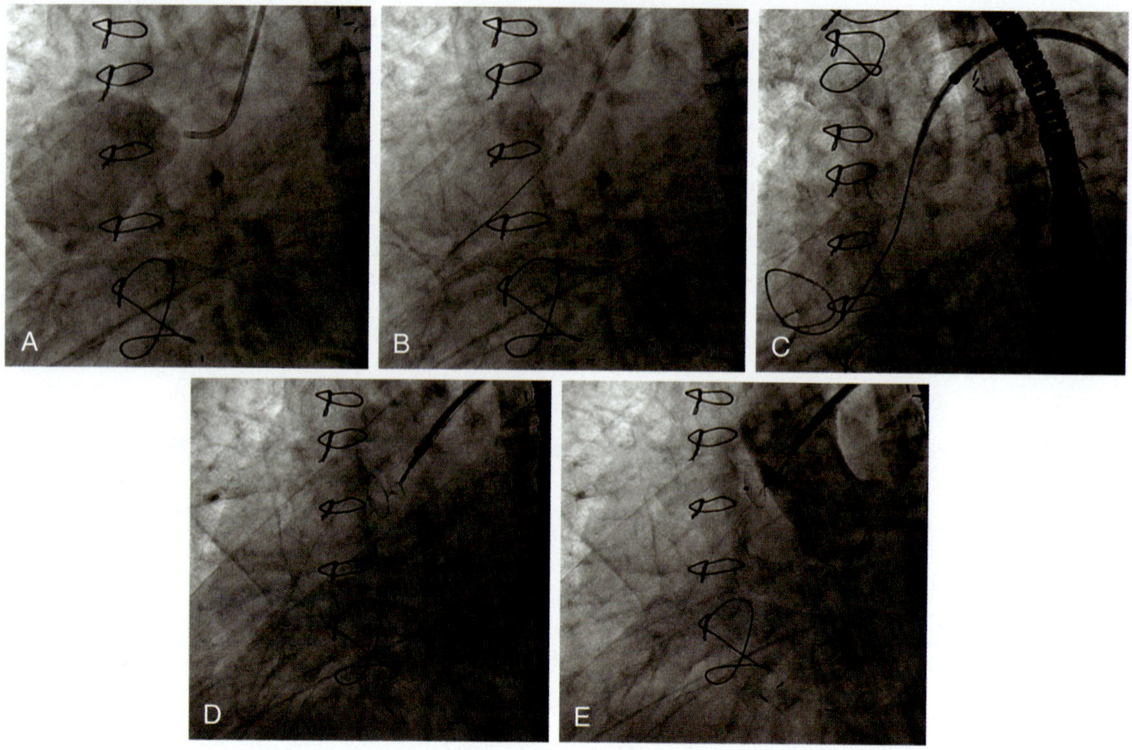

FIG. 3.8 Angiography and Closure of Aneurysm in Shallow Left Anterior Oblique View. (A) Angiogram of aneurysm cavity. (B) Use of coronary balloon to "size" the neck of aneurysm. (C) Stiff wire with formed J and Amplatzer delivery sheath (AGA Medical, Golden Valley, Minnesota). (D) Device deployment. (E) The aortogram after implantation shows absent flow into the aneurysm.

is unknown but may be increasing with increasing use of advanced imaging techniques.[1–3] They often present as a mediastinal mass. Symptoms can be nonspecific and include dyspnea, chest discomfort, and hemoptysis. Aneurysm rupture is associated with a high mortality rate. Such lesions are usually treated surgically, although secondary thrombosis owing to coil implantation has been described.[2,4]

References

1. Aslam A, Chaudhry M, Fox J, Gadhavi P, Wanahita N. Aortocoronary saphenous vein graft aneurysms: a systematic review of published cases. *Catheter Cardiovasc Interv.* 2009;73 Suppl:s68.
2. Pulling TM, Uyesugi W. Aneurysm of an autologous aorta to right coronary artery reverse saphenous vein graft presenting as a mediastinal mass: a case report. *Cases J.* 2008;1:340.
3. Garcia-Lara J, Pinar-Bermudez E, Hurtado JA, Valdez-Chavarri M. Giant true saphenous vein graft aneurysm. *J Am Coll Cardiol.* 2009;54:1899.
4. Cruden NL, Turnbull C, Starkey IR. Saphenous vein graft aneurysm. *Eur Heart J.* 2007;28:1071.

Percutaneous Luminal Reconstruction of Giant Saphenous Vein Graft Aneurysm

Tiffany Patterson, MBBS BSs, Ian Webb, MD, Simon R. Redwood, MD

A 77-year-old woman had a large contrast-enhancing paracardiac mass localized to the right atrium (Fig. 3.9A–B) on screening computed tomography after colonic carcinoma surgery. She had a history of coronary artery bypass grafting with left internal mammary artery to left anterior descending and saphenous vein grafts (SVG) to the obtuse marginal and right coronary artery (RCA) vessels after a myocardial infarction 20 years previously, which was followed by symptom-driven angioplasty to the ostial RCA-SVG.

Diagnostic angiography demonstrated a large contrast-filling aneurysmal segment of the RCA-SVG, with reduced distal flow (Fig. 3.9C, Online Video 3.10). The expanding aneurysm was at risk of possible rupture; however, resternotomy was unfavorable and percutaneous management was sought after heart team discussion.

The SVG was intubated with an 8F multipurpose guiding catheter, and the distal vessel beyond the aneurysm was accessed using a hydrophilic guidewire introduced through a microcatheter. Dilation of the preexisting ostial stents enabled delivery of overlapping pericardial-covered stents in the proximal and mid vessel (4 × 27 mm Aneugraft stent, ITGI Medical, Or Akiva, Israel) covering the aneurysm origin, creating a new tract (Fig. 3.9D). Poor support

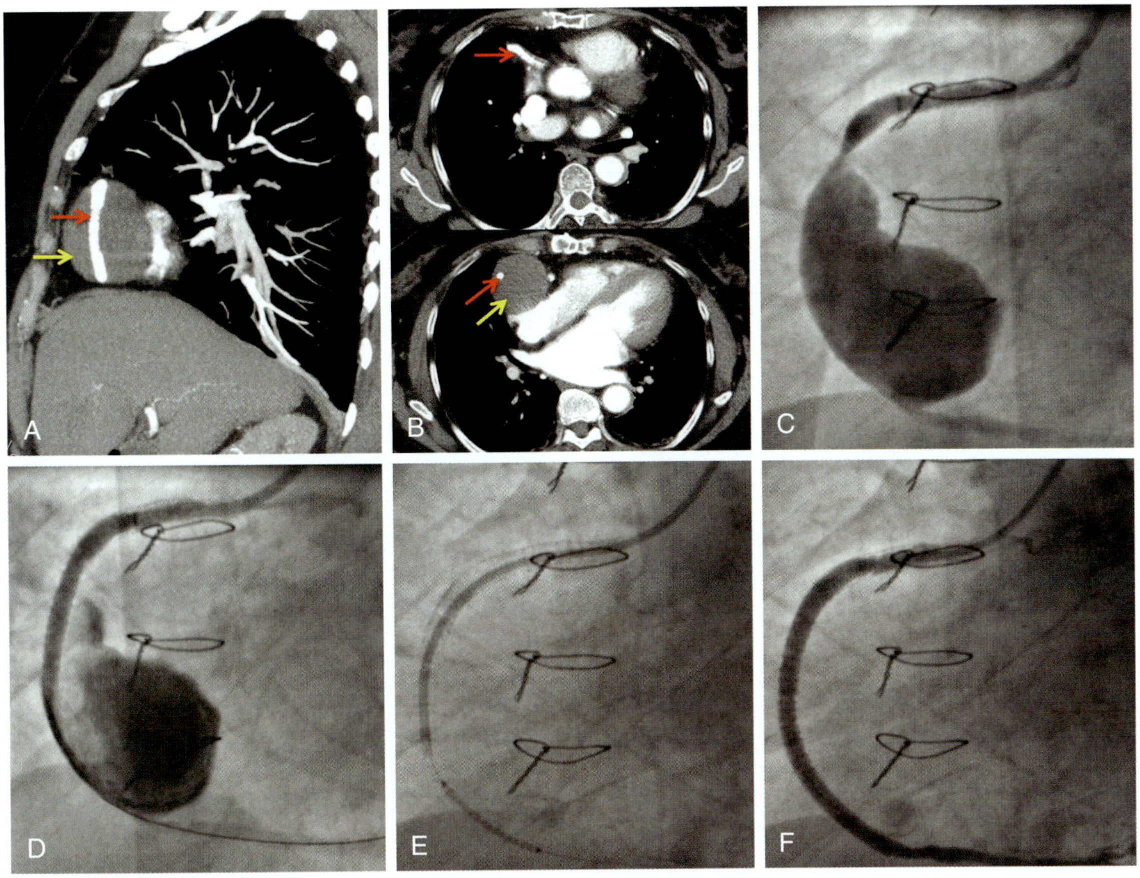

FIG. 3.9 Percutaneous Reconstruction of Giant Saphenous Vein Graft Aneurysm: Before, During, and After Images. Contrast-enhanced mediastinal computed tomography of the (A) sagittal and (B) axial planes shows the course of right coronary artery–saphenous vein graft (RCA-SVG) (*red arrow*) and a paracardiac mass (*yellow arrow*) through which it passes. (C) The lumen of the RCA-SVG aneurysm filling with contrast (see Online Video 3.10). (D) Luminal reconstruction with covered stents. (E) Deep intubation of the guide catheter to implant the final stent and (F) final result (see Online Video 3.11).

precluded further stent delivery distally despite use of a GuideLiner catheter (Vascular Solutions, Minneapolis, Minnesota). A downgrade in guide catheter size to 6F with anchor balloon use distally enabled the advancement of the guide and delivery of final 4.0 × 26 mm GraftMaster polytetrafluoroethylene stent (Abbott Vascular, Santa Clara, California) (Fig. 3.9E) successfully sealing the aneurysm (Fig. 3.9F, Online Video 3.11). The patient had an uneventful recovery.

Aneurysmal dilation of aortocoronary SVG remains rare but widely reported. Although it is often treated with surgical and percutaneous closure techniques, we describe luminal reconstruction as a novel technique to seal the aneurysm and restore distal flow.

Reconstruction of Right Coronary Artery With Two Giant Aneurysms in Series Using Three Overlapped Covered Stents

Alfonso Jurado-Román, MD, PhD, Fernando Lozano-Ruíz-Poveda, MD, María T. López-Lluva, MD, Ignacio Sánchez-Pérez, MD

A 50-year-old man with an inferior myocardial infarction was admitted after successful fibrinolysis. Coronary angiography showed two giant coronary aneurysms in series in the right coronary artery with a high thrombus burden (Fig. 3.10A, Online Video 3.12), a severe ostial lesion, and ecstatic left coronary tree (Fig. 3.10B). Because the patient remained asymptomatic, dual-antiplatelet therapy and heparin were maintained for 1 week when a slight reduction of thrombus was observed (Fig. 3.10C). After three more months of dual-antiplatelet therapy and anticoagulation, the thrombus had almost disappeared. Intravascular ultrasound imaging confirmed a vessel

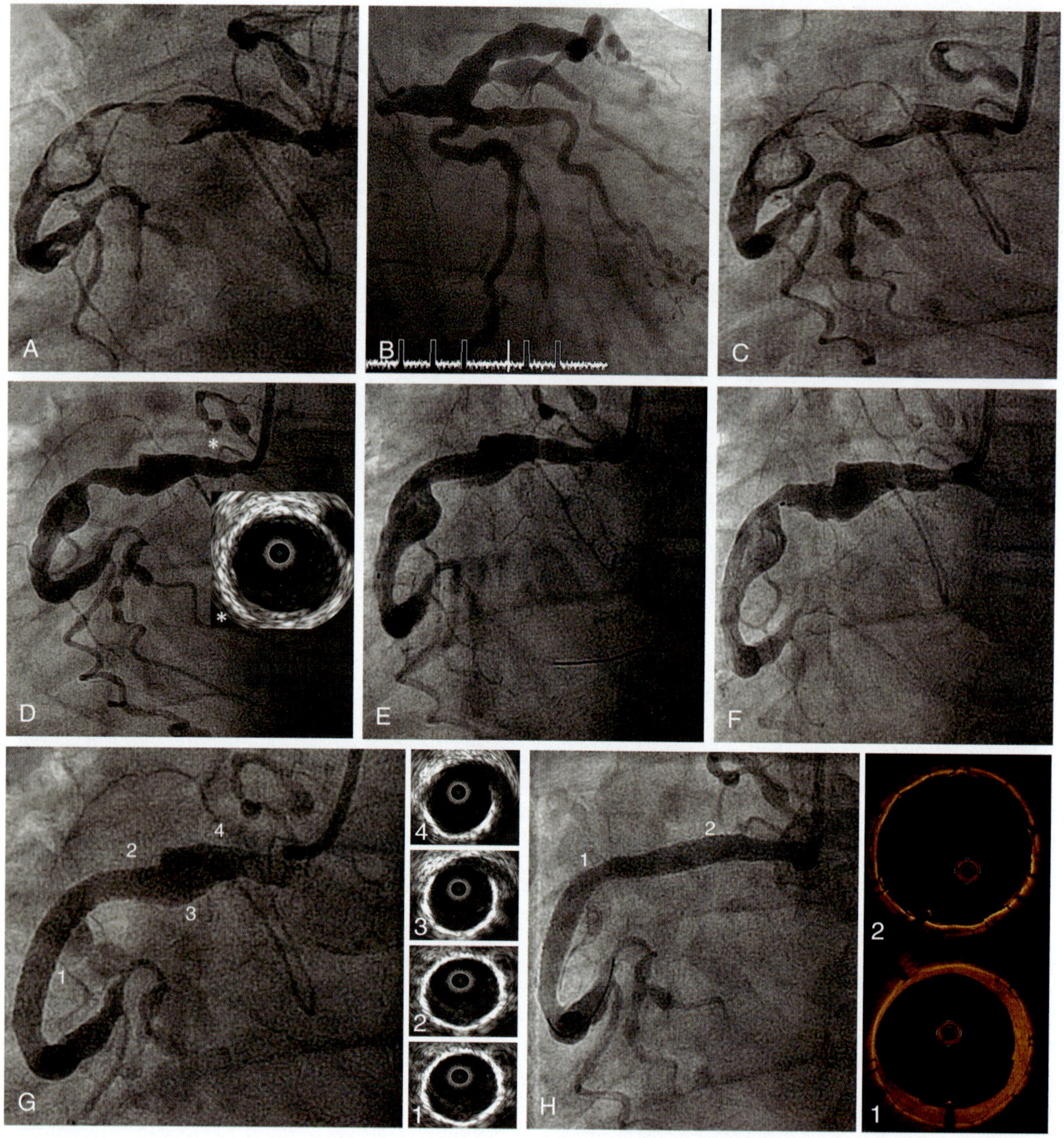

FIG. 3.10 Percutaneous Coronary Intervention of Giant Coronary Aneurysms With Overlapped Covered Stents. (A and B) Initial coronary angiography (CA) (Online Video 3.12). (C) CA after 1 week of dual-antiplatelet therapy (DAPT) and heparin. (D) CA after 3 months of DAPT and anticoagulation. Intravascular ultrasound imaging confirmed a vessel ostial diameter of 4 mm and of 6 mm at the adjacent segments to the aneurysms (*asterisk*). (E and F) Exclusion of both aneurysms with two overlapped 5 × 26 mm PK Papyrus (Biotronik, Berlin, Germany) polyurethane-covered stents (PCSs). (G) Complete sealing of the distal aneurysm (*1*) and the distal edge of the proximal one (2) with incomplete sealing of the proximal aneurysm's proximal edge (*3* and *4*). (H) Complete sealing of the proximal aneurysm after implantation of a third overlapped PCS (5 × 15 mm) in the proximal right coronary artery. Optical coherence tomography showed comparative images of the PCS implanted 3 months before (*1*), with slight neoatherosclerosis without significant restenosis, and the most recently implanted stent (2).

ostial diameter of 4 mm and of 6 mm at the adjacent segments to the aneurysms (Fig. 3.10D). We planned to exclude both aneurysms with two overlapped 5 × 26 mm PK Papyrus polyurethane-covered stents (PCSs) (Biotronik, Berlin, Germany), postdilated with a 6-mm noncompliant balloon (Fig. 3.10E–F). However, the proximal aneurysm's proximal edge was not completely sealed (Fig. 3.10G). Because we did not have more PCSs with the proper dimensions, we programmed a subsequent procedure to implant a third PCS (5 × 15 mm) in the proximal right coronary artery, also post-dilated with a 6-mm noncompliant balloon. Afterward, complete sealing of the proximal aneurysm was achieved, and another zotarolimus-eluting stent (4 × 18 mm) was implanted in the ostial right coronary artery. Optical coherence tomography showed comparative images of the PCS implanted 3 months previously (slight neoatherosclerosis without significant restenosis) and the stent most recently implanted (Fig. 3.10H). Indefinite dual-antiplatelet therapy was prescribed. To the best of our knowledge, this is the first description of a successful exclusion of giant coronary aneurysms in series with overlapped PCSs.

Optimal management of giant coronary aneurysm remains uncertain.[1,2] Some reported experience exists with covered stents to exclude coronary aneurysms.[1,2] However, the majority of cases present difficult deliverability and potential risk for restenosis and thrombosis.[1] The PCS has been designed to improve its deliverability and may expand indications of covered stents to treat coronary aneurysms.[2] Careful follow-up of long-term potential complications is necessary.

References

1. Dhakam S, Rahman N. Myocardial infarction in a youngster due to giant coronary aneurysm. *Catheter Cardiovasc Interv.* 2011;77:528-529.
2. Lattuca B, Schmutz L, Cornillet L, et al. New polyurethane covered stent with low profile for treatment of a large aneurysm after left anterior descending artery stenting: first experience. *Int J Cardiol.* 2015;201:208-209.

Coronary Fistulae

Percutaneous Coronary Intervention for Control of Postoperative Bleeding in Patients With Cardiac Angiosarcoma

María Cristina González-Cambeiro, MD, Diego López-Otero, MD, José Rubio-García, MD, Alejandro Virgós-Lamela, MD, Marino Vega-Fernández, MD, Ramiro Trillo-Nouche, MD, José Ramón González-Juanatey, MD

A 32-year-old man was seen with a primary angiosarcoma of the right atrium, which debuted with palpitations and febrile syndrome, had disseminated bone metastases at the time of diagnosis. The presumptive diagnosis was established by imaging techniques (echocardiography and cardiac magnetic resonance). These images indicated the presence of a mass of 5 × 3 cm, with infiltrative aspect, attached to the lateral wall of the right atrium and the tricuspid annulus, with medium density and a possible hematic-necrotic component, causing pericardial fat and atrioventricular groove infiltration and encompassing the right coronary artery. The presence of a moderate pericardial effusion, without hemodynamic compromise data, was visible in the echocardiogram (Fig. 3.11).

Coronary angiography identified an extensive microvascular feeder grid emerging through the proximal and medium right coronary artery segments, which was also compressed at this level (Fig. 3.12A). After an incomplete mass resection and closure of the right atrial wall by a bovine pericardium implantation, the presence of a continuous arterial bleeding into the pericardial cavity was

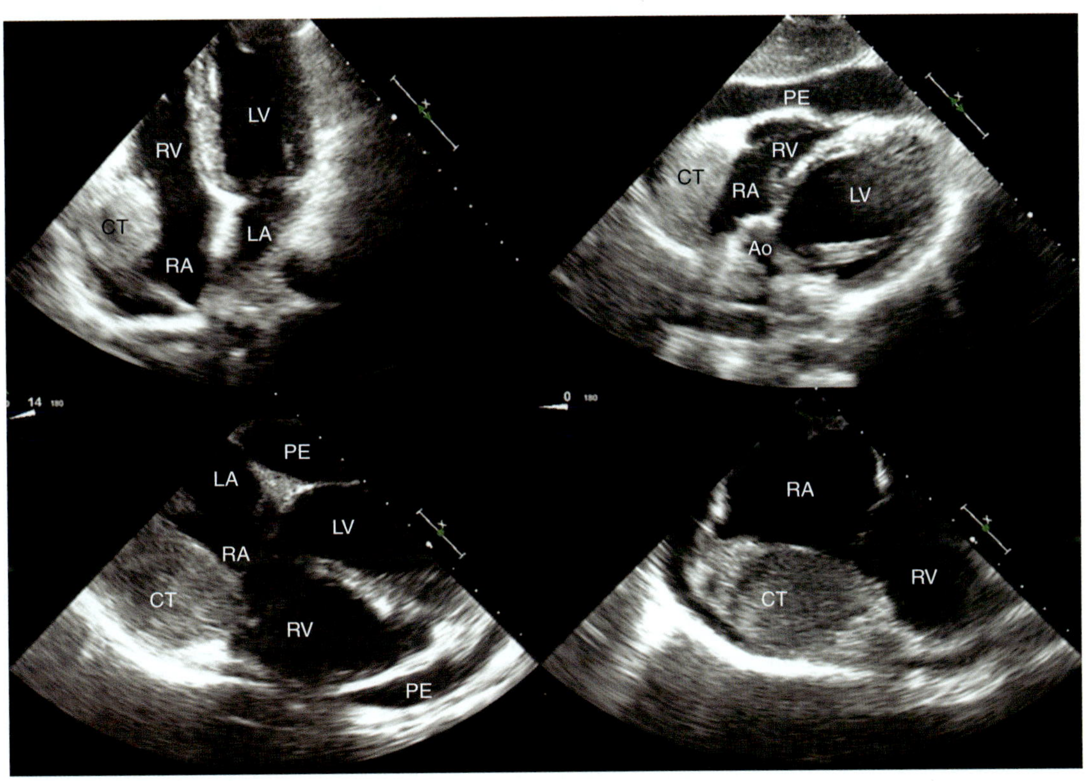

FIG. 3.11 Images of Transthoracic (Superior) and Transesophageal Echocardiogram (Inferior). The images show the presence of a mass of 5 × 3 cm, with infiltrative aspect, attached to the lateral wall of the right atrium and the tricuspid annulus, with medium density and a possible hematic-necrotic component, causing pericardial fat and atrioventricular groove infiltration and encompassing the right coronary artery. Also in the echocardiogram, the presence of a moderate pericardial effusion, without hemodynamic compromise data, was described. *Ao,* aorta; *CT,* cardiac tumor; *LA,* left atrium; *LV,* left ventricle; *PE,* pericardial effusion; *RA,* right atrium; *RV,* right ventricle.

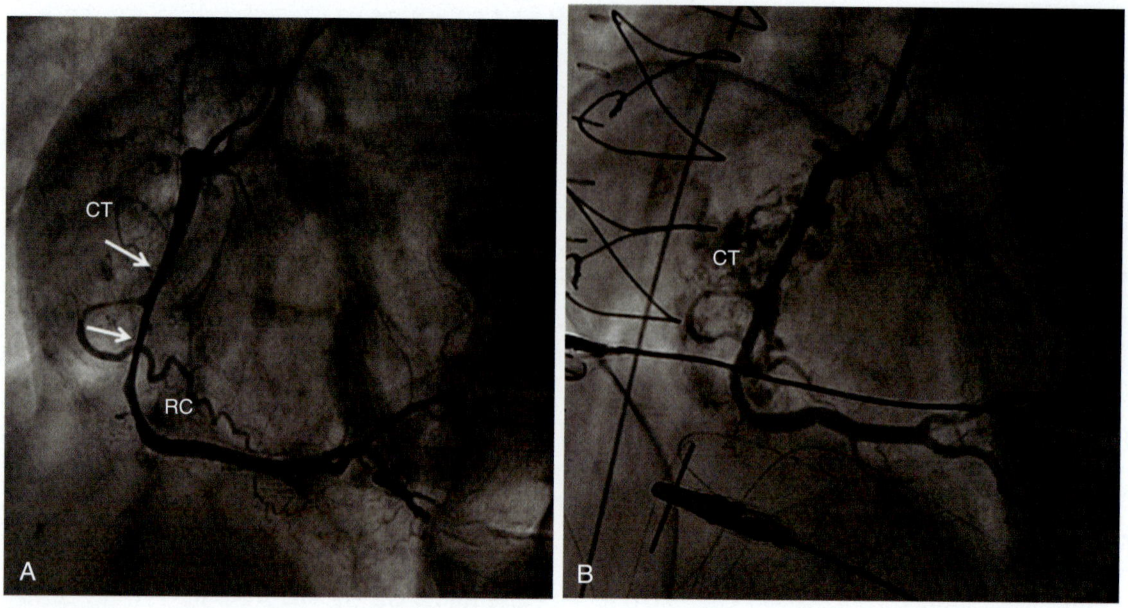

FIG. 3.12 Preoperative and Postpperative Coronary Angiography. (A) In a preoperative coronary angiography, an extensive microvascular feeder grid was identified emerging through the proximal and medium right coronary artery segments, which was also compressed at this level. (B) An immediate postoperative coronary angiography shows a significant extravasation of contrast from the right coronary artery to the pericardial cavity. *CT,* cardiac tumor; *RC,* right coronary.

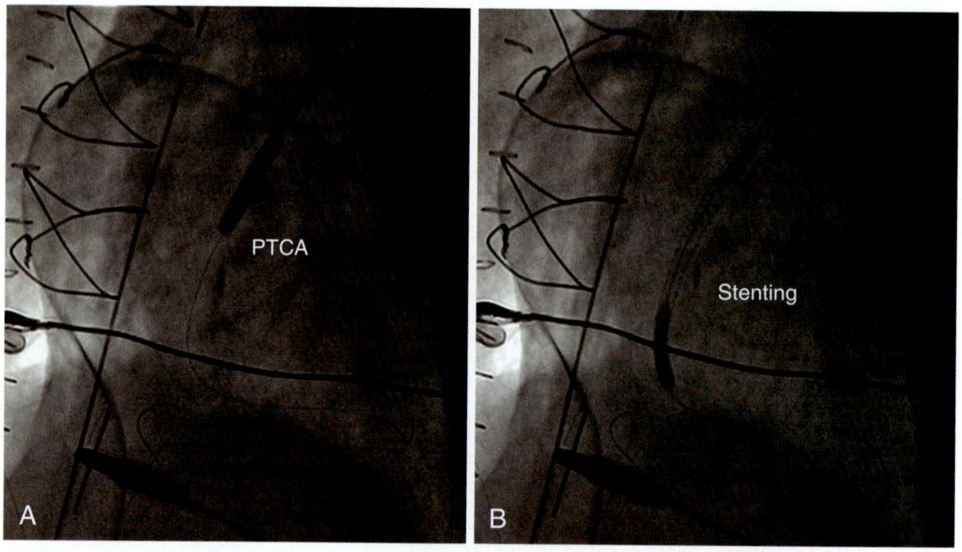

FIG. 3.13 Percutaneous Coronary Intervention. We proceeded to occlude the tumor microvasculature by implanting 5 overlapping polytetrafluoroethylene-covered stents from the proximal to the distal segments. *PTCA,* percutaneous transluminal coronary angioplasty.

shown, from the remaining tumor, with ineffective surgical hemostasis methods. For this reason, we decided to perform urgent coronary angiography, which showed a significant extravasation of contrast from the right coronary artery to the pericardial cavity (Fig. 3.12B). We proceeded to occlude the tumor microvasculature by implanting five overlapping polytetrafluoroethylene-covered stents from the proximal to the distal segment, thus excluding the bleeding area (Figs. 3.13A–B and 3.14). Subsequently, the patient had a favorable outcome and left the recovery unit early. Finally, he underwent four cycles of anthracycline-like palliative chemotherapy. Eight months after neoplasia treatment, the patient remains free of symptoms with stability in local and systemic disease.

The implantation of polytetrafluoroethylene-covered coronary stent after resection of cardiac tumor with a feeder grid emerging from coronary arteries may be an effective measure to treat bleeding caused by the remaining tumor.

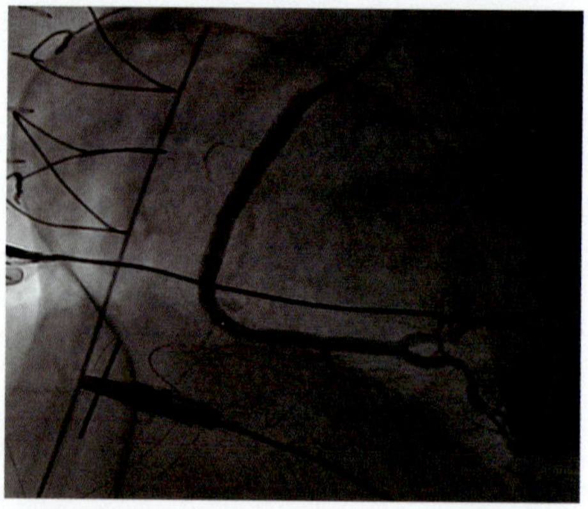

FIG. 3.14 Final Result. After the coronary intervention, the bleeding area was finally excluded.

Anterograde Percutaneous Coronary–Cameral Fistula Closure Employing a Guide-in-Guide Technique

Todd L. Kiefer, MD, John Vavalle, MD, Sharif Halim, MD, Prashant Kaul, MD, J. Larry Klein, MD, Lynne H. Hurwitz, MD, Jeffrey G. Gaca, MD, J. Kevin Harrison, MD

A 33-year-old woman was evaluated for palpitations and a continuous murmur. Echocardiography demonstrated a dilated vascular structure posterior to the aortic root. Coronary angiography revealed a coronary–cameral fistula originating from the left main coronary artery emptying into the right atrium (RA) via a kidney-shaped vascular cistern (Fig. 3.15, Online Video 3.13). The left dominant coronary gave rise to the left anterior descending (LAD) and circumflex (LCx) arteries within 10 mm of the left coronary ostium. The pulmonary artery pressure was 60/30 mm Hg, and the Qp/Qs ratio was 1.5.

Because of atrial arrhythmias and the pulmonary hypertension associated with the left-to-right shunt, fistula closure was advised.

Procedural planning employing computed tomographic angiography (CTA) (Fig. 3.16, Online Video 3.14) suggested multiple fistula exit sites into the RA; anatomy was confirmed by transesophageal echocardiography. Therefore, retrograde closure was not pursued.

An anterograde approach from the right femoral artery using a telescoping dual-guide catheter system was employed. An 8F extra-backup 3.5 guide catheter (Cordis, Miami, Florida) was cut to a length that would just reach the left coronary origin. A 7F Terumo sheath (Terumo Medical, Somerset, New Jersey) applied to the adulterated end afforded hemostasis. A 0.035-inch Terumo Glidewire was advanced into the coronary fistula, coiling the distal wire within the cistern (Fig. 3.17). Over this guidewire, a 100-cm length, 6F Judkins right 4.0 guide catheter was advanced within the 8F guide, with the distal tip reaching the entrance of the vascular cistern. Based on the CTA centerline analysis of the diameter (Fig. 3.18), a 12-mm

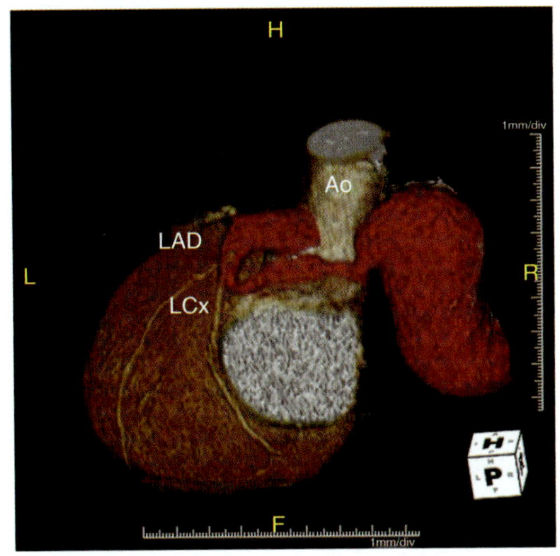

FIG. 3.16. Computed Tomographic Angiography (CTA) With Three-Dimensional (3D) Reconstruction. CTA with 3 D reconstruction shows the course of the fistula (shaded in *red*) from the dilated left main coronary, coursing posterior to the aortic root (*Ao*), then entering the right atrium. Note the position of the origins of the left anterior descending (*LAD*) and circumflex (*LCx*) coronary arteries. *F*, feet; *H*, head; *L*, left; *P*, posterior; *R* one-quarter right (Online Video 3.14).

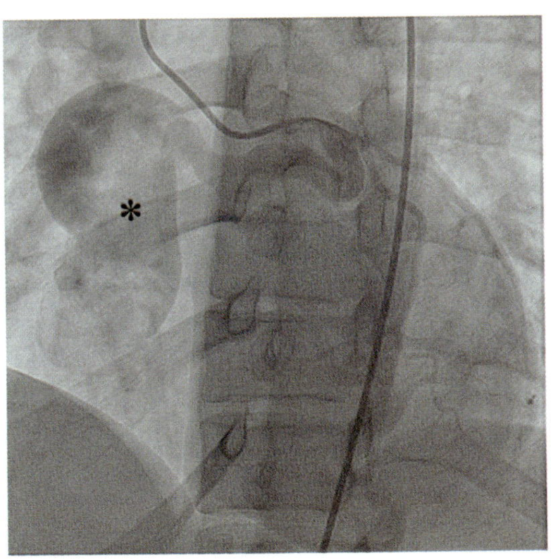

FIG. 3.15. Coronary Angiogram Showing a Coronary–Cameral Fistula. The coronary angiogram (left anterior oblique 28°, cranial 9°) shows a coronary–cameral fistula from the left main emptying via a vascular, kidney-shaped, cistern (*asterisk*) into the right atrium (Online Video 3.13).

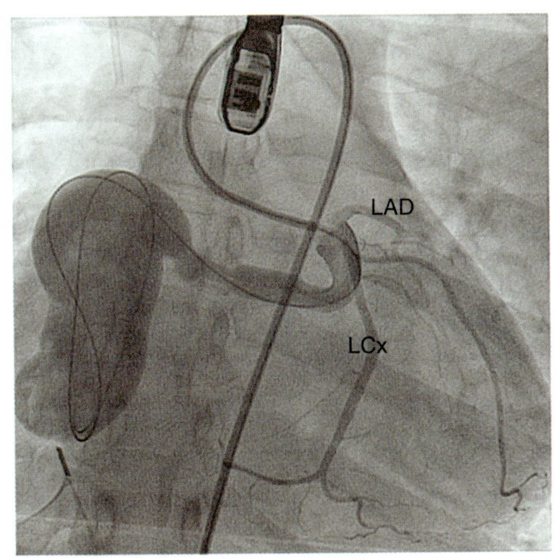

FIG. 3.17. Left Coronary Angiography Using the Shortened 8F Guide Catheter. Left coronary angiography used the shortened 8F guide catheter (left anterior oblique 5°, caudal 19°). Note the course of the Terumo Glidewire with the distal segment coiled in the dilated segment of the coronary fistula. *LAD*, left anterior descending artery; *LCx*, circumflex coronary artery.

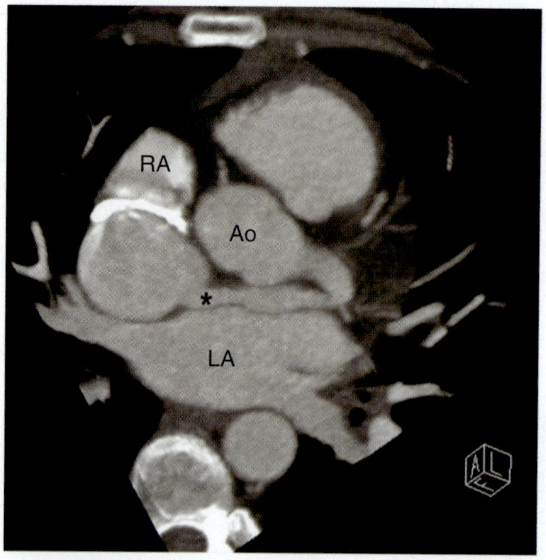

FIG. 3.18. Axial Oblique Computed Tomographic Angiography (CTA) Image. The CTA image was used to measure the coronary fistula diameter with centerline analysis, thus affording vascular device size selection. The *asterisk* indicates the coronary fistula. *Ao*, aortic root; *LA*, left atrium; *RA*, right atrium.

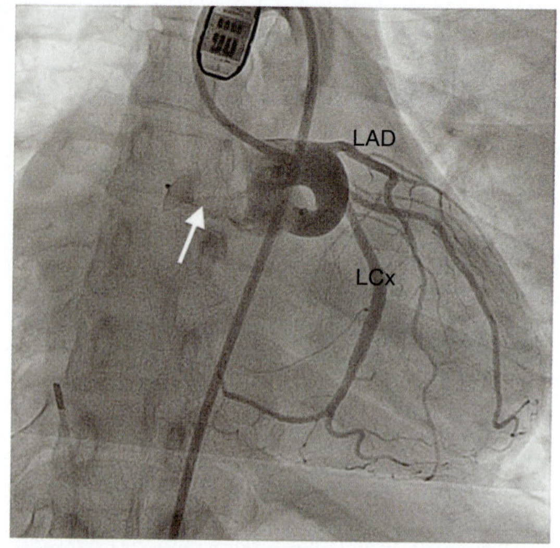

FIG. 3.19. Left Coronary Angiography After Deployment of the Amplatzer Vascular Occlusion Plug II (AVPII). Left coronary angiography (left anterior oblique 5°, caudal 19°) after deployment of the 12-mm-diameter AVPII is shown. Note the absence of flow beyond the AVPII (*arrow*) and improved angiographic filling of the left anterior descending (*LAD*) and circumflex (*LCx*) coronary arteries (Online Video 3.15).

Amplatzer vascular plug II (St. Jude Medical, Plymouth, Minnesota) was deployed via the 6F guide.

Angiography demonstrated complete cessation of fistula flow (3.19, Online Video 3.15) and improved angiographic filling of the LAD and LCx coronary arteries. The patient did well, was discharged the following morning, and was well at the 30-day postoperative re-evaluation.

Large coronary fistulae are uncommon, observed in 225 of 126,595 consecutive angiograms.[1] The associated shunt may lead to volume loading, arrhythmias, pulmonary hypertension, heart failure, and/or coronary steal.

Treatment options include open surgical and catheterization-based fistula closure. The latter is associated with good procedural success in selected cases.[2] Attention to anatomic detail, procedural planning, and the ability to improvise from standard catheter techniques are important to catheterization-based success. For anterograde closure in particular, it is critical that the operator ensure that fistula closure is distal to the origin of all native coronary branches.

References

1. Yamanaka O, Hobbs RE. Coronary artery anomalies in 126,595 patients undergoing coronary arteriography. *Cathet Cardiovasc Diagn.* 1990;21:28-40.
2. Jama A, Barsoum M, Bjarnason H, Holmes DR Jr, Rihal CS. Percutaneous closure of congenital coronary artery fistulae: results and angiographic follow-up. *JACC Cardiovasc Interv.* 2011;4:814-821.

Percutaneous Closure of Left Main Coronary Artery Fistula Using the Amplatzer Vascular Plug II and the Amplatzer Duct Occluder I

Pritish K. Bagul, MD, DM, Milind S. Phadke, MD, DM, Prafulla G. Kerkar, MD, DM

A coronary artery (CA) fistula is a rare entity reported in 0.1% to 0.2% of patients undergoing angiography. A 3-year-old asymptomatic child was diagnosed with a large coronary artery fistula arising from the left main CA, leading to coronary steal. We report our experience of successful transcatheter closure of the coronary arterial fistula arising from the left main CA and draining into the superior vena cava–right atrium (SVC-RA) junction using two devices: the Amplatzer vascular plug II (AVP II) and the Amplatzer duct occluder I (ADO I) (St. Jude Medical, St. Paul, Minnesota).

A 3-year-male child presented with an incidentally detected continuous murmur during evaluation for respiratory tract infection. Two-dimensional echocardiography showed an aneurysmally dilated left main CA with the presence of large coronary–cameral fistula originating from the left main CA (Fig. 3.20).[1]

The procedure was done with the patient under general anesthesia. Bilateral femoral arterial access were secured. Unfractionated heparin, 100 U/kg, was administered before the procedure. An aortic root angiogram was obtained to profile the CAs and demonstrate the coronary steal. An angiogram of the fistula was obtained using a 5F Berman catheter (Arrow Berman angiographic catheter; Teleflex, Morrisville, North Carolina) with distal balloon occlusion. The fistula showed two constrictions: one proximal and one distal before it opened into the SVC-RA junction (Fig. 3.21, Online Video 3.16). Through a 5F end-hole catheter, a 0.035-inch exchange-length angle-tipped guidewire (Terumo Corporation, Tokyo, Japan) was passed to the distal end of the fistula into the SVC (Fig. 3.22, Online Video 3.17). The distal end of this angled-tip guidewire was snared in the SVC and exteriorized from the right femoral venous sheath, using a 15-mm gooseneck snare (Online Video 3.18). A continuous atrioventricular (AV) loop was hence created (Fig. 3.23). Additional angiographic images were taken with the help of a 5F pigtail catheter via the right arterial access (Online Video 3.19). A 6F Amplatzer patent ductus arteriosus sheath was passed over the Terumo guidewire from the venous side and positioned in the fistula just proximal to (on the arterial side of) the proximal constriction. The AV loop circuit was broken. A 12-mm AVP II was deployed in the proximal constriction (Fig. 3.24, Online Video 3.20). The distal constriction was occluded with the help of an ADO I device (Fig. 3.25). An additional angiogram showed that the device was in a good position with no residual shunt and better opacification of the CAs (Fig. 3.26, Online Video 3.21). The procedure was uneventful. An electrocardiogram showed no abnormality. The patient was started on aspirin 5 mg/kg per day for 6 months and annual follow-up. A follow-up angiogram done after 2 years showed complete occlusion of the fistula and good flow in the left anterior descending and circumflex arteries (Figs. 3.27 and 3.28, Online Video 3.22).

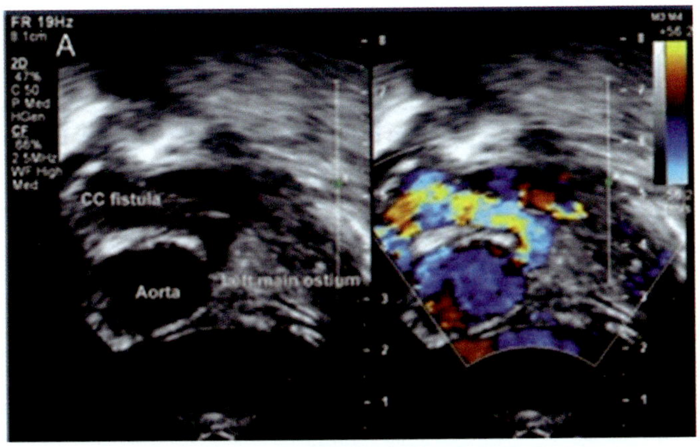

FIG. 3.20. Two-Dimensional (2D) Echocardiogram (Short Axis View) Demonstrating the Fistula. A 2D (short axis view) showing an aneurysmally dilated left main coronary artery (CA) with the presence of a large coronary–cameral (*CC*) fistula originating in the left main CA. Reprinted with permission from Bagul P, Phadke M, Lanjewar C, Nabar A, Kerkar P. Left main trunk connecting to superior vena cava via aneurysmal coronary artery fistula. *Eur Heart J Cardiovasc Imaging*. 2014;15:752.

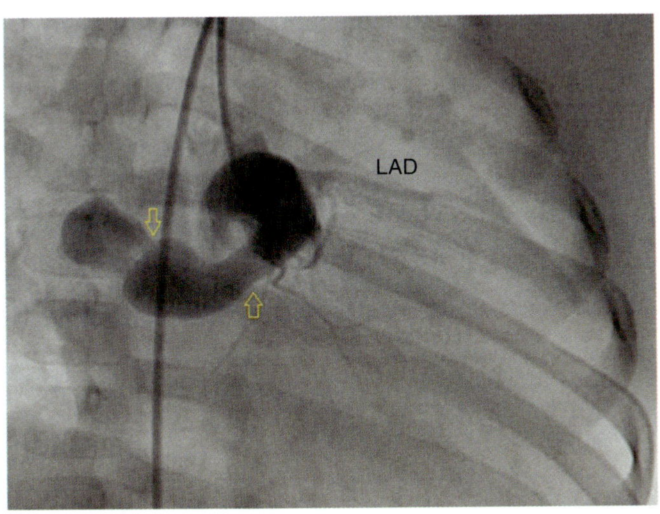

FIG. 3.21. Fistula Angiogram. Angiogram (right anterior oblique view) done with the help of a 5F Berman catheter showing two constrictions: one proximal and one distal before the fistula opened into the superior vena cava–right artery junction. Constrictions are marked by *arrows*. *LAD*, left anterior descending artery (Online Video 3.16).

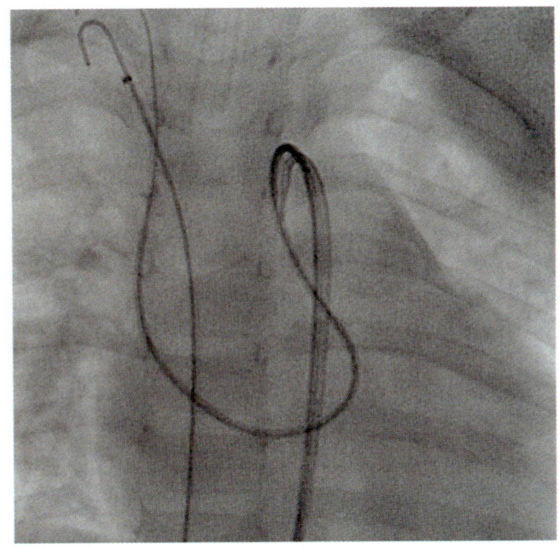

FIG. 3.22. Snaring the Terumo Wire. A 0.035-inch exchange-length angle-tipped guidewire (Terumo Corporation) passed over a 5F end-hole catheter to the distal end of the fistula into the superior vena cava and the guidewire being snared with 15-mm gooseneck snare passed through the venous end (Online Video 3.17).

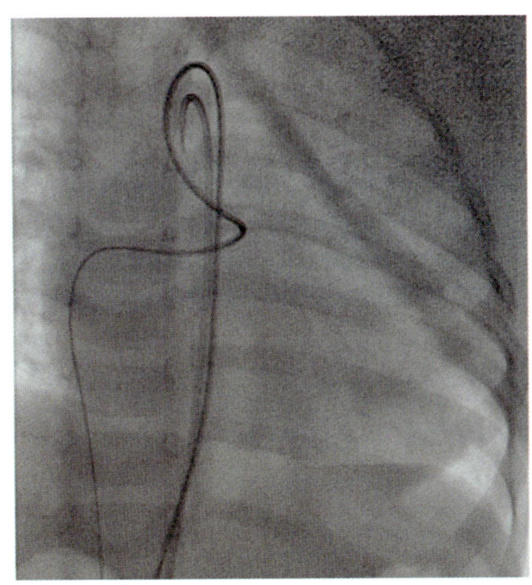

FIG. 3.23. Formation of Continuous Arteriovenous Loop. Fluoroscopy image showing continuous arteriovenous loop and Berman catheter placed in the aortic root.

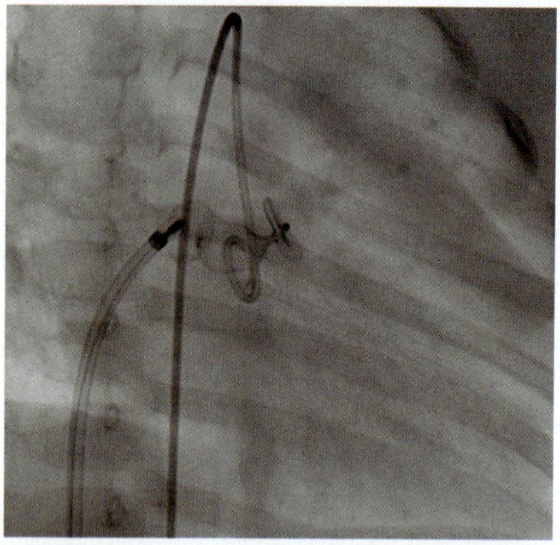

FIG. 3.24. Delivery of Amplatzer Vascular Plug II in Proximal Constriction. Amplatzer vascular plug II delivered with the help of Amplatzer patent ductus arteriosus (St. Jude Medical) sheath across the proximal constriction of the fistula (Online Video 3.20).

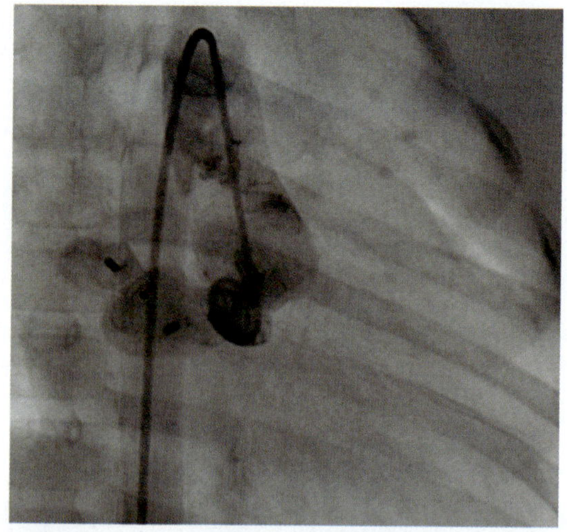

FIG. 3.26. Postprocedure Angiogram. Postprocedure angiogram showing the device in a good position with no residual shunt and better opacification of the coronary arteries (Online Video 3.21).

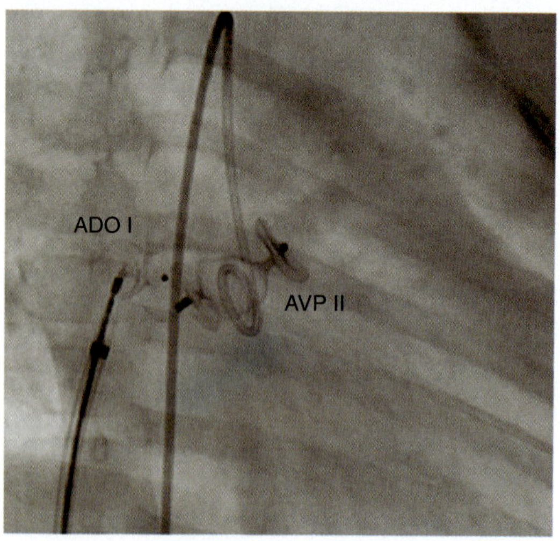

FIG. 3.25. Delivery of Amplatzer Duct Occluder in Distal Constriction. Amplatzer duct occluder I (*ADO I*) delivered via the same sheath across the distal constriction. *AVP II*, Amplatzer vascular plug II.

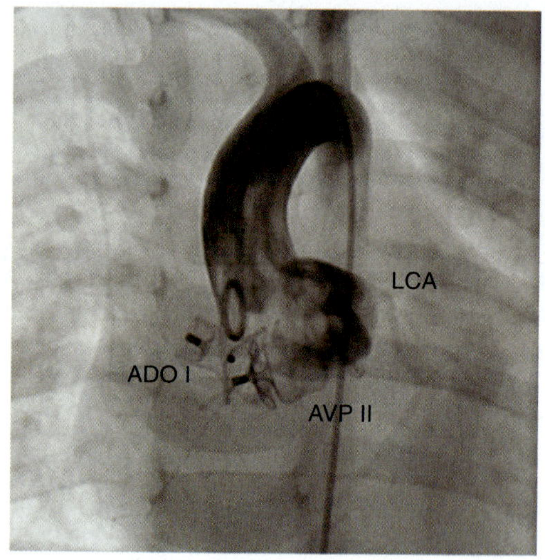

FIG. 3.27. Follow-Up Angiogram After 2 Years. Follow-up angiogram after 2 years showing good opacification of the coronary arteries with complete occlusion of the fistula. *ADO I*, Amplatzer duct occluder I; AVP II, Amplatzer vascular plug II; *LCA*, left coronary artery (Online Video 3.22).

We report this case because a proximal fistula arising from the left main CA is a very rare entity,[2] as is the percutaneous closure of such a defect. To the best of our knowledge, this is the first case of a left main CA fistula being closed percutaneously. We would also like to highlight the precise selection of the devices: the AVP II in the proximal part of the fistula and the ADO I in the distal constriction. Intermediate-term follow-up, both clinically and angiographically, was satisfactory.

References

1. Bagul P, Phadke M, Lanjewar C, Nabar A, Kerkar P. Left main trunk connecting to superior vena cava via aneurysmal coronary artery fistula. *Eur Heart J Cardiovasc Imaging.* 2014;15:752.
2. Ekonomou CK, Papadopoulos DP, Dalianis NV, Stratigis NG, Benos J, Votteas VE. Coronary fistula from left main stem to main pulmonary artery. *J Invasive Cardiol.* 2003;15:600-601.

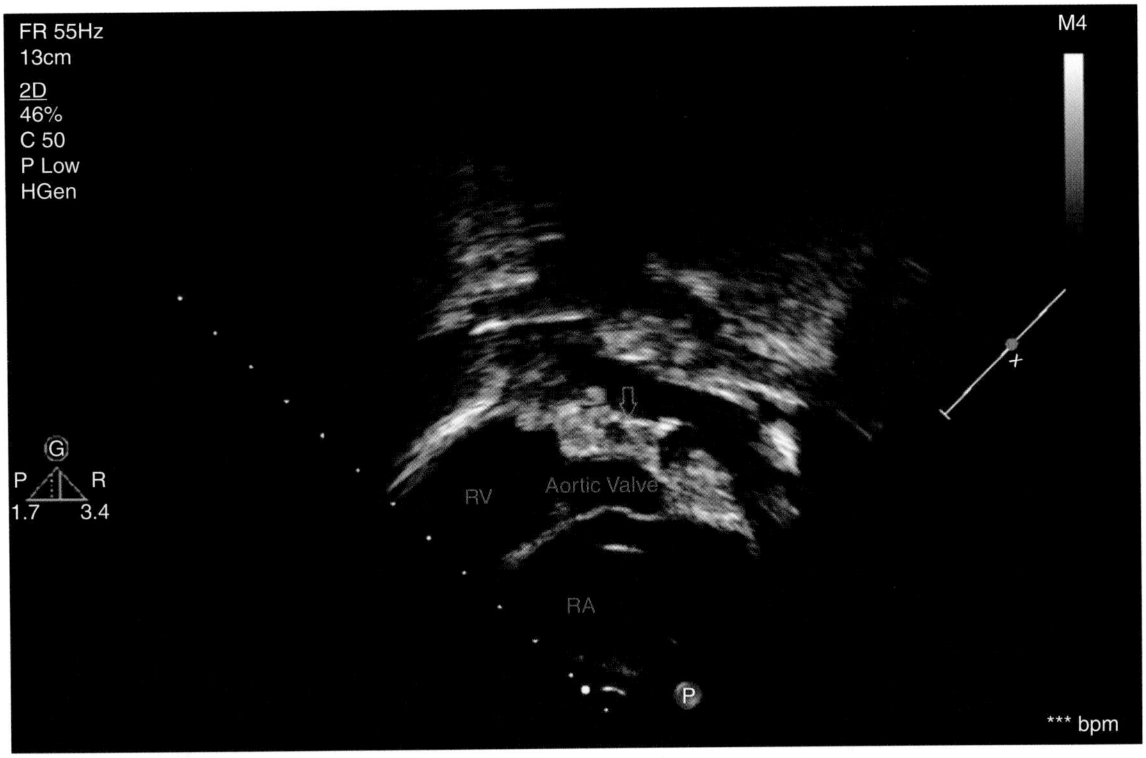

FIG. 3.28. Two-Dimensional (2D) Echocardiogram (Short Axis View). A 2D echocardiogram (short axis view) showing complete occlusion of the fistula and well-placed devices. *Arrow* showing the device in situ. *RA*, right atrium; *RV*, right ventricle (Online Video 3.22).

Percutaneous Intervention to Large Left Anterior Descending Artery Fistula After Right Ventricular Biopsy in a Transplant Recipient

Chris Anthony, MD, Roberto Spina, MD, Meenal Sharma, MD, Christopher Hayward, MD, Anne Keogh, MD, PhD, Peter Macdonald, MD, PhD, David Roy, MD

Endomyocardial biopsy through the right internal jugular vein is the gold standard to screen for rejection in orthotopic heart transplant recipients.[1] Complications associated with the procedure are mainly related to vascular access; however, coronary artery fistulae to the right ventricle are rare and have been anecdotally described.[2–4] Coils and Amplatzer plugs (St. Jude Medical, St. Paul, Minnesota) have been used to achieve closure in congenital fistulae[2,3]; however, in the much larger diameter iatrogenic fistulae, one case has been described in which covered stents were used for closure.[4] We describe a case of a large left anterior descending fistula to the right ventricle after endomyocardial biopsy that was successfully closed using percutaneous coronary stenting.

A 44-year-old woman underwent orthotopic cardiac transplantation in 2011 for end-stage heart failure due to anthracycline-induced cardiomyopathy in the context of breast cancer. During screening endomyocardial biopsy via the right internal jugular approach, she developed a large left anterior descending fistula in the mid- to distal segment draining into her right ventricle (Fig. 3.29). There was a significant shunt as a consequence, resulting in echocardiographic features of right ventricular strain, and a stress echocardiogram performed demonstrated significant inducible ischemia in the anterior myocardial wall.

The decision was made to attempt percutaneous closure of this hemodynamically significant fistula, and the procedure was performed using the right femoral approach with a 7F extra-backup guiding catheter to cannulate the left main coronary artery. A bare-metal wire and an extra support wire were placed in the distal left anterior descending artery. At this time, intravascular ultrasonography and ChromaFlo intravascular ultrasonography were used to better visualize the ostium of the fistula and for accurate sizing of the vessel for stenting (Figs. 3.30 and 3.31). The distal vessel measured 2.7 mm just distal to the fistula. The vessel proximal to the fistula measured 3.8 × 4.4 mm.

A 2.8 × 19-mm Graftmaster covered stent (Abbott Vascular, Abbott Park, Illinois) was placed at the fistula os, but because of residual flow from the distal segment, a second 2.8 × 19-mm stent was placed distally to the first. Both stents were postdilated with a 4-mm noncutting balloon to high pressure. There remained some proximal entry into the stent extraluminal plane with flow into the fistula, so a third 4.5 × 16-mm stent was placed proximally with excellent closure result achieved (Fig. 3.32).

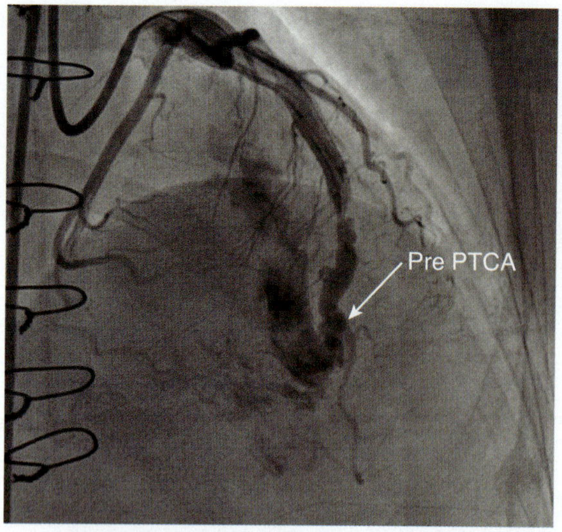

FIG. 3.29. Left Anterior Oblique Cranial Coronary Angiogram of the Left Coronary Artery Before Percutaneous Transluminal Coronary Angioplasty (PTCA).

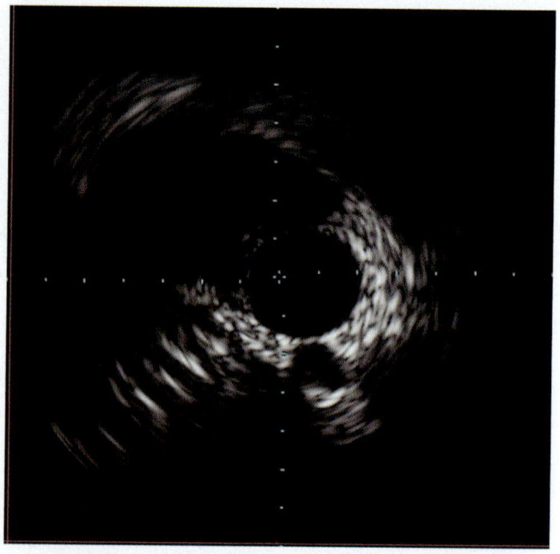

FIG. 3.30. Intravascular Ultrasound of the Left Anterior Descending Artery.

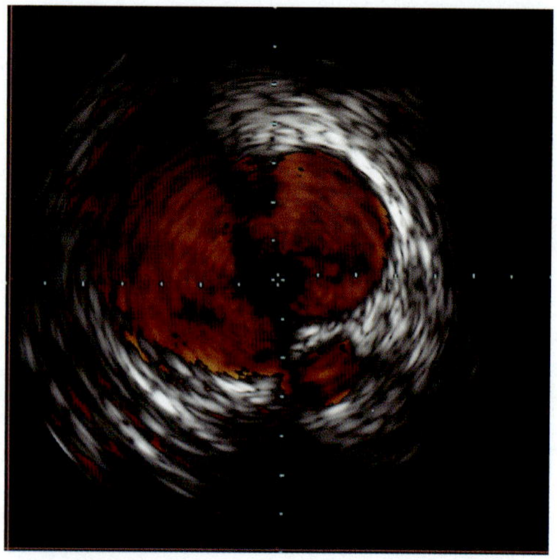

FIG. 3.31. ChromaFlo Intravascular Ultrasound of the Left Anterior Descending Artery.

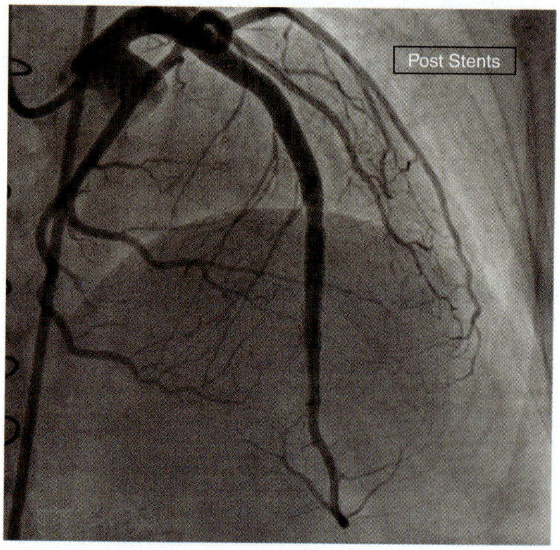

FIG. 3.32. Left Anterior Oblique Cranial Coronary Angiogram of the Left Coronary Artery After Stent Placement.

References

1. Baraldi-Junkins C, Levin HR, Kasper EK, Rayburn BK, Herskowitz A, Baughman KL. Complications of endomyocardial biopsy in heart transplant patients. *J Heart Lung Transplant* 1993;12:63-67.
2. Henzlova MJ, Nath H, Bucy RP, Bourge RC, Kirklin JK, Rogers WJ. Coronary artery to right ventricle fistula in heart transplant recipients: a complication of endomyocardial biopsy. *J Am Coll Cardiol* 1989;14:258-261.
3. Díaz de la Llera LS, Fournier Andray JA, Gómez Moreno S, et al. Percutaneous occlusion with coils of coronary artery fistulas in adults [in Spanish]. *Rev Esp Cardiol.* 2005;58:93-96.
4. Oreglia JA, Bruschi G, Klugmann S. Percutaneous treatment of iatrogenic left-anterior descending artery to right ventricle fistula. *Catheter Cardiovasc Interv.* 2010;76:975-977.

Chronic Total Occlusions

Follow-up Improvement of Distal Vessel Diameter After Successful Chronic Total Coronary Occlusion Recanalization

Gabriele L. Gasparini, MD, Marco L. Rossi, MD, Patrizia Presbitero, MD

Chronic total occlusion (CTO) of a coronary artery promotes negative remodeling in distal reference segments by negative vascular wall remodeling and plaque growth. Restoring blood flow by recanalization potentially leads to positive vascular remodeling.

We present the case of a 53-year-old man, a heavy smoker with dyslipidemia, hypertension, and family history of cardiac disease, who underwent percutaneous coronary intervention (PCI) of a CTO of the proximal right coronary artery (Fig. 3.33A).

CTO recanalization was attempted via a retrograde approach through a septal collateral (Fig. 3.33B–D). PCI was successful with implantation of one drug-eluting stent, 3.0 × 38 mm, in the ostio-proximal segment (Fig. 3.34A–C). At the end of the procedure, the angiography showed thrombolysis in myocardial infarction flow grade 3, with evidence of a severe and diffuse distal bed disease (Fig. 3.34D, Online Video 3.23). A 6-month angiographic follow-up showed a significant improvement in the diameter of the distal vessel, with no evidence of stenotic lesions (Fig. 3.35, Online Video 3.24).

In the setting of CTOs, we have learned not to overtreat distal lesions, particularly small vessels; the distal bed disease, which has been chronically underperfused, tends to be overestimated, and the vessel frequently vasodilates and remodels with restoration of antegrade flow, as previously shown.

Few data have been published to investigate the role of blood flow restoration in the remodeling process.[1] Galassi et al.[2] have suggested that the improvement of distal vessel diameter size detected at follow-up after CTO recanalization can theoretically be explained by three different mechanisms: (1) impaired endothelium-dependent and/or endothelium-independent vasomotion immediately after CTO recanalization (hibernated vascular wall) and/or an intense vasoconstriction that improves at follow-up, (2) positive remodeling, or (3) a combination of both.

References

1. Sianos G, Werner GS, Galassi AR, et al. Recanalisation of chronic total coronary occlusions: 2012 consensus document from the EuroCTO club. *EuroIntervention.* 2012;8:139-145.
2. Galassi AR, Tomasello SD, Crea F, et al. Transient impairment of vasomotion function after successful chronic total occlusion recanalization. *J Am Coll Cardiol.* 2012;59:711-718.

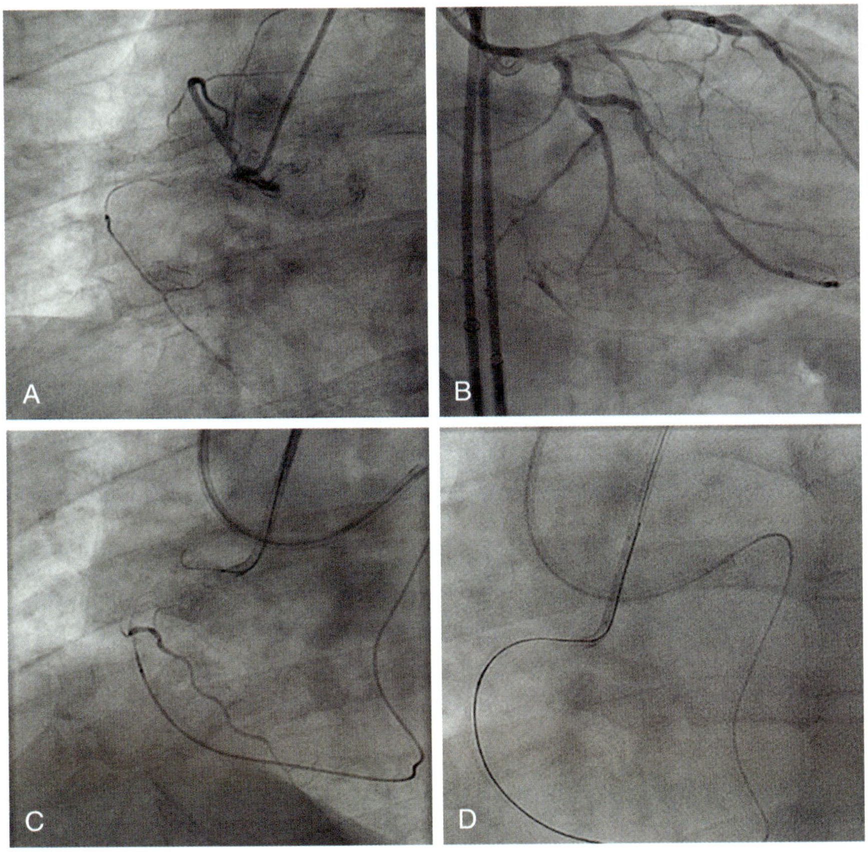

FIG. 3.33. Images of Coronary Angiography: Setting Up the Procedure, Retrograde Collateral Channel Access, Crossing the Chronic Total Occlusion (CTO), and Externalization. (A) Diagnostic coronary angiography demonstrated paraostial CTO of the right coronary artery. (B) Because of the ostial localization, CTO recanalization was attempted via a retrograde approach through a septal collateral. (C) After septal collateral channel crossing, the Corsair microcatheter (Asahi Intecc, Aichi, Japan) was advanced and positioned near the distal end of the occlusion. (D) After successful crossing into the proximal true lumen, the retrograde wire was then externalized into the antegrade guiding catheter.

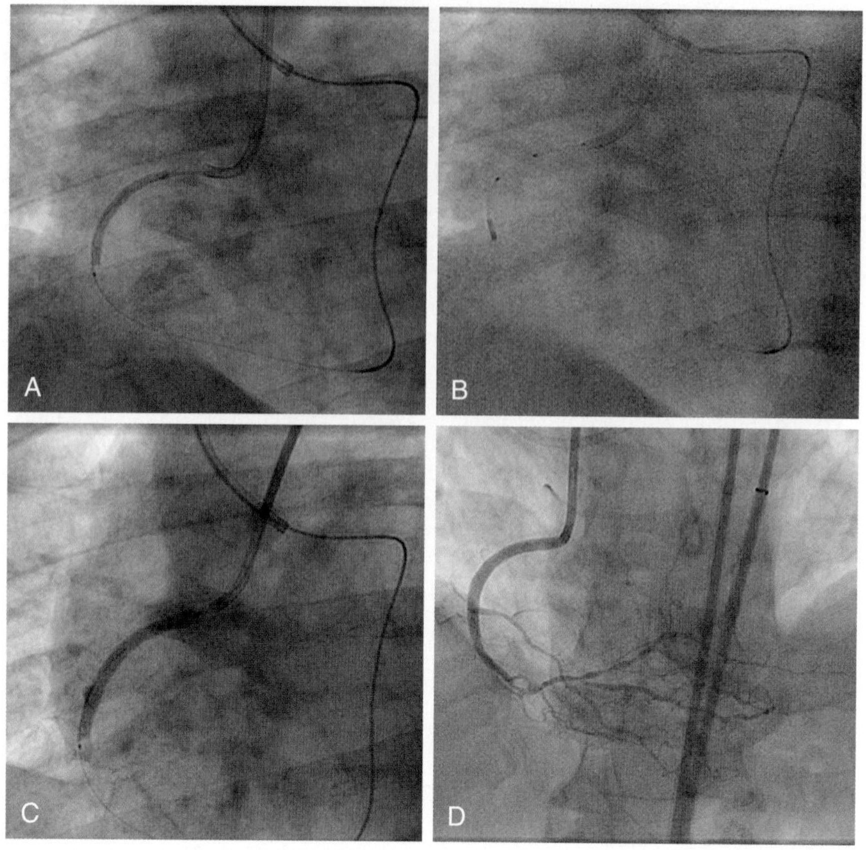

FIG. 3.34. Images of Coronary Angiography: Opening the Occlusion, Stent Implantation, and Final Result. (A) An antegrade rapid exchange balloon was inflated in the occlusion. (B) An intravascular ultrasound control was performed to identify the length of atherosclerotic disease and the vessel diameter to avoid an underestimation of the vessel size. (C) A 3.0 × 38 mm drug-eluting stent was implanted in the ostioproximal segment of the right coronary artery. (D) Final result after stent implantation with angiographic evidence of severe and diffuse distal bed disease (Online Video 3.23).

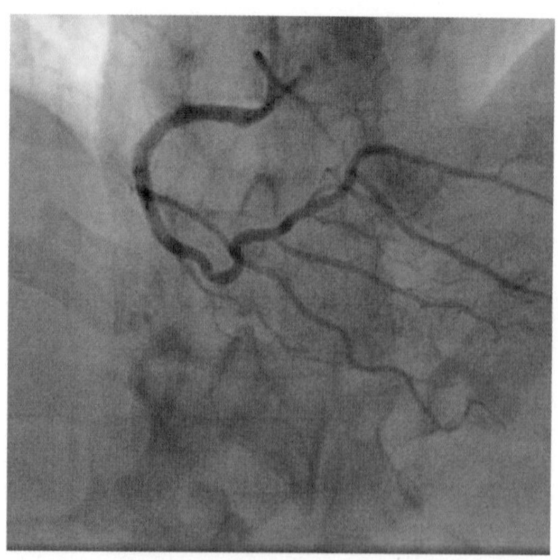

FIG. 3.35. Six-Month Angiographic Follow-Up. A 6-month angiographic follow-up showed a significant improvement in the diameter of the distal vessel, with no evidence of stenotic lesions (Online Video 3.24).

Subintimal Crush of an Occluded Stent to Recanalize a Chronic Total Occlusion Due to In-Stent Restenosis: Insights From a Multimodality Imaging Approach

Giuliana Capretti, MD, Satoru Mitomo, MD, Manuela Giglio, MD, Mauro Carlino, MD, Antonio Colombo, MD, Lorenzo Azzalini, MD, PhD, MSc

A 46-year-old man underwent percutaneous coronary intervention with a drug-eluting stent on the distal right coronary artery. Six years later he was diagnosed with in-stent chronic total occlusion of the right coronary artery causing inferior wall ischemia and was scheduled for percutaneous coronary intervention.

The occlusion was long, with an ambiguous proximal cap and interventional epicardial collateral channels from the circumflex (Fig. 3.36A). An antegrade true-to-true attempt failed to cross the lesion, so a retrograde approach was undertaken. A Sion guidewire (Asahi Intecc, Nagoya, Japan) over a Corsair microcatheter (Asahi Intecc) was successfully advanced across the lesion and into the antegrade guiding catheter (Fig. 3.36B). It was later noticed that the wire crossed the occlusion completely outside the stent, through the subintimal space (Fig. 3.36C). The decision was made to crush the occluded stent and to implant a new drug-eluting stent in the subintimal space (Fig. 3.36D). Three additional overlapping drug-eluting stents were subsequently deployed with good angiographic result (Fig. 3.36E).

Two months later, coronary angiography (Fig. 3.37A–B), multidetector computed tomography (Fig. 3.37C–D), intravascular ultrasound and optical coherence tomography (Fig. 3.37E) were performed, showing persistent optimal result in the right coronary artery and particularly at the site of subintimal crush of the occluded stent. The patient remained asymptomatic throughout follow-up.

Although in-stent chronic total occlusion is usually recanalized using a true-to-true lumen approach,[1] subintimal crush of the occluded stent represents an alternative strategy. Invasive imaging in this setting is useful to confirm optimal crush of the occluded stent, and good expansion and apposition of the newly implanted stent in the subintimal space.[2]

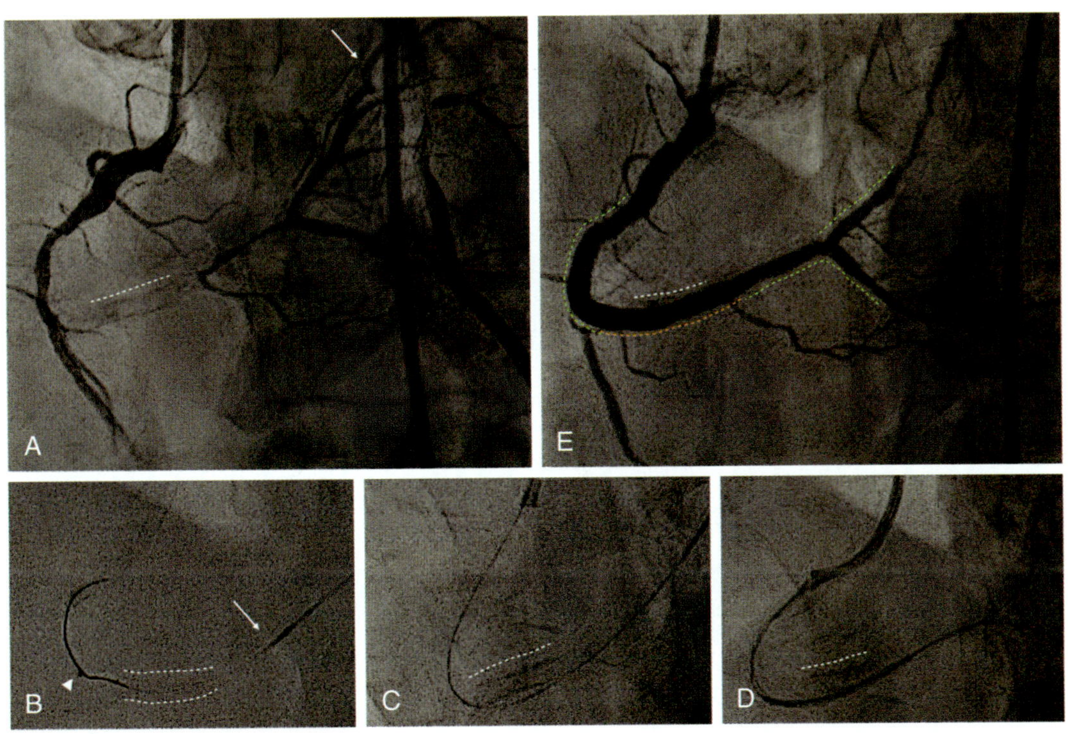

FIG. 3.36. Subintimal Crushing and Recanalization of the Occluded Stent in the Distal Right Coronary Artery *(RCA)*. (A) In-stent chronic total occlusion in the distal RCA (*dashed line*). Epicardial collateral channels from the circumflex are shown (*arrow*). (B) Retrograde approach: a Sion guidewire over a Corsair microcatheter (*arrow*) crosses the occluded stent and enters the antegrade guiding catheter. *Arrowhead* shows the antegrade microcatheter, used as a marker. (C) A different fluoroscopic projection shows that the wire tracked completely outside the stent, through the subintimal space. (D) The occluded stent was then crushed and a new drug-eluting stent (DES) was implanted subintimally. (E) Final result after implantation of four DESs: mid-RCA (*green*), distal RCA (subintimal stent) (*orange*), and T-stenting across the crux (*green*). The crushed stent is also shown (*white*).

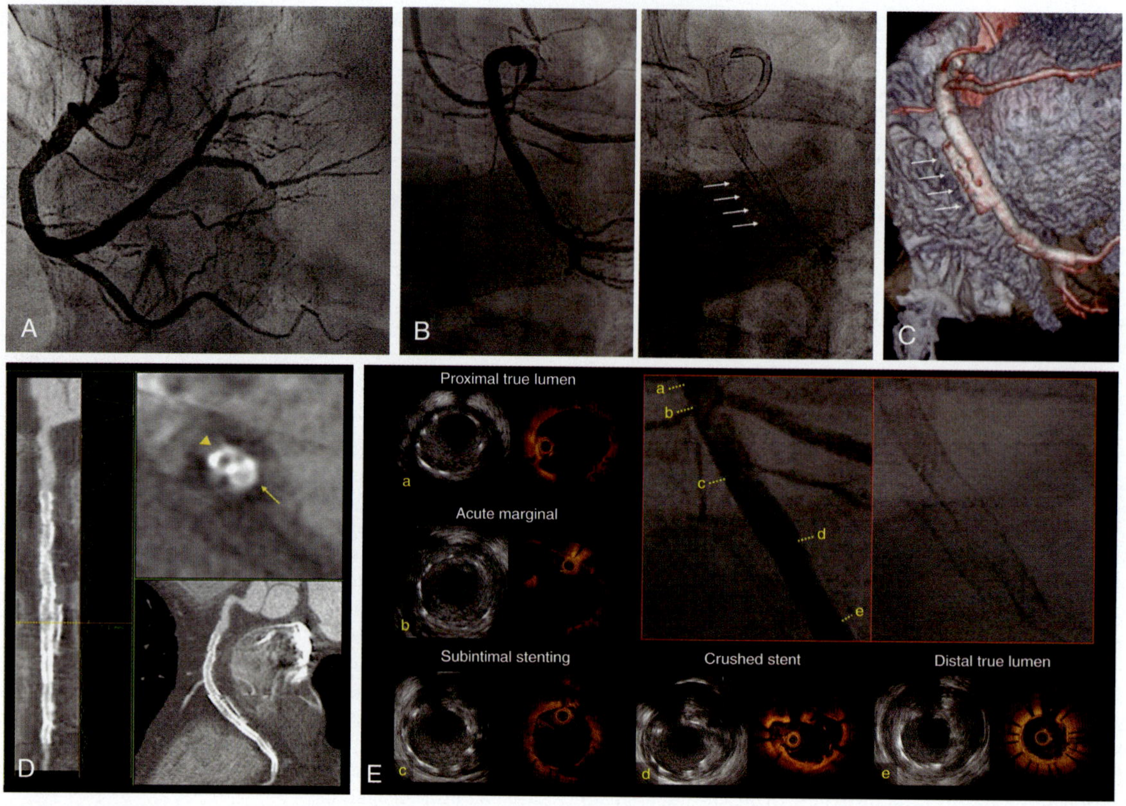

FIG. 3.37. Two-Month and 6-Year Follow-Up With a Multimodality Approach. (A and B) Two-month follow-up shows persistent optimal angiographic result. *Arrows* in (B) indicate the crushed stent. (C) Multidetector computed tomography (MDCT) shows displacement and exclusion of the crushed stent from the right coronary artery (RCA) circulation. *Arrows* indicate the crushed stent. (D) MDCT curved multiplanar reconstructions highlight the crushed/occluded stent (*arrowhead*), and the newly implanted patent stent (*arrow*). (E) At 6-years intravascular ultrasound and optical coherence tomography images of the RCA at several points including the crushed/occluded stent. Invasive imaging confirms optimal crush of the occluded stent, and good expansion and apposition of the newly implanted stent, partially in the subintimal space (*c* and *d*).

References

1. Azzalini L, Dautov R, Ojeda S, et al. Procedural and long-term outcomes of percutaneous coronary intervention for in-stent chronic *JACC Cardiovasc Interv*. 2017;10:892-902.
2. Roy J, Lucking A, Strange J, Spratt JC. The difference between success and failure: subintimal stenting around an occluded stent for treatment of a chronic total occlusion due to in-stent restenosis. *J Invasive Cardiol*. 2016;28:E136-E138.

Intervention for Spontaneous Coronary Dissections

Successful Stenting With Optical Frequency Domain Imaging Guidance For Spontaneous Coronary Artery Dissection

Keisuke Satogami, MD, Yasushi Ino, MD, PhD, Takashi Kubo, MD, PhD, Yasutsugu Shiono, MD, Tsuyoshi Nishiguchi, MD, Yoshiki Matsuo, MD, PhD, Makoto Orii, MD, Takashi Yamano, MD, Tomoyuki Yamaguchi, MD, Kumiko Hirata, MD, PhD, Atsushi Tanaka, MD, PhD, Takashi Akasaka, MD, PhD

A 51-year-old woman was urgently admitted because of chest pain. Emergent coronary angiography revealed diffuse stenosis from the proximal to distal portion of the right coronary artery (RCA) with thrombolysis in myocardial infarction (TIMI) flow grade 2 (Fig. 3.38). No stenosis was seen in the left coronary artery. Intravascular ultrasound (IVUS) images revealed an intracoronary hematoma from the posterior descending artery (PDA) to the ostium of the RCA, but could not show the entry point of the hematoma (Fig. 3.38A2–D2). Optical frequency domain imaging (OFDI) (Terumo, Tokyo, Japan) images clearly demonstrated not only intracoronary hematoma from the PDA to the ostium of the RCA, but also the entry point of the hematoma (Fig. 3.38A1–D1). A 4.0 × 12-mm Multi-Link 8 stent (Abbott Vascular, Santa Clara, California) was deployed in the ostium of the RCA to close the entry of the hematoma, and TIMI flow grade 3 was obtained (Fig. 3.39). The patient had no elevation of cardiac enzymes and no chest pain after the

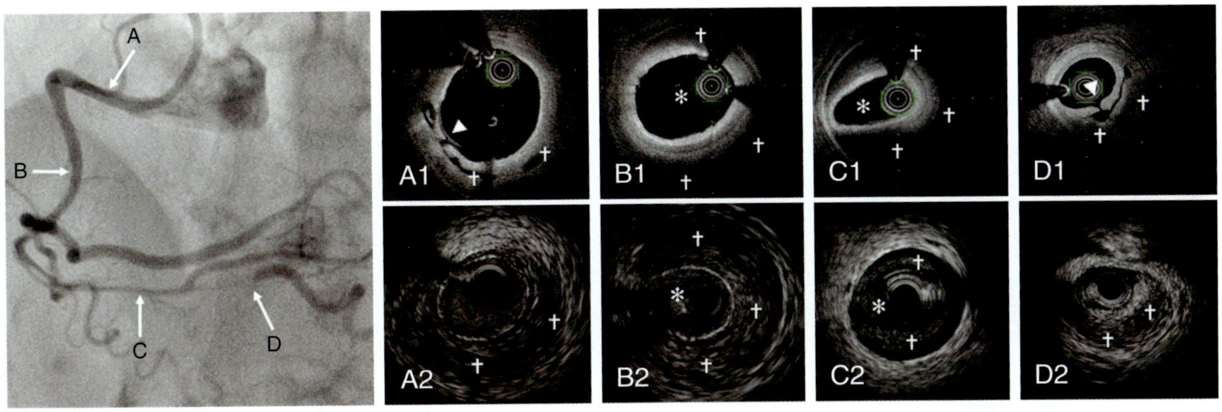

FIG. 3.38. Coronary Angiography, Optical Frequency Domain Imaging, and Intravascular Ultrasound Images Before Angioplasty. Coronary angiography showed diffuse lumen narrowing in the mid to distal portion of the right coronary artery. (A–D) Optical frequency domain imaging (OFDI) ([A1]–[D1]) and intravascular ultrasound (IVUS) ([A2]–[D2]) demonstrated coronary dissection including a small true lumen (*asterisks*) compressed by a large intramural false lumen (*daggers*). OFDI clearly demonstrated intimal tearing (*arrowheads*)([A1] and [D1]), but IVUS could not detect it ([A2] and [D2]).

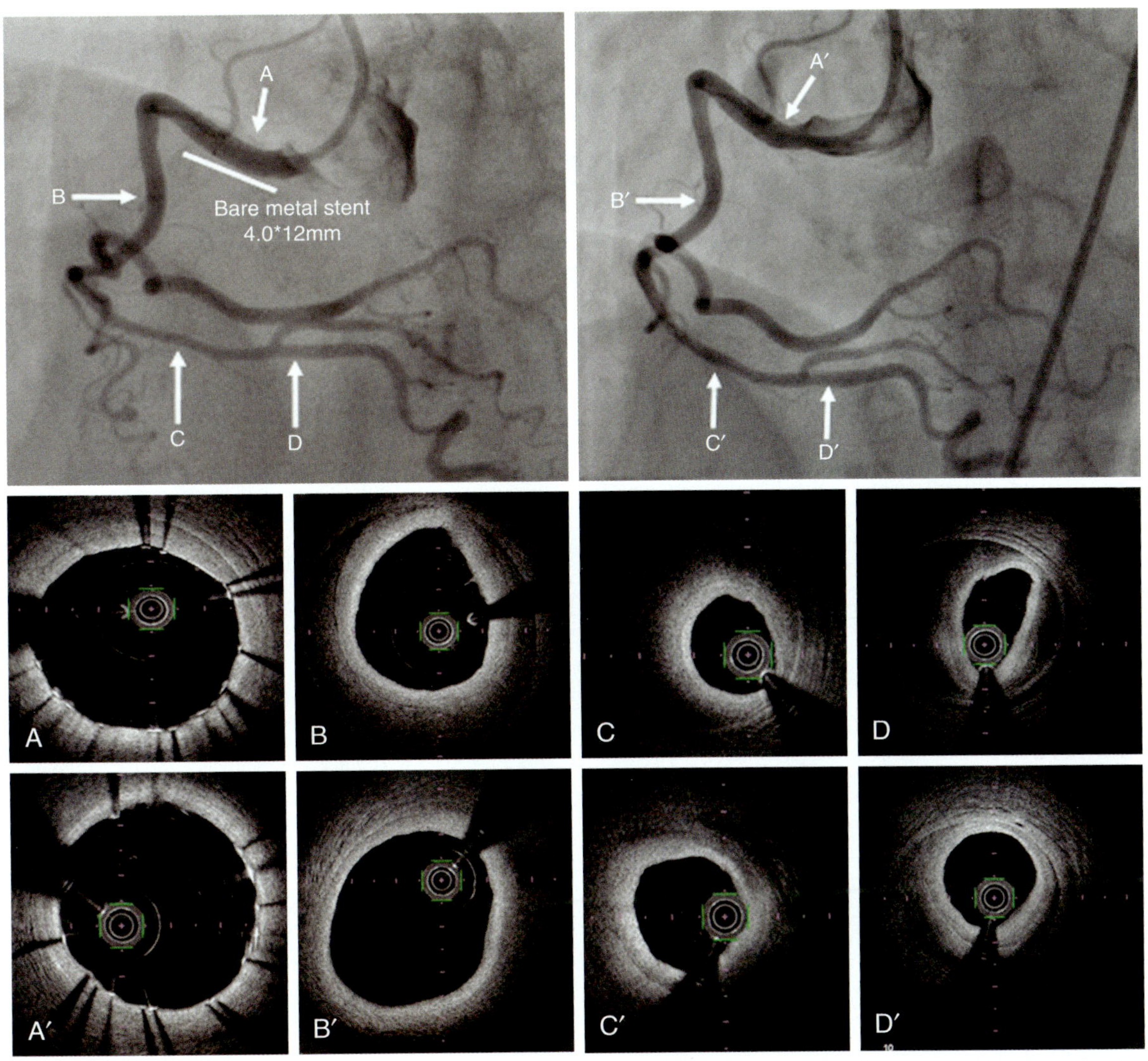

FIG. 3.39. Coronary Angiography and Optical Frequency Domain Imaging (OFDI) Images After Stent Implantation. (*Left*) Coronary angiography showed thrombolysis in myocardial infarction flow grade 3 after bare-metal stent implantation in the ostium of the right coronary artery (RCA) (*white line*). OFDI demonstrated good expansion of the stent (A) and the remaining of coronary dissection (B–D). (*Right*) Follow-up coronary angiography 3 weeks later revealed good patency of the RCA. OFDI showed that vessel lumen size became larger compared with that immediately after stent implantation despite the intracoronary hematoma that remained from the ostium to the distal portion of the RCA (B′–D′).

procedure. Follow-up coronary angiography 3 weeks later revealed no significant stenosis, and OFDI showed that the vessel lumen size became larger compared with immediately after the procedure, and the entry of the hematoma resolved despite intracoronary hematoma remaining (Fig. 3.39A′–D′).

Diagnosis and management of spontaneous coronary artery dissection are very challenging. Previous reports have suggested the value of optical coherence tomography (OCT) in this situation.[1-3] Although a forceful, power injection of contrast medium necessary to clear the artery of blood has a possibility of hydraulic propagation of a dissection in a dissected artery, OCT can visualize the double-lumen morphology and identify the entry tear as well as the circumferential and longitudinal extent of the hematoma. Furthermore, OCT was useful to confirm that the guidewire was located in the true lumen and that adequate stent coverage for the entry tear, expansion, and apposition was achieved. In this case, IVUS could not detect the entry tear. Therefore, long stenting, which has the potential risk of stent thrombosis, might be required for revascularization with IVUS or angiography guidance. OFDI/OCT is useful to diagnose and determine the strategy of percutaneous coronary intervention in spontaneous coronary artery dissection.

References

1. Alfonso F, Paulo M, Gonzalo N, et al. Diagnosis of spontaneous coronary artery dissection by optical coherence tomography. *J Am Coll Cardiol.* 2012;59:1073-1079.
2. Nishiguchi T, Tanaka A, Ozaki Y, et al. Prevalence of spontaneous coronary artery dissection in patients with acute coronary syndrome. *Eur Heart J Acute Cardiovasc Care.* 2016;5(3):263-270.
3. Alfonso F, Paulo MG, Lennie V, et al. Spontaneous coronary artery dissection: long-term follow-up of a large series of patients prospectively managed with a "conservative" therapeutic strategy. *JACC Cardiovasc Interv.* 2012;5:1062-1070.

Successful Treatment of Spontaneous Coronary Artery Dissection With Cutting Balloon Angioplasty as Evaluated With Optical Coherence Tomography

Kazuhiko Yumoto, MD, PhD, Hojo Sasaki, MD, Hajime Aoki, MD, Kenichi Kato, MD

A previously healthy 47-year-old premenopausal woman with no risk factors was admitted to our hospital with severe chest pain. Urgent coronary angiography showed a totally occlusive lesion in the middle of the left anterior descending (LAD) coronary artery with thrombolysis in myocardial infarction (TIMI) flow grade 0. The other coronary arteries appeared normal. Immediate percutaneous coronary intervention (PCI) was performed because of ongoing chest pain and persistent ST-segment elevation. Intravascular ultrasonography showed an extensive intramural hematoma (Fig. 3.40) and confirmed the presence of spontaneous coronary artery dissection (SCAD). We performed a cutting balloon angioplasty to create communications between the true and false lumens, reduce the compression, and restore the distal coronary flow. We used a 2.5-mm cutting balloon dilated to 2 atm in the distal segment and 4 atm in the proximal segment. After ballooning, coronary flow was immediately restored to TIMI flow grade 3. Optical coherence tomography (OCT) confirmed that the incisions on the dissected intima corresponded with the blade shape and that communications were successfully made between the false and true lumens (Fig. 3.41). The patient recovered uneventfully with no complications. Follow-up coronary angiography at 6 months revealed good patency of the LAD. OCT showed healing of the dissection with adequate intimal thickness, although a residual partial false lumen remained in the distal segment (Fig. 3.42). The use of PCI for the treatment of SCAD is generally associated with a high complication rate.[1] In this case, cutting balloon angioplasty was effective to immediately restore coronary flow, and good healing was documented at follow-up.

References

1. Tweet MS, Hayes SN, Pitta SR, et al. Clinical features, management, and prognosis of spontaneous coronary artery dissection. *Circulation.* 2012;126:579-588.

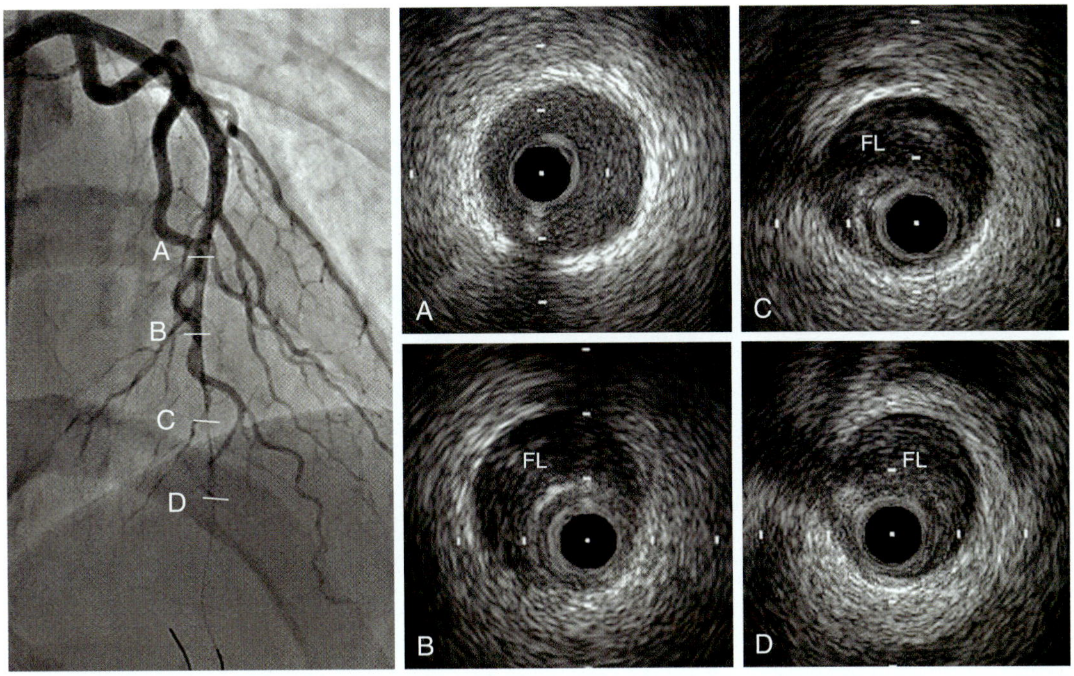

FIG. 3.40. Coronary Angiography and Intravenous Ultrasound Images of the Left Anterior Descending (LAD) Coronary Artery Before Angioplasty. Emergent coronary angiography shows total occlusion in the middle of the LAD. Normal proximal LAD is shown in (A). IVUS shows an extensive intramural hematoma that compresses the true lumen of the LAD throughout the length of the middle to distal LAD (B–D). *FL*, false lumen.

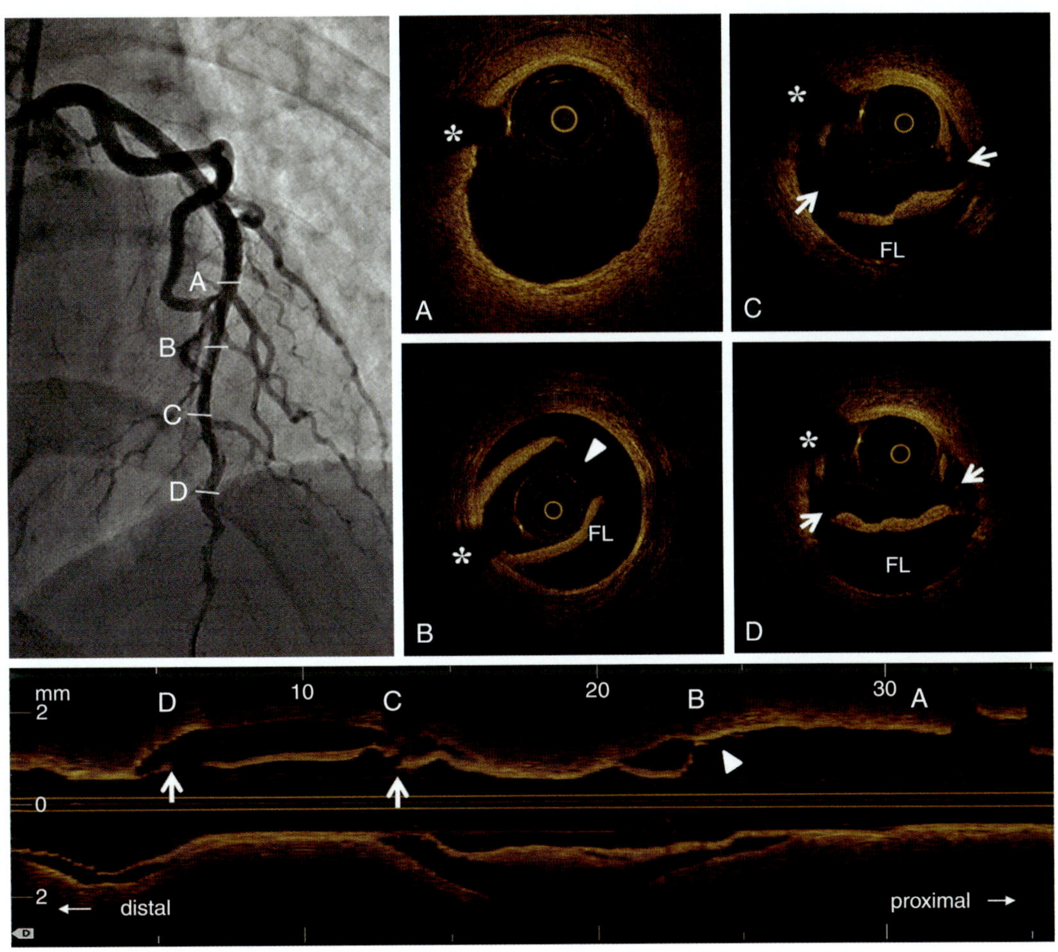

FIG. 3.41. Coronary Angiography and Optical Coherence Tomography (OCT) Images of the Left Anterior Descending (LAD) Coronary Artery After Cutting Balloon Angioplasty. Normal proximal LAD is shown in (A). OCT shows the true and false lumens (*FL*) beginning with the intimal tear (*arrowhead* in [B]) and clearly shows the communication created by the incision (*arrows* in [C] and [D]). These incision sites coincide with the blades of the cutting balloon. *Asterisks* indicate wire artifact.

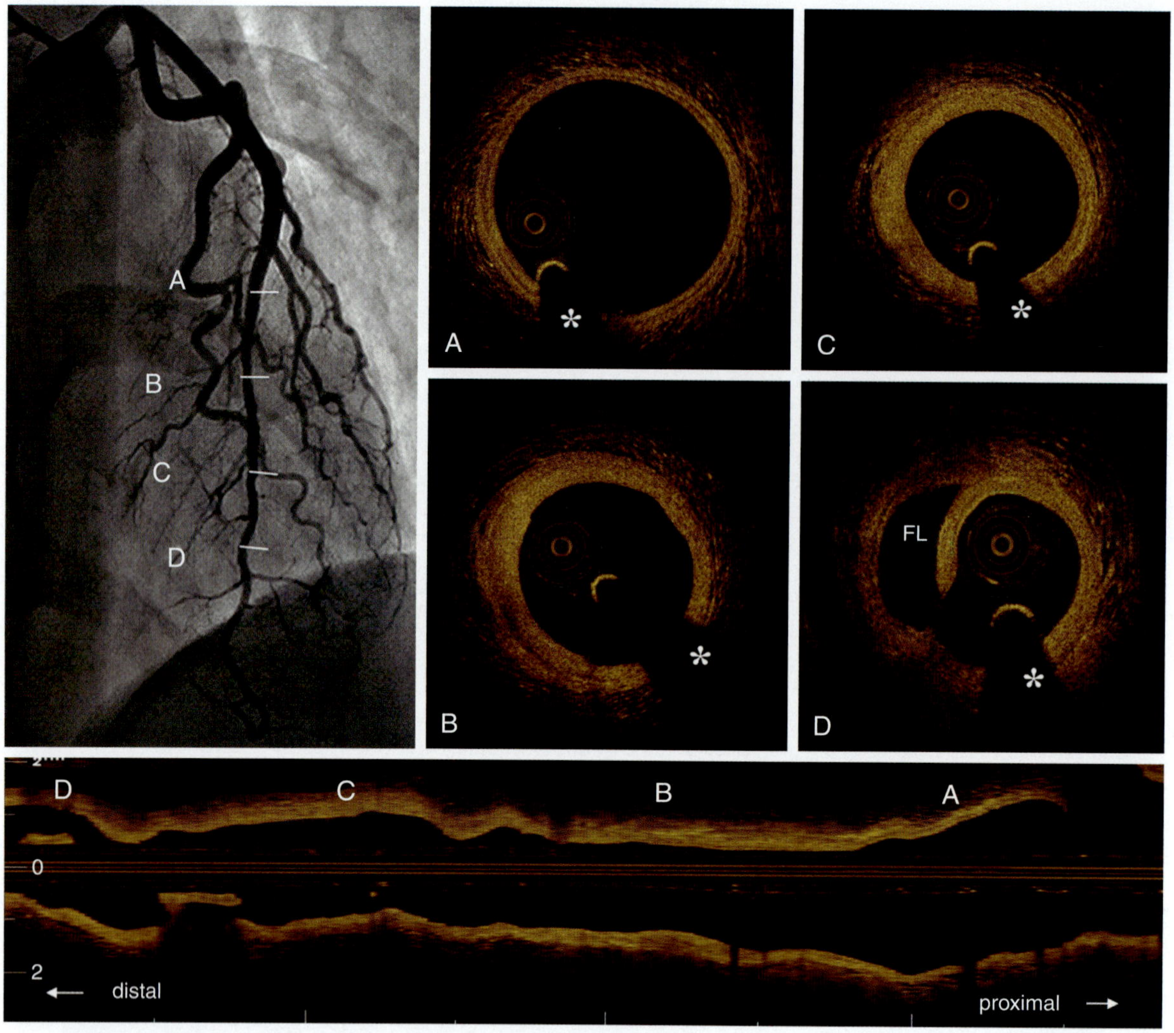

FIG. 3.42. Coronary Angiography and Optical Coherence Tomography (OCT) Images at Follow-Up. Normal proximal left anterior descending coronary artery is shown in (A). OCT shows healing of the dissection; the healed intima appears relatively thick (B and C). A small partial false lumen (*FL*) remains distally (D). *Asterisks* indicate wire artifact.

CHAPTER 4

STRUCTURAL HEART DISEASE: COMPLICATIONS AND TECHNIQUES

Aortic Valve

ACUTE ARTERY OCCLUSION DURING TRANSCATHETER AORTIC VALVE REPLACEMENT IN A PATIENT WITH AN ANOMALOUS ORIGIN OF THE LEFT CIRCUMFLEX CORONARY ARTERY

Juan Gabriel Acosta-Vélez, MD, Bruno García del Blanco, MD, Josep Guindo, MD, Jose Montiel Serrano, MD, Hug Cuellar Calabria, MD, Gerard Martí Aguasca, MD, Teresa Gonzalez-Alujas, MD, Ignasi Durán, MD, Pilar Tornos, MD, PhD

The images presented are of an 86-year-old woman with severe aortic stenosis in whom a transcatheter aortic valve replacement (TAVR) was performed (Fig. 4.1, Online Videos 4.1–4.3). Preprocedural angiography revealed an anomalous origin of the left circumflex coronary artery (LCx) from the right coronary sinus below the ostium of the right coronary artery with a retroannular trajectory, as shown by a computed tomography scan. As a preventive measure, an intracoronary catheter and a 0.014-inch guidewire were positioned in the LCx at the beginning of the TAVR procedure. After balloon inflation and liberation of the 26-mm SAPIEN XT valve (Edwards

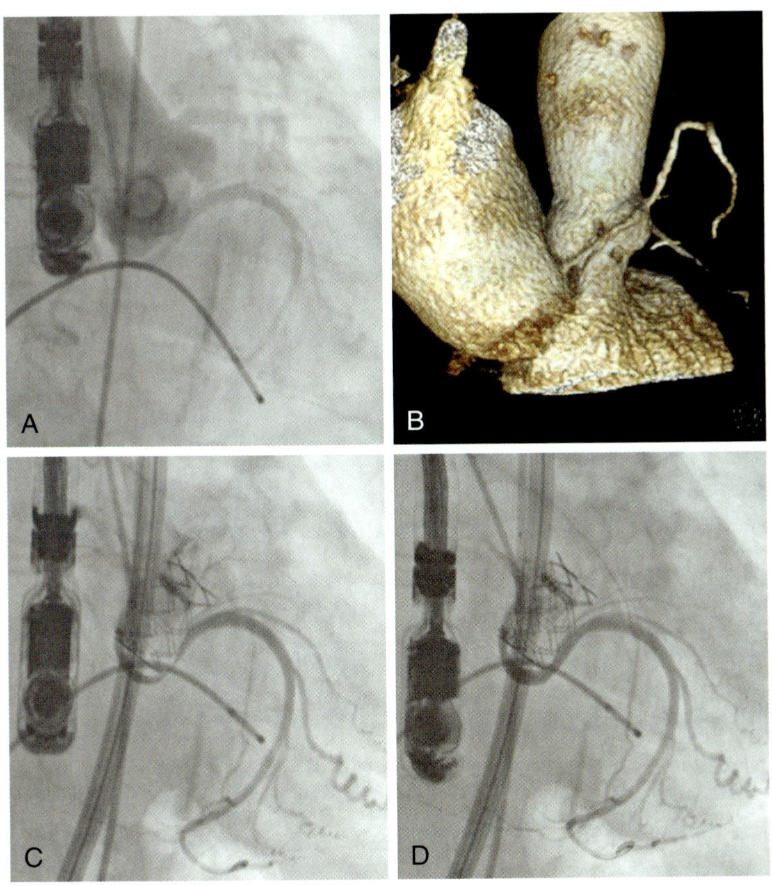

FIG. 4.1 Acute Occlusion of Anomalous Left Circumflex Coronary Artery (LCx) During Transcatheter Aortic Valve Replacement (TAVR). (A) Preprocedural angiography showing an anomalous origin of the LCx from the right coronary sinus (Online Video 4.1). (B) Coronary computed tomography scan shows the relationship between the anomalous LCx and the aortic annulus. (C) LCx compression after balloon inflation during the TAVR procedure (Online Video 4.2). (D) Final result after stent implantation in the LCx (Online Video 4.3).

Lifesciences, Irvine, California), severe narrowing of the LCx was documented with no immediate evidence of hemodynamic or electrocardiographic repercussions. Administration of intracoronary nitroglycerin showed no luminal improvement, which supports the hypothesis of extrinsic compression. It was, therefore, treated with an uneventful implantation of a bare-metal stent in the LCx. Computed tomography-adapted cover index was 17%, and relative oversizing was 20%. We can speculate that the use of a smaller prosthesis size may have resulted in a lesser degree or absence of coronary compression. The left coronary artery (LCA) is the most commonly involved artery in reported cases of acute arterial occlusion during TAVR. Most of these cases are due to ostial compression.[1–4] Nevertheless, when the LCx originates from the right coronary sinus, compression at the posterior aortic annulus should also be considered to undertake preventive measures, as highlighted by our case.

References

1. Ribeiro HB, Nombela-Franco L, Urena M, et al. Coronary obstruction following transcatheter aortic valve implantation: a systematic review. *JACC Cardiovasc Interv.* 2013;6:452-461.
2. Ribeiro HB, Webb JG, Makkar RR, et al. Predictive factors, management and clinical outcomes of coronary obstruction following transcatheter aortic valve implantation: insights from a large multicenter registry. *J Am Coll Cardiol.* 2013;62:1552-1562.
3. Gogas BD, Zacharoulis AA, Antoniadis AG. Acute coronary occlusion following TAVI. *Catheter Cardiovasc Interv.* 2011;77:435-438.
4. Binder RK, Webb JG, Willson AB, et al. The impact of integration of a multidetector computed tomography annulus area sizing algorithm on outcomes of transcatheter aortic valve replacement: a prospective, multicenter, controlled trial. *J Am Coll Cardiol.* 2013;62:431-438.

Anterior Mitral Leaflet Perforation During Transcatheter Aortic Valve Replacement in a Patient With Mitral Annular Calcification

Mike Saji, MD, Gorav Ailawadi, MD, Michael Ragosta, MD, Dale E. Fowler, MD, RDCS, John M. Dent, MD, D. Scott Lim, MD

A 71-year-old man with symptomatic severe aortic stenosis was referred for transcatheter aortic valve replacement (TAVR). His medical history included paroxysmal atrial fibrillation, mild mitral regurgitation, and moderate mitral stenosis with a 10 mm Hg mean transmitral gradient determined using transthoracic echocardiography. Computed tomography (CT) showed mitral annular calcification (MAC) mainly distributed on the anteromedial side of the mitral valve (Fig. 4.2A–B). The aortic annulus area, as evaluated using CT, was 600 cm^2, and a 29-mm Edwards SAPIEN XT valve (Edwards Lifesciences, Irvine, California) was implanted in the optimal position without difficulty (Fig. 4.2C). However, intraoperative transesophageal echocardiography showed a perforation on the medial side of the anterior mitral leaflet (AML) (Fig. 4.2D–G, Online Videos 4.4 and 4.5). On fluoroscopy, the edge of the SAPIEN XT valve reached the MAC (Fig. 4.2H). The postprocedural course was uneventful except for transitional atrial fibrillation, and the patient was discharged on the third postoperative day. Transthoracic echocardiography at the 1-month follow-up did not show evidence

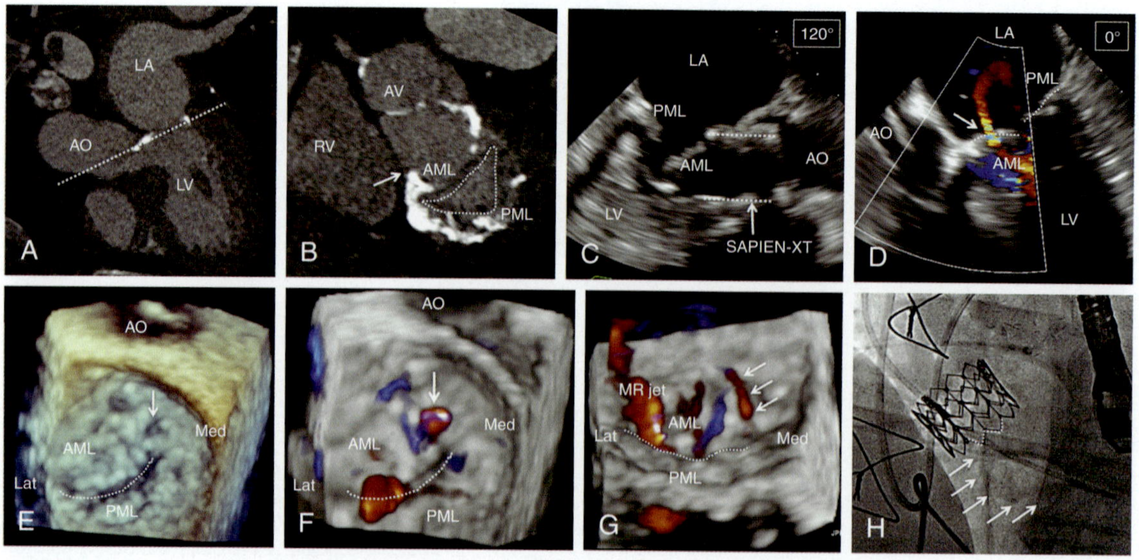

FIG. 4.2 Images of Anterior Mitral Leaflet Perforation. (A and B) Three-dimensional (3D) computed tomography showing significant mitral annular calcification (MAC) (*arrow*). (C) Transesophageal echocardiography (TEE) showing the SAPIEN XT (Edwards Lifesciences, Irvine, California) in the optimal position. (D) Anterior mitral leaflet perforation (*arrow*) (Online Video 4.4). (E–G) Mitral leaflet perforation on 3D TEE (*arrows*) (Online Video 4.5). (H) SAPIEN XT reaching the MAC on fluoroscopy (*arrow*). *AML*, anterior mitral leaflet; *AO*, aorta; *AV*, aortic valve; *LA*, left atrium; *Lat*, lateral; *LV*, left ventricle; *Med*, medial; *MR*, mitral regurgitation; *PML*, posterior mitral leaflet; *RV*, right ventricle.

of heart failure, infective endocarditis, or deterioration of the transmitral gradient.

Acute AML perforation is a rare complication of TAVR.[1] Mitral valve involvement is more likely with the CoreValve prosthesis (Medtronic, Minneapolis, Minnesota) than with the SAPIEN XT valve because it has a larger component extending into the left ventricular outflow tract.[2] However, in this case, the edge of the expanded SAPIEN XT valve impinged the calcification around the mitral valve, resulting in AML perforation. MAC is considered a risk factor for mitral leaflet perforation, which can lead to heart failure and infective endocarditis. Further follow-up is required in this case, and precise CT assessment for MAC is warranted before TAVR.

References

1. Raschpichler M, Seeburger J, Strasser RH, Misfeld M. Corevalve prosthesis causes anterior mitral leaflet perforation resulting in severe mitral regurgitation and subsequent endocarditis. *Eur Heart J.* 2014;35:1587.
2. Franco E, de Agustín JA, Hernandez-Antolin R, et al. Acute mitral stenosis after transcatheter aortic valve implantation. *J Am Coll Cardiol.* 2012; 60:e35.

Aortic Root Intussusception During Transcatheter Aortic Valve Replacement

Ayman Jubran, MD, Moshe Y. Flugelman, MD, Nader Khader, MD, Ronen Jaffe, MD

Accurate valve positioning during transcatheter aortic valve replacement (TAVR) is crucial. Valve migration into the left ventricle during deployment can be treated by pulling the valve toward the aortic root or by implanting a second valve.

An 83-year-old woman with severe symptomatic aortic stenosis (valve area 0.80 cm^2) was referred for TAVR. Computed tomographic angiography revealed a mildly calcified tricuspid aortic valve (960 Agatston units), minimal calcification within the ascending aorta, and aortic annular dimensions of 21 × 25 mm. A 29-mm CoreValve (Medtronic, Minneapolis, Minnesota) was implanted without predilation.

Implantation was initiated after optimal valve position had been achieved (Fig. 4.3, Online Video 4.6), but the valve descended significantly into the ventricle during deployment, resulting in severe aortic regurgitation (Fig. 4.4, Online Video 4.7). Attempts to pull the valve proximally resulted in intussusception of the aortic annulus into the aorta, with deformation of the aortic root (Fig. 4.5, Online Video 4.8). The deformity resolved after tension on the delivery system was released. Despite the deep final position of the valve (12 mm below the aortic annulus), contact between the distal sealing skirt and the annulus prevented paravalvular leak (Fig. 4.6, Online Video 4.9). The temporary aortic root deformation did not result in adverse clinical outcomes, and the patient made an uneventful recovery without need for permanent pacemaker implantation.

This case highlights the need for new-generation retrievable and repositionable valves with improved control of positioning.

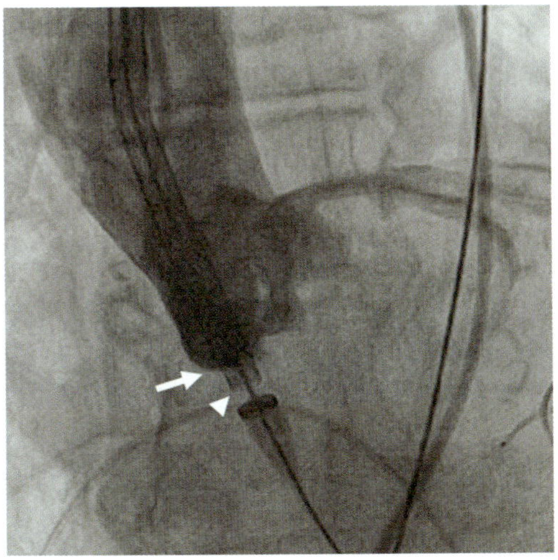

FIG. 4.3 Initial Valve Position. Valve implantation was initiated with the distal valve edge (*arrowhead*) positioned 4 mm below the aortic annulus (*arrow*) (Online Video 4.6).

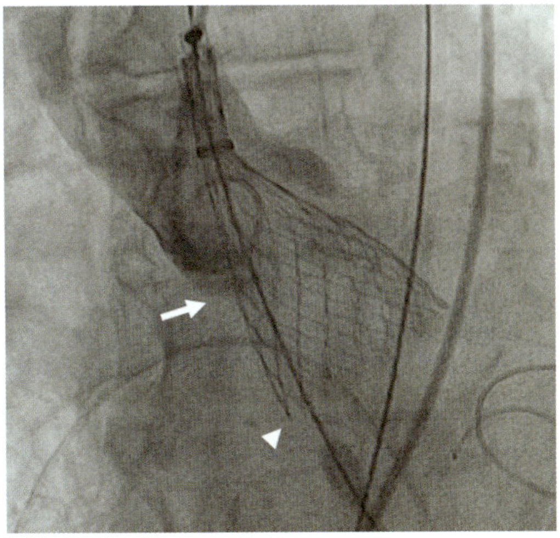

FIG. 4.4 Valve Descent Into the Ventricle. The valve descended into the ventricle during deployment, with the distal valve edge (*arrowhead*) positioned 24 mm below the aortic annulus (*arrow*) (Online Video 4.7).

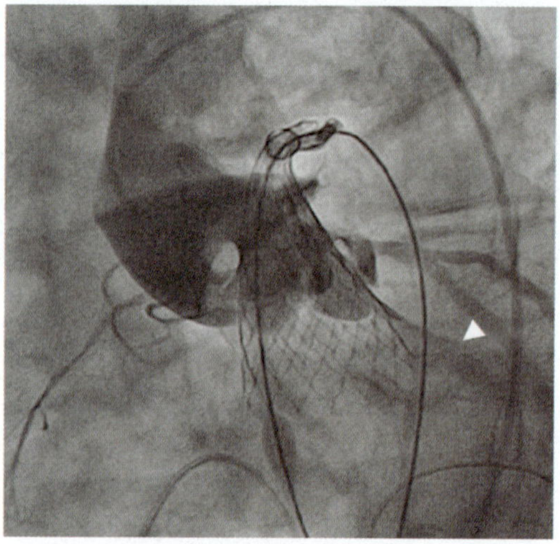

FIG. 4.5 Intussusception of the Aortic Annulus Into the Aorta. Attempts to pull the valve proximally resulted in intussusception of the aortic annulus into the aorta, with deformation of the aortic root anatomy and continued severe aortic regurgitation (*arrowhead*) (Online Video 4.8).

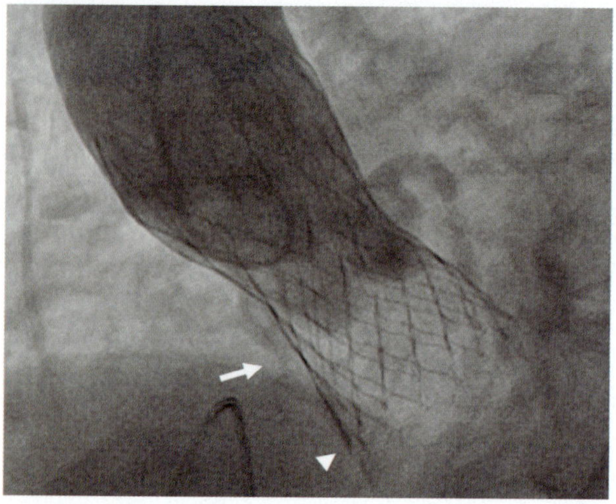

FIG. 4.6 Final Valve Position. Final valve position with the distal valve edge (*arrowhead*) positioned 12 mm below the aortic annulus (*arrow*) (Online Video 4.9).

Conservative Management and Resolution of a Contained Rupture of Aortic Annulus Following Transcatheter Valve Replacement

Vijayakumar Subban, MBBS, MD, DM, Alexander Incani, MBBS, Andrew Clarke, MBBS, Constantine Aroney, MBBS, MD, Gregory M. Scalia, MBBS, MMSc, James A. Crowhurst, BSc, Owen Christopher Raffel, MBChB, Darren L. Walters, MBBS, MPhil

An 87-year-old woman with symptomatic severe aortic stenosis, logistic EuroSCORE (European System for Cardiac Operative Risk Evaluation) of 20.94%, and Society of Thoracic Surgeons estimated surgical mortality of 27.4%, underwent transcatheter aortic valve implantation (TAVI). Her transesophageal echocardiogram (TOE) showed a valve area of 0.7 cm^2 (peak velocity: 5.3 m/s), an annular diameter of 19 mm, and good left ventricular systolic function. The computed tomography aortogram showed heavily calcified aortic root, leaflets, and annulus (Fig. 4.7A–C), a descending thoracic aortic aneurysm, and small-caliber access vessels. The total volume of aortic leaflet calcium was 1444 mm^3. The annulus transverse diameters were a minimum of 20 mm and a maximum of 23 mm, the perimeter was 63 mm, and the area was 290 mm^2 (3mensio valves, Pie Medical Imaging BV, Bilthoven, the Netherlands). The patient underwent TAVI via the transaortic root with a 23-mm Edwards SAPIEN XT valve (Edwards Lifesciences, Irvine, California). The immediate postdeployment TOE and aortogram showed an expanding hematoma of the posterior aortic root below the left main coronary artery (Fig. 4.7D–E). There was no pericardial effusion or hemodynamic compromise; hence, she was managed conservatively with local digital compression, packing of the mediastinal space with surgical sponges, reversal of anticoagulation, and lowering of systolic blood pressure. She was monitored on the table for 1 h. There was no further expansion of the hematoma (Fig 4.7F–G). The packing was removed and the sternum closed. She was transferred to the postoperative ward. The patient remained stable and serial echocardiograms showed resolution of the hematoma (Fig. 4.7H).

Annular rupture is a catastrophic complication of TAVI that occurs in 0.1% to 1% of the patients undergoing this procedure.[1] Extensive annular, leaflet, and aortic calcification and implantation of oversized valve prosthesis predispose individuals to rupture, which has exclusively been reported with balloon-expandable prosthesis. Careful evaluation of the severity of the calcification and selecting an appropriately sized self-expanding valve in patients with extensive calcification might prevent this serious complication. Intraprocedural TOE may be of great value in the timely recognition of this serious adverse event. Frank rupture results in immediate tamponade and requires urgent surgical intervention. In cases with a transaortic approach where the sternum is open, a contained rupture may be managed with a conservative wait-and-watch policy.[2,3]

References

1. Hayashida K, Bouvier E, Lefèvre T, et al. Potential mechanism of annulus rupture during transcatheter aortic valve implantation. *Catheter Cardiovasc Interv.* 2013;82(5):E742-E746. doi:10.1002/ccd.24524. [Epub 2013 Jun 25.].
2. Stortecky S, Buellesfeld L, Wenaweser P, Windecker S. Transcatheter aortic valve implantation: prevention and management of complications. *Heart.* 2012;98(suppl 4):iv52-64.
3. Généreux P, Reiss GR, Kodali SK, Williams MR, Hahn RT. Periaortic hematoma after transcatheter aortic valve replacement: description of a new complication. *Catheter Cardiovasc Interv.* 2012;79:766-776.

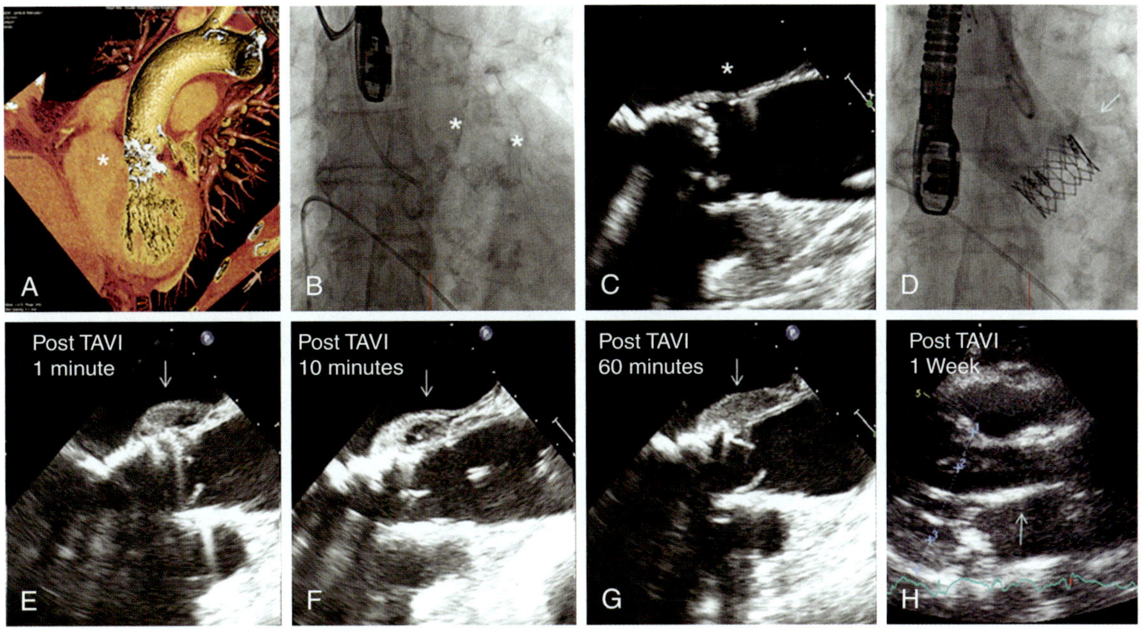

FIG. 4.7 Developments of Contained Aortic Annulus Rupture During Transcatheter Aortic Valve Implantation (*TAVI*) and Its Resolution With Conservative Management. Computed tomography aortogram with 3mensio (Pie Medical Imaging BV, Bilthoven, the Netherlands) three-dimensional reconstruction (A), fluoroscopy (B), and transesophageal echocardiogram (TOE) (C) showing extensive aortic annular and outflow tract calcification (*asterisk*). (D) Aortogram revealing contained rupture below the left main coronary artery. (E) to (G) TOE in esophageal long axis view showing aortic root hematoma at various time intervals. (H) Follow-up transthoracic echocardiogram in parasternal long axis view showing resolved hematoma (*arrow*).

Coronary Ostia Stenosis After Transcatheter Aortic Valve Implantation

Rodrigo Bagur, MD, Eric Dumont, MD, Daniel Doyle, MD, Eric Larose, DVM, MD, Jerôme Lemieux, MD, Sébastien Bergeron, MD, Sylvie Bilodeau, MD, Olivier F. Bertrand, MD, PhD, Robert De Larochellière, MD, Josep Rodés-Cabau, MD

A frail 85-year-old woman with symptomatic severe aortic stenosis was evaluated for transcatheter aortic valve implantation (TAVI). The Society of Thoracic Surgeons risk score and the logistic EuroSCORE (European System for Cardiac Operative Risk Evaluation) were 7.2% and 13.3%, respectively. Based on her extreme frailty and severe chronic kidney disease, the patient was considered nonsuitable for conventional surgery. Cardiac computed tomography and coronary angiography are shown in Fig. 4.8. Because of the patient's calcified and small (<7 mm) iliofemoral arteries, the procedure was performed by transapical approach.[1] A 26-mm Edwards SAPIEN valve (Edwards Lifesciences, Irvine, California) was successfully implanted, although the valve was situated in a high position with respect to the aortic annulus (Online Videos 4.10–4.13). Twenty-four hours after TAVI, the patient had chest pain with transient ST-segment changes. A coronary angiography showed significant stenosis of the left main coronary artery (LMCA) and right coronary artery (RCA) ostia secondary to the displacement of the calcified native aortic leaflets toward the coronary ostia (Fig. 4.9A–B, Online Videos 4.14 and 4.15). Percutaneous coronary intervention was successfully performed in both LMCA and RCA ostia (Fig. 4.9C–D, Online Videos 4.16 and 4.17). A predischarge cardiac computed tomography and echocardiography are shown in Fig. 4.10 and Online Video 4.18, respectively. At 6-month follow-up the patient was in functional class II without cardiovascular events.

LMCA stenosis is a potential complication of TAVI.[2,3] This case shows that this complication can affect the two coronary ostia and become clinically evident in the subacute phase after TAVI. It also supports the feasibility of percutaneous coronary intervention through the struts of the implanted valve. The presence of a bulky calcified valve has been recognized as a risk factor for LMCA stenosis after TAVI, especially in those cases with a short distance (<8 mm) between the aortic leaflets and the coronary ostia.[3,4] In these cases, dye injection at the time of balloon valvuloplasty might be useful to determine the relation of the extended leaflets to coronary ostia.[3]

References

1. Rodés-Cabau J, Dumont E, De Larochellière R, et al. Feasibility and initial results of percutaneous aortic valve implantation including selection of the transfemoral or transapical approach in patients with severe aortic stenosis. *Am J Cardiol.* 2008;102:1240-1246.
2. Webb JG, Chandavimol M, Thompson CR, et al. Percutaneous aortic valve implantation retrograde from the femoral artery. *Circulation.* 2006;113:842-850.
3. Kapadia SR, Svensson L, Tuzcu EM. Successful percutaneous management of left main trunk occlusion during percutaneous aortic valve replacement. *Catheter Cardiovasc Interv.* 2009;73:966-972.
4. Akhtar M, Tuzcu EM, Kapadia SR, et al. Aortic root morphology in patients undergoing percutaneous aortic valve replacement. *J Thorac Cardiovasc Surg.* 2009;137:950-956.

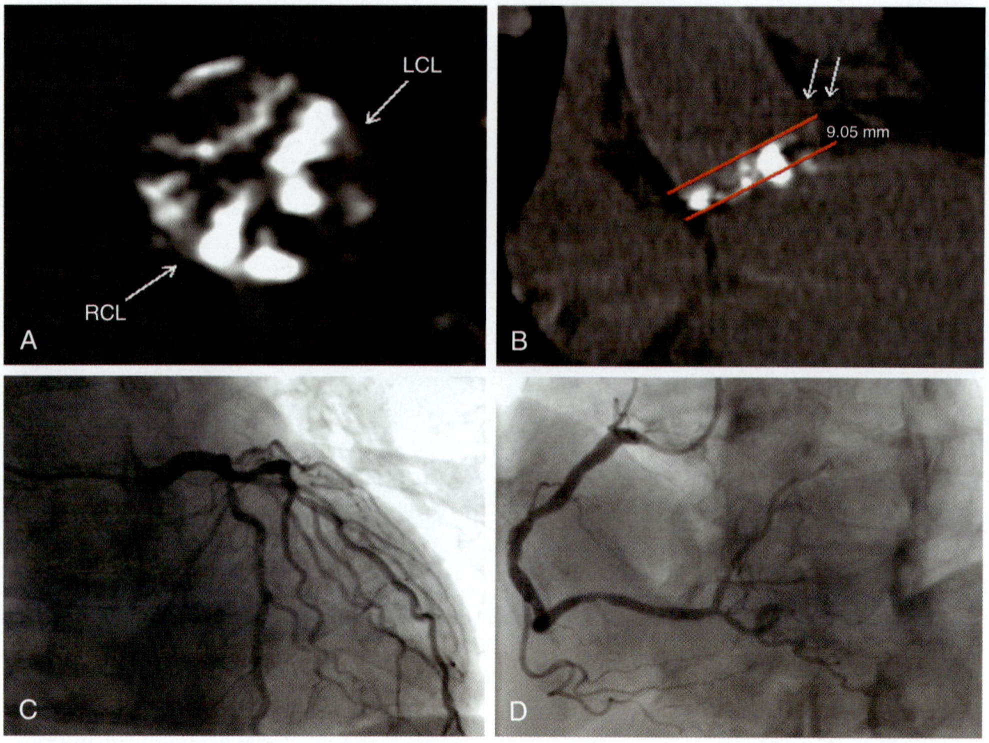

FIG. 4.8 Baseline Computed Tomography and Coronary Angiography. (A) Computed tomography image showing the severity of aortic valve calcification (left coronary leaflet [*LCL*], right coronary leaflet [*RCL*]). (B) Computed tomography image showing the distance (*red lines*) between the insertion of the aortic leaflets and the origin of the left main coronary artery (*white arrows*). The distance between the insertion of the aortic leaflets and the origin of the right coronary artery was 11.5 mm. (C) Left coronary angiography showing the absence of left main coronary artery disease. (D) Right coronary angiography showing a moderate lesion (34% diameter stenosis by quantitative coronary angiography) at the origin of the right coronary artery.

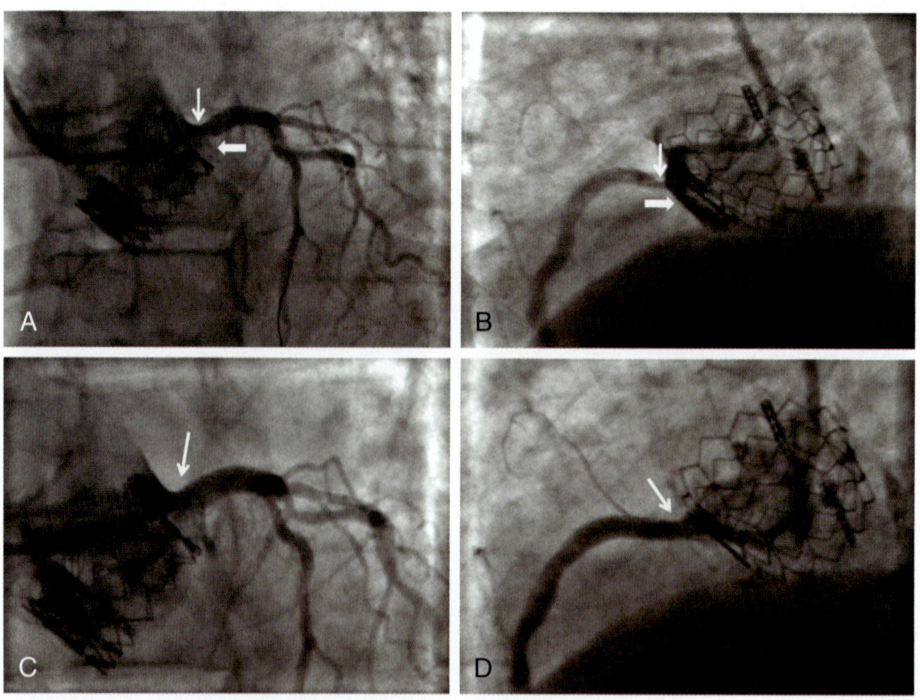

FIG. 4.9 Coronary Angiography at 24 h After Transcatheter Aortic Valve Implantation. Coronary angiography images showing significant stenosis (*thin arrows*) of the left main coronary artery (LMCA) (A) and right coronary artery (RCA) (B) ostia secondary to the displacement of the calcified native aortic leaflets (*thick arrows*) toward the coronary ostia. Coronary angiography images after percutaneous coronary intervention and stent implantation showing the absence of residual stenosis (*thin arrows*) at the LMCA (C) and RCA (D) ostia. The distance between the LMCA and RCA ostia and the struts of the valve were 1.89 mm and 1.29 mm, respectively. The transcatheter aortic valve implantation procedure and immediate echocardiographic results are shown in Online Videos 4.10–4.13. Coronary angiography and intervention are shown in Online Videos 4.14–4.17.

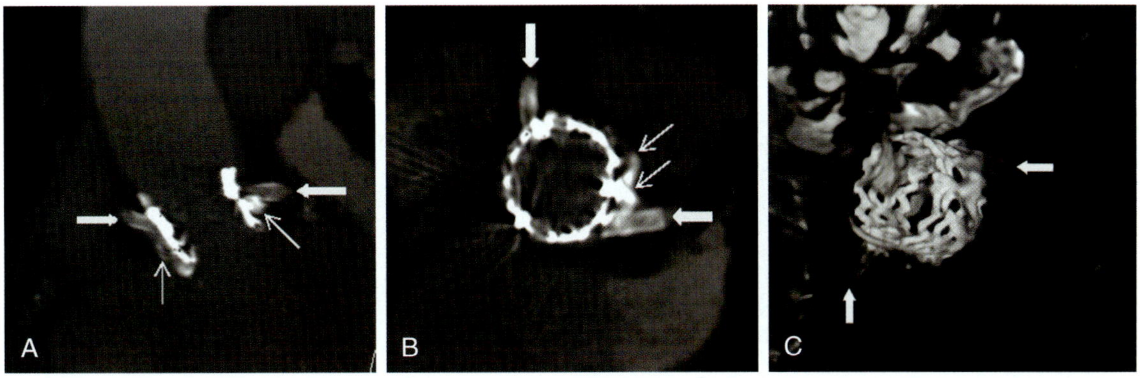

FIG. 4.10 Computed Tomography at Hospital Discharge. (A and B) Cardiac computed tomography images of the Edwards SAPIEN valve and the two coronary stents (*thick arrows*) through the struts of the Edwards SAPIEN valve stent; *thin arrows* highlight the calcified native aortic leaflets. (C) Three-dimensional reconstruction of the Edwards SAPIEN valve with the two coronary stents (*thick arrows*) through the struts of the valve. A complementary transthoracic echocardiogram is shown in Online Video 4.18.

Cutaneopericardial Fistula After Transapical Approach for Transcatheter Aortic Valve Replacement

Karthiek Narala, MD, Sandeep Banga, MD, Sajjan Gayam, BS, Sudhir Mungee, MD

A 77-year-old man with severe aortic stenosis, previous coronary artery bypass graft, recurrent infective endocarditis, and chronic Q fever (taking hydroxychloroquine and doxycycline) underwent a transcatheter aortic valve replacement (TAVR) by the transapical (TA) approach via left thoracotomy. A 29-mm Edwards SAPIEN XT valve (Edwards Lifesciences, Irvine, California) was successfully deployed using the Ascendra 2 delivery system (Edwards Lifesciences). Purse-string sutures were placed at the left ventricular (LV) apex. Postprocedure development of a hemorrhagic pericardial effusion necessitated surgical reexploration; bleeding from the LV apex was controlled with placement of pledgeted purse-string sutures. Further postprocedure recovery was complicated by gram-negative pneumonia (*Serratia marcescens* and *Klebsiella pneumoniae*) that improved with levofloxacin.

Two months later, the patient complained of swelling above the incision site. Chest computed tomography demonstrated a hematoma that was managed conservatively (Fig. 4.11A).

Four months after TAVR, the patient developed a necrotic skin lesion with wound drainage (Fig. 4.11B). Computed tomography showed extravasation of contrast through the LV apex into the surrounding soft tissue and a fluid collection within the chest wall consistent with an LV apical pseudoaneurysm and cutaneopericardial fistula (Fig. 4.11C–D). The patient underwent a left thoracotomy with rib resection, removal of the epicardial pacemaker lead, fistula repair, and replacement of the pledgets (Fig. 4.12A–C). Cultures from the surgical specimen demonstrated no growth. The patient received prophylactic vancomycin and was subsequently discharged.

Unusual complications of a TA approach, including ventricular septal defect, apical pseudoaneurysm, and LV rupture, have been reported.[1] In TAVR, TA access site infections have an occurrence rate of 3.2%.[2] One of the rarest complications is cutaneopericardial fistula, with only one reported case; pledgeted sutures were attributed as the source of infection.[3]

To our knowledge, this is the first reported case in the United States. The immunocompromised status of our patient (due to long-term hydroxychloroquine) possibly increased the risk of infection. Furthermore, chronic doxycycline therapy possibly obscured the search for causative organisms. Potential sources of infection were the presence of an epicardial pacemaker lead, need for surgical reexploration, and the development of nosocomial pneumonia. Prior reports have implicated BioGlue (CryoLife Inc., Kennesaw, Georgia) as a source of infection[4]; however, it was not used in this case.

Cutaneopericardial fistula is a rare but clinically significant complication of the TA approach in TAVR. Infection control, meticulous procedural technique, heightened clinical suspicion, early recognition, and prompt treatment are all important measures in reducing adverse clinical outcomes.

References

1. Al-Attar N, Ghodbane W, Himbert D, et al. Unexpected complications of transapical valve implantation. *Ann Thorac Surg.* 2009;88:90-94.
2. Baillot R, Fréchette E, Cloutier D, et al. Surgical site infections following transcatheter apical aortic valve implantation: incidence and management. *J Cardiothorac Surg.* 2012;7:122-127.
3. Scheid M, Grothusen C, Lutter G, Petzina R. Cutaneo-pericardial fistula after transapical aortic valve implantation. *Interact Cardiovasc Thorac Surg.* 2013;16:558-559.
4. Pasic M, Unbehaun A, Drews T, Hetzer R. Late wound healing problems after use of BioGlue for apical hemostasis during transapical aortic valve implantation. *Interact Cardiovasc Thorac Surg.* 2011;13:532-534.

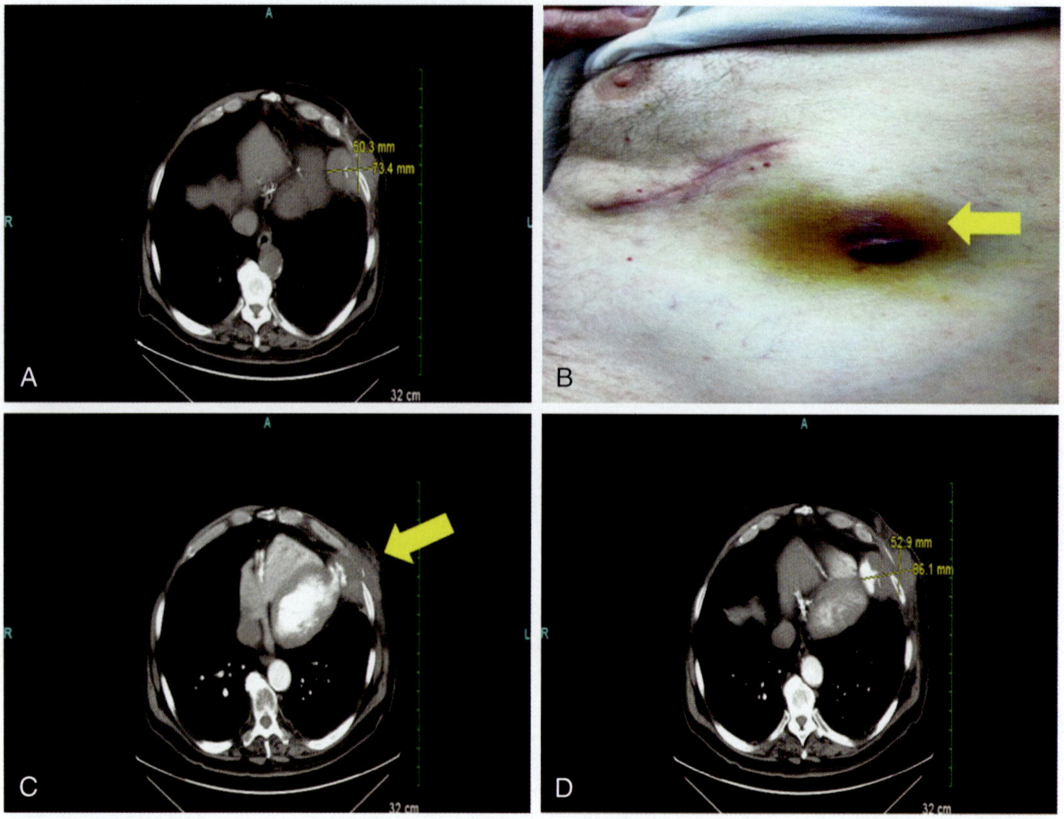

FIG. 4.11 Presentation and Imaging. (A) Computed tomography (CT) of the chest shows a hematoma of 73.4 × 50.3 mm in the left chest wall. (B) Left lateral chest wall demonstrates a healed thoracotomy scar and a necrotic 1- × 2-cm abscess along the anterior axillary line (*arrow*). (C) CT showing extravasation of contrast from the left ventricular cavity into the pseudoaneurysm and fistula formation extending to the chest wall (*arrow*). (D) CT showing the contrast in left ventricle draining in the abscess under the chest wall of 86.1 × 52.9 mm.

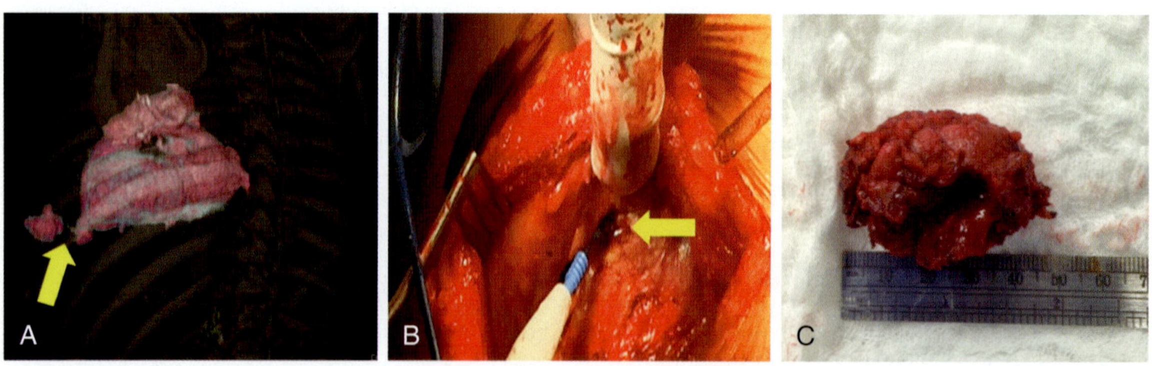

FIG. 4.12 Surgical Evacuation. (A) Left lateral view three-dimensional reconstruction of computed tomography images showing the connection (*arrow*) between the left ventricle and the pseudoaneurysm. (B) Fistula opening (*arrow*) in the chest wall during surgical excision. (C) Excised pseudoaneurysm and clot, approximately 45 mm.

FAILED VALVE-IN-VALVE TRANSCATHETER AORTIC VALVE IMPLANTATION

Stefan Klotz, MD, Michael Scharfschwerdt, PhD, Doreen Richardt, MD, Hans H. Sievers, MD

In 2004, a 68-year-old man received aortocoronary bypass surgery and a 23-mm Hancock porcine bioprosthesis (Medtronic, Minneapolis, Minnesota). Six years later, in January 2011, cardiac reevaluation was performed due to progressive dyspnea. Invasive angiography showed open bypass grafts and severe stenosis of the porcine aortic bioprosthesis. Because of significant comorbidities, a 23-mm SAPIEN XT (Edwards Lifesciences, Irvine, California) transcatheter aortic valve implantation (TAVI) was performed as valve-in-valve. The procedure was uneventful. Initial angiography and echocardiography showed a good function of the valve with no insufficiency and a mean gradient of 20 mm Hg (Online Video 4.19).

In March 2011, 3 months after the procedure, the patient was readmitted with cardiac decompensation. Reangiography showed open bypass grafts, but an invasive gradient of 50 mm Hg over the SAPIEN valve. Echocardiography confirmed the severe stenosis of the SAPIEN valve with a maximum gradient of 66 mm Hg, a mean of 43 mm Hg, and a valve opening area of 0.6 cm^2. Because of the patient's dyspnea, reoperation was scheduled after recompensation. In May 2011, both the SAPIEN valve and the 2004 implanted Hancock bioprosthesis were explanted (Fig. 4.13) and replaced with a 21-mm Trifecta (St. Jude Medical, Inc., St. Paul, Minnesota) bioprosthesis. The postoperative course was uneventful.

Postexplantation assessment of the valves showed the implanted 23-mm SAPIEN valve incompletely expanded within the stents of the 23-mm Hancock bioprosthesis. This leads to asymmetrical commissural distances and wrinkles of the leaflets (Fig. 4.14). In vitro investigation of the valves under pulsatile conditions showed folding and uneven leaflet coaptation in the diastolic state and a severely limited opening of the valve in systole, with a visual orifice area of 0.54 cm^2 (Online Video 4.20). Pressure gradients were 24.2 mm Hg (mean) and 42.2 mm Hg (maximum) at a cardiac output of 4.3 L/min. Even though TAVI shows promising results in high-risk patients,[1] the concept of valve-in-valve in degenerated aortic bioprostheses is quite new.[2] Reports successfully demonstrated the feasibility of this approach.[3] However, experimental studies could show the rigidity of the bioprosthesis can constrain the TAVI valve and prevent full expansion of the stents.[4] Because the inner diameter of a 23-mm Hancock bioprosthesis is only 19 mm, a circumferential part of 12.5-mm is missing to unfold the 23-mm Edwards SAPIEN transcatheter valve. This leads to uneven commissural distances that might affect leaflet coaptation and leaflet folding, which could severely restrict the opening of the valve. Our case emphasizes the difficulties of valve-in-valve TAVI for degenerated aortic bioprosthesis. These procedures should be done with caution.

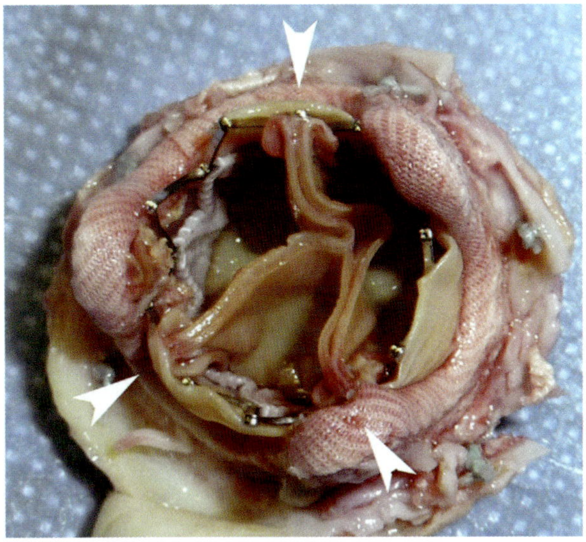

FIG. 4.13 The Explanted 23-mm Hancock Bioprosthesis With the Implanted 23-mm SAPIEN Transcatheter Valve. The *arrowheads* show the uneven commissures in the Hancock valve (Online Video 4.19).

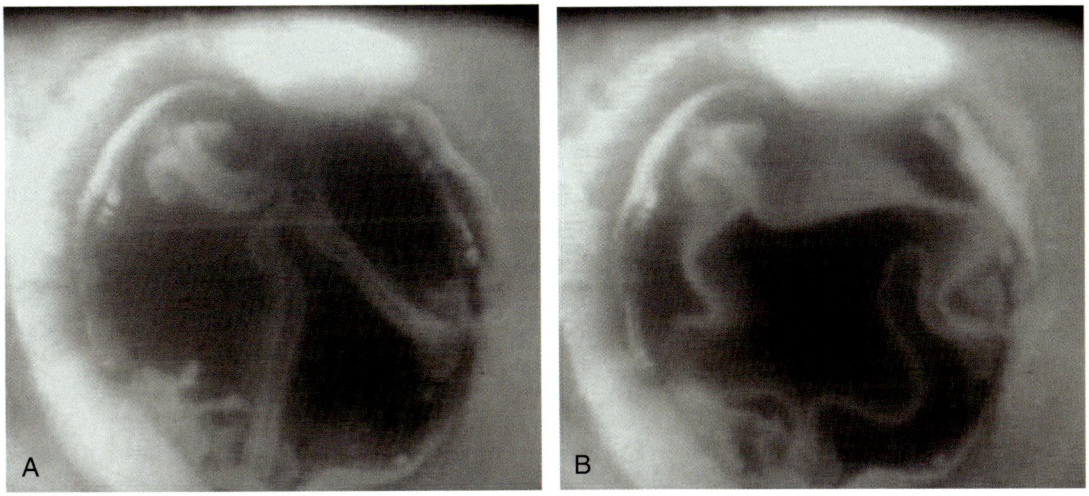

FIG. 4.14 In Vitro Assessment in Diastole and Systole. (A) Diastole. (B) Systole (Online Video 4.20).

REFERENCES

1. Lefèvre T, Kappetein AP, Wolner E, et al., for the PARTNER EU Investigator Group. One year follow-up of the multi-centre European PARTNER transcatheter heart valve study. *Eur Heart J.* 2011;32:148-157.
2. Walther T, Falk V, Dewey T, et al. Valve-in-a-valve concept for transcatheter minimally invasive repeat xenograft implantation. *J Am Coll Cardiol.* 2007;50:56-60.
3. Ferrari E, Marcucci C, Sulzer C, von Segesser LK. Which available transapical transcatheter valve fits into degenerated aortic bioprostheses? *Interact Cardiovasc Thorac Surg.* 2010;11:83-85.
4. Azadani AN, Jaussaud N, Matthews PB, Ge L, Chuter TA, Tseng EE. Transcatheter aortic valves inadequately relieve stenosis in small degenerated bioprostheses. *Interact Cardiovasc Thorac Surg.* 2010; 11:70-77.

GLUING AN AORTIC PERFORATION DURING TRANSCATHETER AORTIC VALVE REPLACEMENT: AN ALTERNATIVE TREATMENT FOR ANNULAR RUPTURE?

Nicolas Piliero, MSc, Fréderic Thony, MD, Gerald Vanzetto, MD, PhD, Gilles Barone-Rochette, MD, PhD

A 96-year-old man was referred to our cardiology center for a transcatheter aortic valve replacement (TAVR). Preimplantation transthoracic echocardiography showed preserved ejection fraction, mean transvalvular pressure gradient at 46 mm Hg, aortic valve area of 1 cm^2, and maximal aortic jet velocity at 4.1 m/s, confirming severe aortic stenosis. Aortic annulus diameter was 25 mm as measured by transesophageal echocardiography, and its surface was 671 mm^2 as observed with three-dimensional multidetector computed tomography (Fig. 4.15A–B). A 29-mm SAPIENS XT valve (Edwards Lifesciences, Irvine, California) was implanted using left transfemoral access. During prosthetic valve deployment, contrast extravasation into the pericardium occurred (Fig. 4.15C), causing cardiac shock and pericardial tamponade demonstrated by transthoracic echocardiography. Percutaneous pericardiocentesis and fluid infusion were immediately performed, allowing hemodynamic stabilization. Tissue glue composed of a 1/1 mixture of *N*-butyl-2-cyanoacrylate (Histoacryl) and Lipiodol (B. Braun, Melsungen, Germany) was injected into the perforation using a Progreat microcatheter (Terumo Corporation, Tokyo, Japan) introduced through a 6F Amplatz left guiding catheter (Medtronic, Dublin, Ireland) (Fig. 4.15D). This successfully stopped the pericardial effusion (Fig. 4.15E) and allowed the procedure to be completed without further complications. The patient was discharged 5 days after the valve deployment.

Aortic rupture occurs in about 1% of all TAVR implantations.[1,2] Potential causes include radial forces during valve deployment inducing tissue overdistention along with calcification of the annulus and/or valve leaflets.[1] Depending on the severity and location of the perforation, treatment can include cardiac surgery, isolated percutaneous pericardiocentesis, or a conservative strategy.[1] *N*-butyl-2-cyanoacrylate is a tissue glue that has the capacity to harden immediately when in contact with blood. The adjunction of oily radiopaque substance (Lipiodol) delays polymerization and allows radiopacity.[3] Thus we report here a novel potential treatment for aortic rupture during TAVR by an endovascular approach.

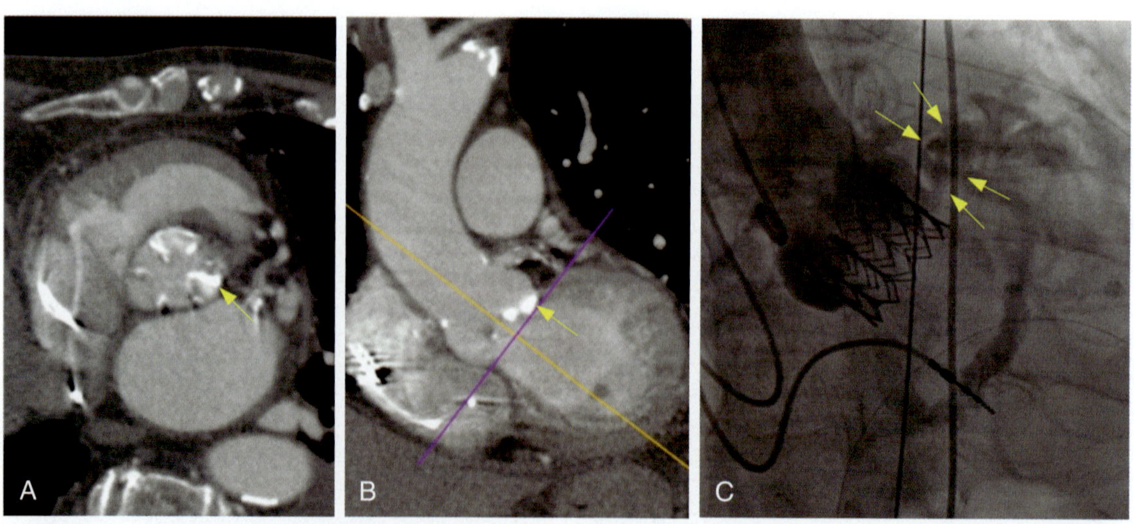

FIG. 4.15 Computed Tomography and Angiography Imagery Before and During Transcatheter Aortic Valve Replacement Procedure. (A and B) Preoperative computed tomography showed massive calcification on the aortic valve annulus and left anterior leaflet (*yellow arrow*). (C) A severe contrast extravasation (*yellow arrows*) was identified during angiography after transcatheter aortic valve implantation.

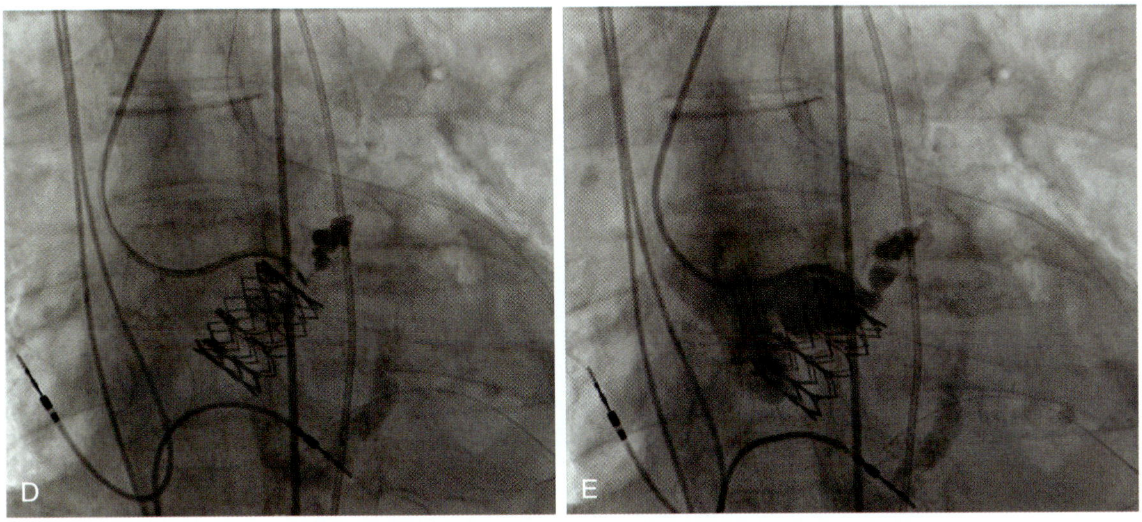

FIG. 4.15, cont'd (D) Tissue glue was injected into the perforation with a microcatheter. (E) Severe contrast extravasation was stopped successfully by liquid embolization mixtures.

ACKNOWLEDGMENT

The authors thank Raphaëlle-Ashley Guerbaai for editorial support.

REFERENCES

1. Pasi M, Unbehaun A, Buz S, Drews T, Hetzer R. Annular rupture during transcatheter aortic valve replacement: classification, pathophysiology, diagnostics, treatment approaches, and prevention. *JACC Cardiovasc Interv.* 2015;8:1-9.
2. Möllmann H, Kim WK, Kempfert J, Walther T, Hamm C. Complications of transcatheter aortic valve implantation (TAVI): how to avoid and treat them. *Heart.* 2015;101:900-908.
3. Stoesslein F, Ditscherlein G, Romaniuk PA. Experimental studies on new liquid embolization mixtures (Histoacryl-Lipiodol, Histoacryl-Pan-thopaque). *Cardiovasc Intervent Radiol.* 1982;5: 264-267.

LEFT ANTERIOR DESCENDING CORONARY ARTERY OBSTRUCTION ASSOCIATED WITH AN APICAL SUTURE AFTER TRANSCATHETER AORTIC VALVE REPLACEMENT

Yutaka Koyama, MD, Masanori Yamamoto, MD, Yasuhide Okawa, MD, Takahiko Suzuki, MD

An 88-year-old woman with symptomatic severe aortic stenosis was referred to our center. She was considered to be at high risk for surgical aortic valve replacement because of comorbidities and advanced age. Our heart team opted for transcatheter aortic valve replacement via transapical access because of issues with the peripheral artery. A pair of pledgeted purse-string sutures was placed around the apex via left anterolateral thoracotomy at the sixth intercostal space. A 23-mm SAPIEN XT prosthesis (Edwards Lifesciences, Irvine, California) was successfully implanted in the target position. However, the recovery of blood pressure was poor, and hypokinetic motion of the apex was noted in the surgical view. Aortography showed trivial aortic regurgitation without obstruction of the left coronary artery orifice (Fig. 4.16A). Additionally, selective angiography of the left coronary artery revealed obstruction of the middle part of left anterior descending artery (LAD) (Fig. 4.16B), whereas previous coronary angiography did not show significant stenosis. The sutures were more than 10 mm away from the LAD in direct vision, which was confirmed in postprocedural computed tomography (Fig. 4.16C). After removing one of the sutures, which was relatively close to the LAD, the obstruction of the LAD improved slightly but remained significant. Therefore a vasodilator was repeatedly infused into the LAD, and the flow of the LAD completely recovered (Fig. 4.16D).

Obstruction of the LAD in the present case was induced by muscle tension and deformation around the apical sutures. In addition to the removal of the apical suture, selective vasodilator infusion for the obstructed LAD might be effective. The present unique case revealed one of the potential etiologies of LAD obstruction after transapical transcatheter aortic valve replacement.

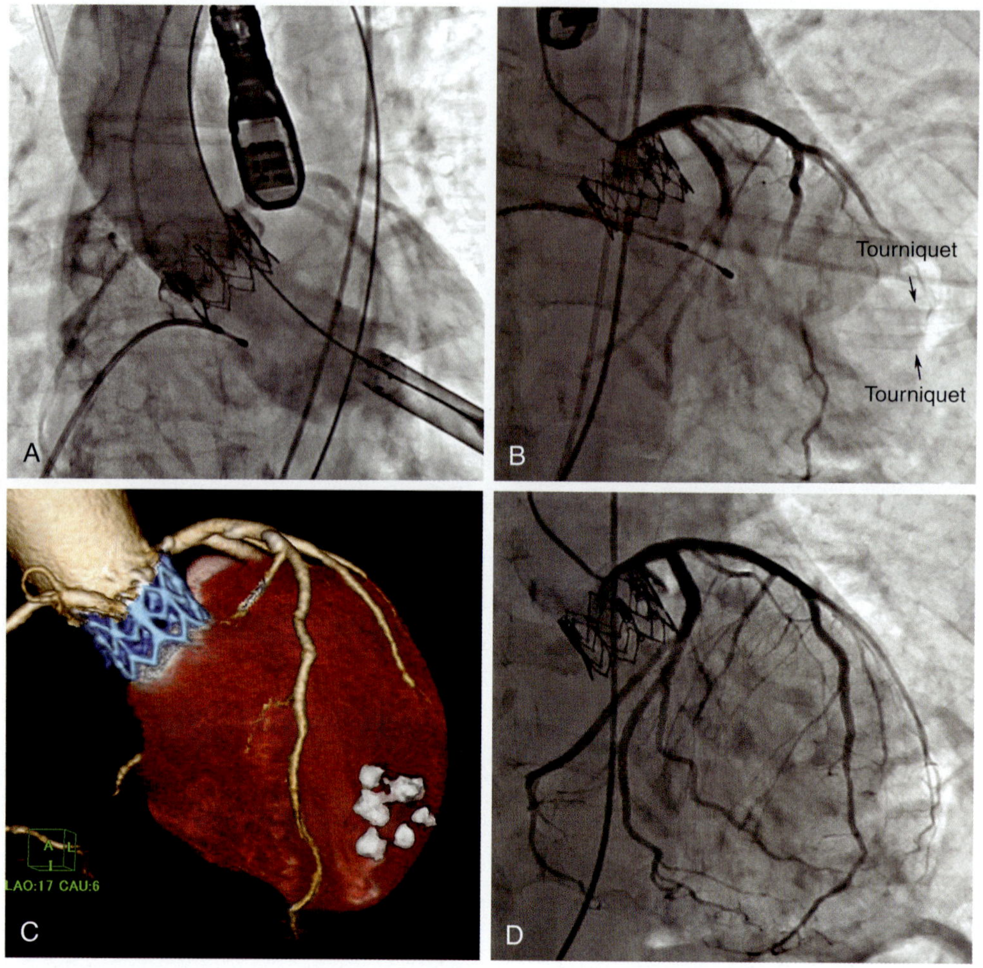

FIG. 4.16 Angiography and Postprocedural Computed Tomography. (A) Aortography shows the target position of the prosthetic valve and the patency of the left coronary orifice. (B) Left coronary angiography shows narrowing of the left anterior descending artery (LAD) after the sheath is removed and the apical sutures are snared with tourniquets. (C) Postprocedural computed tomography shows that the apical sutures are away from the LAD. (D) Angiography shows complete recovery of LAD flow after infusion of a vasodilator.

Left-to-Right Interventricular Shunt as a Late Complication of Transapical Aortic Valve Implantation

Pierre Massabuau, MD, Nicolas Dumonteil, MD, Pierre Berthoumieu, MD, Bertrand Marcheix, MD, PhD, David Duterque, MD, Gérard Fournial, MD, Didier Carrié, MD, PhD

An 86-year-old man was referred to our institution for a symptomatic severe aortic stenosis (New York Heart Association [NYHA] functional dyspnea class III; indexed effective orifice area [EOA] 0.3 cm^2/m^2; mean gradient [MG] 54 mm Hg; left ventricular ejection fraction [LVEF] 56%). He had a history of dyslipidemia, prostate cancer, and coronary artery bypass graft (saphenous vein graft on left anterior descending coronary artery [LAD] and right coronary artery) 26 years previously.

A transcatheter aortic valve implantation (TAVI) was proposed because this patient was considered a high surgical risk candidate (logistic EuroSCORE [European System for Cardiac Operative Risk Evaluation] 28%, Society of Thoracic Surgeons score 7%). A transapical approach was chosen, because both the iliofemoral and subclavian arteries were not suitable for transarterial access. The aortic annulus measured by transesophageal echocardiography was 22.6 mm.

The procedure was performed under general anesthesia, through a left minithoracotomy, as previously described.[1] A 26-mm Edwards SAPIEN valve (Edwards Lifesciences, Irvine, California) was implanted under fluoroscopy and transesophageal echocardiography guidance with good procedural outcome. The postimplantation period was marked by an increase of cardiac troponin I (peak,

12.9 ng/mL) and a transient renal failure. At discharge (day 10), the patient was in NYHA functional class II and heart sounds were normal. Transthoracic echocardiography (TTE) showed LVEF at 63%, prosthesis MG at 11 mm Hg, indexed EOA at 0.91 cm^2/m^2, stable mild paravalvular leak, and pulmonary artery systolic pressure at 47 mm Hg.

Clinical and TTE data were similar at 1-month and 6-month follow-up. At 1-year follow-up, the patient declined to NYHA functional class III. He described no chest pain since his last visit. Clinical examination revealed a loud continuous systolic and diastolic murmur. There was no change of the electrocardiogram. The TTE revealed a moderate enlargement of the right ventricular cavity. The apical part of the interventricular septum appeared less echogenic than the rest of the myocardium (Fig. 4.17). Color Doppler showed a continuous left-to-right flow through the apical part of the interventricular septum with a Doppler peak systolic gradient of 89 mm Hg (Fig. 4.18A–B). The LVEF, prosthetic mean gradient, and indexed EOA were 63%, 11 mm Hg, and 0.90 cm^2/m^2, respectively. Pulmonary artery systolic pressure was 65 mm Hg. An echocardiographic contrast agent (SonoVue, Bracco Imaging, Milan, Italy) failed to reach the apex of the right ventricle. It seemed to be "washed" by the shunt flow (Fig. 4.19, Online Video 4.21). After a few cardiac cycles, contrast agent appeared into the left cardiac cavities and at last into the right ventricle apex through the septal communication.

After considering the age and will of the patient, a moderate cognitive impairment, a progressive prostate cancer, and despite the worsening of his functional status, we decided against any invasive treatment.

Various transapical TAVI complications have been described, mostly observed during initial procedure or short-term follow-up.[2,3]

In this case, we can reasonably argue that puncture through the septum at the time of the procedure did not cause this late septal defect, because we can expect that it would have been observed before discharge or during initial follow-up. It is likely that this complication was caused by late rupture of scar tissue due to periprocedural injury. The potential mechanisms of this injury could be (1) occlusion of the distal LAD or a side branch by the purse-string suture, resulting in a periprocedural myocardial infarction, or (2) a pressure

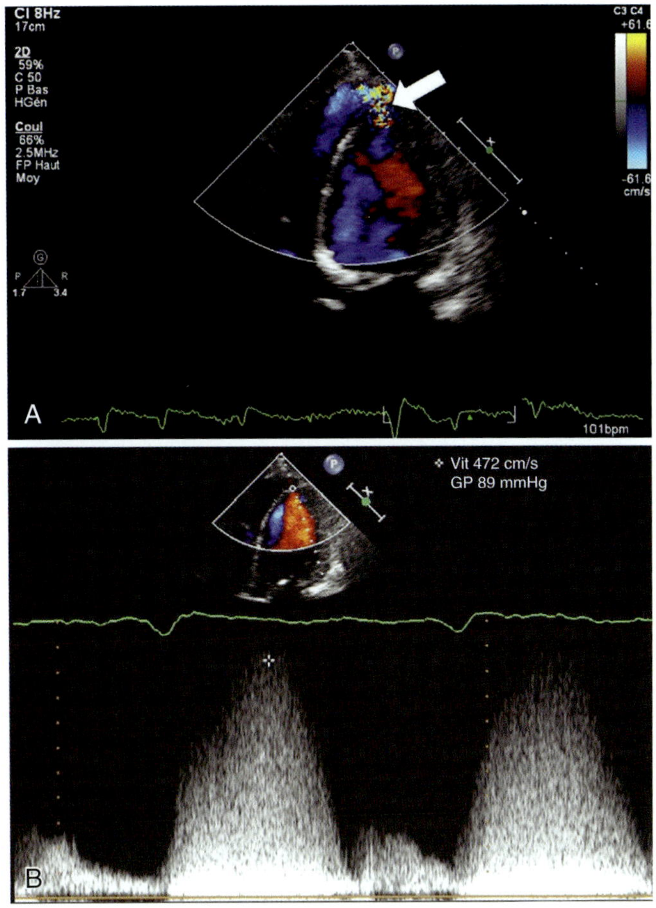

FIG. 4.18 Color Doppler Imaging of the Left-to-Right Flow. (A) Color Doppler imaging of the left-to-right flow through the apical part (*white arrow*) of the interventricular septum. (B) Continuous-wave Doppler of the left-to-right flow through the apical part of the interventricular septum. *GP*, maximal pressure gradient; *Vit*, peak velocity.

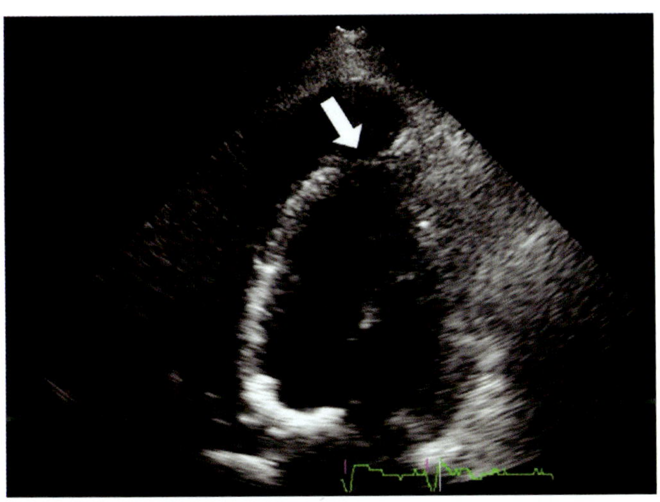

FIG. 4.17 Two-Dimensional Transthoracic Echocardiography Apical View of the Left Ventricle and Right Ventricle. The echogenicity of the apical segment (*white arrow*) of interventricular septum is less pronounced than the basal and medial segments. The right ventricle apex is enlarged.

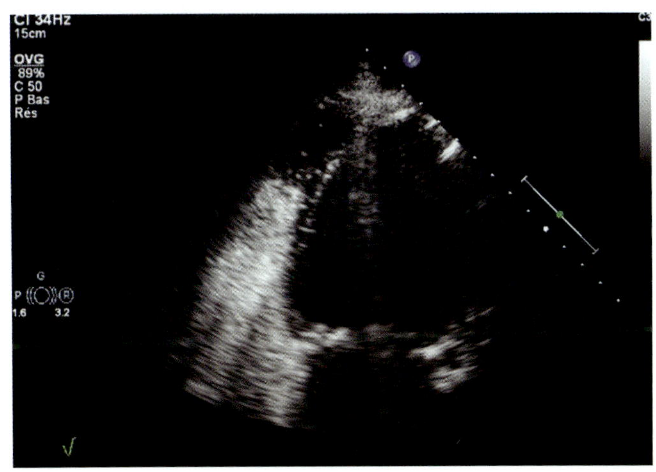

FIG. 4.19 Intravenous Injection of an Echocardiographic Contrast Agent. During the first cardiac cycles, microbubbles cannot reach the right ventricular apex because of "washing effect" of left-to-right flow (Online Video 4.21).

necrosis caused by an apical puncture and then an insertion of the sheath too close to the distal septum.

To our best knowledge, this is the first report of late apical interventricular communication after transapical TAVI. Considering the possible causes just discussed, periprocedural echocardiographic guidance of the left ventricle apical puncture and subsequent sheath insertion could be proposed to prevent this complication. Particular attention should also be given to the location of the distal LAD before making the purse-string suture.

This case emphasizes the role of systematic regular follow-up to detect late complications after such procedures. It might also improve our awareness of the wide range of potential complications of TAVI.

References

1. Ye J, Cheung A, Lichtenstein SV, et al. Transapical aortic valve implantation in humans. *J Thorac Cardiovasc Surg.* 2006;131:1194-1196.
2. Al-Attar N, Ghodbane W, Himbert D, et al. Unexpected complications of transapical aortic valve implantation. *Ann Thorac Surg.* 2009;88:90-94.
3. Tzikas A, Schultz C, Piazza N, et al. Perforation of the membranous interventricular septum after transcatheter aortic valve implantation. *Circ Cardiovasc Interv.* 2009;2:582-583.

Novel Percutaneous Apical Exclusion of a Left Ventricular Pseudoaneurysm After Complicated Transapical Transcatheter Aortic Valve Replacement

Soraya Merchan, MD, Chi-Hion Li, MD, Francisco Javier Martinez, MD, Chad Kliger, MD, Vladimir Jelnin, MD, Gila Perk, MD, Derek Brinster, MD, Itzhak Kronzon, MD, Carlos E. Ruiz, MD, PhD

A 78-year-old woman with a history of coronary artery bypass grafting underwent transapical transcatheter aortic valve replacement with a SAPIEN XT (Edwards, Irvine, California) prosthesis that was complicated by an apical left ventricular pseudoaneurysm (LVPA). Unsuccessful attempts at closure included percutaneous retrograde transaortic placement of a 12-mm Amplatzer ventricular septal defect occluder (St. Jude Medical, Minneapolis, Minnesota) and surgical CorMatrix (CorMatrix Cardiovascular, Roswell, Georgia) patch repair on cardiopulmonary bypass, both with residual expanding and/or recurrent LVPA. A novel transcatheter approach was performed to exclude the left ventricular apex and flow into the LVPA. Using computed tomography–fluoroscopy fusion imaging (HeartNavigator, Philips, Best, the Netherlands), percutaneous transapical access was performed adjacent to the true apical site of the LVPA. The 26-mm Amplatzer septal and 35-mm Amplatzer cribriform occluders were positioned and deployed with the distal disks overlapping, excluding the apical cavity, and the proximal disks positioned on the epicardial surface. Residual flow was noted through the polyester fabric of the devices, and an additional percutaneous transapical access through the LVPA exit site was performed with placement of a 4F sheath. Three 0.052-inch 10 × 15-mm coils (Cook Medical, Bloomington, Indiana) soaked in thrombin were placed within the excluded apical segment. Echocardiography revealed no further flow into the LVPA, with increased echogenicity of the sac suggesting thrombosis. Computed tomography performed before discharge confirmed total occlusion of the LVPA with complete apical exclusion (Fig. 4.20).

Apical left ventricular pseudoaneurysm is an infrequent complication after transapical transcatheter aortic valve replacement (TAVR). They have been traditionally surgically repaired[1]; however, patients who undergo TAVR have high operative risk with multiple comorbidities, increasing significantly the risk of surgical repair.

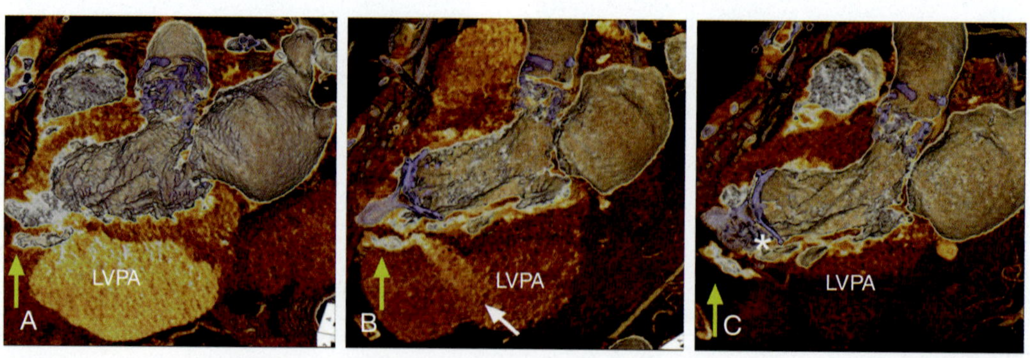

FIG. 4.20 Computed Tomographic Angiography (CTA) With Three-Dimensional (3D) Volume-Rendered Images and Fluoroscopy With CT Fluoroscopy Fusion Imaging Illustrate This Novel Percutaneous Approach. (A) to (C) CTA with 3D volume-rendered images. (D) to (F) Fluoroscopy with computed tomography–fluoroscopy fusion imaging. (A) After unsuccessful surgical patch (*yellow arrows*) closure, a large recurrent left ventricular pseudoaneurysm (*LVPA*) was identified. (B) Complete apical exclusion was next noted with the placement of two overlapping Amplatzer occluders (St. Jude, Minneapolis, Minnesota) adjacent to the true apical site of the LVPA, and residual flow was identified. (C) Percutaneous transapical placement of three 0.052-inch 10 × 15-mm coils (Cook Medical, Bloomington, Indiana) soaked in thrombin were placed into the excluded apical space (*asterisks*) with total occlusion of the LVPA shown.

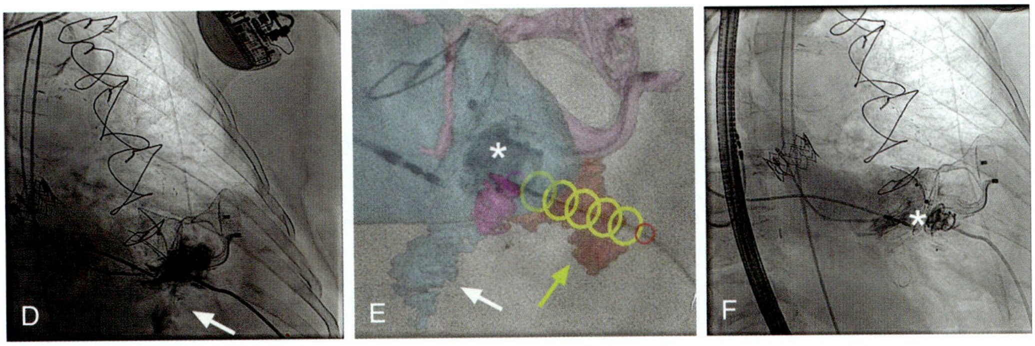

FIG. 4.20, cont'd (D) A percutaneous transapical sheath can be identified within the excluded apical segment created by Amplatzer devices; contrast injection revealed flow through the device. (E) Placement of coils with the aid of fusion imaging can be seen, and (F) final left ventriculography confirmed complete apical exclusion and no residual contrast into the LVPA. *White arrows* indicate residual leak.

Some cases of percutaneous closure have been reported,[2] but the experience with this procedure is limited. We describe the first case of percutaneous closure guided by a novel system of image fusion using computed tomography and fluoroscopy.

References

1. Collier P, Phelan D, Soltesz E, Aljaroudi W. Left ventricular pseudoaneurysm: "to-and-fro" flow. *J Am Coll Cardiol.* 2013;61:896.
2. Acharya D, Nagaraj H, Misra VK. Transcatheter closure of left ventricular pseudoaneurysm. *J Invasive Cardiol.* 2012;24:E111-E114.

Percutaneous Management of Mitral Perforation During Transcatheter Aortic Valve Replacement

Asma Bourezg, MD, Cyril Prieur, MD, Gérard Finet, MD, PhD, Gilles Rioufol, MD, PhD

A New York Heart Association functional class III symptomatic 90-year-old man with severe aortic stenosis had a 519-mm^2 annulus aortic area estimated by computed tomography (sinus of Valsalva 710 mm^2 and sinotubular junction 540 mm^2) (Fig. 4.21A and A′). He underwent an uneventful femoral access transcatheter aortic valve replacement (26-mm Edwards SAPIEN 3, Edwards Lifesciences, Irvine, California) (Fig. 4.21B) and 1 h later experienced intractable cardiogenic shock with intense holosystolic murmur. By transesophageal echocardiography, aortic prosthesis showed no anomaly, and a massive mitral regurgitation by perforation of the mitral-aortic curtain was diagnosed (Fig. 4.21C [*arrow*] and C′). Mitral-aortic curtain calcifications were a posteriori thought to be causative (Fig. 4.21A′, *arrow*). A rescue percutaneous repair was decided upon and, under transesophageal echocardiography control after transseptal catheterization, the mitral perforation could be crossed (Fig. 4.21D) with a 5F coronary hooked catheter (Bartorelli-Cozzi, Johnson & Johnson, New Brunswick, New Jersey) and a hydrophilic 0.035-inch wire. Using the standard technique, an 8-mm Amplatzer septal occluder (St. Jude Medical, St. Paul, Minnesota) was then successfully deployed across the anterior leaflet (Fig. 4.21D′ and E) and dramatically decreased the mitral regurgitation (Fig. 4.21E′). Mitral valve functioning was not significantly impaired (Fig. 4.21F and F′, Online Video 4.22) by the plug, and no anterograde gradient was noted. Hemodynamics rapidly recovered, and inotropic support as well as the assisted ventilation could be stopped 6 h later. The patient was discharged 5 days later. Mild hemolytic anemia was observed during the first 6 months; this was corrected by episodic blood transfusions and ultimately resolved. At 2-year-follow-up, the patient is doing well without aortic or mitral valve abnormalities.

The mitral apparatus is vulnerable and could be badly impaired in transcatheter aortic valve replacement patients. Albeit rare, mitral perforation is a complication that physicians should be aware of because percutaneous management may be lifesaving.

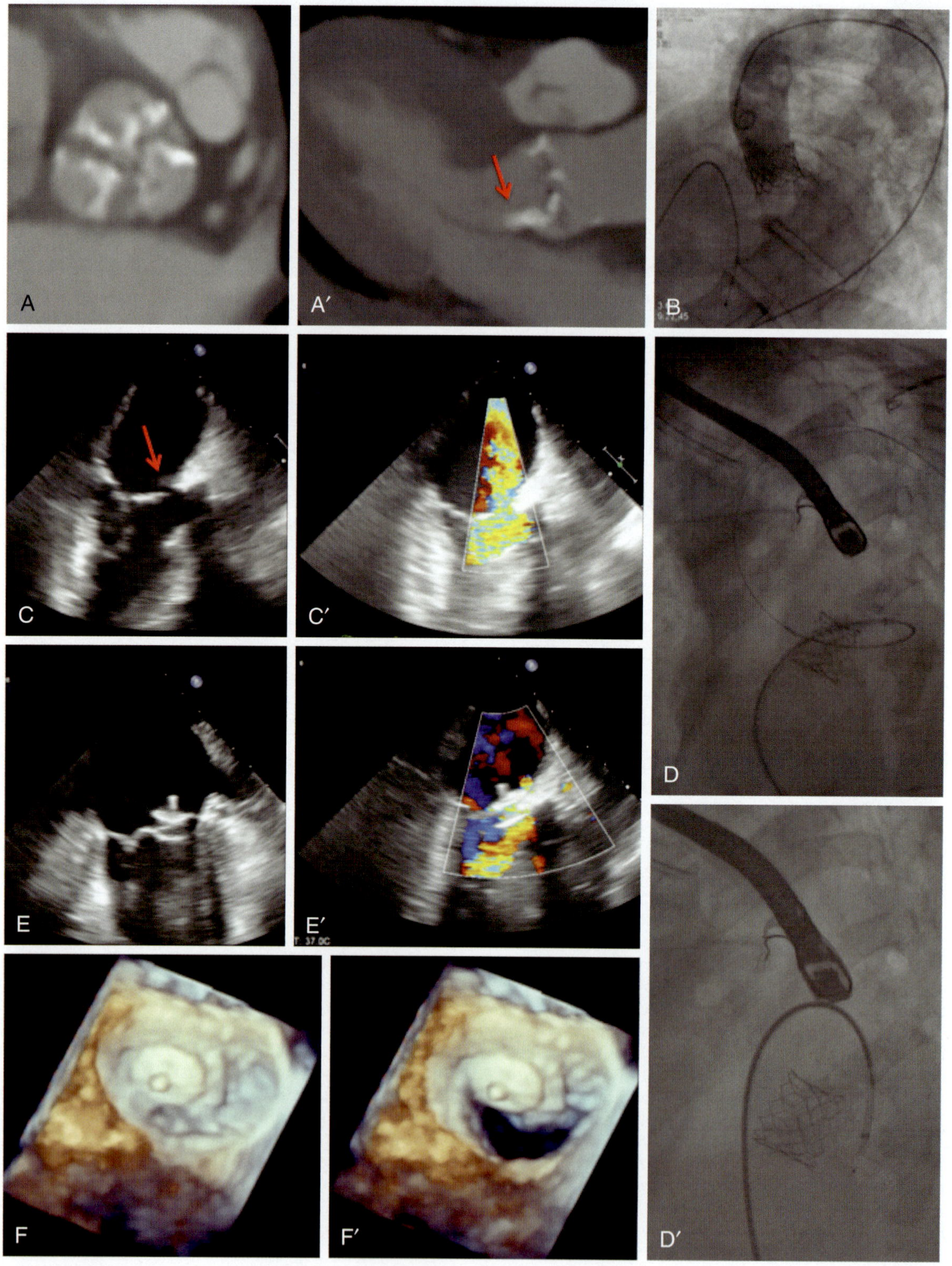

FIG. 4.21 Images of Mitral Aortic Curtain Perforation Management. (A and A′) Three-dimensional computed tomography showing aortic stenosis and calcification developing on mitral-aortic curtain (A′, *arrow*). (B) Final angiogram of the transcatheter aortic valve replacement. (C and C′) Transesophageal echocardiography (TEE) showing severe mitral regurgitation (MR) by perforation of the mitral-aortic curtain (C, *arrow*). (D and D′) Percutaneous management with an 8-mm Amplatzer septal occluder (St. Jude Medical, St. Paul, Minnesota). (E and E′) Postprocedure TEE showing the plug and near disappearance of the MR. (F and F′) Three-dimensional TEE of the mitral valve in systole (F) and diastole (F′) (Online Video 4.22).

Percutaneous Treatment of Severe Aortic Insufficiency in a Patient With a Left Ventricular Assist Device: Friend or Foe?

Michael Zacharias, DO, Ravi Dhingra, MD, MPH

A 29-year-old man with congenitally corrected transposition of the great arteries underwent implantation of a HeartMate II left ventricular assist device (LVAD) (Thoratec Corp., Pleasanton, California) as a result of worsening systemic right ventricular failure and New York Heart Association class IV symptoms, as a bridge to transplant. After 6 months, he presented with atrial arrhythmias and abdominal bloating. Transthoracic echocardiogram was repeated and showed severe continuous aortic insufficiency, which previously had been mild. The patient was referred to the cardiac catheterization laboratory for a hemodynamic assessment and possible use of an Amplatzer septal occluder (AGA Medical, Plymouth, Minnesota) for closure of his aortic valve. Right-sided heart catheterization hemodynamics showed a right atrial pressure of 16 mm Hg, pulmonary artery pressure of 49/22 mm Hg, and pulmonary wedge pressure of 18 mm Hg. Via the right femoral artery, a 30-mm Amplatzer atrial septal cribriform device was advanced across the aortic valve and positioned under transesophageal echocardiogram guidance. To-and-fro motion was performed to test stability, and the device appeared secure with minimal residual aortic insufficiency. The device was released and stayed in a stable position, which was also confirmed by chest x-ray (Fig. 4.22A). This technique has been previously described with success through a femoral[1] and subclavian[2] approach. The following day, a chest x-ray showed that the device had migrated into the left ventricle (Fig. 4.22B). An emergent computed tomography scan of the chest was performed that showed that the occluder device had migrated to the orifice of the LVAD inflow cannula (Fig. 4.23). The LVAD speed was reduced to prevent the device from completely obstructing the LVAD inflow cannula. Coincidentally, a donor heart became available on the same night, and the patient successfully received the transplant without any complications. Although a septal occluder device has previously been described to improve aortic insufficiency; it does so with potential risk.

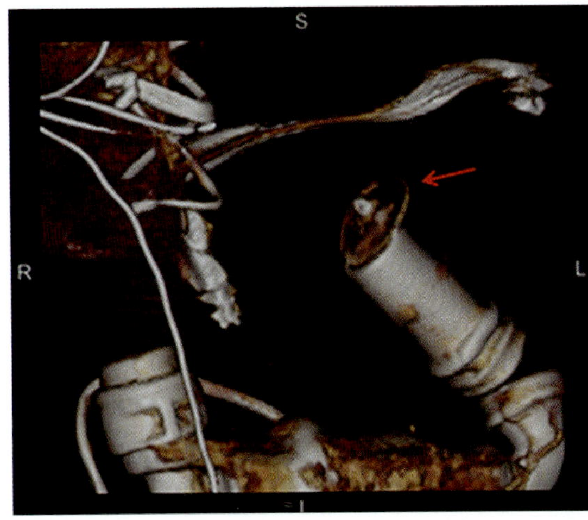

FIG. 4.23 Computed Tomography (CT) Scan of the Chest. CT scan of the chest shows the Amplatzer septal occluder (*red arrow*) partially overlying the left ventricular assist device inflow cannula.

References

1. Parikh KS, Mehrotra AK, Russo MJ, et al. Percutaneous transcatheter aortic valve closure successfully treats left ventricular assist device–associated aortic insufficiency and improves cardiac hemodynamics. *JACC Cardiovasc Interv.* 2013;6:84-89.
2. Grohmann J, Blanke P, Benk C, Schlensak C. Trans-catheter closure of the native aortic valve with an Amplatzer Occluder to treat progressive aortic regurgitation after implantation of a left-ventricular assist device. *Eur J Cardiothorac Surg.* 2011;39:e181-e183.

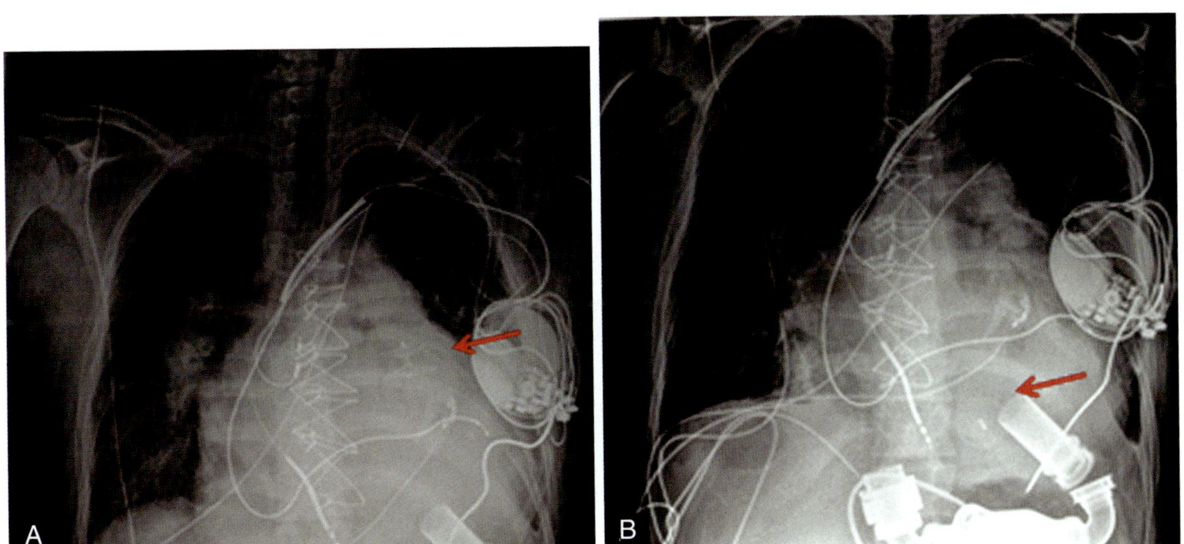

FIG. 4.22 Chest X-Ray. The chest x-ray shows (A) stable position postdeployment and (B) migration the following day. *Red arrows* indicate septal occluder position.

Perforation of Anterior Mitral Leaflet Due to Mechanical Stimulation Late After Transcatheter Aortic Valve Replacement

Mizuki Miura, MD, Akihiro Isotani, MD, Kenichiro Murata, MD, Tomohiro Kawaguchi, MD, Masaomi Hayashi, MD, Yoshio Arai, MD, Shinichi Shirai, MD, Michiya Hanyu, MD, Kenji Ando, MD

An 82-year-old man underwent transcatheter aortic valve replacement (TAVR) for symptomatic severe aortic stenosis (AS) using a 23-mm balloon-expandable SAPIEN XT valve (Edwards Lifesciences, Irvine, California) deployed via a transapical approach (Fig. 4.24A). He was referred to our center for dyspnea (New York Heart Association functional class IV) 6 months after TAVR. Transthoracic echocardiography revealed new mitral regurgitation from the middle of the anterior mitral leaflet (AML) to the posterior wall (Fig. 4.24B, Online Video 4.23). Transesophageal echocardiography revealed perforation of the AML where it made contact with the bottom of the implanted valve (Fig. 4.24C–D, Online Videos 4.24 and 4.25). He could not undergo open-heart surgery because of a history of coronary artery bypass surgery, poor general health, and frailty. Despite intensive heart failure treatment for a month, he died of progressive low-output syndrome and worsening renal failure. According to the results of autopsy, the AML had been perforated by mechanical stimulation from the implanted valve; however, mitral valve destruction by infectious endocarditis (IE) was not recognized macroscopically (Fig. 4.24E). Microscopically, well-defined disruption of elastic fiber in the mitral valve was found in elastica Masson stain, suggesting mechanical stimulation, rather than infectious endocarditis (Fig. 4.24F).

TAVR is an alternative option for patients with severe AS considered inoperable or at high risk for surgical aortic valve replacement. Although the number of TAVR procedures has rapidly increased worldwide, there are few reports about perforation of the AML because of mechanical stimulation late after TAVR without IE. It is important to note this point and avoid low implantation during the TAVR procedure.

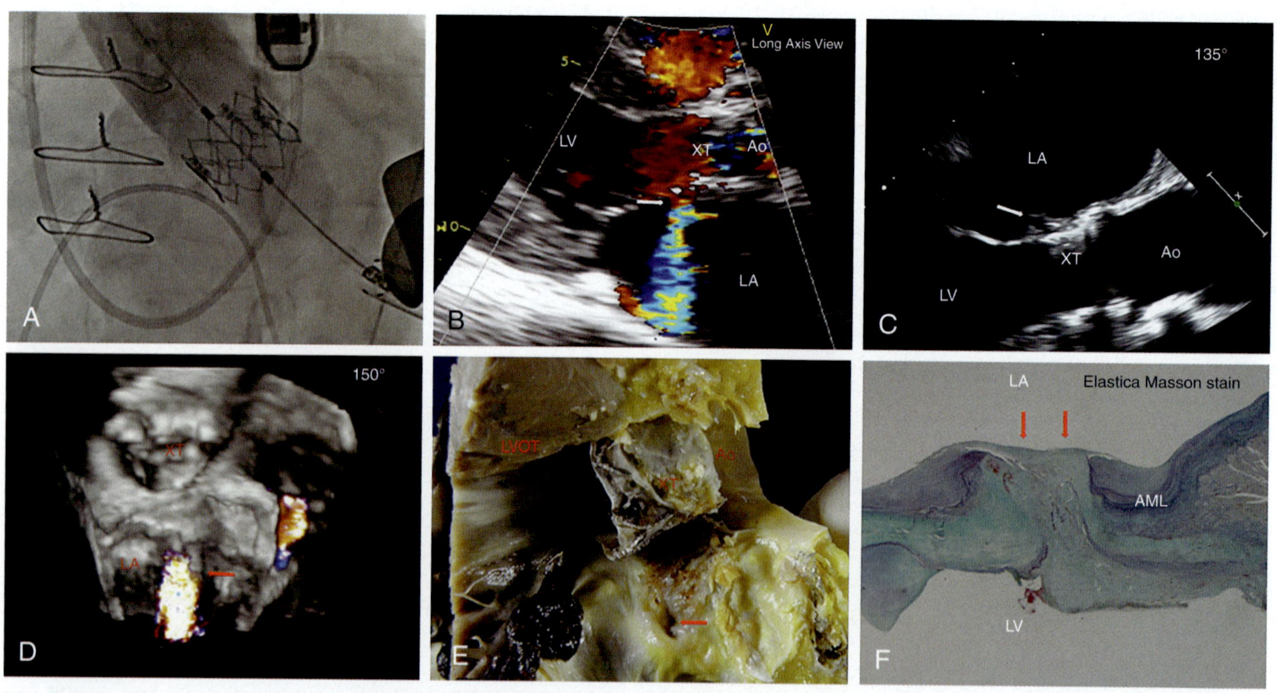

FIG. 4.24 Transcatheter Aortic Valve Replacement (TAVR), Transthoracic Echocardiography (TTE), Transesophageal Echocardiography (TEE), and Pathologic Images. (A) A 23-mm SAPIEN XT deployed via a transapical approach. (B) TTE showing new mitral regurgitation (MR) (*arrow*) (Online Video 4.23). (C) TEE showing perforation of the anterior mitral leaflet (AML) where it made contact with the bottom of the implanted valve (*arrow*) (Online Video 4.24). (D) Three-dimensional TEE showing perforation of the AML and severe MR (*arrow*) (Online Video 4.25). (E) Macroscopic findings showing the AML perforated by mechanical stimulation from the implanted valve (*arrow*). (F) Microscopic findings showing elastic fiber cut by mechanical stimulation (*arrow*). *AML*, anterior mitral leaflet; *Ao*, aorta; *LA*, left atrium; *LV*, left ventricle; *LVOT*, left ventricular outflow tract; *XT*, SAPIEN XT valve.

Severe Valve Deformation Following Cardiopulmonary Resuscitation in a Patient With a Transcatheter Aortic Valve

Creighton W. Don, MD, PhD, James M. McCabe, MD, Corinne L. Fligner, MD

An 87-year-old patient with severe aortic stenosis underwent transapical transcatheter aortic valve replacement with a 26-mm Edwards SAPIEN valve (Edwards Lifesciences, Irvine, California). Preoperative imaging was notable for severe asymmetric calcification along the posterolateral aspect of the left ventricular outflow tract (LVOT) involving the intravalvular fibrous curtain (Fig. 4.25). The aortic annulus area measured 430 mm^2 by computed tomographic imaging, allowing for 23% oversizing. Valve deployment was appropriate but was remarkable for moderate paravalvular regurgitation at the site of the LVOT calcification. The valve was redilated with an additional 1 mL of fluid added to the delivery balloon, modestly reducing the regurgitation. The patient recovered well and experienced mild heart failure symptoms. On hospital day 4, the patient experienced a cardiac arrest and underwent 48 min of cardiopulmonary resuscitation without return of spontaneous circulation. Autopsy demonstrated that the SAPIEN valve was crushed, with deformation of the valve at the site of the LVOT calcium (Fig. 4.26, Online Video 4.26). Such severe valve distortion would have significantly impaired leaflet coaptation and function, and it is likely that successful resuscitation was impossible once the valve was crushed.[1] The LVOT calcium caused significant paravalvular leak and likely contributed to valve deformation during chest compressions (Fig. 4.27, Online Video 4.26). Care must be taken when providing cardiopulmonary resuscitation to patients with balloon-expandable transcatheter aortic valve prostheses, and follow-up imaging to evaluate valve deformation is crucial.

References

1. Gunning PS, Vaughan TJ, McNamara LM. Simulation of self-expanding transcatheter aortic valve in a realistic aortic root: implications of deployment geometry on leaflet deformation. *Ann Biomed Eng.* 2014; 42:1989-2001.

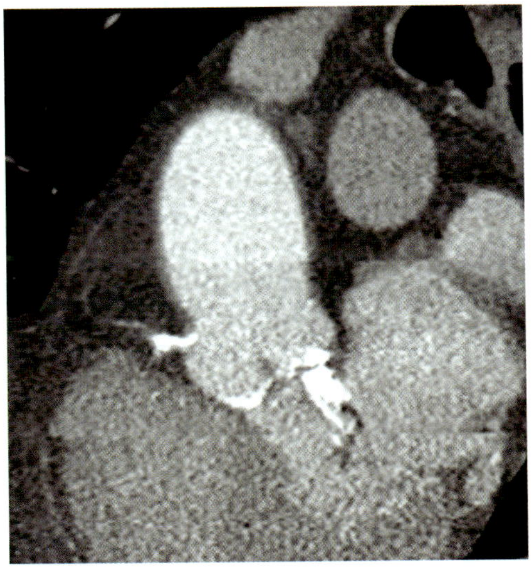

FIG. 4.25 Severe Calcification of the Left Ventricular Outflow Tract (LVOT). Computed tomography angiogram showing severe calcification of the LVOT along the intravalvular fibrous curtain.

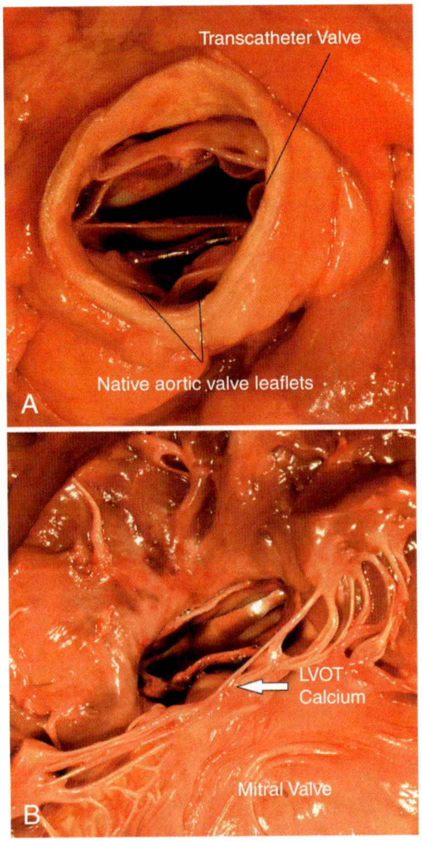

FIG. 4.26 Autopsy Images of the Transcatheter Valve After Cardiopulmonary Resuscitation. (A) Crushed transcatheter valve shown from the aortic side. (B) Crushed transcatheter valve shown from the ventricular side (Online Video 4.26). *LVOT*, left ventricular outflow tract.

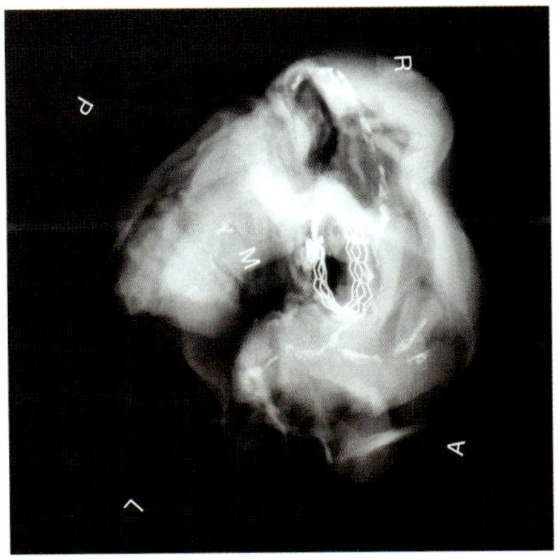

FIG. 4.27 Left Ventricular Outflow Tract (LVOT) Calcium Deforming the Transcatheter Valve Frame. Postmortem radiograph showing left ventricular outflow tract (LVOT) calcium deforming the transcatheter valve frame (Online Video 4.26).

ST-Elevation Myocardial Infarction After Transcatheter Aortic Valve Replacement: Procedural Challenge and Catastrophic Outcome

Ahmed Harhash, MD, Julia Ansari, MD, Leonid Mandel, MD, Robert Kipperman, MD

An 82-year-old woman with severe aortic stenosis, 6 months posttranscatheter aortic valve replacement (TAVR) with a 29-mm CoreValve Evolut system (Medtronic, Minneapolis, Minnesota), presented with an anterior ST-segment elevation myocardial infarction. Coronary angiography (CA) using an extra-backup (EBU) 3.5 guide catheter (Medtronic, Minneapolis, Minnesota) via radial access was unfeasible because the stent frame interfered with the guide catheter. Using a 4.0 Judkins left guide catheter (Cordis, Fremont, California) via femoral access, left CA revealed complete occlusion of the distal left anterior descending coronary artery (LAD) (Fig. 4.28A). Percutaneous coronary intervention (PCI) using an EBU 3.5 catheter with deployment of a drug-eluting stent was successful (Fig. 4.28B). Balloon and guidewire were removed, but guide catheter recovery was not feasible because of its entrapment within the stent frame. Multiple maneuvers to retrieve the catheter failed and resulted in dissection of the left main coronary artery and the LAD (Fig. 4.28C–D). Surgical extraction of the catheter was recommended, but the patient and her family declined further intervention. With the catheter in place, the patient developed cardiogenic shock and her family requested withdrawal of care.

PCI after TAVR is increasing as indications for TAVR expand. Technical difficulties of coronary intervention with supracoronary valves have been described.[1] With ex vivo simulation of our case, we concluded that catheter entrapment within the stent frame is more likely if: (1) the guide catheter crosses the stent frame at an acute angle (Fig. 4.28E–F, Online Video 4.27), (2) a preshaped double-curved catheter is used (e.g., EBU), and (3) crossing of the stent frame through a diamond lower than the ostium occurs. We recommend the following for CA/PCI with supracoronary prostheses: (1) crossing the stent frame perpendicularly through a diamond at the same

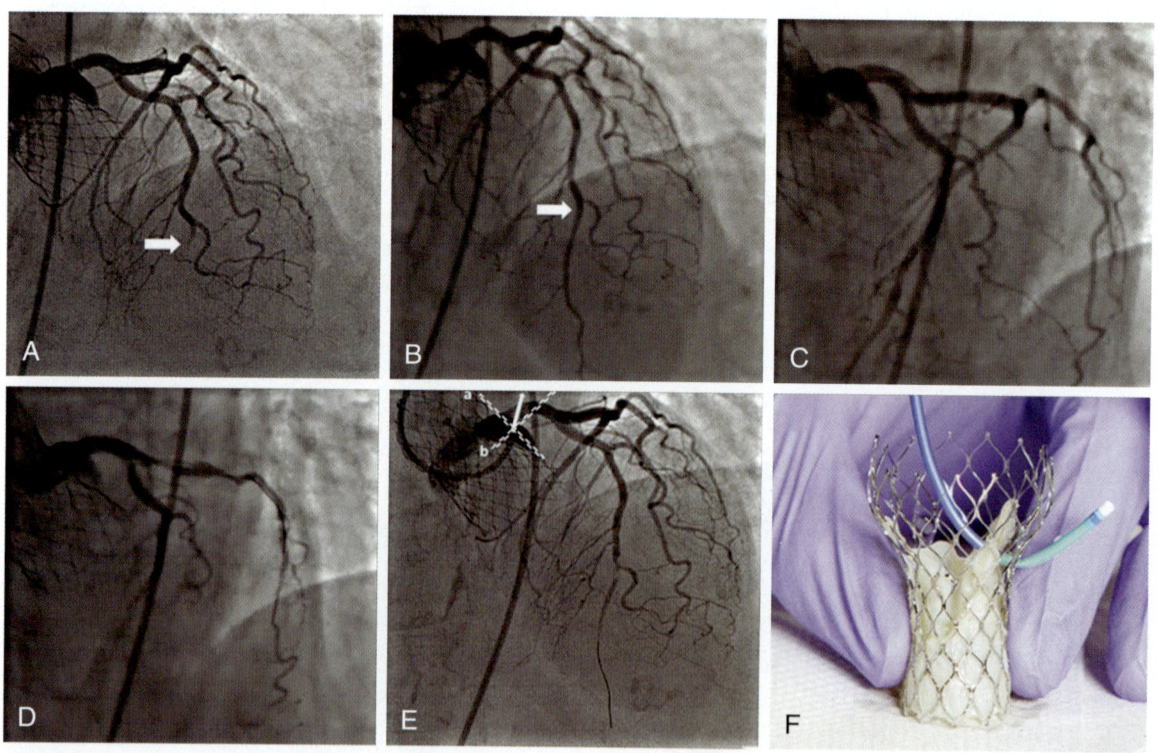

FIG. 4.28 Left Coronary Angiography and Ex Vivo Simulation. (A) Left coronary angiography showing total occlusion of the distal left anterior descending coronary artery (*arrow*). (B) Left coronary angiography postpercutaneous coronary intervention and drug-eluting stent deployment (*arrow*). (C and D) Dissection of the left main and left anterior descending coronary arteries. (E) (*a*) Interrupted line showing guide catheter engagement into the left coronary ostium at an acute angle with the vertical axis of the stent frame. (*b*) Interrupted line showing crossing of the stent frame at a perpendicular angle. (F) Ex vivo simulation using an extra-backup 3.5 guide catheter, showing catheter entrapment within the stent frame when crossed at an acute angle (Online Videos 4.27 and 4.28).

level of the coronary ostium (Online Video 4.28), (2) using catheters with favorable geometry (e.g., left Judkins for left and right Amplatz [Boston Scientific, Marlborough, Massachusetts] for right CA/PCI),[1] and (3) using a balloon and/or a guidewire to back the catheter out of the coronary ostium.

Reference

1. Blumenstein J, Kim W, Liebetrau C, et al. Challenges of coronary angiography and intervention in patients previously treated by TAVI. *Clin Res Cardiol.* 2015;104:632-639.

Stroke With Valve Tissue Embolization During Transcatheter Aortic Valve Replacement Treated With Endovascular Intervention

Amornpol Anuwatworn, MD, Amol Raizada, MD, Shawn Kelly, MD, Tomasz Stys, MD, Orvar Jonsson, MD, Adam Stys, MD

A 78-year-old man presented with progressive dyspnea on exertion and syncope. His relevant history included coronary bypass surgery twice. Severe aortic stenosis with left ventricular ejection fraction of 65% was evident on echocardiography. Coronary angiogram showed patent left internal mammary artery and saphenous vein grafts with severe three-vessel disease. Transesophageal echocardiogram revealed heavily calcified, poorly opening aortic valve leaflets, and a mobile echodense mass measuring 1 cm × 0.4 cm attached to the valve (Fig. 4.29, Online Videos 4.29 and 4.30). Transfemoral transcatheter aortic valve replacement (TAVR) was performed with a CoreValve system (Medtronic, Minneapolis, Minnesota) because the patient was deemed high risk for open-heart surgery. After the procedure, most of the mobile aortic valve mass was no longer seen on the transesophageal echocardiogram. When the patient awakened from sedation, right hemiplegia was noted (one-fifth strength). Head computed tomographic angiography showed narrowing involving the distal M1 segment of the left middle cerebral artery (MCA) with diminished enhancement suggestive of early infarction. Emergent cerebral angiography showed a partially occlusive defect in the M1 segment of the left MCA that was limiting the distal flow (Fig. 4.30). Endovascular mechanical extraction of the mass responsible for these findings was performed with a Penumbra ACE catheter (Penumbra, Inc., Alameda, California), achieving complete recanalization (Figs. 4.31 and 4.32). Subsequently, the patient's strength improved significantly (four-fifths strength). Brain magnetic resonance imaging revealed a large acute infarct of the left MCA territory (Fig. 4.33). Histopathology of the extracted mass was consistent with heart valve tissue (Fig. 4.34).

Stroke is a well-known complication of TAVR. The incidence rate of major strokes at 30 days in the PARTNER (Placement of Aortic Transcatheter Valves) A trial was 3.8%.[1] Svensson et al.[1] found that 51% of strokes occurred during the procedure, and 38% of strokes occurred within 2 days; however, the mortality rate in patients with stroke was 43%. Of patients undergoing TAVR, 0.56% developed valve embolization.[2] One case report of a TAVR patient demonstrated the successful endovascular retrieval of an embolized calcium fragment that may have derived from the aortic wall or the valve.[3] In our case, the valve tissue recovery from the MCA resulted in significant neurologic improvement. To our knowledge, this case demonstrates the first successful endovascular recanalization of acute ischemic stroke caused specifically by valve tissue embolization. Endovascular intervention should be considered as emergency

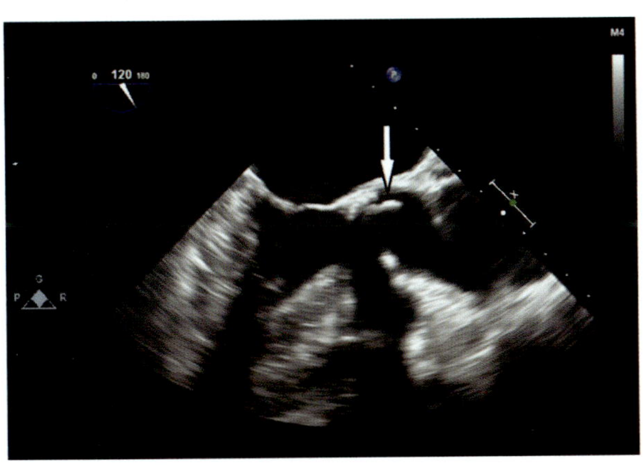

FIG. 4.29 Mobile Echodense Mass Attached to Aortic Valve. Transesophageal echocardiography shows mobile echodense mass (*white arrow*), which measured 1 cm × 0.4 cm, attached to the aortic valve (Online Videos 4.29 and 4.30).

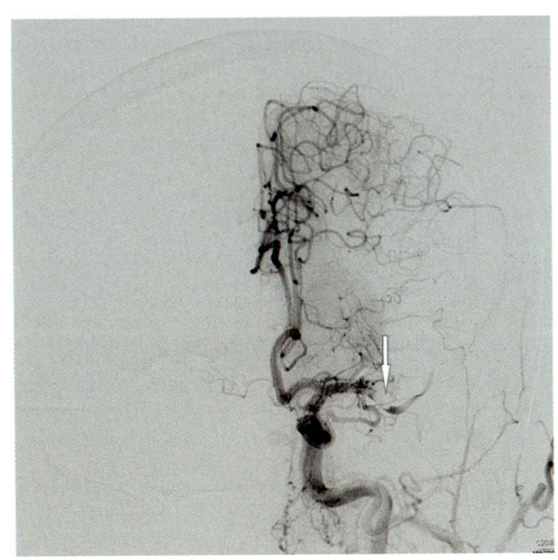

FIG. 4.30 Filling Defect in the Distal M1 Segment of the Left Middle Cerebral Artery. Cerebral angiogram shows filling defect in the distal M1 segment of the left middle cerebral artery (*white arrow*) with minimal contrast distally.

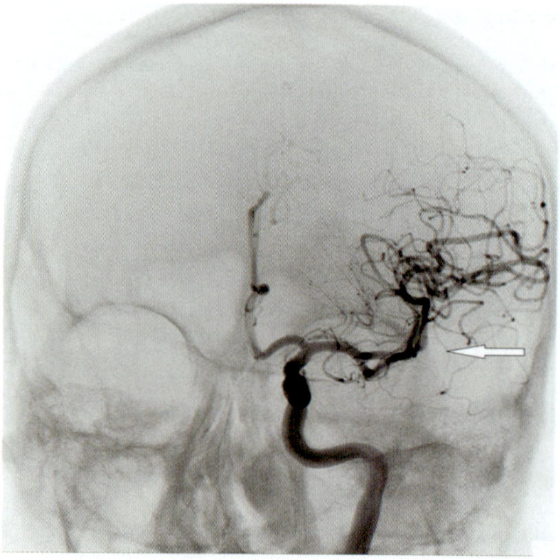

FIG. 4.31 Good Flow After Retrieval of Embolic Material. Cerebral angiogram after retrieval of embolic material from left middle cerebral artery (*white arrow*) shows good subsequent flow.

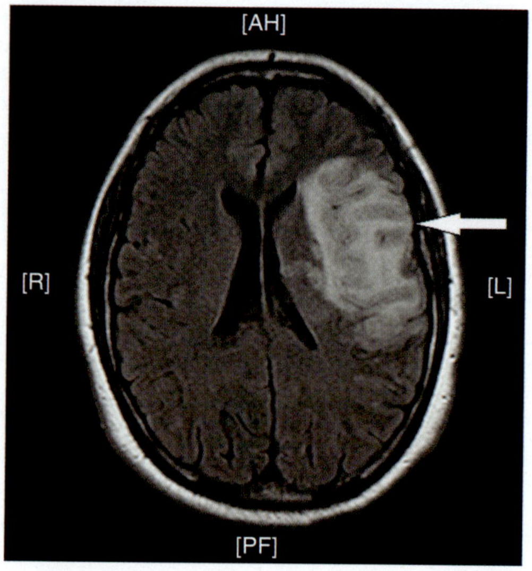

FIG. 4.33 Brain Magnetic Resonance Imaging (MRI) Reveals Middle Cerebral Artery (MCA) Acute Infarct. Brain MRI reveals a large MCA acute infarct (*white arrow*).

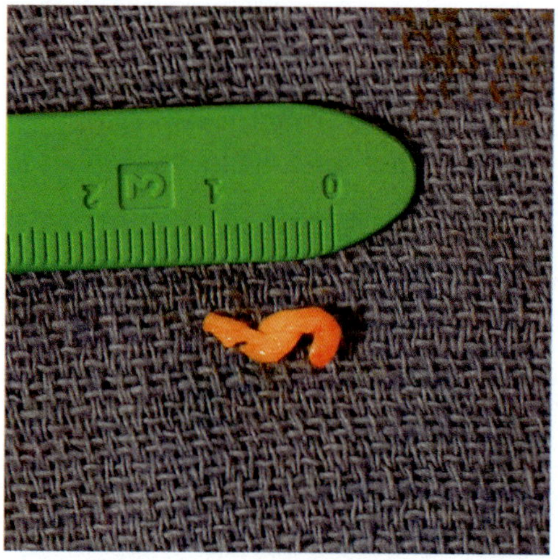

FIG. 4. 32 Gross Specimen of the Embolic Valvular Tissue. Gross specimen of the embolic valvular tissue retrieved from the left middle cerebral artery.

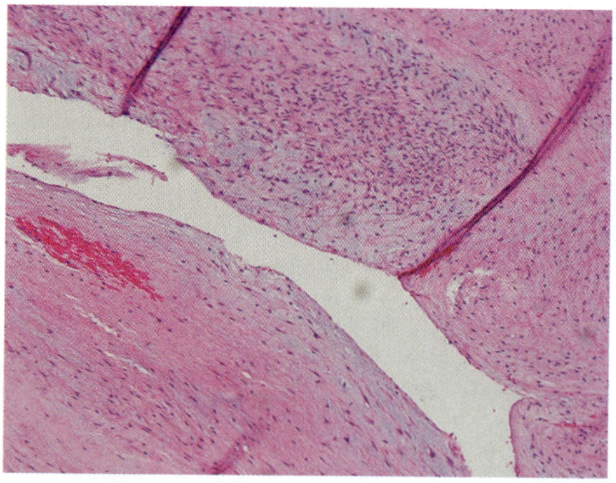

FIG. 4.34 Connective Tissue Core of a Heart Valve With Endothelial Lining. Histopathology demonstrates the typical dense connective tissue core of a heart valve with endothelial lining. There is evidence of mild myxoid change and fibrous proliferative activity within the tissue.

rescue therapy for acute ischemic stroke resulting from valve tissue emboli.

Acknowledgments

The authors thank Dr. Jitendra Sharma for providing advanced interventional neurology care and postprocedure photographs of retrieved valvular tissue. Special thanks to Dr. David W. Ohrt and Dr. Usama Yusef for providing the histopathology slide.

References

1. Svensson LG, Tuzcu M, Kapadia S, et al. A comprehensive review of the PARTNER trial. *J Thorac Cardiovasc Surg.* 2013;145(suppl 3): S11-S16.
2. Jilaihawi H, Chakravarty T, Weiss RE, Fontana GP, Forrester J, Makkar RR. Meta-analysis of complications in aortic valve replacement: comparison of Medtronic-CoreValve, Edwards-Sapien and surgical aortic valve replacement in 8,536 patients. *Catheter Cardiovasc Interv.* 2012;80: 128-138.
3. Fassa AA, Mazighi M, Himbert D, et al. Successful endovascular stroke rescue with retrieval of an embolized calcium fragment after transcatheter aortic valve replacement. *Circ Cardiovasc Interv.* 2014;7:125-126.

Successful Management of Annulus Rupture in Transcatheter Aortic Valve Implantation

Kentaro Hayashida, MD, PhD, Erik Bouvier, MD, Thierry Lefèvre, MD

An 82-year-old woman with severe aortic stenosis was referred to our center. Transcatheter aortic valve implantation (TAVI) was scheduled because of her high surgical risk (logistic EuroSCORE [European System for Cardiac Operative Risk Evaluation] 25.8%). The annulus diameter measured by transesophageal echocardiography (TEE) was 22.2 and 23.6 mm by multidetector computed tomography (CT). A 26-mm Edwards valve (Edwards Lifesciences, Irvine, California) was subsequently implanted via the transfemoral approach. After implantation, sudden hemodynamic collapse occurred, and aortography revealed contrast protrusion from the aortic cusp (Fig. 4.35A, Online Video 4.31). Fluoroscopic detection of restricted heart motion with surrounding white area (Online Video 4.31) facilitated immediate diagnosis of tamponade before echocardiography. After percutaneous pericardial drainage via the subxiphoid approach and heparin neutralization, blood autotransfusion was performed via a circuit connecting the drainage catheter and the femoral vein sheath. Hemodynamics were stabilized within 30 min, and contrast protrusion disappeared (Online Video 4.32). Preprocedural CT showed a calcified nodule (5 × 7.5 mm) at the epicardial fat segment between the interventricular septum and left atrium (Fig. 4.35B, *arrow*), and contrast leakage was observed in postprocedural CT (Fig. 4.35C, *arrow*). The patient was discharged on day 8 with no complications. We successfully treated a similar case (with a 26-mm valve for the 22-mm TEE-measured annulus diameter) with contrast protrusion (Fig. 4.35D, Online Videos 4.33 and 4.34) and similar pre- and post-CT findings (Fig. 4.35E–F). Annulus rupture is a rare complication of TAVI, reported in about 1% of cases.[1,2] However, when it occurs, acute hemodynamic collapse frequently causes catastrophic outcomes. Immediate diagnosis by fluoroscopy and echocardiography, percutaneous drainage, autotransfusion of drained blood, and heparin neutralization may save lives.

References

1. Pasic M, Unbehaun A, Dreysse S, et al. Rupture of the device landing zone during transcatheter aortic valve implantation: a life-threatening but treatable complication. *Circ Cardiovasc Interv.* 2012;5:424-432.
2. Hayashida K, Bouvier E, Lefevre T, et al. Potential mechanism for annulus rupture in transcatheter aortic valve implantation. *Catheter Cardiovasc Interv.* 2013;82(5):E742-E746. doi:10.1002/ccd.24524. [Epub 2013 Jun 25.]

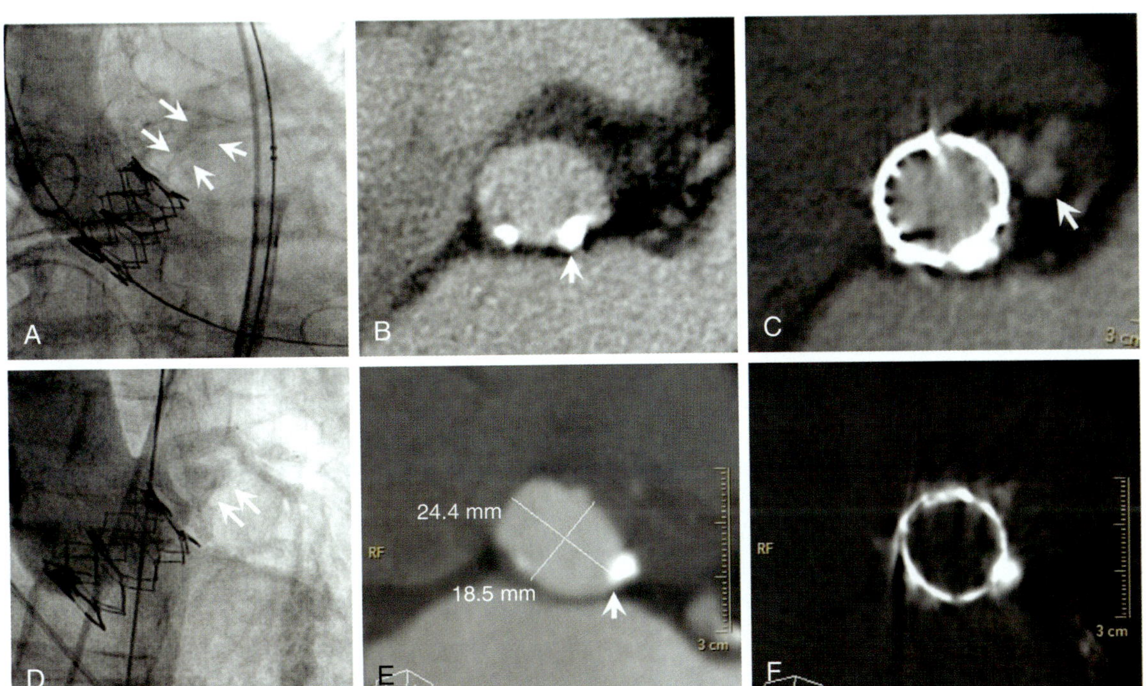

FIG. 4.35 Angiographic and Computed Tomography (CT) Images of Annulus Rupture in Patient No. 1 and Patient No. 2. (A) Aortography showed contrast protrusion from the aortic cusp (anteroposterior view) (Online Video 4.31). (B) Preprocedural CT scan showed a huge calcified nodule (5 × 7.5 mm) on the annulus (*arrow*). (C) Postprocedural CT scan showed contrast leakage due to annulus rupture (*arrow*). (D) Contrast protrusion from the aortic cusp in another case of annulus rupture (left anterior oblique 20°) (Online Video 4.33). (E) A calcified nodule on the annulus on preprocedural CT scan (*arrow*). (F) Postprocedural CT scan (Online Videos 4.31–4.34).

Valve Migration Into the Left Ventricular Outflow Tract Managed by Coaxial Double-Valve Alignment

Annamaria Nicolino, MD, Massimo Vischi, MD, Shahram Moshiri, MD, Antonio Salsano, MD, Giancarlo Passerone, MD, Francesco Chiarella, MD, Francesco Santini, MD

The efficacy and overall safety of transcatheter aortic valve implantation (TAVI) in patients with severe aortic stenosis at high risk for conventional surgery is validated. Nevertheless, infrequent but severe intraprocedural complications, often necessitating intraoperative bail-out maneuvers, are reported. Among these, valve migration into the left ventricle is particularly dismal and requires conversion to an emergent surgical procedure with a reported disproportionally high mortality rate.[1]

We report herein a case in which valve migration into the left ventricular outflow tract (LVOT) was successfully managed by repositioning a second prosthesis, thus avoiding emergent surgery.

An 81-year-old woman with severe symptomatic aortic stenosis and a logistic EuroSCORE (European System for Cardiac Operative Risk Evaluation) of 26% was admitted for transfemoral TAVI. At computed tomography (CT) scan, aortic valve and root measurements showed an annulus diameter of 21 × 23 mm (mean 22 mm), a perimeter of 7.1 cm, an area of 3.7 cm^2 (Fig. 4.36A–B), an aortic root at the level of the sinus of Valsalva of 26 × 28 mm, and a sinotubular junction of 23 × 25 mm.

Interestingly, calcifications were present only on two valve leaflets and very scarcely on the annulus (Fig. 4.36C). Because of the borderline annular size, a calibrated balloon aortic valvuloplasty was performed, with the evidence that a 20-mm size completely occluded the annulus. A 23-mm Edwards SAPIEN XT valve (Edwards Lifesciences, Irvine, California) was therefore deployed as for a routine procedure during rapid pacing at the proper annular position (Fig. 4.37, Online Video 4.35).

Immediately after valve implantation, however, a self-limiting ventricular tachycardia occurred, and fluoroscopy showed the valve had migrated into the LVOT (Fig. 4.38, Online Video 4.36). In view of the rapidly deteriorating hemodynamics with marked hypotension (90/60 mm Hg) and bradycardia requiring inotropic support, tracheal intubation, and ventricular pacing, having excluded by transesophageal echocardiography (TEE) any involvement of the mitral valve, the heart team decided on an emergency, lifesaving, second aortic valve deployment with the concurrent intent of repositioning the previous prosthesis. The decision was made in view of the patient's prohibitive overall clinical conditions for surgery, including a very high frailty score (Geriatric Status Scale).[1]

Again, a second 23-mm Edwards SAPIEN XT valve was deployed, slightly overinflated by means of a balloon prepared with 2 mL of extradilute contrast medium, and in a higher position than the previous valve in the aortic annulus (Fig. 4.39A–B, Online Video 4.37). Furthermore, after balloon deflection and without rapid pacing, by using the delivery system tip of the second valve balloon catheter, the lower-edge mesh frame of the first inserted valve was engaged and carefully pulled back to a stable position in the LVOT, coaxial to the second deployed prosthesis (Fig. 4.40, Online Video 4.38). The patient regained hemodynamic stability, allowing rapid withdrawal of inotropic support. TEE excluded any mitral regurgitation or restriction of the anterior mitral leaflet motion. The patient was discharged on day 7 after permanent pacemaker implantation for persistent complete atrioventricular block.

At 12 months of follow-up, the patient is stable in New York Heart Association functional class I and has had no adverse events in the interim period. The electrocardiogram shows sinus rhythm and normal atrioventricular conduction, with no pacemaker intervention. Serial echocardiograms, radiographic controls, and CT angiography (Fig. 4.41, Online Video 4.39) showed stable valve positions and no mitral dysfunction.

Transcatheter heart valve migration is a largely, but not entirely, preventable complication with current balloon-expandable valves. An asymmetrically calcified aortic valve and a borderline annular size may have favored prosthesis migration by preventing proper annular anchoring. A 23-mm prosthesis was chosen to minimize complications of a smallish aortic root and after calibrated measurements. It is conceivable that a more aggressive valve dilation in the first instance might have prevented valve migration. During the procedure, the position of the pigtail was higher than recommended but still deemed satisfactory to visualize the annulus during aortography. We chose to inflate the valve according to the "two-step implantation technique" to be able to adjust the position should it have become necessary. Retrospectively, the potential impact of the two-step technique on valve migration cannot be excluded. Nevertheless, the evidence that the valve prosthesis stayed in position for a given time seems to underscore that the applied radial forces rather than the application time might have had more of an impact on the final result.

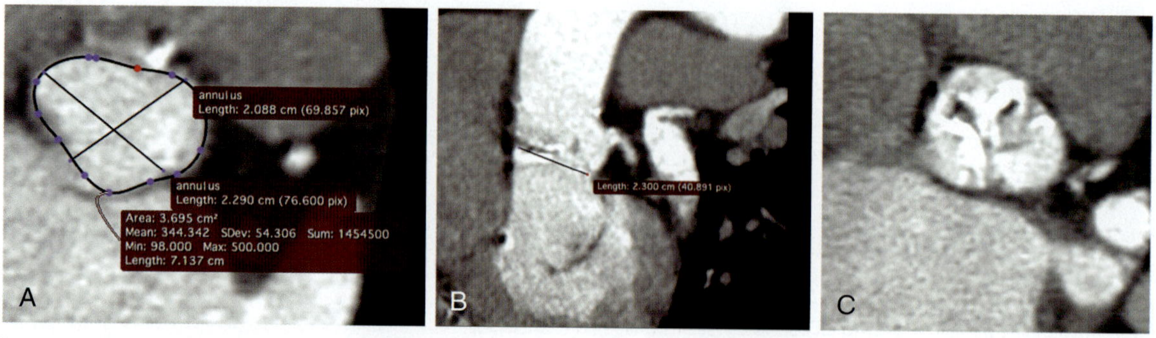

FIG. 4.36 Computed Tomography Scan of the Aortic Valve and Root Measurements. Aortic valve (A) and annular (B) measures. (C) Aortic valve calcifications involving mainly two leaflets and scarcely the annulus.

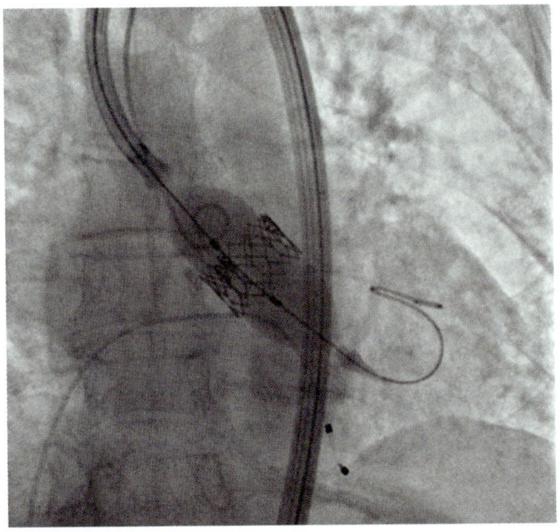

FIG. 4.37 First Valve After Deployment at the Annular Level. Fluoroscopic view showing the first 23-mm Edwards SAPIEN XT valve deployed in the correct position (Online Video 4.35).

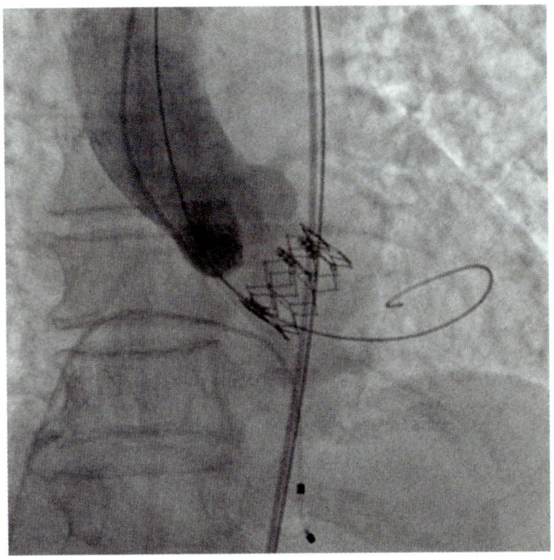

FIG. 4.38 Migrated Valve at the Subannular Level. Fluoroscopic view showing the 23-mm Edwards SAPIEN XT valve migrated into the left ventricular outflow tract (Online Video 4.36).

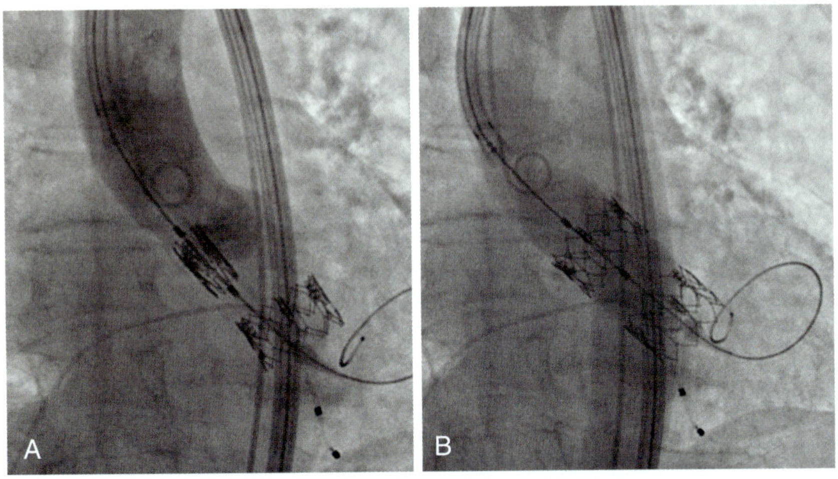

FIG. 4.39 Deployment of the Second Valve. Fluoroscopic view showing the second 23-mm Edwards SAPIEN XT valve in position before (A) and after (B) balloon dilation (Online Video 4.37).

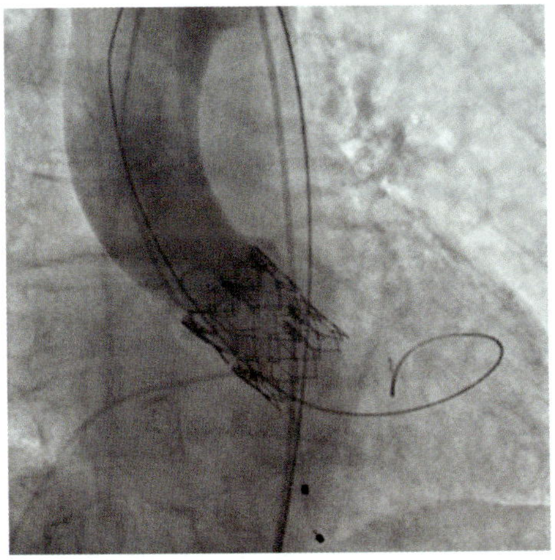

FIG. 4.40 Coaxial Position of the Two Valves. Fluoroscopic view showing the coaxial double-valve left ventricular outflow tract alignment achieved after balloon catheter retrieval (Online Video 4.38).

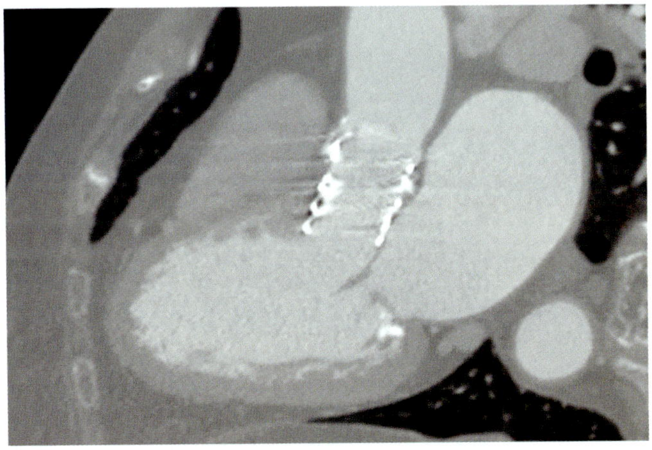

FIG. 4.41 Cine Computed Tomographic (CT) Scan at Follow-Up. Contrast material–enhanced electrocardiographically gated CT angiography showing the stable coaxial alignment of the two deployed valves at 9 months follow-up (Online Video 4.39).

Although prevention with meticulous image analysis and sizing remains the key to success, the prompt availability of an interdisciplinary surgical and interventional safety net to manage bail-out maneuvers in potentially fatal complications is confirmed to be mandatory. In our case, excluded any mitral valve involvement, the decision to proceed with a second deployment was made in view of the patient's prohibitive clinical conditions, further worsened by the casualty, and by the reported evidence of poor surgical results in an emergency setting.[1,2]

Although our approach was successful, the potential for a disastrous outcome and therefore the need for extensive planning should never be underestimated.

References

1. Hein R, Abdel-Wahab M, Sievert H, et al. Outcome of patients after emergency conversion from transcatheter aortic valve implantation to surgery. *EuroIntervention.* 2013;9:446-451.
2. Makkar RR, Jilaihawi H, Chakravarty T, et al. Determinants and outcomes of acute transcatheter valve-in-valve therapy or embolization: a study of multiple valve implants in the U.S. PARTNER trial (Placement of AoRTic TraNscathetER Valve Trial Edwards SAPIEN Transcatheter Heart Valve). *J Am Coll Cardiol.* 2013;62:418-430.

Vascular Injury Caused by Retrieval of Ruptured and Detached Balloon Valvuloplasty Catheter During Transcatheter Aortic Valve Replacement

Shunsuke Kubo, MD, Yasushi Fuku, MD, Takeshi Shimamoto, MD, PhD, Akimune Kuwayama, MD, Masanobu Ohya, MD, Hidewo Amano, MD, Takeshi Maruo, MD, Tsuyoshi Goto, MD, Tatsuhiko Komiya, MD, PhD, Kazushige Kadota, MD, PhD

An 88-year-old woman underwent transcatheter aortic valve implantation using a SAPIEN 3 valve (Edwards Lifesciences, Irvine, California) for symptomatic severe aortic stenosis. Preprocedural examinations showed an aortic valve area of 0.39 cm^2 and severe calcification of the leaflets. During predilatation using a 20-mm balloon valvuloplasty catheter (Edwards Lifesciences), balloon rupture occurred at the calcified leaflet (Fig. 4.42). We pulled the balloon catheter back to the eSheath (Edwards Lifesciences) and removed it together with the eSheath through the right femoral artery. The ruptured balloon was, however, completely detached and a part of the balloon remained in the artery (Fig. 4.43A). Iliac angiography showed the right external iliac artery occluded with the detached balloon (Fig. 4.43B–C). After heart team discussion, we cut down the groin and successfully retrieved the detached ruptured balloon (Fig. 4.43D–E). Then, a

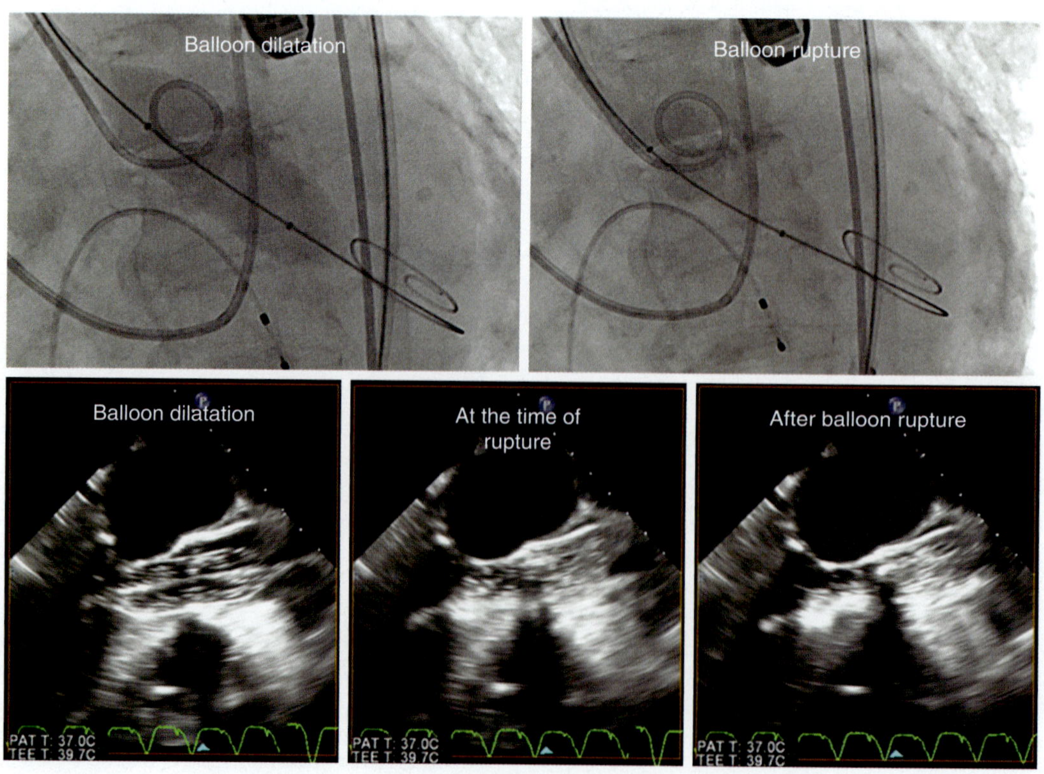

FIG. 4.42 Fluoroscopic and Echocardiographic Findings of Balloon.

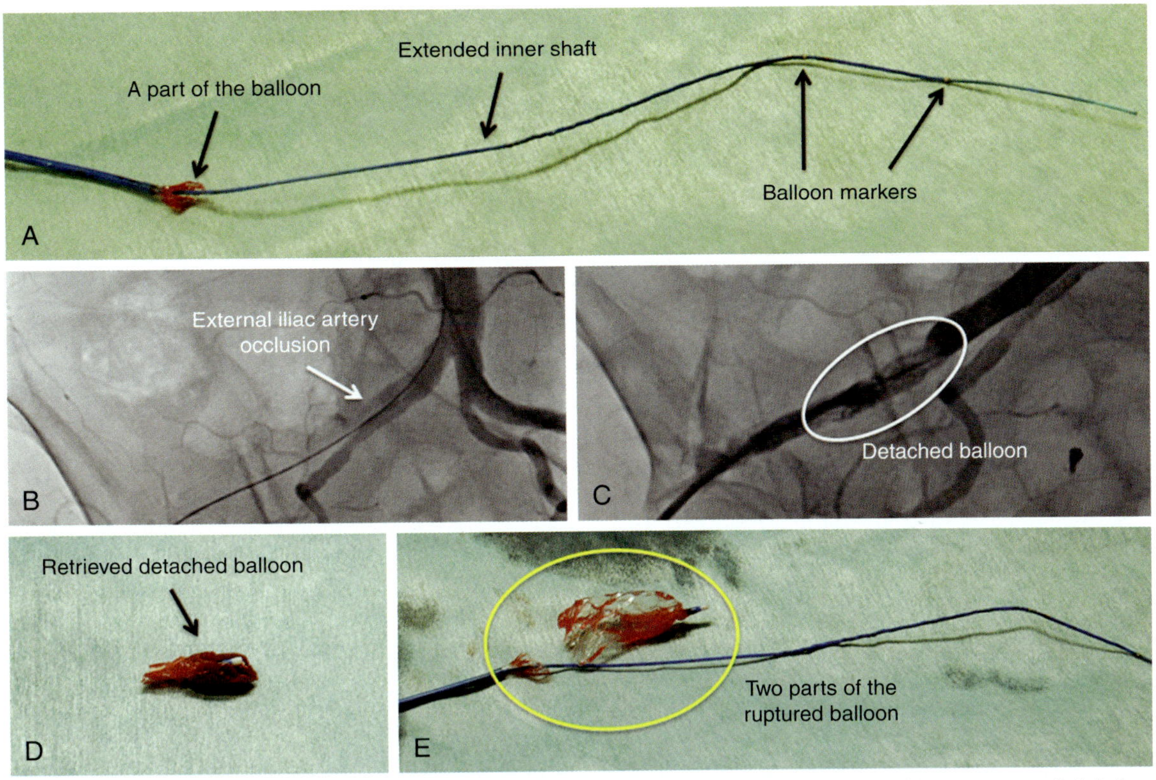

FIG. 4.43 Retrieved Ruptured Balloon Valvuloplasty Catheter. (A) The initially retrieved balloon catheter showing an extended shaft and a part of the balloon. Iliac angiography showing the occlusion of the external iliac artery (B) with a detached ruptured balloon (*white circle*) (C). (D) Retrieval of the detached balloon by cutting down the groin. (E) Successful retrieval of two parts of the ruptured balloon (*yellow circle*).

23-mm SAPIEN 3 valve was implanted via left femoral access. After percutaneous closure of the left femoral access site, the right limb appeared to have developed cyanosis. Right limb angiography revealed that the superficial femoral artery was occluded due to embolization (Fig. 4.44A). After removal of the embolized material through the cutdown site, the right superficial femoral artery was recanalized (Fig. 4.44B) and the cyanosis improved. The retrieved material was pathologically proved to be an arterial intima (Fig. 4.44C). This finding indicates that a ruptured balloon caused vascular injury in the process of retrieval, and the dissected free arterial intima embolized the right femoral artery.

Balloon rupture can occur during valvuloplasty of a severely calcified aortic valve.[1] In this case, we tried to pull out the ruptured balloon catheter, which resulted in complete detachment of the balloon, arterial injury, and subsequent embolization with a resected arterial intima. Retrieval of a ruptured balloon valvuloplasty catheter is occasionally challenging, and careful management is required to prevent serious vascular complications.

Reference

1. Percutaneous balloon aortic valvuloplasty. Acute and 30-day follow-up results in 674 patients from the NHLBI Balloon Valvuloplasty Registry. *Circulation*. 1991;84:2383-2397.

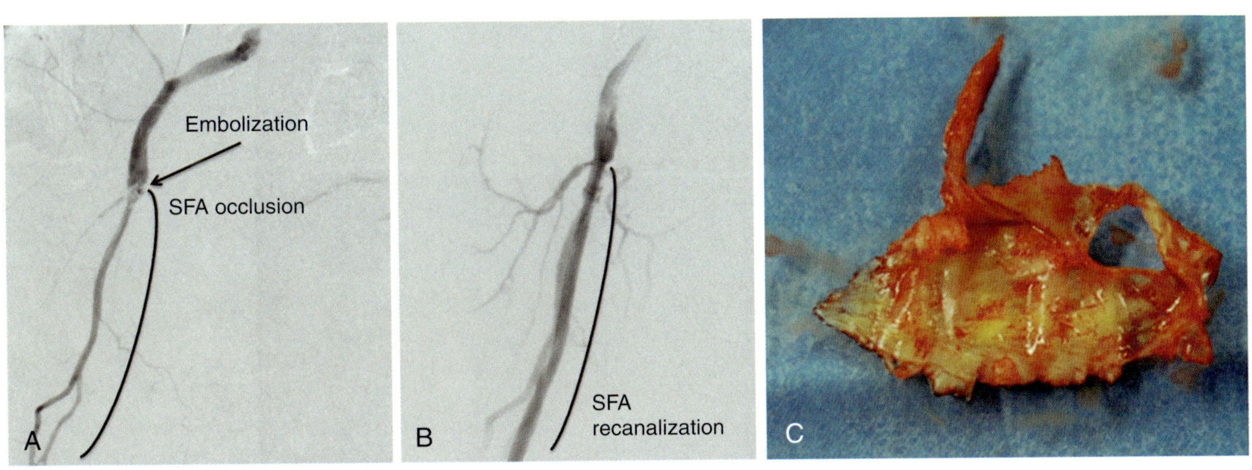

FIG. 4.44 Superficial Femoral Artery (SFA) Occlusion Due to Arterial Intimal Embolization. (A) Right femoral angiography showing SFA occlusion due to embolization. (B) After removal of the embolized material, the SFA was successfully recanalized. (C) Removed embolized material indicating an arterial intima.

Very Late Thrombosis of a Transcatheter Aortic Valve-in-Valve

David Martí, MD, PhD, Miguel Rubio, MD, Natalia Escribano, MD, Ramón de Miguel, MD, Ignacio Rada, MD, PhD, César Morís, MD, PhD

An 85-year-old man presented with dyspnea (New York Heart Association functional class IV) 4 years after implantation of a 26-mm CoreValve transcatheter aortic valve (TAV) (Medtronic, Minneapolis, Minnesota). Angiography revealed severe aortic regurgitation because of the deep position of the prosthesis (Online Video 4.40), and a 23-mm SAPIEN XT (Edwards Lifesciences, Irvine, California) valve-in-valve implantation was performed. Midterm follow-up was favorable; clopidogrel was discontinued 15 months after the SAPIEN XT valve implantation, and aspirin monotherapy continued thereafter.

Two months after clopidogrel discontinuation, the patient required three visits to the emergency department with overt heart failure. Echocardiography showed high transvalvular gradients (peak, 55 mm Hg; mean, 31 mm Hg; dimensionless valve index, 0.25), thickened leaflets, and mild to moderate central aortic regurgitation (Fig. 4.45, Online Videos 4.41 and 4.42). The heart team decided to perform a surgical aortic valve replacement. Operative and pathology findings revealed a diffuse fibrin-platelet thrombus adhered to the aortic surface on the three SAPIEN XT valve cusps (Figs. 4.46 and 4.47). This valve was partially denuded and easily extracted from within the CoreValve prosthesis. Both TAVs were explanted via a longitudinal aortotomy, and a 21-mm bioprosthesis was sutured to the well-preserved aortic annulus.

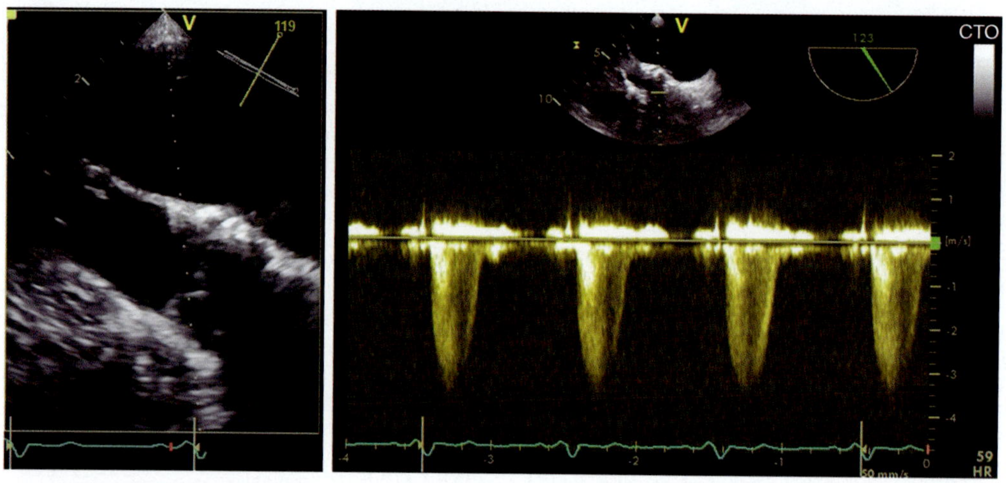

FIG. 4.45 Multiplane Transesophageal Echocardiography. (Left) Homogeneous thickening of the SAPIEN XT (Edwards Lifesciences, Irvine, California) cusps, with neither significant calcification nor mobile images. (Right) Elevated transvalvular velocities (Online Videos 4.40–4.42).

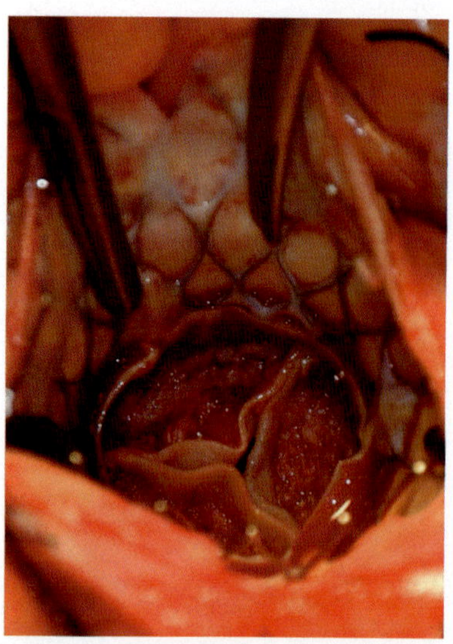

FIG. 4.46 Operative Findings Revealing Thrombotic Material Adhered to the Three Aortic Cusps. Note the endothelialization of the CoreValve (Medtronic, Minneapolis, Minnesota) frame and the proper expansion of the SAPIEN XT valve (Edwards Lifesciences, Irvine, California).

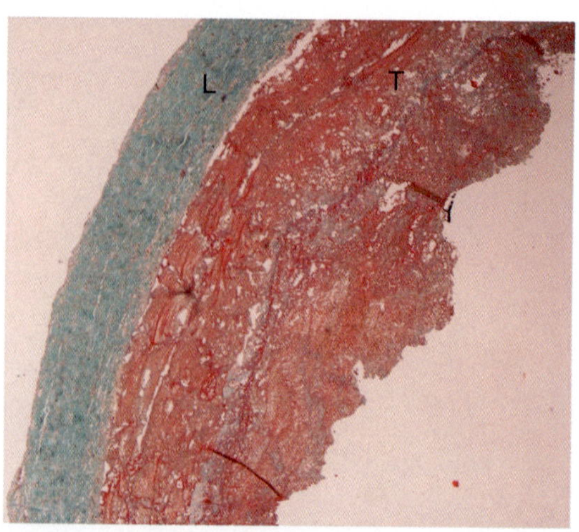

FIG. 4.47 Pathologic Sample of a Thrombosed Leaflet. Masson trichrome-stained section of a thrombosed leaflet, with lines of Zahn present and without fibrosis or calcification within the thrombus (magnification ×4). *L*, leaflet; *T*, thrombus.

Unfortunately, the patient died of cardiac arrest in the postoperative period.

Valve thrombosis is a rare but increasingly recognized complication of transcatheter heart valves. Indeed, a systematic review has shown that thrombosis is the major cause of valve stenosis in the early years after implantation.[1] As in this case, TAV thrombosis is usually not associated with typical thrombus images on transesophageal echocardiography, and operators must be cautious when handling catheters in the vicinity of a stenotic TAV.[1,2]

Balloon-expandable prostheses are sometimes used to reduce aortic regurgitation after CoreValve implantation.[3] Our findings suggest that in this setting, internal prosthesis endothelialization may be delayed or incomplete, representing an additional risk factor for late thrombosis. Therefore TAV-in-TAV therapies with balloon-expandable valves might require longer duration of dual-antiplatelet therapy.

References

1. Mylotte D, Andalib A, Thériault-Lauzier P, et al. Transcatheter heart valve failure: a systematic review. *Eur Heart J.* 2015;36:1306-1327.
2. De Backer O, Ihlemann N, Olsen NT, Vejlstrup N, Søndergaard L. Intracardiac echocardiography unveils large thrombus on a restenotic TAVR prosthesis more than 6 years after implantation. *Eur Heart J.* 2016;37(28): 2271. doi:10.1093/eurheartj/ehv064. [Epub 2015 Mar 22.]
3. Diemert P, Lange P, Greif M, et al. Edwards Sapien XT valve placement as treatment option for aortic regurgitation after transfemoral Core Valve implantation: a multicenter experience. *Clin Res Cardiol.* 2014;103: 183-190.

Balloon "Valvuloplasty" for Mechanical Valve Dysfunction

David E. Kandzari, MD, Harold Carlson, MD, John P. Gott, MD, Prashant Kaul, MD, W. Morris Brown, MD

A 46-year-old woman with a history of Marfan syndrome experienced witnessed cardiac arrest with persistent shock requiring circulatory support with extracorporeal membrane oxygenation (ECMO). In 2000, the patient underwent ascending aortic root replacement and mechanical bileaflet valve replacement followed by second sternotomy in 2012 with bypass grafting to the left anterior descending artery and left main artery patch closure for progressive coronary aneurysmal enlargement.

Coronary angiography demonstrated no significant right coronary artery disease but severe stenosis at the origin of the single venous bypass graft to the left coronary anatomy (Fig. 4.48). During successful percutaneous revascularization of the bypass graft, a fixed, immobile leaflet of the mechanical valve was identified (Fig. 4.49A–B, Online Video 4.43). The international normalized ratio was within therapeutic range upon admission. After surgical consultation, the risk of a third operation was considered prohibitive. Furthermore, given prolonged cardiopulmonary resuscitation and ECMO cannulation, fibrinolytic therapy for possible valve thrombosis represented at least a relative contraindication.

With no alternative therapeutic options, we hypothesized that balloon expansion between the leaflet struts may free the fixed leaflet and restore mobility. The method was initially tested with a valve model in the catheterization laboratory. A coronary guidewire was then passed across the valve between the struts followed by advancement of a 2.5- × 20-mm angioplasty catheter (Fig. 4.50A, Online Video 4.44). Inflation of the balloon immediately resulted in recovery of leaflet mobility (Fig 4.50B) with functional aortic regurgitation and no clinical or radiographic evidence of an embolic event (Fig. 4.51A–B, Online Video 4.45).

Treatment options for prosthetic valve dysfunction are limited to surgery or fibrinolytic therapy, both of which were unfavorable in this situation. After reviewing the medical literature, we find that this case represents the first description of balloon "valvuloplasty" for mechanical valve dysfunction.

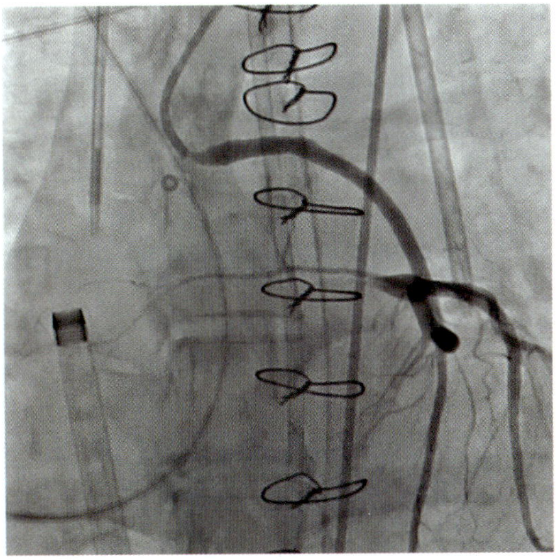

FIG. 4.48 Bypass Graft Angiography to Left Coronary Anatomy. Angiography demonstrating severe stenosis of solitary venous bypass graft to left coronary arteries.

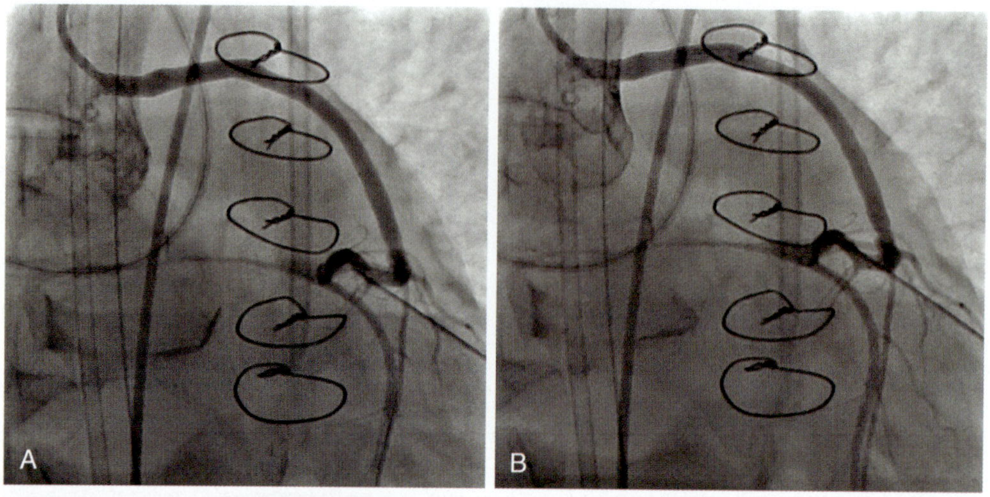

FIG. 4.49 Fluoroscopy of Immobile Prosthetic Valve Leaflet. After successful revascularization, fluoroscopy indicates a single, fixed, immobile valve leaflet during diastole (A) and systole (B) (Online Video 4.43).

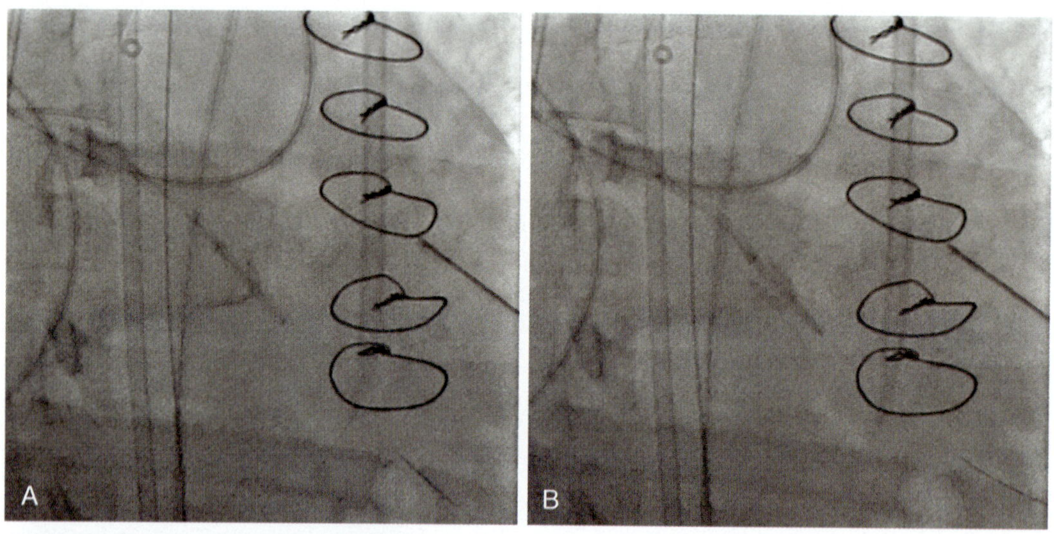

FIG. 4.50 Balloon "Valvuloplasty" of Fixed Prosthetic Valve Leaflet. Advancement of a coronary balloon angioplasty catheter between the valve struts (A) and recovery of leaflet mobility (B) (Online Video 4.44).

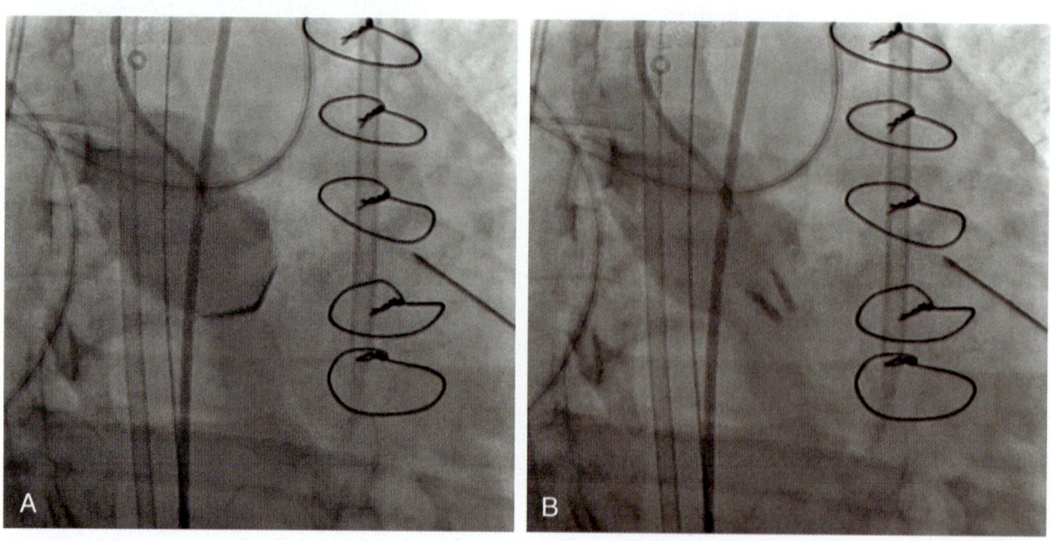

Fig 4.51 Recovery of Normal Prosthetic Valve Bileaflet Function. Supravalvular angiography confirming leaflet mobility in diastole (A) and systole (B) (Online Video 4.45).

Transesophageal Echocardiography-Guided, Bedside Bail-Out Aortic Valvuloplasty

Mathias C. Busch, MD, Sigrun Friesecke, MD, Klaus Empen, MD, Stephan B. Felix, MD

A 73-year-old man developed hemodynamic deterioration in the context of bilateral pneumonia, despite treatment of septic shock according to guidelines. Transthoracic echocardiography was of poor quality because of the patient's obesity but revealed severely reduced left ventricular (LV) function. Significant coronary heart disease had previously been ruled out angiographically. With hemodynamic status deteriorating further (intermittently requiring cardiopulmonary resuscitation), implantation of a percutaneous LV assist device (Impella, Abiomed, Danvers, Massachusetts) was planned. Because current circumstances made transfer to the catheterization laboratory impossible, transesophageal echocardiography (TEE)-guided implantation in the intensive care unit was initiated. The ultrasound image, however, revealed severe aortic valve (AV) stenosis (Fig. 4.52A), inaudible on auscultation. A transfemoral AL1-shaped 5F catheter was placed in the ascending aorta. The AV was passed under TEE guidance with a straight-tip hydrophilic guidewire (Fig. 4.52B). After advancement of the catheter into the LV, pressure measurement with the intensive care unit monitor showed a peak-to-peak gradient of approximately 50 mm Hg. A J-tipped extra-stiff guidewire was placed into the LV. A NuMed NuCLEUS (Hopkington, New York) 23-mm balloon was advanced across the AV with TEE guidance (Fig. 4.52C). Valvuloplasty was performed (Fig. 4.52D) without rapid ventricular pacing in the setting of low-output cardiac failure, immediately leading to dramatic hemodynamic improvement. After further stabilization, transcatheter aortic valve implantation (CoreValve, Medtronic, Minneapolis, Minnesota) was performed several days later. Over the following days LV function recovered to ejection fraction 45%, and hemodynamic status stabilized without the need of vasopressors.

The images demonstrate the pitfalls of nondiagnostic imaging in an emergency situation and how an innovative strategy can help in an unexpected difficult situation.

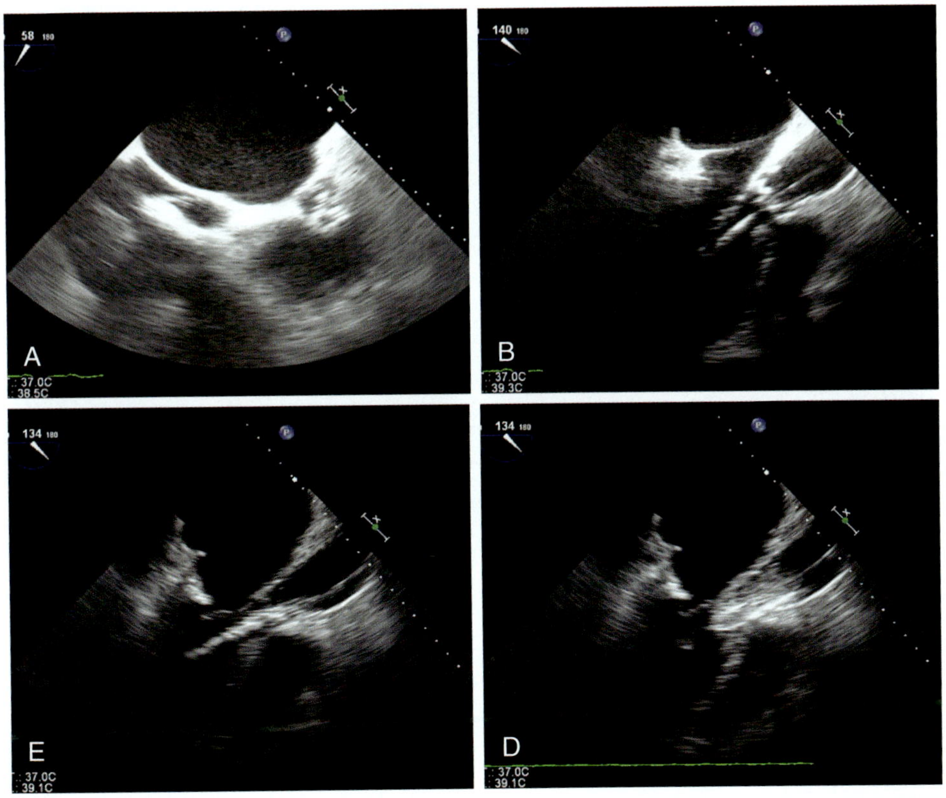

FIG. 4.52 Transesophageal Echocardiography (TEE). (A) Heavily calcified, highly stenosed aortic valve in cross-sectional TEE view. (B) TEE-guided wire placement. (C) TEE-guided placement of valvuloplasty balloon. (D) Balloon inflation.

First Successful Management of Aortic Valve Insufficiency Associated With HeartMate II Left Ventricular Assist Device Support by Transfemoral CoreValve Implantation: Columbus' Egg?

Francesco Santini, MD, Alberto Forni, MD, Rajesh Dandale, MD, Flavio Ribichini, MD, Andrea Rossi, MD, Gianluigi Franchi, MD, Francesco Onorati, MD, Corrado Vassanelli, MD, Alessandro Mazzucco, MD, Giuseppe Faggian, MD

Left ventricular assist device (LVAD) support has offered many individuals with end-stage heart failure an improved quality of life and enhanced survival. Prolonged mechanical assistance, however, has shown the potential to induce hemodynamic and structural changes in the native heart. One such dismal drawback is the development of de novo aortic valve lesions leading to aortic insufficiency (AI). Significant AI can lead to ineffective LVAD output and end-organ malperfusion, and may hamper the success of recovery attempts. If AI at the time of LVAD implantation can be proactively managed by replacement or closure of the aortic valve, later development of aortic valve dysfunction may pose a difficult management issue.

A 53-year-old male patient (height, 190 cm; weight, 90 kg) with end-stage dilated cardiomyopathy was uneventfully implanted with a Thoratec HeartMate II LVAD (Thoratec Corporation, Pleasanton, California) intended as a bridge to transplantation. Ten months postoperatively, he showed progressively worsening AI, requiring hospital readmissions for increased exercise intolerance, desaturation, and arrhythmia. In view of the unfavorable anthropometric characteristics, any attempt to anticipate transplantation was unsuccessful for lack of appropriate donors. Ineffective LVAD output, pulmonary edema with desaturation, and arrhythmia ultimately required endotracheal intubation and cardiopulmonary resuscitation. Because neither optimal medical therapy nor LVAD adjustments provided hemodynamic stability, the heart team decided on emergency lifesaving aortic valve implantation (Fig. 4.53, Online Video 4.46). Transcatheter aortic valve implantation was undertaken with a percutaneous approach through the right femoral artery. Through an 18F introducer, an extra-stiff guidewire was positioned in the left ventricle, and a 29-mm CoreValve (Medtronic, Minneapolis, Minnesota) was implanted under fluoroscopy and echo control. Because of a moderate periprosthetic regurgitation (Fig. 4.54, Online Video 4.47), a second 29-mm CoreValve was deployed within the previous valve prosthesis (Fig. 4.55), with minimal residual leak (Fig. 4.56, Online Video 4.48) and no complications. The femoral access was repaired by the Prostar XL closure device (Abbott Vascular, Santa Clara, California). The patient's hemodynamics improved immediately and led to a successful extubation by postoperative day 1. At the time of discharge, echocardiography displayed very little residual regurgitation. The patient is currently in New York Heart Association functional class II, waiting for heart transplantation.

De novo AI tends to develop and progress with the duration of LVAD support, has a multifactorial etiology, and can lead to ineffective LVAD output and end-organ malperfusion. In our case, transfemoral transcatheter CoreValve implantation resulted in a lifesaving reproducible procedure to manage an acutely developed hemodynamic instability. A longer follow-up and further experience are needed to find out the durability of this combination therapy.

ACKNOWLEDGMENT

The authors wish to thank Francesco Bedogni, MD, Department of Interventional Cardiology, S. Ambrogio Clinical Institute, Milan, Italy, for his technical assistance during the procedure.

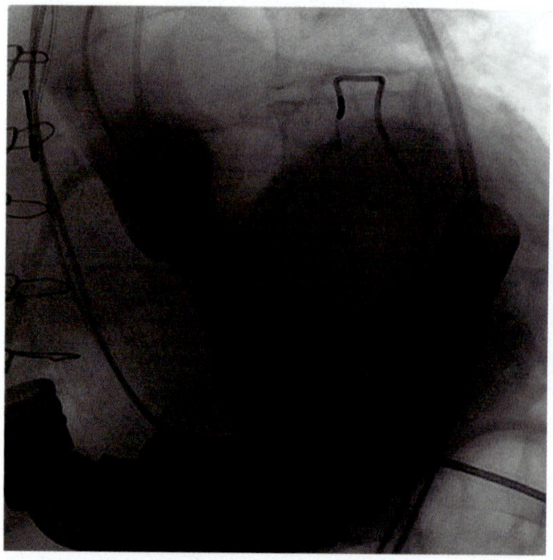

FIG. 4.53 Fluoroscopic View Showing Severe Aortic Valve Regurgitation Along With the HeartMate II Device. See also Online Video 4.46.

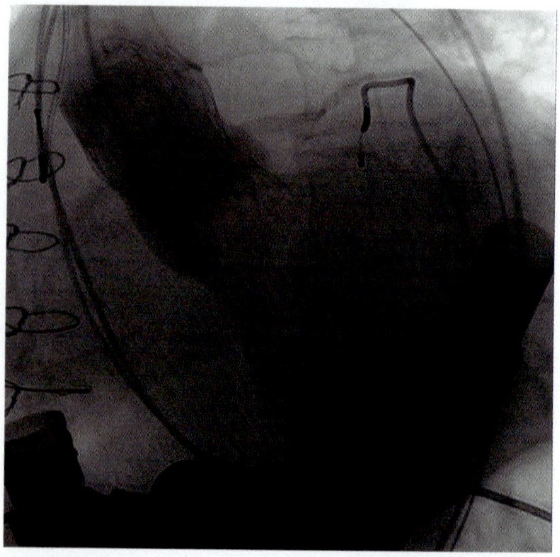

FIG. 4.54 Fluoroscopic View Showing Moderate Periprosthetic Aortic Valve Regurgitation. See also Online Video 4.47.

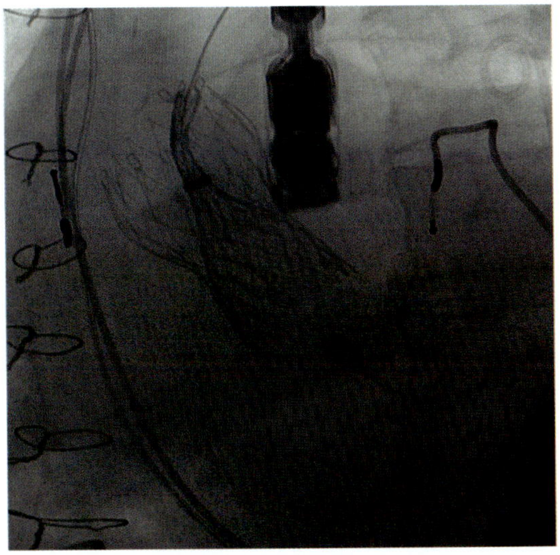

FIG. 4.55 Fluoroscopic View Showing Second 29-mm CoreValve Deployment Within the Previous Valve Prosthesis.

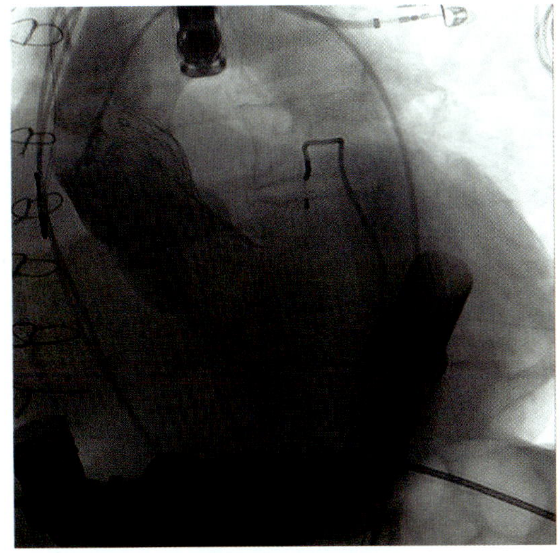

FIG. 4.56 Fluoroscopic View Showing Reduced Periprosthetic Aortic Valve Regurgitation. See also Online Video 4.48.

Hyperacute Valve Thrombosis After Transapical Transcatheter Aortic Valve Replacement in a Patient With Polycythemia Vera

Augusto D'Onofrio, MD, PhD, Stefania Rizzo, MD, PhD, Laura Besola, MD, Giambattista Isabella, MD, Valerio Rancitelli, MD, Maria Luigia Randi, MD, PhD, Elena Campello, MD, Gianclaudio Falasco, MD, Cristina Basso, MD, PhD, Gaetano Thiene, MD, Gino Gerosa, MD

An 86-year-old woman with polycythemia vera (high allele burden of JAK2 V617F mutation, 95.3%) was referred for pulmonary edema due to severe aortic valve stenosis and was scheduled for transapical transcatheter aortic valve replacement. Because hydroxyurea administration was interrupted because of retromalleolar ulcers, preoperative blood examinations showed severe thrombocytosis (1500 $\times 10^9$/L) and neutrophilic leukocytosis (24.6 $\times$ 10^9/l). Multiplate impedance aggregometry showed a slight increase in platelet aggregation with the ASPItest and the ADPtest and aggregation within normal limits with the TRAPtest (all by Roche Diagnostics, Rotkreuz, Switzerland); thromboelastometry showed increased maximal cloth firmness with the FIBTEM test and normal maximal cloth firmness with the EXTEM and with the INTEM tests (TEM International GmbH, Basel, Switzerland). The patient was not receiving anticoagulant agents or antiplatelet drugs, because an extremely high platelet count may lead to hemorrhagic complications because of acquired von Willebrand disease.[1] Transapical transcatheter aortic valve replacement with a SAPIEN 3 valve bioprosthesis (Edwards Lifesciences, Irvine, California) was performed with a good final result. Six hours later, the patient's hemodynamic status suddenly deteriorated, necessitating cardiopulmonary resuscitation. Transesophageal echocardiography showed massive thrombosis of the aortic valve bioprosthesis with severely reduced leaflet excursion (Fig. 4.57A, Online Video 4.49). Percutaneous femorofemoral extracorporeal membrane oxygenation was positioned, but in a few minutes, acute thrombosis of the oxygenator occurred, necessitating complete heparinization and emergency replacement of the whole circuit. Coronary angiography was performed and showed patent coronary ostia with distal coronary embolization in the left anterior descending coronary artery (Fig. 4.57B, Online Video 4.50). Despite maximal support, the patient died a few hours later of massive cerebral hemorrhage. At autopsy, the leaflets of the SAPIEN 3 bioprosthesis were blocked by massive white thrombosis, on both the aortic and ventricular sides[2–4] (Fig. 4.57C). The bioprosthesis was well seated in the aortic root, without either coronary ostia obstruction or paravalvular leaks. On histologic examination, the thrombus consisted predominantly of platelet aggregates in a fibrin network (Fig. 4.57D). Occluding platelet emboli were found in the distal intramural small vessels of the anteroseptal ventricular myocardium.

References

1. Federici AB. Acquired von Willebrand syndrome: an underdiagnosed and misdiagnosed bleeding complication in patients with lymphoproliferative and myeloproliferative disorders. *Semin Hematol.* 2006;43:S48-S58.
2. Makkar RR, Fontana G, Jilaihawi H, et al. Possible subclinical leaflet thrombosis in bioprosthetic aortic valves. *N Engl J Med.* 2015;373:2015-2024.
3. Lima B, Soltesz E. Management of extensive intracardiac thrombosis in a patient with polycythemia vera undergoing coronary artery bypass grafting. *J Card Surg.* 2012;27:320-322.
4. Thiene G, Bortolotti U, Panizzon G, et al. Pathological substrates of thrombus formation after heart valve replacement with the Hancock bioprosthesis. *J Thorac Cardiovasc Surg.* 1980;80:414-423.

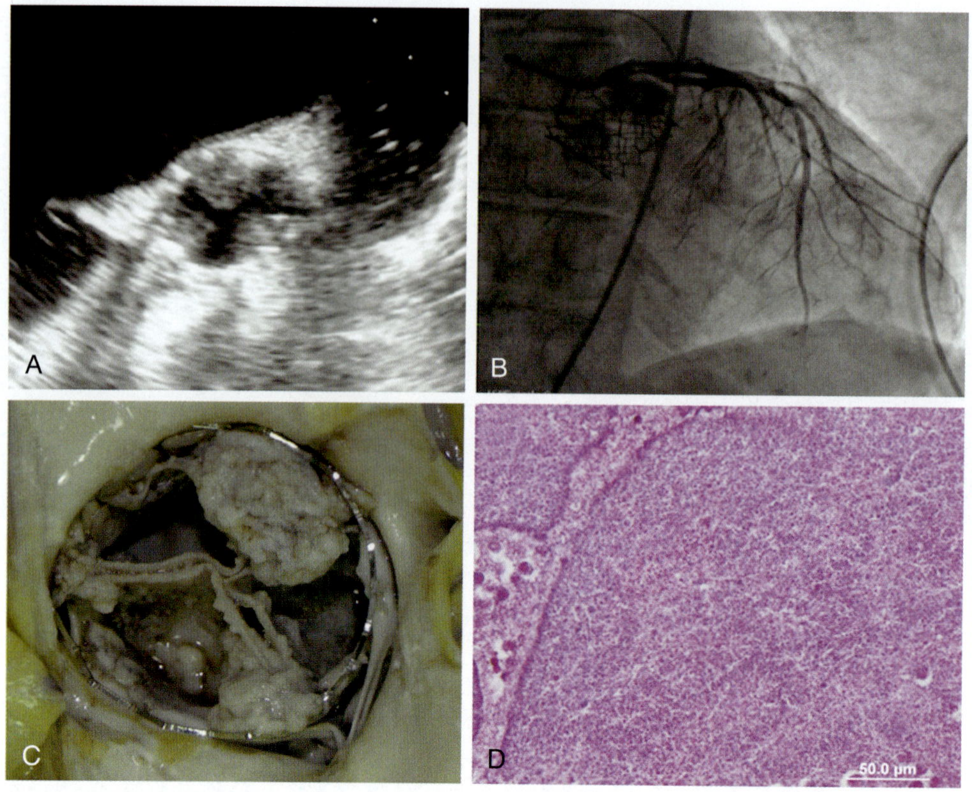

FIG. 4.57 Postoperative Imaging and Postmortem Heart Findings. (A) Short axis view of the aortic valve with transesophageal echocardiography showing severe thrombosis of the three leaflets of the SAPIEN 3 valve (Edwards Lifesciences, Irvine, California) (Online Video 4.49). (B) Coronary artery angiography showing distal embolic occlusion of the left anterior descending coronary artery (Online Video 4.50). (C) Arterial view of the aortic bioprosthesis showing massive white thrombotic vegetations blocking the valve leaflets. (D) On histologic examination, the thrombotic material was composed of an admixture of fibrin with abundant platelets aggregates (trichrome stain).

Left Ventricular Embolization of an Aortic Balloon-Expandable Bioprosthesis: Balloon Capture and Reimpaction as an Alternative to Emergent Conversion to Open-Heart Surgery

Nicolas Dumonteil, MD, Bertrand Marcheix, MD, PhD, Etienne Grunenwald, MD, Jérôme Roncalli, MD, PhD, Pierre Massabuau, MD, Didier Carrié, MD, PhD

An 83-year-old man with severe symptomatic aortic stenosis, deemed to be at high risk for conventional surgery (Logistic EuroSCORE [European System for Cardiac Operative Risk Evaluation] 26.63%, Society of Thoracic Surgeons score 7.2%) was referred to our institution for a transcatheter aortic valve implantation. A transapical approach was chosen because his anatomic features were not suitable for transarterial access. The aortic annulus measured by transesophageal echocardiography (TEE) was 23.8 mm (Fig. 4.58).

A 26-mm Edwards SAPIEN valve (Edwards Lifesciences, Irvine, California) was implanted with fluoroscopy and TEE guidance with one-step inflation, as previously described.[1] Although there were no technical problems during deployment, the prosthesis embolized into the left ventricle a few seconds after hemodynamic recovery (Fig. 4.59A, Online Video 4.51). The stiff wire was kept in place, preventing the prosthesis from rotating and obstructing the left ventricular outflow tract (Fig. 4.59B). Because conventional surgery had been declined for this patient, we tried to find an interventional solution.

An oversized 28-mm aortic valvuloplasty balloon was placed over the stiff wire and partially inflated during rapid-pacing bursts once its distal part was in the prosthesis. After a few attempts the prosthesis was captured. It was then pushed into the aortic annulus, and because it was possible to reposition it, it was fixed by a full 5-s inflation in a stable, high position (Fig. 4.60A–B, Online Video 4.52) but with a severe paravalvular regurgitation (Fig. 4.60C). A second 26-mm SAPIEN valve was then implanted deeper into the first one with an overlay of four-fifths to the previous prosthesis (Fig. 4.61A). Final TEE showed a good prosthesis function, with a mild

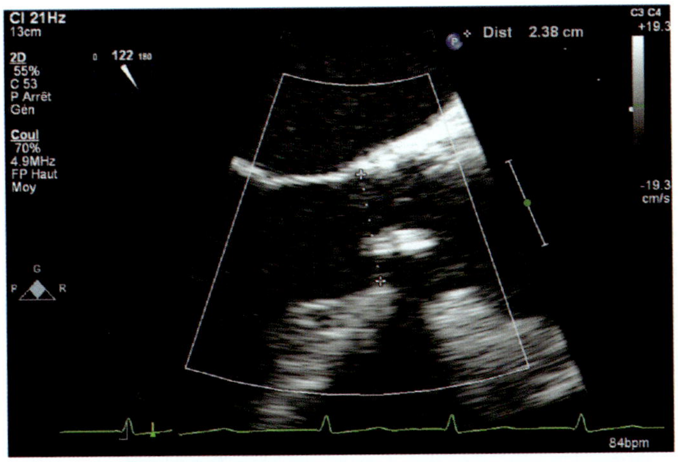

FIG. 4.58 Preprocedural Transesophageal Echocardiography (TEE) Aortic Annulus Measurement. Two-dimensional 120° TEE view, aortic annulus measured at 23.8 mm.

paravalvular leak (Fig. 4.61B). Postoperative course was uneventful. At the 1-month follow-up, the patient was in New York Heart Association functional class II. Transthoracic echocardiography showed an effective orifice area of 1.3 cm^2, a mean gradient of 12 mm Hg, and a mild paravalvular leak.

To the best of our knowledge, this is the first case that demonstrates the feasibility of recapturing a balloon-expandable prosthesis after left ventricular embolization. Among various potential causes of such a complication,[2] mild valve calcifications and a possible underestimation of the true annular size by TEE are the most likely. A multimodal annulus sizing with a computed tomography scan[3] could have been helpful but was not included in our selection process at this time before balloon-expandable prosthesis implantation.

References

1. Walther T, Dewey T, Borger MA, et al. Transapical aortic valve implantation: step by step. *Ann Thorac Surg.* 2009;87:276-283.
2. Al Ali AM, Altwegg L, Horlick EM, et al. Prevention and management of transcatheter balloon-expandable aortic valve malposition. Catheter *Cardiovasc Interv.* 2008;72:573-578.
3. Jilaihawi H, Kashif M, Fontana G, et al. Cross-sectional computed tomographic assessment improves accuracy of aortic annular sizing for transcatheter aortic valve replacement and reduces the incidence of paravalvular aortic regurgitation. *J Am Coll Cardiol.* 2012;59:1275-1286.

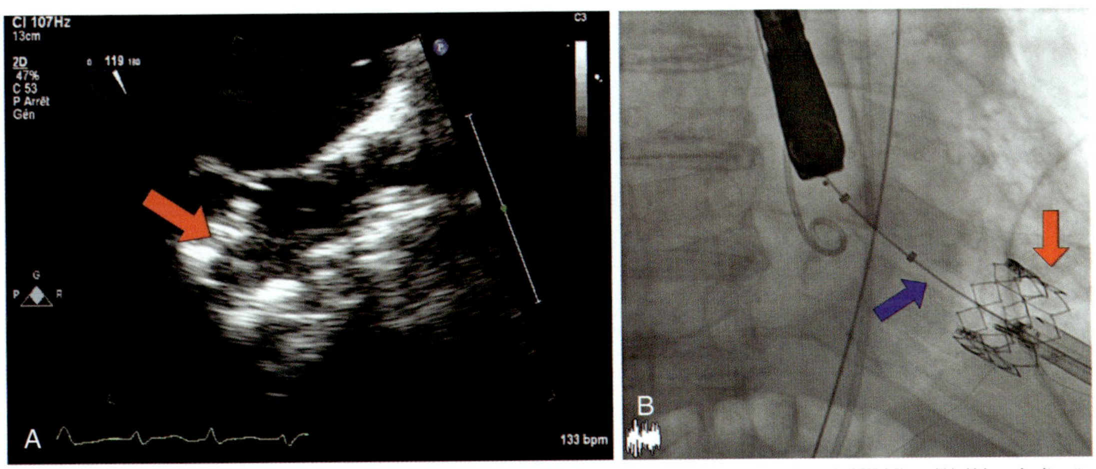

FIG. 4.59 Left Ventricular (LV) Embolization of Prosthesis and Prosthesis Stabilized With Stiff Wire (A) LV embolization of the prosthesis. Two-dimensional 120° transesophageal echocardiography view showing the balloon-expandable prosthesis (*red arrow*) after embolization in the LV. (B) Prosthesis stabilized with stiff wire. Fluoroscopic screen capture showing the balloon-expandable prosthesis (*red arrow*) stabilized in the LV by stiff wire (*blue arrow*) (Online Video 4.51).

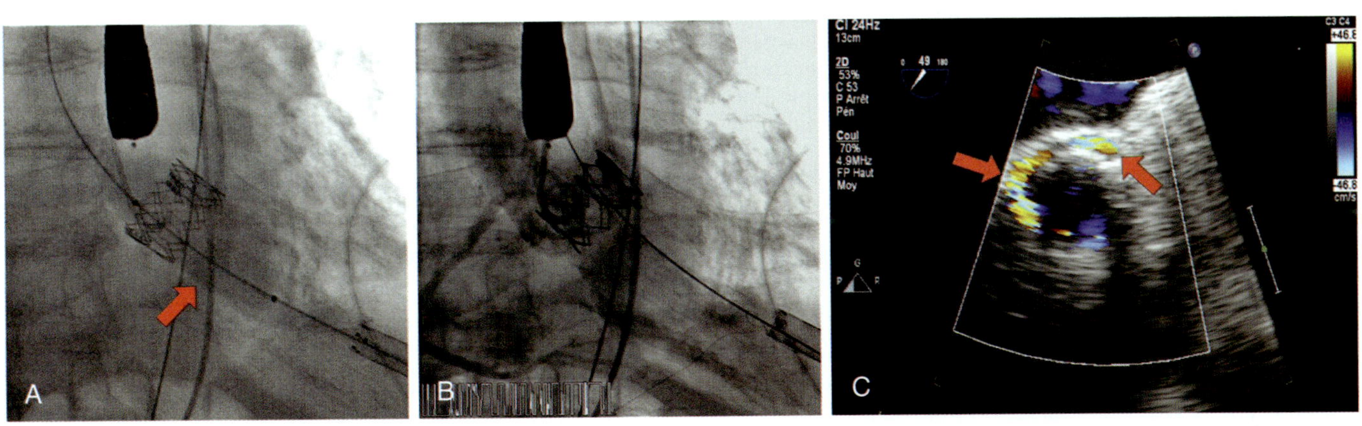

FIG. 4.60 Balloon Capture and Aortography and Paravalvular Aortic Regurgitation (PAR) Assessment After Repositioning of Prosthesis. (A) Balloon capture of the prosthesis. Capture of the prosthesis with a 28-mm aortic valvuloplasty balloon (*red arrow*) inflated during rapid-pacing bursts to push and reposition the prosthesis into the aortic annulus. (B) Aortography after the repositioning of the prosthesis. Repositioning of the prosthesis in a final high position, with severe paravalvular regurgitation. (C) PAR assessment after repositioning the prosthesis. Short axis transesophageal echocardiography view with color Doppler imaging showing a severe PAR with a >20% circumferential extent of the regurgitant flow (*red arrows*) (Online Video 4.52).

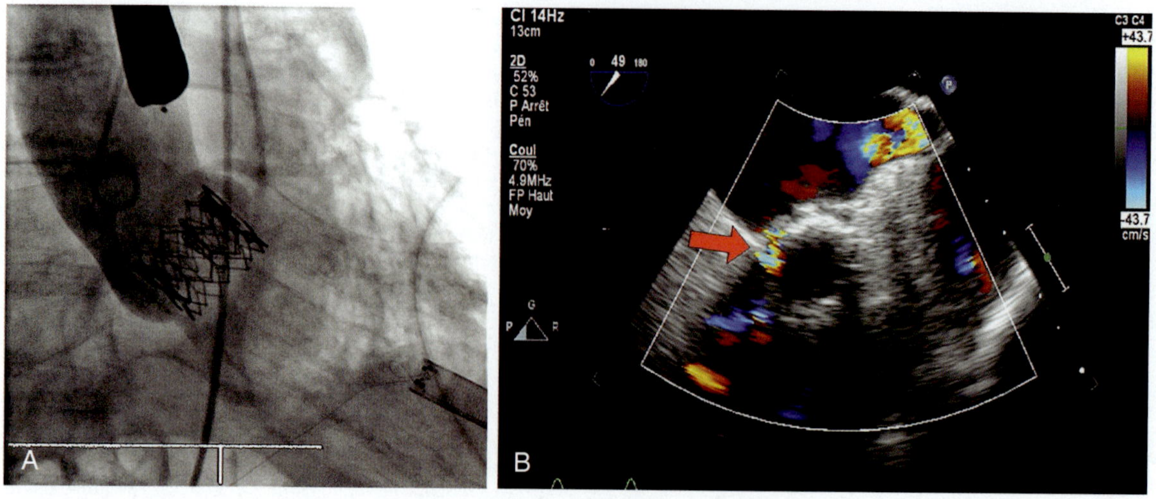

FIG. 4.61 Final Aortography and Paravalvular Aortic Regurgitation (PAR) Assessment After Second Prosthesis Deployment. (A) Final aortography after the second prosthesis deployment. Second prosthesis deployed deeper, with a four-fifths overlay to the first one. Good final position with mild regurgitation. (B) PAR assessment after deployment of the second prosthesis. Short axis transesophageal echocardiography view with color-Doppler imaging showing final mild PAR with a <10% circumferential extent of the regurgitant flow (*red arrow*).

Transcatheter Treatment of Subaortic Stenosis via Transcaval Access

Norihiko Kamioka, MD, Ateet Patel, MD, Stamatios Lerakis, MD, Ioannis Parastatidis, MD, Jessica Forcillo, MD, Frank Corrigan, MD, Vinod Thourani, MD, Peter Block, MD, Vasilis Babaliaros, MD

A 34-year-old woman with Down syndrome with a history of an atrioventricular canal repair and a mechanical mitral valve replacement came to our hospital because of worsening symptoms of heart failure. Echocardiography and computed tomography imaging revealed a thickened bicuspid aortic valve without significant stenosis and discrete subaortic stenosis (SAS) (mean pressure gradient, 67.4 mm Hg) despite resection of subvalvular membrane at her last surgery 11 years prior (Fig. 4.62A–B, Online Video 4.53). Because of her significant cognitive impairment and two prior sternotomies, she was deemed a poor surgical candidate. Transcatheter treatment, using the same technique as transcatheter aortic valve replacement, was planned for SAS. Multidetector computed tomography revealed her arterial access was inadequate for traditional transfemoral access or transsubclavian access. Again because of her cognitive impairment, other surgical alternative access options (transaortic, transapical, and transcarotid) were not attempted, and therefore the procedure was performed via transcaval access.[1,2]

The procedure was performed under general anesthesia in the catheterization laboratory. A Confianza Pro wire (Abbott Vascular, Santa Clara, California) was crossed into the aorta (Fig. 4.62C–D, Online Video 4.54) and subsequently exchanged to a Lunderquist wire (Cook Medical, Bloomington, Indiana). After the establishment of transcaval access, a 14F sheath was advanced from the right femoral vein into the aorta. After balloon valvuloplasty with a 20-mm Z-MED balloon (NuMED, Hopkinton, New York) to confirm the position of the stenosis (Fig. 4.62E, Online Video 4.55), a 23-mm SAPIEN 3 valve (Edwards Lifesciences, Irvine, California) was deployed covering the stenosis with neither paravalvular leakage nor interference of the mitral valve (Fig. 4.62F, Online Video 4.56). Aortocaval fistula was closed with a 10/8-mm Amplatzer duct occluder (St. Jude Medical, St. Paul, Minnesota) (Fig. 4.62G–H, Online Video 4.57). The mean gradient had improved to 12.6 mm Hg (Fig. 4.62G–H, Online Video 4.58). The patient was discharged with symptom relief on postoperative day 1.

SAS is often observed in patients with congenital heart disease. Although surgical treatment for SAS remains the gold standard for therapy, reoperation rates are high.[3–5] We demonstrated the feasibility of transcatheter treatment as an alternative therapy for SAS in patients with very high surgical risk.

References

1. Lederman RJ, Babaliaros VC, Greenbaum AB. How to perform transcaval access and closure for transcatheter aortic valve implantation. *Catheter Cardiovasc Interv.* 2015;86:1242-1254.
2. Greenbaum AB, O'Neill WW, Paone G, et al. Caval-aortic access to allow transcatheter aortic valve replacement in otherwise ineligible patients: initial human experience. *J Am Coll Cardiol.* 2014;63:2795-2804.
3. Erentug V, Bozbuga N, Kirali K, et al. Surgical treatment of subaortic obstruction in adolescent and adults: long-term follow-up. *J Card Surg.* 2005;20:16-21.
4. Dorobantu DM, Sharabiani MT, Martin RP, et al. Surgery for simple and complex subaortic stenosis in children and young adults: results from a prospective, procedure-based national database. *J Thorac Cardiovasc Surg.* 2014;148:2618-2626.
5. Stassano P, Di Tommaso L, Contaldo A, et al. Discrete subaortic stenosis: long-term prognosis on the progression of the obstruction and of the aortic insufficiency. *Thorac Cardiovasc Surg.* 2005; 53:23-27.

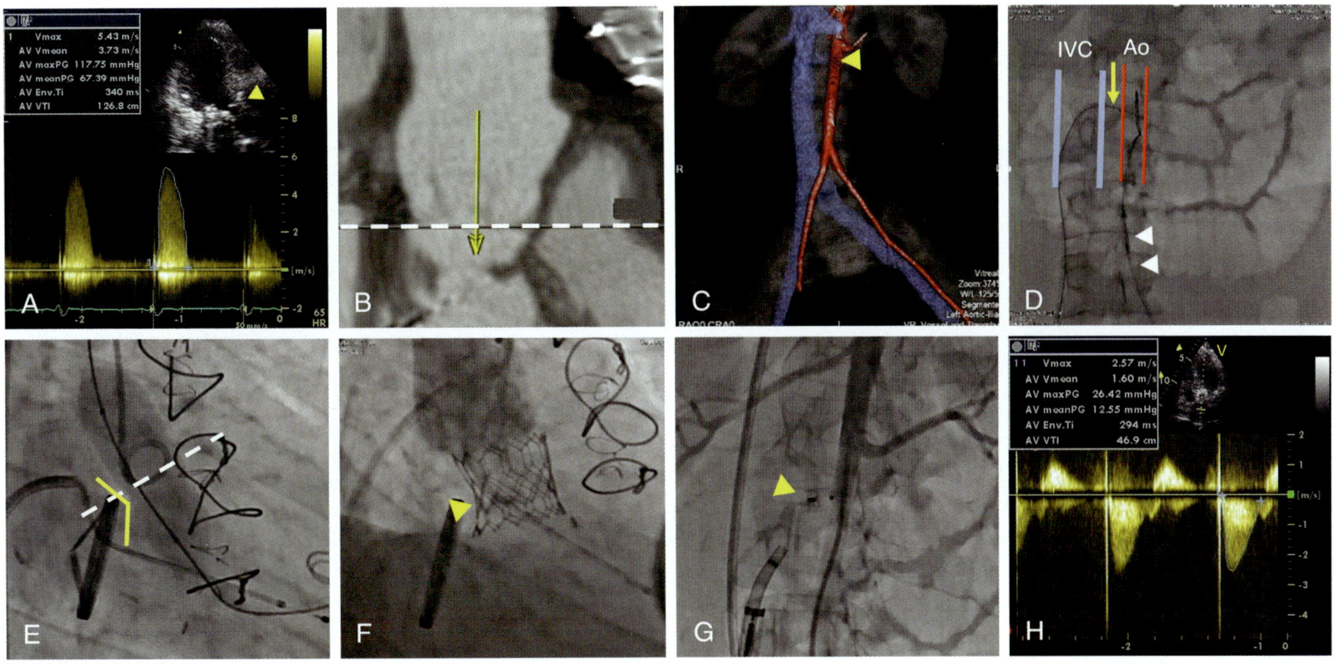

FIG. 4.62 Transcatheter Treatment of Subaortic Stenosis via Transcaval Access. (A) The mean gradient had improved to 67.4 mm Hg. Transthoracic echocardiography identified subaortic stenosis (*arrowhead*) (Online Video 4.53). (B) Multidetector computed tomography revealed subaortic stenosis (*arrow*) under the annulus plane (*dashed line*). (C) Puncture point was located near the top of the second lumbar vertebrae (*arrowhead*). (D) A Confianza Pro guidewire (Abbott Vascular, Santa Clara, California) (*arrow*) was crossed from the inferior vena cava (*IVC*) into the aorta (*Ao*) toward a snare catheter (*arrowheads*) (Online Video 4.54). (E) Remaining indentation of the balloon indicated location of the subaortic stenosis (along with *yellow line*) under annulus plane (*dashed line*) (Online Video 4.55). (F) A SAPIEN 3 valve (Edwards Lifesciences, Irvine, California) was deployed covering the stenosis (*arrowhead*) without paravalvular leakage (Online Video 4.56). (G) Aortocaval fistula was closed with an Amplatzer duct occluder (St. Jude Medical, St. Paul, Minnesota) (*arrowhead*) (Online Video 4.57). (H) The mean gradient had improved to 12.6 mm Hg without interference of the mitral valve (Online Video 4.58).

Transfemoral Transcatheter Aortic Valve Implantation in the Presence of Mitral and Tricuspid Prostheses

Iraj Nazeri, MD, Seifollah Abdi, MD, Mohammad Hossein Mandegar, MD, Farideh Roshanali, MD, Payman Shahabi, MD

A 53-year-old woman presented to our center with progressive fatigue and dyspnea on exertion (New York Heart Association functional class III). The patient's medical history was significant for multiple cardiac interventions: open mitral commissurotomy for the treatment of rheumatic mitral stenosis 30 years earlier, mitral valve replacement for the treatment of severe mitral regurgitation at age 25 years, and tricuspid valve implantation for the treatment of rheumatic tricuspid valve regurgitation and stenosis 5 years earlier. She had also undergone several noncardiac surgeries: trauma-related splenectomy 30 years earlier, partial meniscectomy 27 years earlier, tibial external fixation 10 years earlier, and Billroth II procedure for the treatment of peptic ulcer 5 years earlier. At the time of presentation, she was also under medical treatment for hypothyroidism and depression.

Transesophageal echocardiographic (TEE) assessment revealed severe aortic stenosis (mean systolic gradient, 47 mm Hg; peak gradient, 98 mm Hg; aortic valve area, 0.7 cm^2; valve annulus, 20 mm), moderate aortic regurgitation, functionally normal mitral and tricuspid prosthetic valves, severe pulmonary hypertension (mean pulmonary artery pressure, 68 mm Hg), and moderately reduced left ventricular function (ejection fraction, 35%). Selective coronary angiogram revealed normal coronaries.

Because of excessive surgical risk with conventional aortic valve replacement (logistic EuroSCORE [European System for Cardiac Operative Risk Evaluation] of 15.23%), the patients was scheduled for transfemoral transcatheter aortic valve implantation. The procedure was performed under general anesthesia and as previously described.[1] Briefly, after aortography, balloon valvuloplasty of the native aortic valve was performed under rapid ventricular pacing; subsequently a 23-mm Edwards SAPIEN aortic valve (Edwards Lifesciences, Irvine, California) was implanted at the aortic annulus (Fig. 4.63). The procedure was performed without any complications, and postprocedure and predischarge TEE revealed normal aortic prosthetic valve function (peak gradient, 12 mm Hg; aortic valve area, 2.2 cm^2) with no residual aortic paravalvular leaks. The patient was discharged on postprocedural day 5; her in-hospital stay had been uneventful.

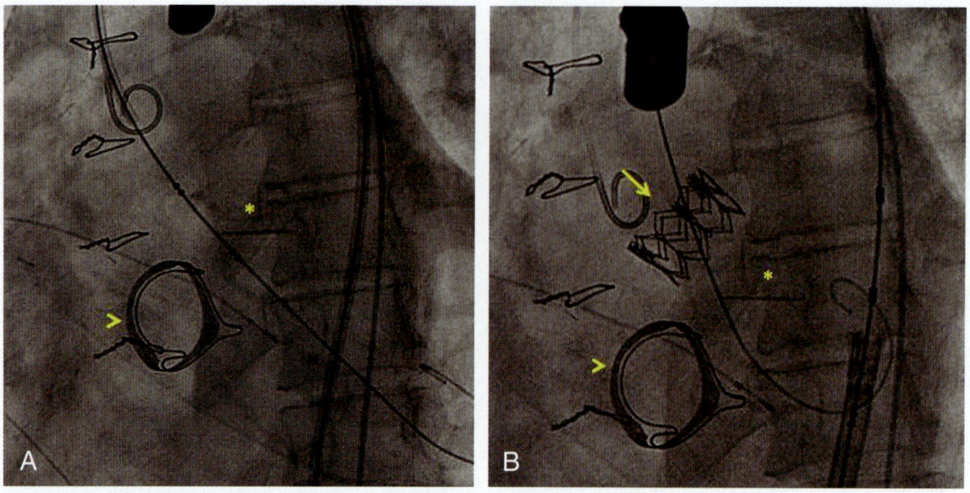

FIG. 4.63 Fluoroscopy Before and After Transfemoral Aortic Valve Implantation. Fluoroscopic images before (A) and after (B) transfemoral aortic valve deployment depicting the prosthetic tricuspid valve (*arrowhead*) and mitral prosthesis (*asterisk*). The *arrow* indicates the prosthetic aortic valve.

At 6-month and 1-year follow-up, echocardiographic evaluation revealed normal left ventricular function (ejection fraction, 55%) and the appropriate position and normal function of all three prosthetic valves. At these times, she was symptom free and was in New York Heart Association functional class I.

Reference

1. Cribier A, Eltchaninoff H, Bash A, et al. Percutaneous transcatheter implantation of an aortic valve prosthesis for calcific aortic stenosis: first human case description. *Circulation.* 2002;106:3006-3008.

Mitral Valve

Backward Migration of a MitraClip Through a Patent Transseptal Orifice: The Salmon Syndrome

Christophe Caussin, MD, Christelle Diakov, MD, Patrice Dervanian, MD, Nicolas Amabile, MD, PhD

A 70-year-old man with severe mitral regurgitation (MR) was referred to our institution for percutaneous mitral valve repair. A MitraClip (Abbott Vascular, Abbott Park, Illinois) was implanted but did not correctly tether the posterior leaflet and was solely attached to the anterior leaflet. A second clip was thus implanted to stabilize the first clip. However, a residual severe eccentric MR was still present on final transesophageal echocardiographic control, after full retraction of the delivery system (Fig. 4.64A–B).

Although the patient was asymptomatic, transthoracic echocardiography revealed dislodgment of clip 1 on day 2. A computed tomography scan without contrast revealed the device's presence within the right renal hilum (Fig. 4.64C). Selective renal arteriography and phlebography localized the detached clip in the right ostial renal vein (Fig. 4.64D–E, Online Videos 4.59 and 4.60). The device was successfully retrieved using a double-snare technique through an 18F sheath (Fig. 4.64F1–F3, Online Videos 4.61 and 4.62).

The patient underwent surgical MR correction. Periprocedural analysis revealed a large interatrial defect, a diffuse hematoma on the anterior leaflet, and a tear on the initial clip tethering zone (Fig. 4.64G1–G2). The patient benefited from a bioprosthesis implantation with a subsequent uneventful clinical course. The most plausible hypothesis explaining this case is a primary leaflet tear induced by the clip, followed by its migration toward the right atrium through the transseptal puncture orifice and, finally, backward migration within the inferior vena cava.

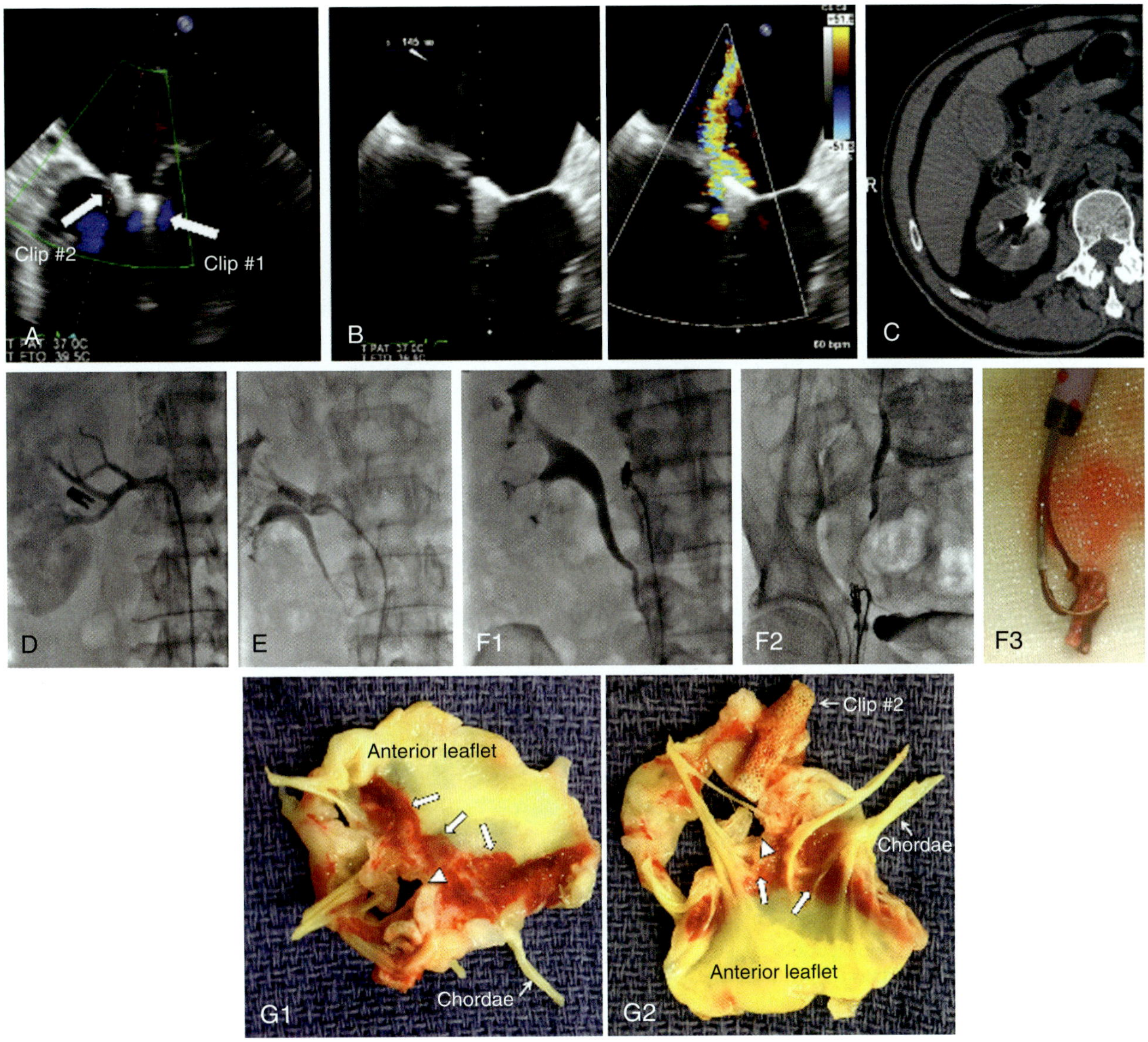

FIG. 4.64 Different Steps in Mitral Clip Implantation and Retrieval. (A and B) Postprocedural transesophageal echocardiographic views showing the presence of two MitraClips (*arrows*). (C) Computed tomography scan localized the detached clip in the right renal hilum. Selective renal arteriography (D) (Online Video 4.59) and phlebography (E) (Online Video 4.60) localized the clip in the right ostial renal vein. (F1–F3) Clip extraction through the venous femoral vein (Online Videos 4.61 and 4.62). Mitral valve gross pathology examination (G1, atrial view; G2, ventricular view) showing a hematoma related to tethering attempts (*white arrows*) and a leaflet tear (*white arrowhead*) on clip 1 at the previous implantation site.

Bioprosthetic Leaflet Erosion After Percutaneous Mitral Paravalvular Leak Closure

Jason H. Rogers, MD, Allen S. Morris, MD, Patricia A. Takeda, MD, Reginald I. Low, MD

Transcatheter closure of prosthetic paravalvular leaks is increasingly performed at experienced centers.[1–3] The lack of devices dedicated to paravalvular leak closure has not deterred the off-label use of various occluder devices. These images illustrate the potential complexity of transcatheter paravalvular leak repair with the need for additional occluder placement, and the development of severe leaflet erosion from occluder contact.

A 72-year-old woman who developed acute mitral regurgitation (MR) and cardiogenic shock in December 2006 underwent emergency mitral valve replacement with a No. 25 Hancock II bioprosthetic valve (Medtronic, Minneapolis, Minnesota) complicated by postoperative adult respiratory distress syndrome, mitral paravalvular leak, hemolytic anemia, and recurrent congestive heart failure. In April 2007, she had transcatheter mitral paravalvular leak closure at

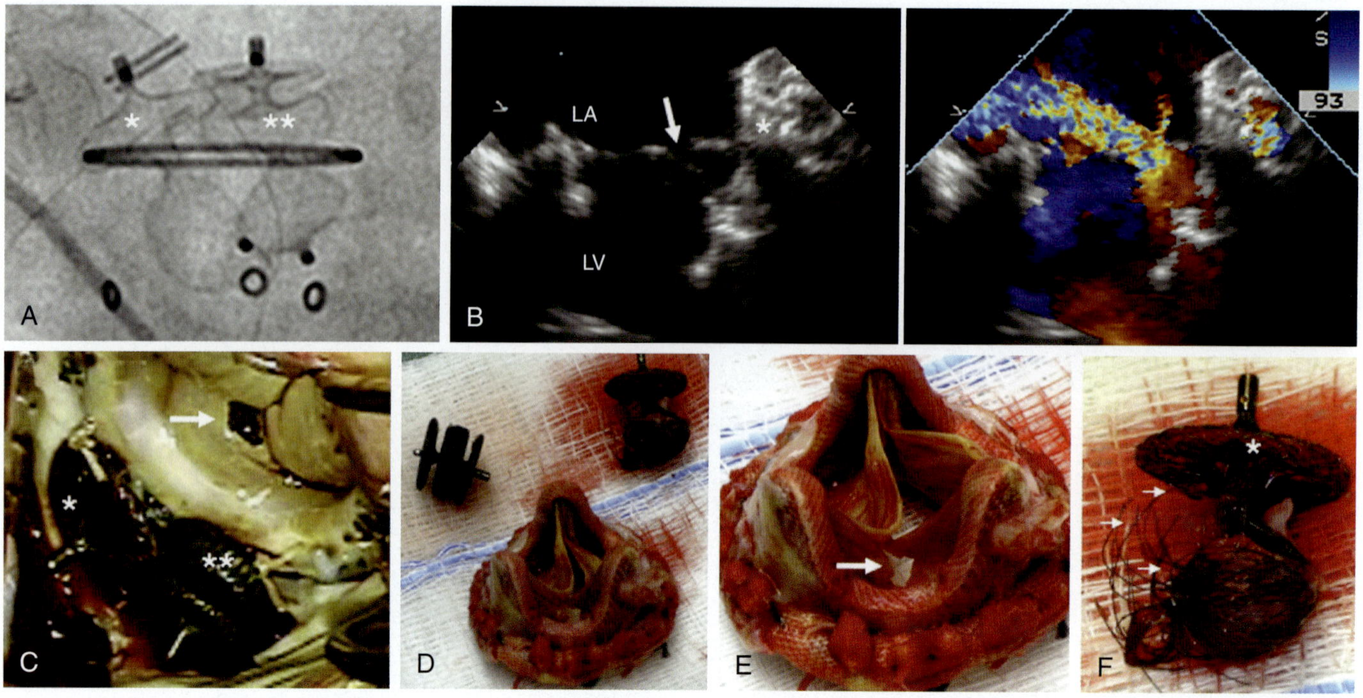

FIG. 4.65 Bioprosthetic Mitral Valvular Leaflet Erosion After Transcatheter Paravalvular Leak Closure. (A) Fluoroscopic view of adjacent Amplatzer atrial septal occluder (*ASO*) (*single asterisk*) and Amplatzer vascular plug II (*AVP*) (*double asterisk*) occluding the mitral paravalvular leak. (B) Transesophageal echocardiographic images demonstrating leaflet perforation (*arrow*) from the ASO (*asterisk*), which protrudes in the left ventricular (*LV*) cavity. Note severe regurgitant jet through the leaflet. *LA*, left atrial. (C) LA intraoperative view of adjacent occluder devices and valve. The ASO (*asterisk*) and AVP *double asterisk* are shown, as is the eroded posterolateral leaflet (*arrow*). The ventricular aspect of the ASO is visible through the defect in the leaflet. (D) Excised valve and devices, showing relative sizes. (E) Close-up of ventricular aspect of excised valve showing large erosion defect in the posterior leaflet (*arrow*). (F) ASO with LA disc (asterisk) and deformed ventricular disk with multiple wire fractures (*small arrows*). See Online Videos 4.63 and 4.64.

an outside facility using an 8-mm Amplatzer atrial septal occluder (AGA Medical Corp., Plymouth, Minnesota), with reduction in the MR as well as improvement in hemolytic anemia and congestive symptoms. In May 2008, she had progressive paravalvular leak adjacent to the original occluder with recurrent congestive heart failure, left pleural effusion, and hemolysis. Because of her high risk for reoperation, she underwent successful percutaneous closure of the remaining lateral paravalvular leak with placement of a 12-mm Amplatzer vascular plug II (AGA Medical Corp.). At that time, transesophageal echocardiography showed that the posterior bioprosthetic leaflet was contacting the previously deployed Amplatzer device during diastole, resulting in moderate valvular MR.

Although the patient was initially well compensated, she developed increasing symptomatic valvular MR and 1 year later underwent open surgical mitral valve replacement with a No. 27 Carpentier-Edwards Magna ThermaFix pericardial valve (Edwards Lifesciences, Irvine, California), as well as bioprosthetic aortic valve replacement for moderate central aortic insufficiency. Intraoperative inspection of the bioprosthetic mitral valve revealed the occluder devices in place, but with significant fractures seen in the first occluder, which was contacting the posterior leaflet, resulting in severe leaflet erosion and perforation (Fig. 4.65, Online Videos 4.63 and 4.64). The patient's recovery was uneventful.

References

1. Kim MS, Casserly IP, Garcia JA, Klein AJ, Salcedo EE, Carroll JD. Percutaneous transcatheter closure of prosthetic mitral paravalvular leaks: are we there yet? *JACC Cardiovasc Interv.* 2009;2:81-90.
2. Pate GE, Al Zubaidi A, Chandavimol M, Thompson CR, Munt BI, Webb JG. Percutaneous closure of prosthetic paravalvular leaks: case series and review. *Catheter Cardiovasc Interv.* 2006;68:528-533.
3. Sorajja P, Cabalka AK, Hagler DJ, et al. Successful percutaneous repair of perivalvular prosthetic regurgitation. *Catheter Cardiovasc Interv.* 2007;70:815-823.

Percutaneous Closure of a Delayed Left Ventricular Pseudoaneurysm After Transseptal Transcatheter Mitral Valve Replacement

Neal Sawlani, MD, MPH, Natalia Berry, MD, MBA, Piotr Sobieszczyk, MD, Tsuyoshi Kaneko, MD, Marc Pelletier, MD, Pinak Shah, MD

A 65-year-old woman underwent transseptal transcatheter mitral valve-in-valve replacement (TMVR) with a 29-mm SAPIEN 3 valve (Edwards Lifesciences, Irvine, California). A hand-curved, Amplatz Super-Stiff wire (Boston Scientific, Marlborough, Massachusetts) was used for valve delivery. The patient was discharged 4 days later and remained free from hospital readmission. However, routine echocardiography 8 months afterward revealed a left ventricle pseudoaneurysm (PSA) that had grown in size to 3.0 cm × 3.4 cm × 2.6 cm with a 1.4-cm × 1.6-cm neck (Fig. 4.66A–D). A multidisciplinary heart team evaluation determined that attempt at percutaneous closure was the most appropriate course of action. The procedure was performed in a hybrid operating room with a plan to convert to open surgery if necessary. An Agilis NxT steerable catheter (St. Jude Medical, St. Paul, Minnesota) was placed through the previous atrial septostomy to deploy a closure device transseptally. However, ventriculography performed through a pigtail catheter suggested that a retrograde approach provided a more favorable deployment angle. Thus, a 9F Amplatzer TorqVue (St. Jude Medical) delivery sheath was inserted across the aortic valve and a 16-mm Amplatzer muscular ventricular septal defect occluder (St. Jude Medical) was deployed in the PSA neck (Fig. 4.66E–F, Online Video 4.65). An echocardiogram 3 months later confirmed successful closure (Fig. 4.66G–H).

Left ventricular PSA is a rare complication after transcatheter valve replacement, with most reports implicating transapical access as the proximate cause.[1–4] Improvements in transcatheter design have allowed for a preliminary experience with TMVR, though procedural and device limitations exist. To our knowledge, this represents the first report of delayed left ventricular PSA after TMVR without transapical access. The use of a prior atrial septostomy for pigtail ventriculography facilitates placement of a closure device and should be considered when attempting percutaneous ventricular PSA closure after transseptal TMVR.

References

1. Feldman T, Pearson P, Smart SS. Percutaneous closure of post TAVR LV apical pseudoaneurysm. *Catheter Cardiovasc Interv.* 2016;88:479-485.
2. Salaun E, Aldebert P, Jaussaud N, et al. Early endocarditis and delayed left ventricular pseudoaneurysm complicating a transapical transcatheter mitral valve-in-valve implantation. *Circ Cardiovasc Interv.* 2016;9:e003886.
3. Narayan RL, Vaishnava P, Goldman ME, et al. Percutaneous closure of left ventricular pseudoaneurysm. *Ann Thorac Surg.* 2012;94: e123-e125.
4. Noack T, Kiefer P, Mohr FW, et al. Late left ventricular pseudoaneurysm following trans-femoral transcatheter aortic valve replacement. *Eur J Cardiothorac Surg.* 2015;48:172-173.

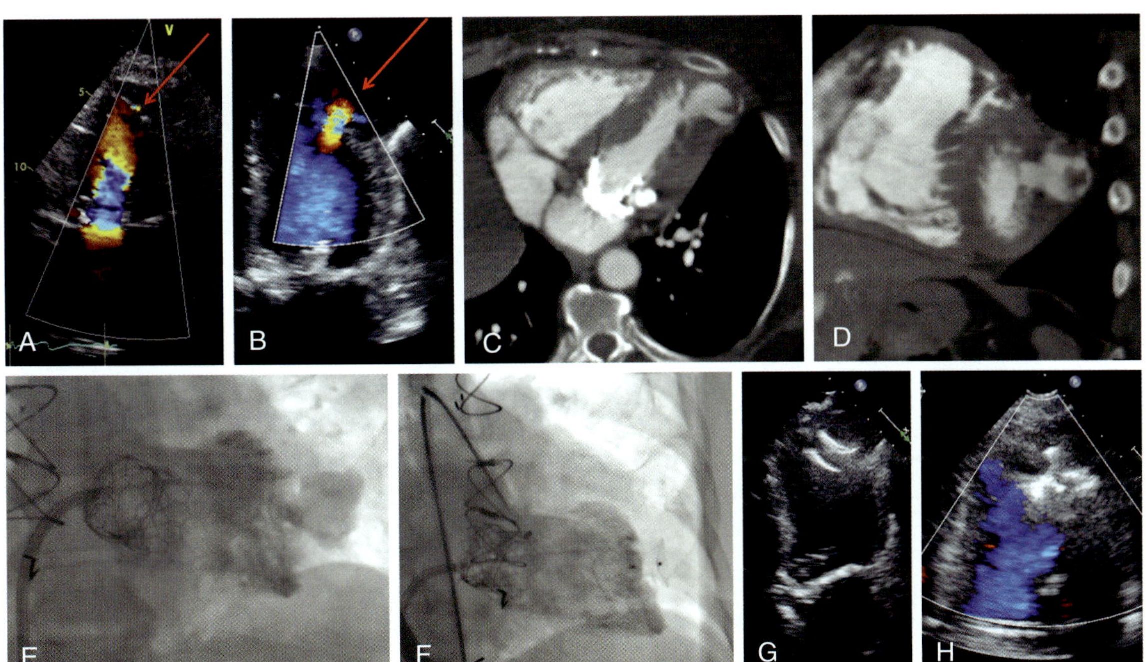

FIG. 4.66 Echocardiogram, Computed Tomography, and Catheterization Imaging of Left Ventricle Pseudoaneurysm and Closure. (A and B) Echocardiogram after transcatheter mitral valve-in-valve replacement and 8 months later demonstrating enlarging left ventricle pseudoaneurysm (*arrows*). (C and D) Computed tomography scan in axial and coronal sections. (E and F) Transseptal pigtail ventriculography–guided successful closure (Online Video 4.65). (G and H) Echocardiogram 3 months later confirmed closure.

Percutaneous Transcatheter Closure for Aortic Puncture and Paravalvular Leak Closure With the New Amplatzer III Device

Bernhard Meier, MD, Bernhard Winkler, MD, Thierry Carrel, MD, Christoph Huber, MD

A 72-year-old woman with a long-standing history of rheumatic heart disease was admitted to our hospital for a severe paravalvular leak (PVL). The patient contracted rheumatic fever in 1953 and received closed mitral commissurotomy in 1965, mechanical aortic valve replacement with open mitral commissurotomy in 1977, and mechanical mitral valve replacement in 1997. In 2014, the patient was medically treated for endocarditis of the mitral valve prosthesis but subsequently developed a severe PVL of the mitral valve prosthesis and important concomitant hemolysis requiring one to two blood transfusions a week. The patient was referred for reoperation in a severely reduced clinical state. Surgical treatment as primarily recommended in this context of endocarditis can be associated with mortality rates approaching 16%.[1] Because of the increased perioperative risk, a percutaneous transcatheter approach was selected to close the PVL with an Amplatzer vascular plug III device (St. Jude Medical, Plymouth, Minnesota) through a transseptal approach.[2]

The procedure was performed from the right femoral vein, under general anesthesia, and guided by transesophageal echocardiography. Accidental perforation and dilation of the ascending aorta next to the right coronary ostium was immediately treated by insertion of a first Amplatzer vascular plug III (Fig. 4.67A–B, Online Video 4.66). After successful transseptal puncture, the atrial septum was dilated, an Amplatz Extra-Stiff guidewire (Cook Medical, Bloomington, Indiana) was positioned in the left ventricle through the paravalvular leak (Fig. 4.68A). An 8- × 4-mm Amplatzer vascular plug III was then successfully implanted within the PVL in the mitral annulus (Fig. 4.68B, Online Video 4.67). Transesophageal echocardiography showed no paravalvular regurgitation and a mean gradient of 4 mm Hg. Hospital stay was uneventful, and the patient was discharged 7 days after the intervention. The patient was in excellent condition without further symptoms and without hemolysis 3 months after the intervention.

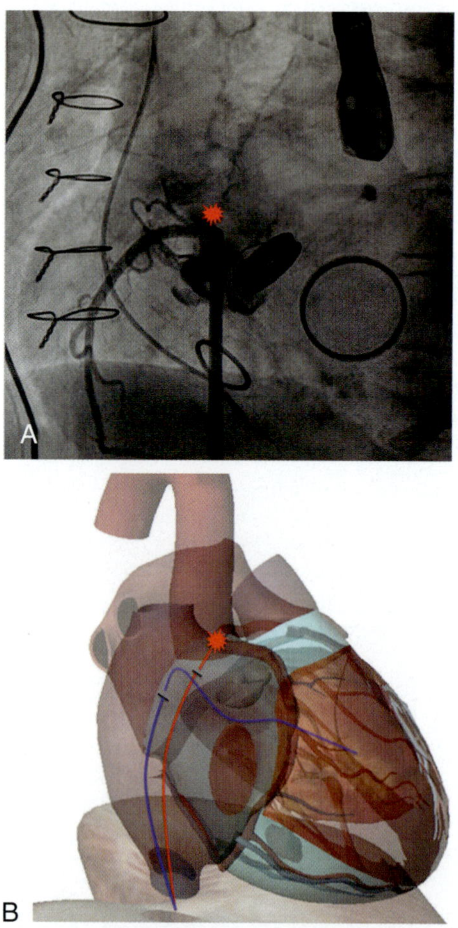

FIG. 4.67 Perforation of the Ascending Aorta. (A) Perforation of the ascending aorta next to the right coronary ostium is indicated by the *red asterisk*. (B) The *red line* indicates the wire route with the aortic puncture, the *blue line* represents the guidewire path through the mitral valve annulus/paravalvular leak after transseptal puncture (Online Video 4.66).

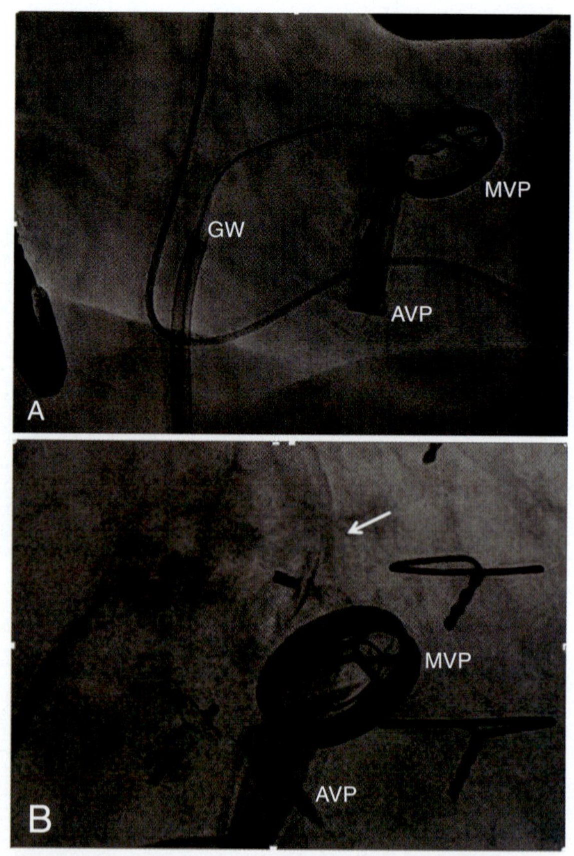

FIG. 4.68 Amplatz Guidewire Positioned in the Left Ventricle. (A) After transseptal puncture, the Amplatz Extra-Stiff guidewire (*GW*) is positioned in the left ventricle (*LV*) through the paravalvular leak. (B) An 8- × 4-mm Amplatzer vascular plug was implanted within the paravalvular leak in the mitral annulus (Online Video 4.67). *AVP*, aortic valve prosthesis; *MVP*, mitral valve prosthesis.

References

1. Echevarria JR, Bernal JM, Rabasa JM, Morales D, Revilla Y, Revuelta JM. Reoperation for bioprosthetic valve dysfunction: a decade of clinical experience. *Eur J Cardiothorac Surg.* 1991;5:523-526.
2. Momplaisir T, Matthews RV. Paravalvular mitral regurgitation treated with an Amplatzer septal occluder device: a case report and review of the literature. *J Invasive Cardiol.* 2007;19:E46-E50.

Bail-Out Alcohol Septal Ablation for Left Ventricular Outflow Tract Obstruction After Transcatheter Mitral Valve Replacement

Pierre Deharo, MD, Marina Urena, MD, Dominique Himbert, MD, Eric Brochet, MD, Frederic Rouleau, MD, Frederic Pinaud, MD, PhD, Stephane Delepine, MD, Jose Luis Carrasco, MD, Walid Ghodbane, MD, Fabrice Extramiana, MD, Phalla Ou, MD, PhD, Marie Pierre Dilly, MD, David Messika-Zeitoun, MD, PhD, Bernard Iung, MD, PhD, Patrick Nataf, MD, Alec Vahanian, MD

A 76-year-old woman with degenerative mitral valve disease was referred for refractory heart failure. An echocardiogram showed the presence of a massive mitral annular calcification with severe stenosis (mitral valve area, 1.0 cm^2; mean gradient, 11 mm Hg) and a small left ventricular cavity with a 23-mm septal bulge without obstruction (Fig. 4.69A–C, Online Video 4.68). Computed tomography (CT) findings were almost circumferential calcification of the mitral annulus; mitral annulus diameter of 22.8 × 30.0 mm and area of 472 mm^2, and mitral annulus-aorta angle of 122° (Fig. 4.69D–F).

The heart team recommended a transcatheter mitral valve replacement (TMVR). The procedure was performed via the transseptal approach using a 26-mm SAPIEN 3 valve (Edwards Lifesciences, Irvine, California) (Online Video 4.69). Immediately after deployment, the patient had severe hypotension requiring hemodynamic support (Fig. 4.70A–B). An echocardiographic assessment showed a satisfactory function of the prosthesis (trace paravalvular leak and a mean gradient of 5 mm Hg), which contacted the septum, leading to a severe left ventricular outflow tract (LVOT) obstruction with a maximal gradient of 100 mm Hg (Online Video 4.70), confirmed by hemodynamic measurements (Fig. 4.70B). Bail-out septal alcohol ablation was performed (Fig. 4.71A–C) with an initial restoration of systemic pressure and a marked decrease in LVOT gradient (Fig. 4.71D–E). A few hours later, a permanent pacemaker was implanted because of a secondary increase in the LVOT gradient. Thereafter the evolution was favorable, and the patient was discharged on day 12. Six months after the procedure, the patient was in New York Heart Association functional class II. Echocardiographic and CT images confirmed an adequate prosthesis placement and function (Online Video 4.71) and a maximal LVOT gradient of 25 mm Hg.

Severe LVOT obstruction is a life-threatening complication of TMVR. A septal bulge with a small left ventricular cavity increases the risk of this complication. Therefore, left ventricular morphology should be carefully evaluated before the procedure, and contraindication to the intervention should be considered if such features are observed. If severe LVOT obstruction occurs, bail-out alcohol septal ablation may be lifesaving.

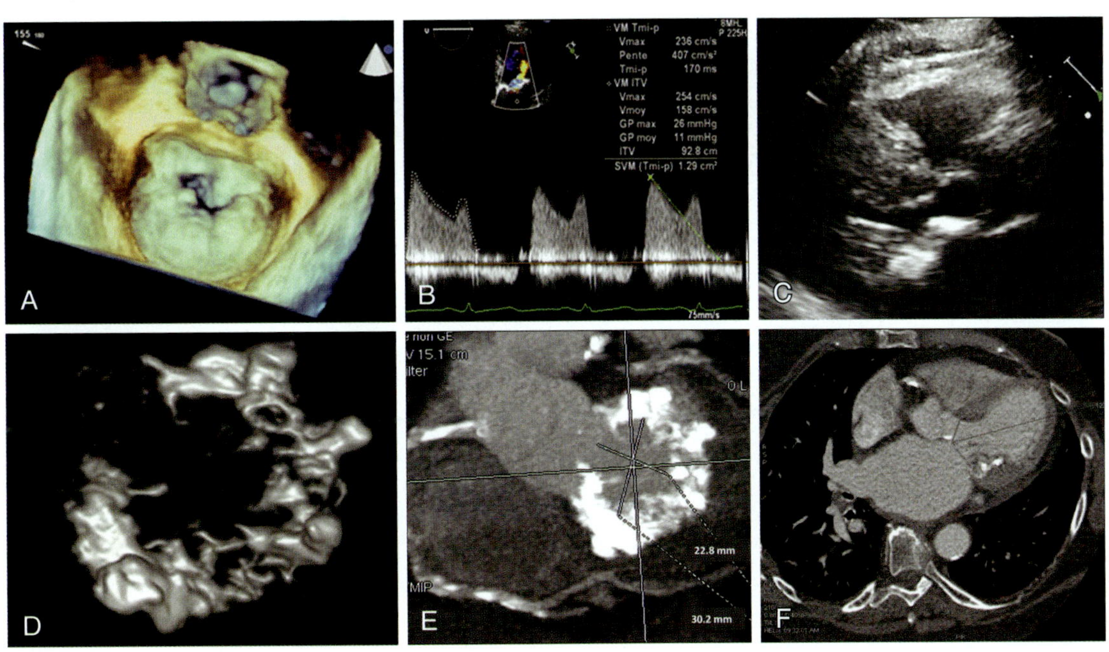

FIG. 4.69 Echocardiographic and Computed Tomography Images of the Mitral Valve and Left Ventricle. Three- and two-dimensional echocardiographic images showing a degenerative mitral valve with massive annular calcification (A), severe mitral stenosis (B), and a small left ventricular cavity with a septal bulge (C) (Online Video 4.68). (D) Three-dimensional volume-rendered computed tomography image showing roughly circumferential calcification of the mitral annulus. (E and F) Oblique reconstruction and sagittal view showing the dimensions of the mitral annulus and the mitral annulus to aorta angle.

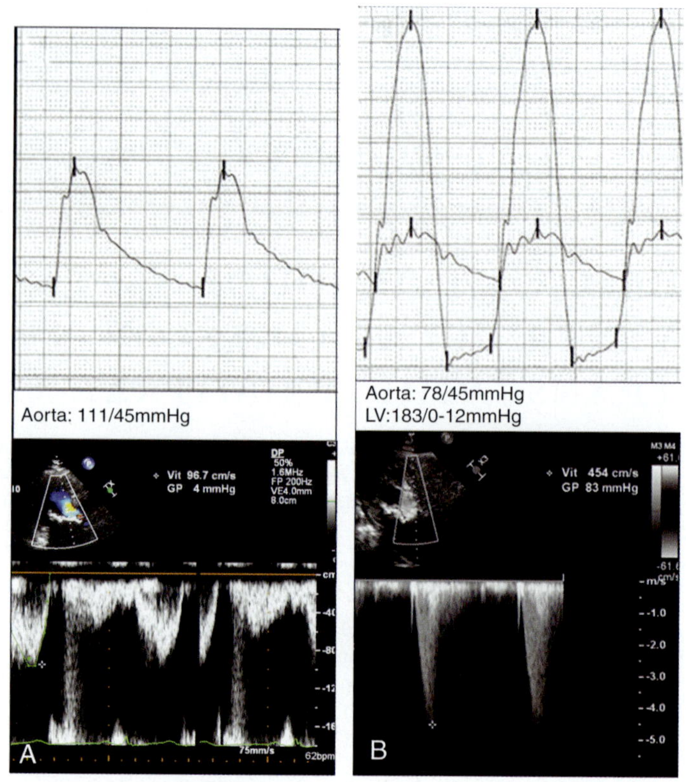

FIG. 4.70 Doppler Echocardiographic Images and Hemodynamic Curves Showing the Changes in the Left Ventricular Outflow Tract (LVOT) Gradient. (A) Before implantation of the prosthesis, the aortic pressure was 111/45 mm Hg, the shape of the aortic pressure wave was normal, and there was not a significant gradient at the LVOT.
(B) Immediately after implantation of the prosthesis, the aortic pressure decreased to 78/45, the shape of the aortic pressure wave changed to a spike-and-dome pattern, and the maximal LVOT gradient was >100 mm Hg (Online Videos 4.69 and 4.70).

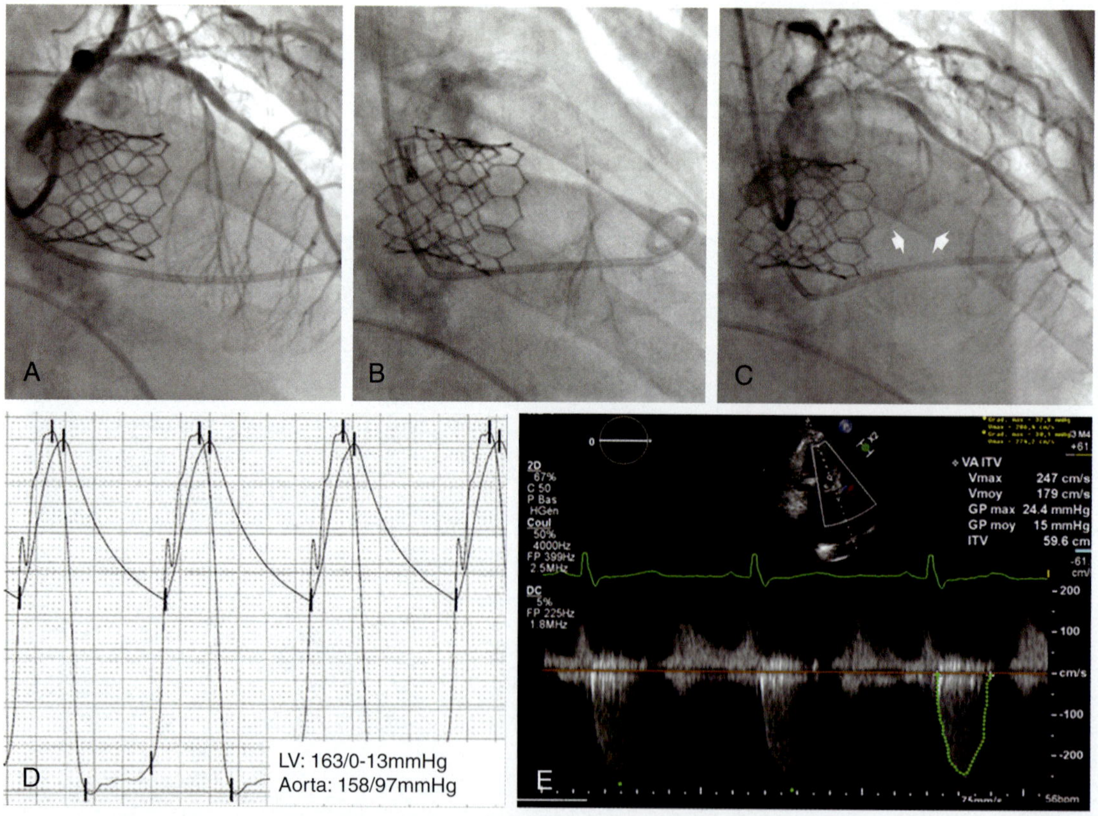

FIG. 4.71 Fluoroscopy Images Showing the Different Steps of the Septal Alcohol Ablation Procedure and Hemodynamic Curves and Echocardiographic Images Showing Acute Results. (A) A coronary angiogram confirmed the presence of a septal artery suitable for alcohol ablation. Two milliliters of pure ethanol were injected in the first septal branch (B), with complete occlusion of the artery (C, *white arrows*). (D) Immediately after injecting the ethanol, a normalization of the shape of the aorta pressure curve and recovery of the pressure were observed. (E) Echocardiographic assessment confirmed the maximal left ventricular outflow gradient of 24 mm Hg (Online Video 4.71). *LV*, left ventricle.

Clipping the Alfieri Stitch

Stefan Buchner, MD, Markus Resch, MD, Reinhard Kobuch, MD, Christoph Birner, MD

A 75-year-old woman underwent surgical correction of severe mitral regurgitation (MR). The valve morphology was characterized by chordae rupture (P2), prolapse (A2), and an unusual small anterior valve area with a restrictive posterior leaflet. The correction comprised chordae replacement P2/A2 without annuloplasty because of a tight annulus. Finally, an Alfieri stitch was performed.

Four weeks later, the patient presented with dyspnea. Echocardiography revealed a rupture of the Alfieri stitch (Fig. 4.72A–B, Online Videos 4.72 and 4.73) with severe MR (Fig. 4.72C, Online Video 4.74) and a mitral valve area of 2.47 cm^2 (Fig. 4.72D). The patient did not prefer to undergo a reoperation, and the heart team's consensus was an interventional strategy with an "edge-to-edge" repair.

To prevent significant mitral stenosis, we performed a thorough hemodynamic monitoring by simultaneous measurements with one pigtail catheter in the left atrium and one in left ventricle (Fig. 4.72E). The initial transvalvular gradient was 6 mm Hg (Fig. 4.72F). Using 3-dimensional echocardiography, the clip was positioned and the grasp was done (Fig. 4.72G, Online Video 4.75). Before final detachment of the clip, simultaneous measurements showed a decrease of the v wave (from 63 to 30 mm Hg) and a mean gradient of 8 mm Hg (Fig. 4.72H). Thus the clip was released. Three-dimensional echocardiography confirmed a significant reduction in MR and the mitral valve area of 1.8 cm^2 (7 mm Hg) (Fig. 4.72I–K, Online Videos 4.76 and 4.77). On follow-up, the patient is doing well.

This case highlights the feasibility and efficacy of MitraClip (Abbott Vascular, Abbott Park, Illinois) therapy as a bail-out strategy after failure of a surgical edge-to-edge repair.

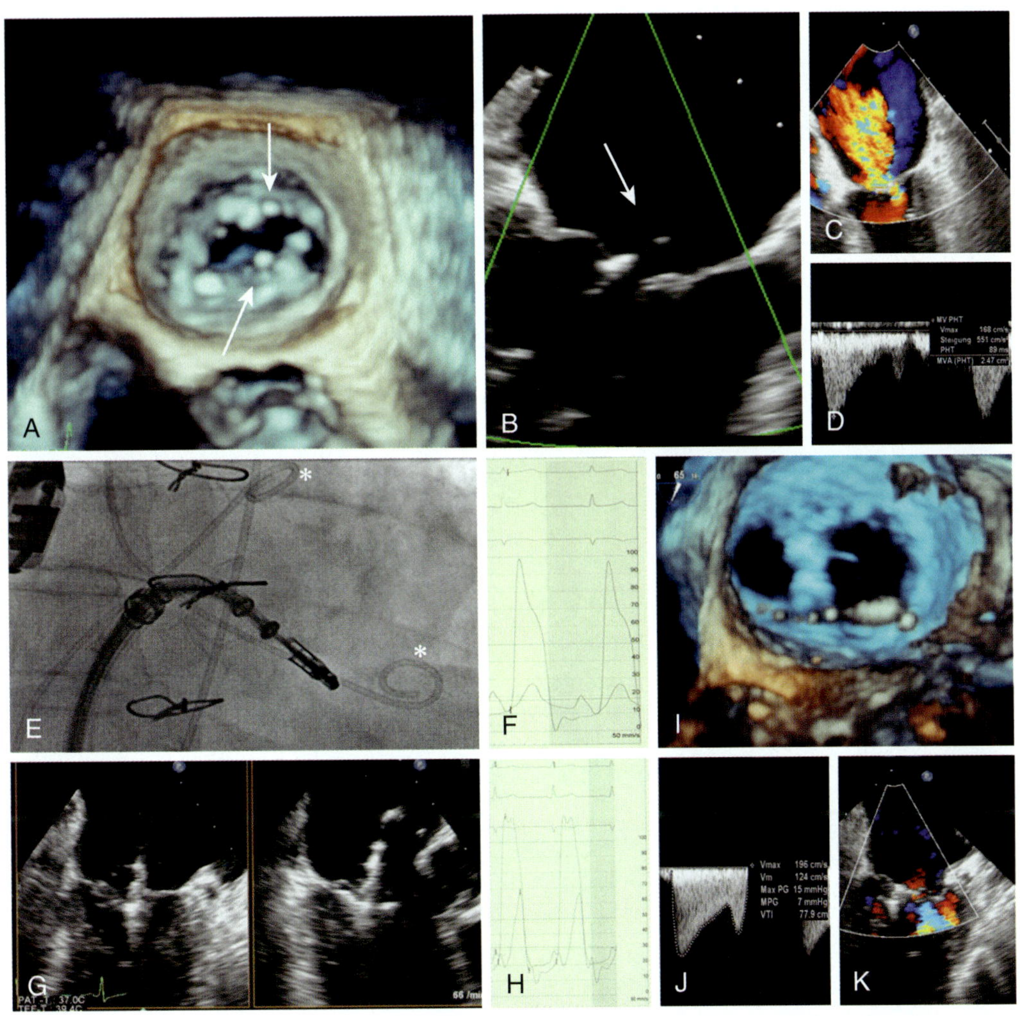

FIG. 4.72 Interventional Edge-to-Edge Repair of the Failed Surgical Edge-to-Edge Repair. Three-dimensional (A) and two-dimensional (B) echocardiography of the failed surgical edge-to-edge repair (*arrows*) (Online Videos 4.72 and 4.73) with severe mitral regurgitation (Online Video 4.74) (C) and mitral valve area by pressure half-time (D). (E) One pigtail catheter in the left atrium (*asterisk*) and one in the left ventricle (*asterisk*) for the transvalvular gradient (F). (G) Echocardiography of the grasp (Online Video 4.75). (H) Transvalvular gradient after the grasp. (I) Three-dimensional echocardiography of the clip with the mitral valve area by pressure half-time (J) and a significant reduction in mitral regurgitation (K) (Online Videos 4.76 and 4.77).

First-in-Human Use of Catheter-Delivered Annuloplasty Ring to Treat Functional Mitral Regurgitation

Gino Gerosa, MD, Laura Besola, MD, Erica Manzan, MD, Eleonora Bizzotto, MD, Fabio Zucchetta, MD, Demetrio Pittarello, MD, Giuseppe Tarantini, MD, PhD, David Meerkin, MD, Andrea Colli, MD, PhD

Restrictive mitral valve annuloplasty with a rigid closed ring has evolved as a surgical alternative to mitral valve replacement[1–3] to correct functional mitral regurgitation (MR).

By reducing the anteroposterior annular diameter, mitral valve annuloplasty facilitates effective leaflet coaptation by directly reducing the MR as well as preventing further annular dilation that could lead to MR recurrence.

We present images of a first-in-human case of implantation of the AMEND transcatheter mitral valve repair system (Valcare Medical, Herzliya, Israel) to treat functional mitral incompetence under a compassionate use approval.

A 74-year-old woman presented with progressive dyspnea and New York Heart Association functional class III. Echocardiography demonstrated severe central MR (Fig. 4.73A–B, Online Video 4.78) and an ejection fraction of 35%. Multislice computed tomography demonstrated an anteroposterior diameter of 30 mm (Fig. 4.73C), compatible with a medium prosthesis (24.5 × 34.0 mm).

The procedure was performed under general anesthesia with standard transapical access, using guidance from 2- and 3-dimensional transesophageal echocardiography and fluoroscopy (Figs. 4.74 and 4.75, Online Videos 4.79–4.88). After introduction into the left ventricle, the 28F AMEND system was advanced through the mitral valve over a wire to the left atrium and the ring was unsheathed and it adopted its closed-D shape. The ring was then oriented appropriately to the annulus using the different adjustment tools, achieving intimate contact with the posterior annulus and fixed to it with anchors. At this point the sheath was steered anteriorly toward the mitroaortic continuity and again when good contact was achieved the anterior anchors were also deployed. The device was then released from the delivery system and retracted from the heart.

The patient was discharged home and at 3-month follow-up, she was asymptomatic (New York Heart Association functional class I) with mild MR, and stable ring position was confirmed by multislice computed tomography (Fig. 4.73D–F, Online Videos 4.89 and 4.90).

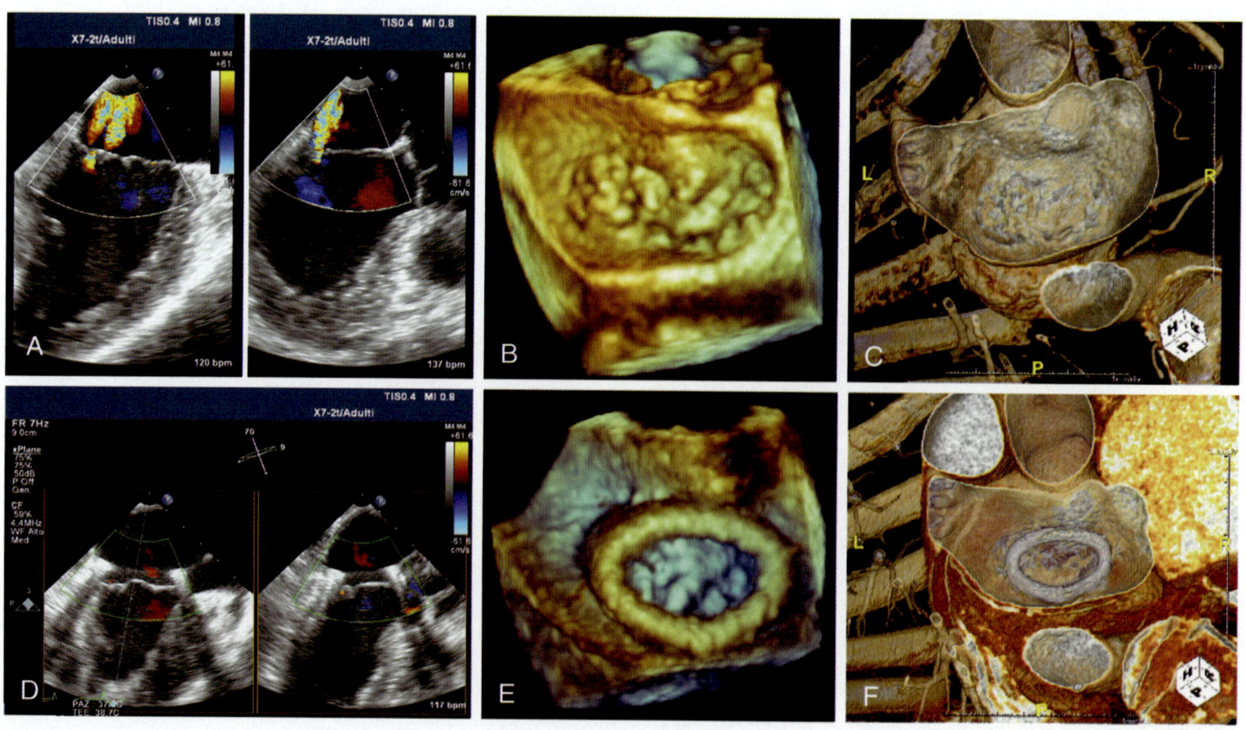

FIG. 4.73 Echocardiographic and Multislice Computed Tomography (CT) Imaging Before and After Implantation of the AMEND Annuloplasty Device. (A) Severe central mitral regurgitation on transesophageal echocardiography. (B) Three-dimensional echocardiographic image of mitral valve. (C) CT evaluation of the mitral valve. (D) Postimplantation echocardiography confirming the presence of mild mitral regurgitation. Three-dimensional echocardiographic image (E) and CT image (F) of the AMEND mitral ring (Online Videos 4.78–4.90).

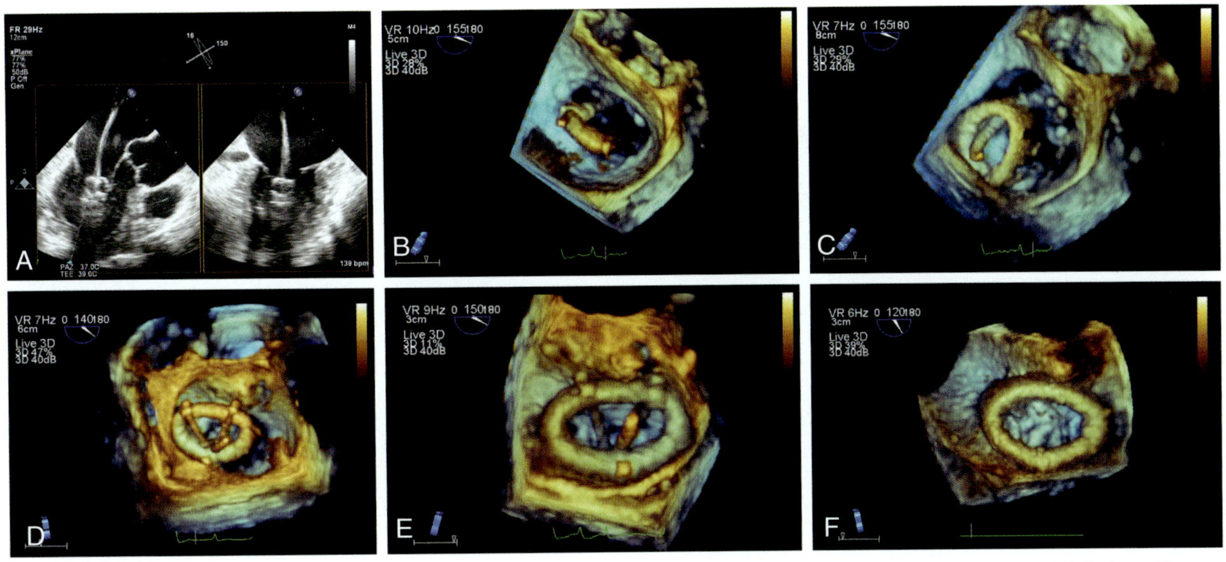

FIG. 4.74 Intraoperative Transesophageal Two- and Three-Dimensional Images Summarizing Procedural Steps. (A) A Swan-Ganz catheter is passed through the mitral valve over the guidewire to assess central valve crossing. (B) The ring is partially unsheathed in the left atrium. (C) The ring is fully unsheathed with closed-D shape. (D) The stabilizing tool is unsheathed and the ring is positioned anatomically. (E) Posterior and anterior anchors have been deployed. (F) Final appearance of the AMEND ring deployed (Online Videos 4.79–4.83).

REFERENCES

1. Nishimura RA, Otto CM, Bonow RO, et al. 2014 AHA/ACC guidelines for the management of patients with valvular heart disease: a report of the American College of Cardiology/American Heart Association Task Force on Practice Guidelines. *J Am Coll Cardiol.* 2014;63:e57-e185.
2. Vahanian A, Alfieri O, Andreotti F, et al. Guidelines on the management of valvular heart disease (version 2012): the Joint Task Force on the Management of Valvular Heart Disease of the European Society of Cardiology (ESC) and the European Association for Cardio-Thoracic Surgery. *Eur Heart J.* 2012;33:2451-2496.
3. Acker MA, Parides MK, Perrault LP, et al. Mitral valve repair versus replacement for severe ischemic mitral regurgitation. *N Engl J Med.* 2014; 370:23-32.

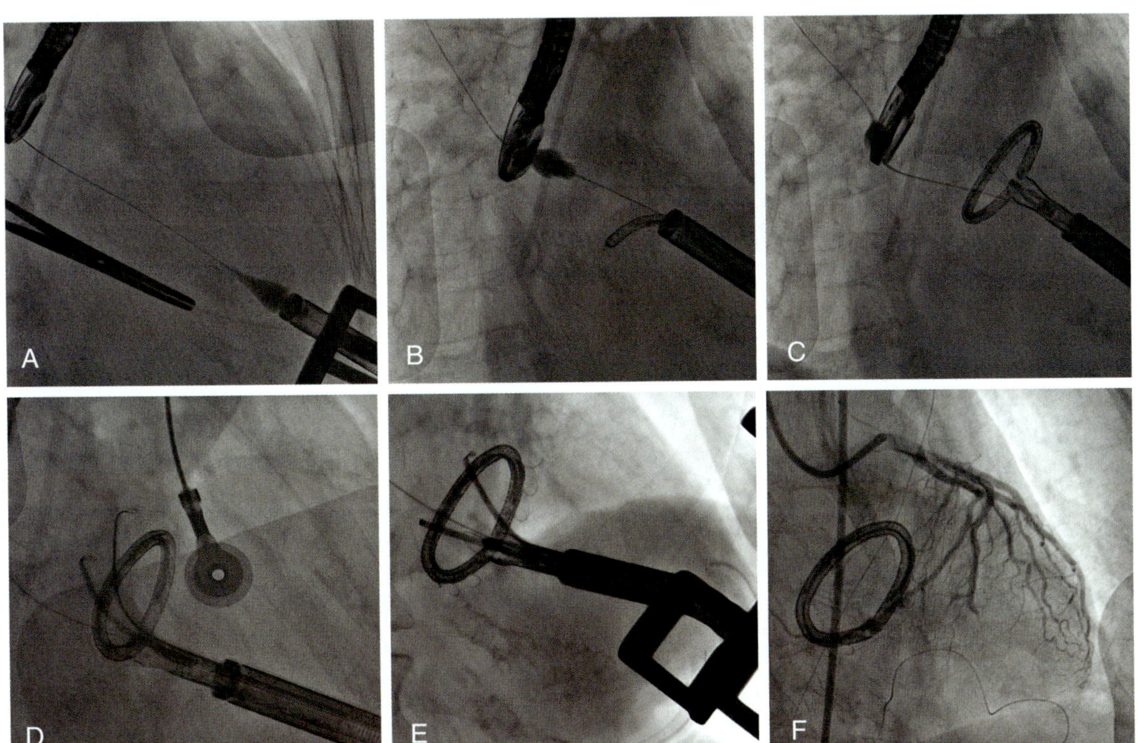

Fig 4.75 Fluoroscopic Images Summarizing Procedural Steps. (A) Ventriculography demonstrating guidewire crossing of the mitral valve and landing in superior pulmonary vein with the tip of the delivery system on the ventricular apex. (B) The ring is partially unsheathed in the left atrium. (C) The ring is fully unsheathed with closed-D shape. (D) The stabilizing tool is unsheathed and the ring is positioned anatomically. (E) Posterior anchors have been deployed. (F) Final appearance of the AMEND ring with all anchors deployed (Online Videos 4.84–4.88).

Leaflet-to-Annuloplasty Ring Clipping for Severe Mitral Regurgitation

Brinder S. Kanda, MD, Desmond Jay, MD, R. Saeid Farivar, MD, PhD, Paul Sorajja, MD

An 86-year-old man presented with recurrent heart failure and severe mitral regurgitation in the setting of previous surgical mitral repair for degenerative valve disease. Surgery had consisted of placement of a 32-mm Carpentier-Edwards Physio II annuloplasty ring (Edwards Lifesciences, Irvine, California). Transesophageal echocardiography demonstrated a large anterior leaflet (Fig. 4.76A, *arrow*), poor coaptation of the anterior leaflet with the annuloplasty ring, a markedly deficient posterior leaflet (Fig. 4.76B, *arrow*), and severe residual mitral regurgitation (Fig. 4.76C, *arrow*) between the tip of the anterior leaflet and the annuloplasty ring (Fig. 4.76D, *arrow*). Using a transfemoral, transseptal approach, a MitraClip (Abbott Vascular, Santa Clara, California) (Fig. 4.76E–F, *arrows*) was implanted to affix the anterior leaflet to the annuloplasty ring (Fig. 4.76G, *arrow*). This implantation led to acute reduction in mitral regurgitation (Fig. 4.76H, *arrows*). The mean left atrial pressure decreased from 28 mm Hg at baseline (Fig. 4.76I) to 21 mm Hg at the end of the procedure (Fig. 4.76J). There was relief of heart failure symptoms, and the MitraClip procedure obviated the need for additional cardiac surgery. To our knowledge, this description represents the first report of MitraClip implantation for fixation of native leaflets onto a surgical annuloplasty ring.

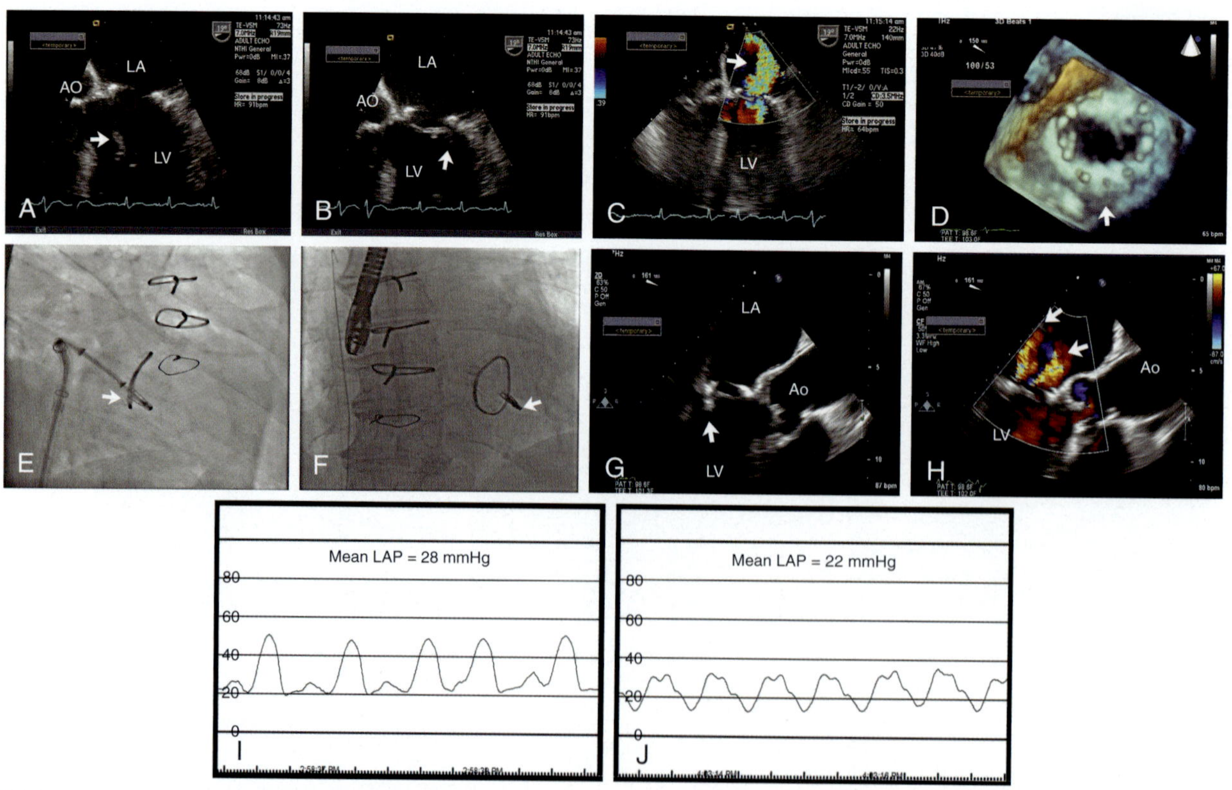

FIG. 4.76 Transcatheter Mitral Valve Repair After Mitral Surgery. (A) Transesophageal echocardiography (TEE) demonstrating a large anterior leaflet (*arrow*) and a deficient posterior leaflet. (B) Poor coaptation of the anterior leaflet with the annuloplasty ring and a markedly deficient posterior leaflet (*arrow*). (C) TEE showing the presence of severe mitral regurgitation after cardiac surgery (*arrow*). (D) Three-dimensional echocardiography showing previously placed surgical annuloplasty ring (*arrow*). (E) Fluoroscopy with right anterior oblique view showing fixation of the MitraClip (Abbott Vascular, Santa Clara, California) to the annuloplasty ring (*arrow*). (F) Fluoroscopy with left anterior oblique view showing fixation of the MitraClip to the annuloplasty ring (*arrow*). (G) TEE showing the final position of the fully deployed MitraClip (*arrow*). (H) TEE showing mild-to-moderate residual regurgitation after MitraClip deployment (*arrows*). (I) Left atrial pressure (*LAP*) recording before transcatheter mitral valve repair. (J) LAP recording after transcatheter mitral valve repair. *Ao*, aorta; *LA*, left atrium; *LV*, left ventricle.

Low-Dose and Slow-Infusion Thrombolysis for Prosthetic Valve Thrombosis After a Transcatheter Valve in the Mitral Position

John Roosen, MD, Peter Haemers, MD, Peter Verhamme, MD, PhD, Koen Ameloot, MD, Herbert De Praetere, MD

An 82-year-old female patient with a history of aortic valve replacement and mitral valve repair was admitted several times with severe heart failure due to severe mitral valve regurgitation (Fig. 4.77A). Given the poor prognosis and the high operative risk of redo surgery (European System for Cardiac Operative Risk Evaluation II, 40.63%), the heart team scheduled the patient for a valve-in-ring procedure. A left anterolateral minithoracotomy was performed, the apex was punctured, and a SAFARI wire (Boston Scientific, Marlborough, Massachusetts) was placed in the left atrium. Using a BOLT sheath (Boston Scientific), a 23-mm LOTUS valve (size based on the preoperative ultrasound with valve diameter of 1.5 mm × 1.8 mm) (Boston Scientific) was smoothly delivered in the mitral annulus and gradually deployed (Fig. 4.77B). In the final position, the grade of mitral regurgitation was reduced to less than grade 1 with only slight obstruction of the left ventricular outflow tract (Fig. 4.77C). Hemodynamics improved immediately after valve implantation, dual-antiplatelet therapy (aspirin, clopidogrel) was started, and the patient was discharged home after 10 days. Six weeks later, the patient presented with pulmonary edema. Ultrasound revealed a severe increase of the mitral valve gradient with confirmation of prosthetic valve thrombosis (Fig. 4.77D). Low-dose alteplase (1 mg/h) in combination with fondaparinux (2.5 mg, given previously positive heparin-induced thrombocytopenia antibodies) was administered. During 38 h of thrombolysis, gradual improvement of the clinical condition and the mitral valve gradient were observed. Echocardiography confirmed resolution of thrombotic material (Fig. 4.77E–H). Patient was discharged with oral vitamin K antagonists in combination with aspirin. To the best of our knowledge, this is the first case of thrombosis of a transcatheter valve in the mitral position. The position of the transcatheter valve is more atrialized compared with the conventional position of a surgical mitral valve. This might cause a worse washout of blood by the flow in the outflow tract. It remains open to discussion whether patients with transcatheter valves in more prothrombotic mitral position would benefit from postoperative anticoagulation as suggested for surgical mitral valve replacement.

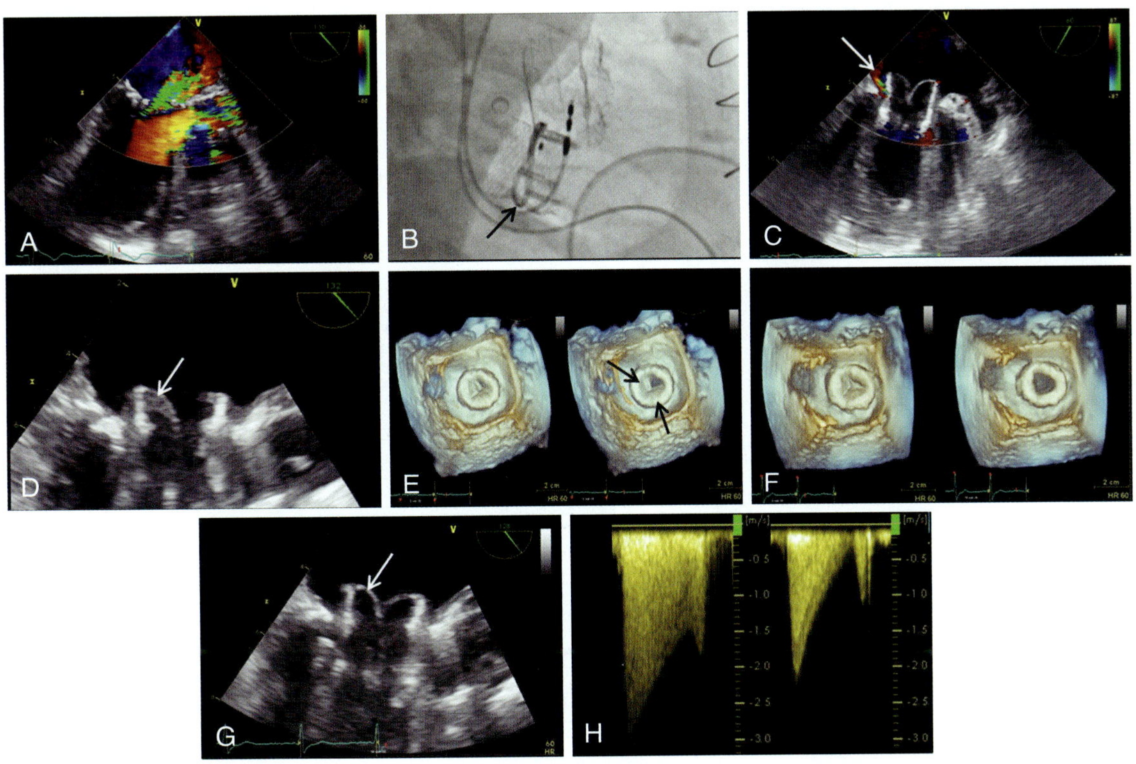

FIG. 4.77 Thrombolysis of a Transcatheter Valve in the Mitral Position. (A) Before mitral intervention there was severe mitral regurgitation. (B) Fluoroscopic image after placement of the transcatheter valve in the mitral position (*arrow*). (C) Transesophageal ultrasound after placement of transcatheter valve in the mitral position showing only a mild paravalvular mitral regurgitation (*arrow*). (D) Six weeks after discharge, ultrasound reveals thrombotic material (*arrow*) at the ventricular side of the LOTUS valve (Boston Scientific, Marlborough, Massachusetts) leaflets. (E) Three-dimensional ultrasound imaging showing a closed valve with three leaflets during systole. During diastole, two of three leaflets are immobilized by thrombotic material (*arrows*), inducing a severe mitral valve stenosis. (F) After low-dose and slow-infusion thrombolytic therapy, 3-dimensional ultrasound imaging demonstrates a recovery of the mobility of all 3 leaflets, with a full opening of the LOTUS valve during diastole. (G) Disappearance of all thrombotic material at the ventricular side of the leaflets (*arrow*) (same view as [D]). (H) After thrombolytic therapy, continuous-wave Doppler ultrasound showing a normalization of the mean mitral valve gradient (before, 15 mm Hg; after, 5 mm Hg) and the calculated mitral valve area (before, 0.93 cm^2; after, 1.69 cm^2).

Needing a Helping Hand: Left Amplatz Catheter to Facilitate Anterior Leaflet Grasping in the MitraClip Procedure

Fausto Castriota, MD, Roberto Nerla, MD, Angelo Squeri, MD, Antonio Micari, MD, PhD, Mauro Del Giglio, MD, Alberto Cremonesi, MD

A 53-year-old man with primitive dilated cardiomyopathy and severe left ventricular dysfunction awaiting cardiac transplantation was referred to our hospital to undergo a MitraClip (Abbott Vascular, Menlo Park, California) procedure as a bridge therapy for his functional mitral regurgitation (MR).

After transseptal puncture (8:44 a.m.), the MitraClip device was easily moved to the central position. Unfortunately, because of asymmetrical leaflet tethering, grasping was particularly challenging. A number of strategies were tried to facilitate approaching the leaflets, including adenosine-induced asystole, ventilation maneuvers, the Trendelenburg position, and ventricular fibrillation induction. Because none of these strategies was effective because of the asymmetrical tethering of anterior leaflet (Fig. 4.78, Online Video 4.91), a left Amplatz catheter (Boston Scientific, Marlborough, Massachusetts) was advanced from the femoral artery (11:21 a.m.) beyond the aortic valve (Fig. 4.78), and, under fluoroscopic and echocardiographic guidance, it was positioned in such a way that the tip pushed the anterior leaflet toward the grasping system (Fig. 4.79, Online Video 4.92). At this point, both leaflets could be simultaneously grasped, and the MitraClip was positioned (12:03 p.m.). A second MitraClip was then placed (12:29 p.m.), with a residual mild MR with two small jets beside the implanted clips (Fig. 4.79, Online Video 4.93).

MitraClips are increasingly used for functional MR as a bridge therapy to cardiac transplantation.[1] However, the unpredictable and often challenging ventricular remodeling of patients with advanced heart failure could significantly increase procedural complexity. In particular, the grasping process is often facilitated by a number of tricks to reduce leaflet mobility,[2,3] including the use of a pigtail catheter to help grasp posterior leaflets.[4]

However, this is the first case showing how a left Amplatz catheter could facilitate the grasping process of the anterior leaflet during a MitraClip procedure. Although technically more difficult, given the tighter angle between the anterior leaflet and the aortic root, this opportunity should be taken into account, even in the earlier phases of more complex grasping processes (i.e., for asymmetrical tethering).

References

1. Garatti A, Castelvecchio S, Bandera F, Medda M, Menicanti L. Mitraclip procedure as a bridge therapy in a patient with heart failure listed for heart transplantation. *Ann Thorac Surg*. 2015;99:1796-1799.
2. Borgia F, Di Mario C, Franzen O. Adenosine-induced asystole to facilitate MitraClip placement in a patient with adverse mitral valve morphology. *Heart*. 2011;97:864.
3. Mayr NP, Martin K, Hausleiter J, Brown A, Tassani P. Ventilation manoeuvres facilitate MitraClip placement. *Heart*. 2011;97:1717, author reply 1717.
4. Jones BM, Tuzcu EM, Kapadia SR. Pushing with the pigtail: a novel approach to placing the MitraClip in a patient with severely restricted posterior mitral leaflet. *Catheter Cardiovasc Interv*. 2015;85:906-908.

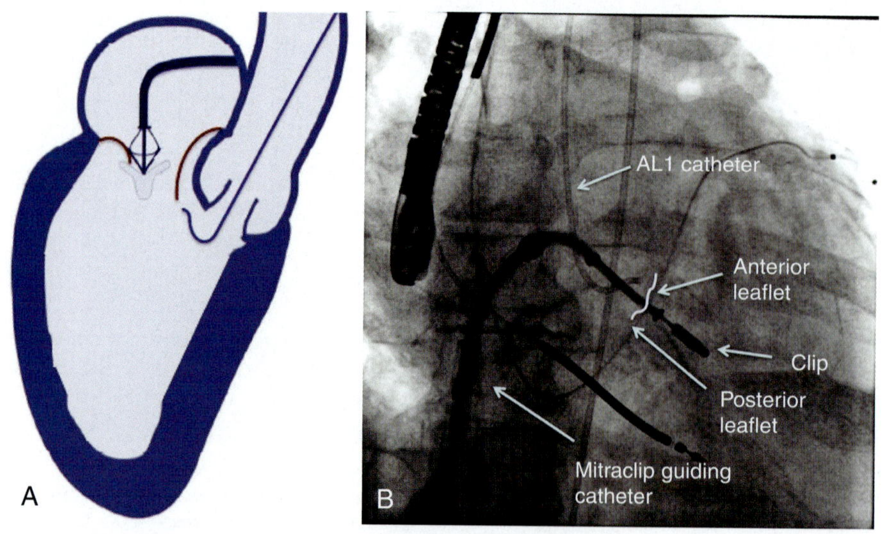

FIG. 4.78 Plan of the Strategy to Facilitate Anterior Leaflet Grasping. A left Amplatz catheter was advanced from the femoral artery beyond the aortic valve (A) to push the anterior mitral leaflet during the grasping phase (B) (Online Video 4.91).

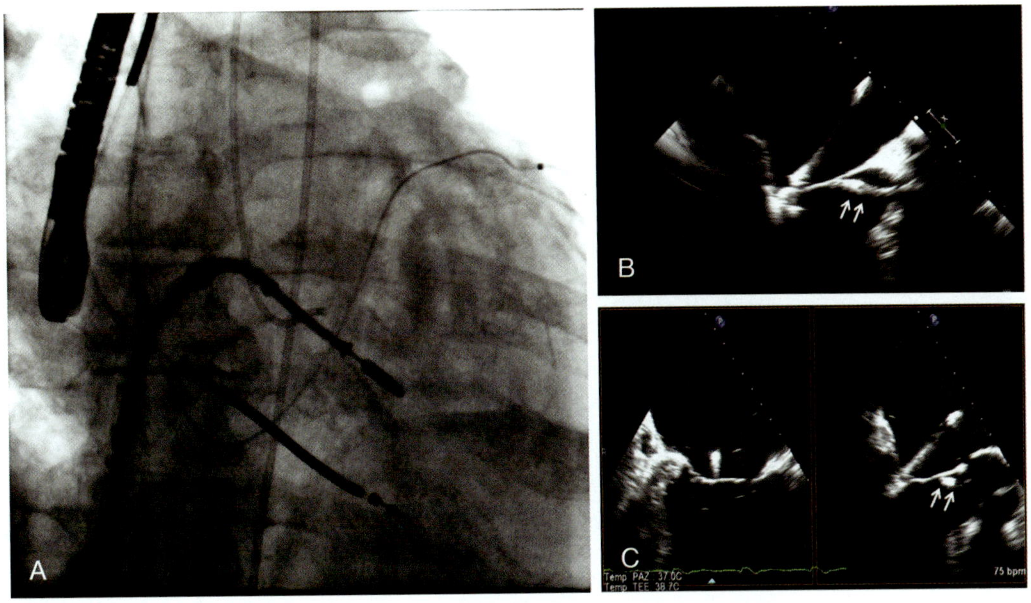

FIG. 4.79 The Grasping Phase During the First Clip Deployment. The Amplatz catheter is clearly visualized by both fluoroscopic (A) and echocardiographic views, as indicated by the *arrows*. (B) Long axis view. (C) Simultaneous bicaval and long axis transesophageal echocardiographic views (Online Videos 4.92 and 4.93).

Novel Treatment of Residual Peri-MitraClip Regurgitation With an Amplatzer Vascular Plug II

Mohamad Alkhouli, MD, Abdallah El Sabbagh, MD, Hector R. Villarraga, MD, Donald J. Hagler, MD, Charanjit S. Rihal, MD, MBA, Mackram F. Eleid, MD

Significant residual mitral regurgitation (MR) may persist after MitraClip (Abbott Vascular, Santa Clara, California) implantation in up to 7% of patients with degenerative MR.[1] Treatment of the residual MR with an adjacent MitraClip may not be feasible, because of commissural location, cleft, or perforation. The feasibility of Amplatzer vascular plug II (AVP-II) (St. Jude Medical, St. Paul, Minnesota) implantation between two MitraClips to treat residual "intraclip" MR has been recently demonstrated.[2,3] However, the use of the AVP-II device to treat commissural "periclip" MR when only one MitraClip is placed has not been reported.

A 69-year-old woman with a history of severe chronic obstructive lung disease (forced expiratory volume in 1 second, 29% of predicted) and remote native mitral valve endocarditis, treated with appropriate antibiotic therapy 3 years previously, presented for evaluation of severe primary MR. She was initially minimally symptomatic but recently developed progressive dyspnea of 6 months' duration. After a multidisciplinary evaluation, transcatheter mitral valve repair was the favored approach given that her surgical risk was deemed prohibitive because of her severe pulmonary disease.

Transesophageal echocardiography revealed severe MR with a regurgitant volume of 100 mL and systolic Doppler flow reversals in the pulmonary veins (Online Video 4.94). There was a small unsupported P1 segment with a cleft-like indentation likely related to previous endocarditis. A MitraClip device was implanted at the lateral aspect of the A2-P2 commissure (Fig. 4.80A, Online Video 4.95). Postprocedure there was a slight reduction in MR severity to moderate to severe and no pulmonary venous systolic flow reversals. The residual regurgitant jet originated lateral to the MitraClip at the unsupported P1 segment.

At 1-month follow-up, the patient had no significant change in her dyspnea or 6-min walk distance compared with her preprocedure baseline. Therefore the decision was made to attempt AVP-II implantation lateral to the MitraClip to reduce the degree of residual regurgitation.

A 14F introducer (Cook Medical, Bloomington, Indiana) was placed in the right femoral vein. Left atrial access was obtained with a Mullins transseptal introducer sheath and a Brockenbrough needle (Medtronic, Minneapolis, Minnesota) through the midposterior fossa ovalis. An Inoue wire was advanced into the left atrium and the septum was dilated with a 14F Inoue dilator (Toray Medical, Tokyo, Japan). A large-curl Agilis steerable introducer (St. Jude Medical) was advanced into the left atrium and steered toward the regurgitant jet. A telescoping system (100-cm 7F multipurpose guide and 120-cm 5F multipurpose catheter) with a 260-cm stiff-angled Glidewire (Terumo, Tokyo, Japan) was used to cross the mitral valve lateral to the MitraClip at the A1/P1 segment. A precurved Amplatz Extra-Stiff wire (Boston Scientific, Marlborough, Massachusetts) was placed in the left ventricle to deliver the AVP-II device. Initially, a 14-mm plug was deployed via the 7F multipurpose guide, resulting in a reduction in MR grade to mild (Online Video 4.96). However, over the next 20 min, there was atrial displacement of the plug with worsening MR noted on transesophageal echocardiographic imaging (Figs. 4.80 and 4.81, Online Video 4.97). Therefore, the device was

FIG. 4.80 Real-Time Transesophageal Echocardiographic (TEE) Images of the Peri-MitraClip Placement of a 14-mm Amplatzer Vascular Plug. (A) Three-dimensional TEE dome view of the mitral valve. (B and C) Two- and 4-chamber 2-dimensional (2D) TEE view showing a stable position of the 14-mm Amplatzer vascular pPlug II (AVP-II). (D) Two-chamber 2D TEE view showing atrial displacement of the AVP-II (Online Videos 4.94–4.96). *AV*, aortic valve; *LAA*, left atrial appendage; *MR*, mitral regurgitation.

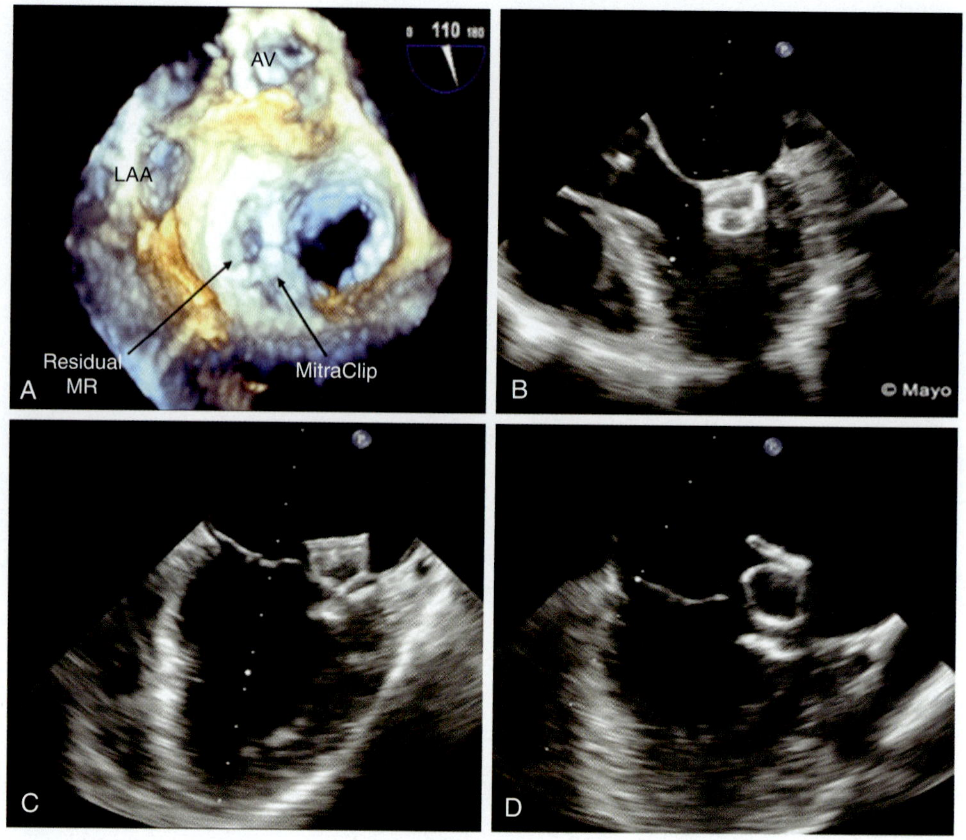

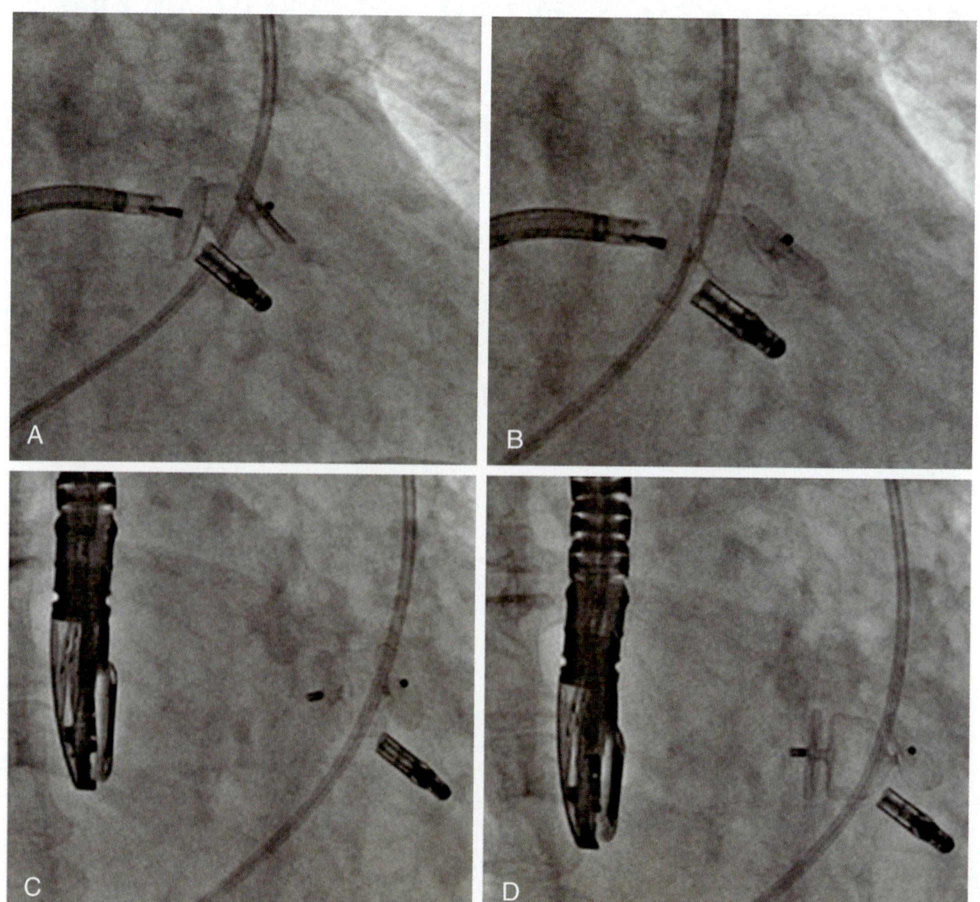

FIG. 4.81 Cine Fluoroscopy Still Frames of the 14-mm Amplatzer Vascular Plug II Implantation. (A and B) Stable initial position plug during systole and diastole. (C and D) Atrial displacement of the Amplatzer vascular plug II.

retrieved with a 6F 30-mm EN Snare (Merit, South Jordan, Utah). The defect was crossed again in the same fashion, and an 18-mm AVP-II was deployed through a 9F 75-cm Mullins sheath, with reduction of MR severity to mild and excellent device stability (Fig. 4.82). After placement of the AVP-II device, the left atrial v wave decreased from 30 to 20 mm Hg (Fig. 4.83). The mean diastolic transmitral gradient was 3 mm Hg. Follow-up transthoracic echocardiography at 24 h showed trivial MR (Online Video 4.98). The patient was discharged home in stable condition the following day. This first-in-human report demonstrates the feasibility of treating residual commissural "peri-MitraClip" MR with an AVP-II device.

References

1. Sorajja P, Mack M, Vemulapalli S, et al. Initial experience with commercial transcatheter mitral valve repair in the United States. *J Am Coll Cardiol.* 2016;67:1129-1140.
2. Taramasso M, Zuber M, Gruner C, Gaemperli O, Nietlispach F, Maisano F. First-in-man report of residual "intra-clip" regurgitation between two MitraClips treated by Amplatzer Vascular Plug II. *EuroIntervention.* 2016;11:1537-1540.

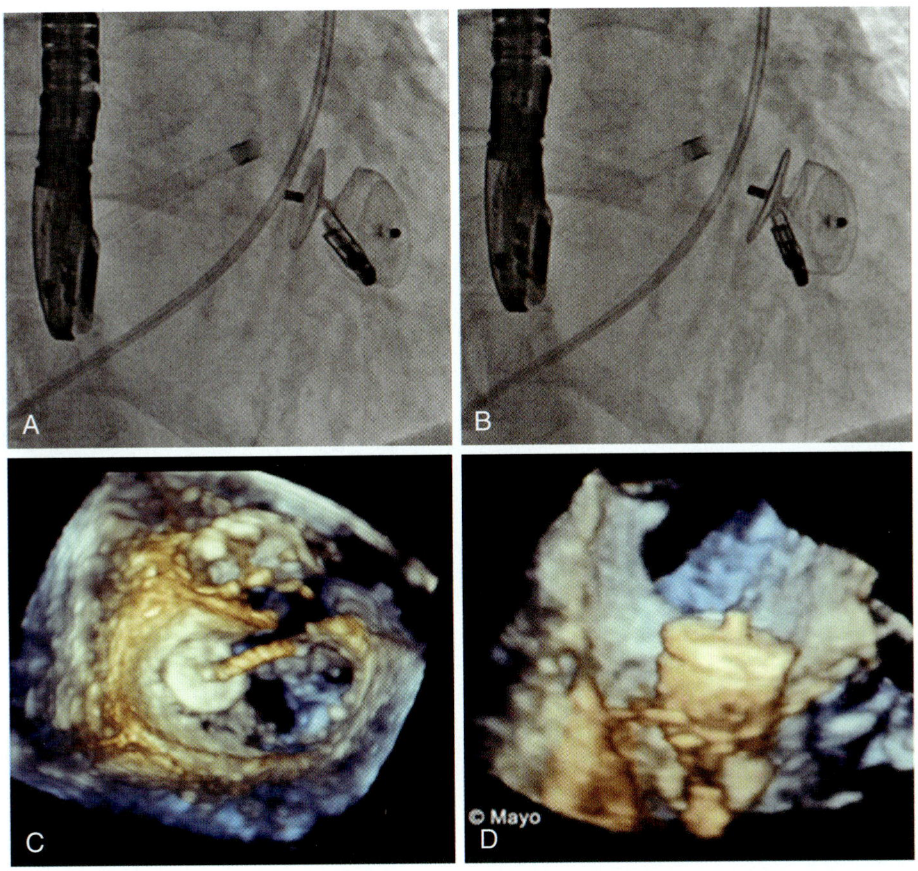

FIG. 4.82 Cine Fluoroscopy and Real-Time 3-Dimensional Transesophageal Echocardiographic (TEE) Still Frames of the 18-mm Amplatzer Vascular Plug II (AVP-II) Implantation Lateral to the MitraClip. (A and B) Stable position of the 18-mm AVP-II during systole and diastole. (C) Three-dimensional (3D) TEE dome view of the AVP-II lateral to the MitraClip. (D) Lateral real-time 3D TEE imaging showing the AVP-II next to the MitraClip (Online Videos 4.97 and 4.98).

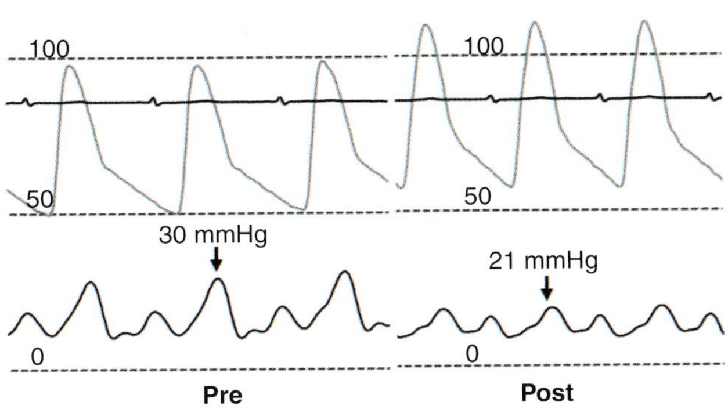

FIG. 4.83 Hemodynamic Tracings Before and After Amplatzer Vascular Plug II Implantation. Left atrial pressure significantly decreased after the Amplatzer vascular plug II implantation. (*Top*) Aortic pressure. (*Bottom*) Left atrial pressure.

Redo Mitral Valve Clipping After Partial Clip Detachment

Ben J. L. Van den Branden, MD, Martin J. Swaans, MD, Martijn C. Post, MD, PhD, Benno J.W. M. Rensing, MD, PhD, Frank D. Eefting, MD, Wybren Jaarsma, MD, PhD, Jan A. S. Van der Heyden, MD

A 45-year-old male patient with a history of ischemic cardiomyopathy, peripheral arterial disease, and renal dysfunction was admitted for percutaneous mitral valve repair. Cardiac magnetic resonance imaging showed an ejection fraction of 18% without viability. Severe mitral regurgitation (MR) occurred due to left ventricular annular dilatation and restriction of the posterior leaflet (Fig. 4.84). Consequently, an important reduction in functional capacity (New York Heart Association class III) was present. He was declined for surgery because of a predicted operative mortality rate of 36% (logistic European System for Cardiac Operative Risk Evaluation) and accepted for the percutaneous approach.

The procedure was performed under general anesthesia and guided with fluoroscopy and three-dimensional transesophageal echocardiography (Philips probe, transducer X7-2t, Philips Healthcare, Best, the Netherlands). Access was gained using the right femoral vein, and after transseptal puncture the clip delivery system was advanced into the left atrium. The clip was successfully delivered into the left ventricle just below the mitral valve annulus and retrieved in the center of the maximal jet of the MR, which was located medial to the center of the annulus. After grasping the mitral valve leaflet edges, the clip was closed and released, creating a double mitral valve orifice. Unfortunately, 24 hours later, transthoracic echocardiography showed clip detachment from the anterior mitral leaflet (Fig. 4.85A) without reduction in MR (Fig. 4.85B). A second clip was placed more centrally to maintain a better coaptation of the two leaflets (Fig. 4.86).

The procedure was uneventful, and echocardiography confirmed adequate positioning of the second clip with substantial reduction in MR (Fig. 4.87). Reviewing the echocardiographic studies, the first clip was positioned too far to the medial (P1-A1) coaptation line. The selection of this position was guided by what we assumed to be the maximum jet of regurgitation. Obviously, the real maximum jet was originating more laterally. Most probably, favoring the medial site, insufficient leaflet insertion was obtained. The patient was discharged 5 days later without clinical events related to the clip detachment. At 1 month, echocardiography showed mild MR (grade 2), unfortunately without clinical improvement. Because of persistent heart failure, the patient received a biventricular implantable cardioverter-defibrillator 3 months later.

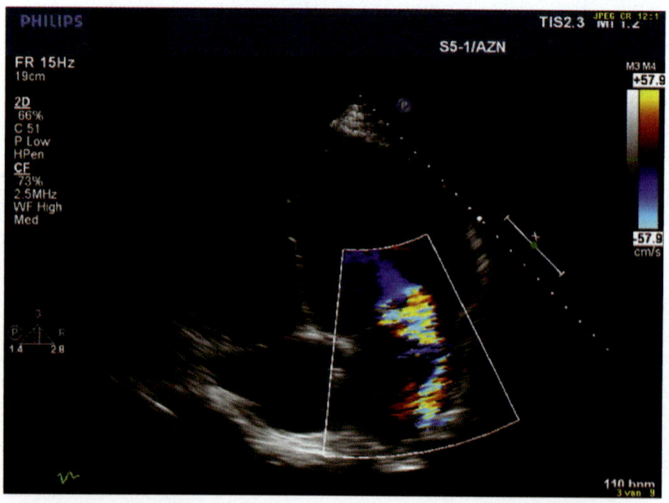

FIG. 4.84 Two-Dimensional Four-Chamber Transthoracic Echocardiographic Image Showing a Severe, Eccentric Mitral Regurgitation Jet. The important mitral regurgitation (MR) (*color jet*) is due to left ventricular annular dilatation and restriction of the posterior mitral valve leaflet. Consequently, the MR jet is oriented to the posterolateral wall of the left atrium and almost reaches the right upper pulmonary vein.

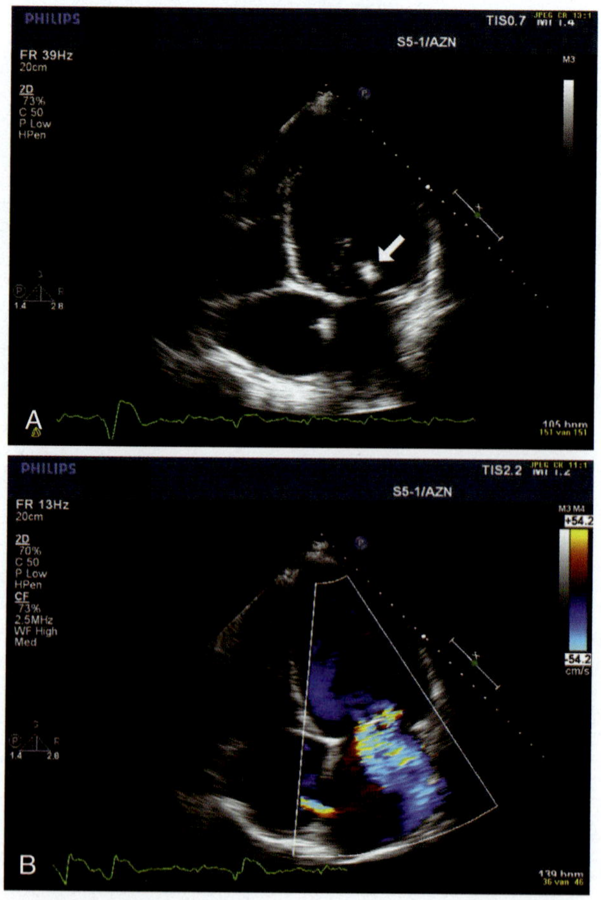

FIG. 4.85 Two-Dimensional Four-Chamber Transthoracic Echocardiographic Image After Partial Clip Detachment. (A) This image shows clip detachment from the anterior mitral valve leaflet. The clip (*arrow*) is only attached to the posterior mitral valve leaflet. (B) With color Doppler imaging, an even more important mitral regurgitation (MR) is recognized, with an MR jet area accounting for more than one-half of the left atrium area. An iatrogenic atrial septum defect is seen after transseptal puncture.

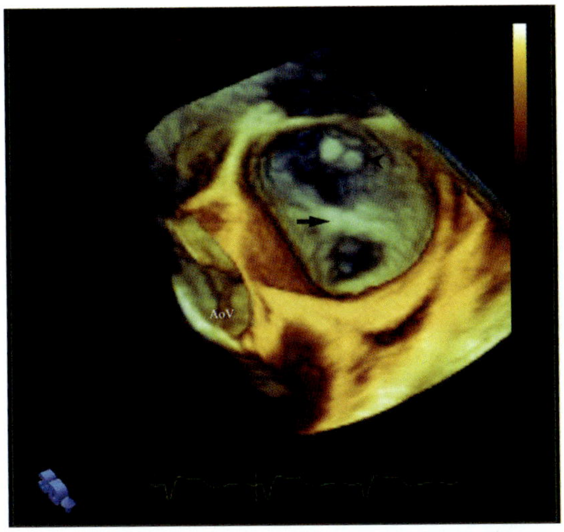

FIG. 4.86 Three-Dimensional Transesophageal Echocardiography Image After Successful Placement of the Second Clip. The first clip (*arrowhead*) is only attached to the posterior mitral valve leaflet. The second clip (*arrow*) was placed more centrally, creating a double-orifice mitral valve. *AoV*, aortic valve.

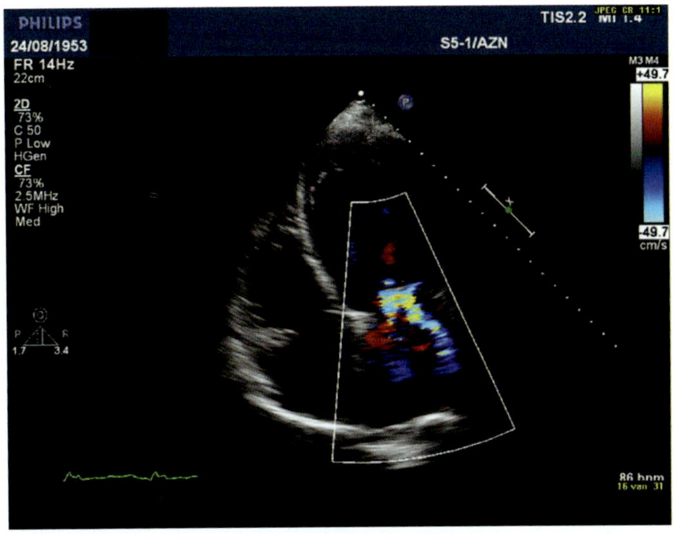

FIG. 4.87 Two-Dimensional Four-Chamber Transthoracic Echocardiographic Image Shows Reduction in Mitral Regurgitation After Second Clip Placement. This figure shows the final result in a four-chamber transthoracic echocardiographic view. There is an obvious reduction in mitral regurgitation (MR). Placement of the second clip has resulted in a central coaptation of the leaflets with a double orifice, creating two small MR jets.

Theoretically, partial clip detachment holds an increased risk of endocarditis, thrombus formation, and clip dislodgment with embolization. Therefore, we treated the patient with warfarin and clopidogrel.

Furthermore, lifelong endocarditis prophylaxis was advised. At 6 months follow-up no such complications did occur, which is in line with recent findings of the Endovascular Valve Edge-to-Edge Repair Study trial investigators.[1]

Reference

1. Feldman T, Kar S, Rinaldi M, et al. Percutaneous mitral repair with the Mitraclip system. *J Am Coll Cardiol.* 2009;54:686-694.

Transjugular Balloon Mitral Valvotomy in a Patient With Inferior Vena Caval Interruption

John Jose, DM, MD, Vipin Kumar, MD, George Joseph, DM, MD

Balloon mitral valvotomy (BMV) is an effective method of relieving severe rheumatic mitral valve stenosis in patients with suitable valve morphology. In most patients, BMV can be successfully performed using femoral venous access; however, certain congenital or acquired anomalies of the inferior vena cava or iliofemoral veins may preclude this option and necessitate the use of alternative access routes. We present a 20-year-old woman with severe symptomatic rheumatic mitral valve stenosis who was referred to our center after an unsuccessful BMV attempt using femoral venous access. Venography revealed inferior vena caval interruption with azygous continuation (Fig. 4.88A) and onward drainage into the superior vena cava (note the "candy cane" appearance; Fig. 4.88B); the hepatic veins drained directly into the right atrium (Fig. 4.88C). Right internal jugular vein access was obtained, and pulmonary angiography was performed in right anterior oblique projection to obtain a levophase image of the left atrium. The atrial septum was punctured using a pediatric transseptal needle (*asterisk* demarcates the intended site of the interatrial septal puncture), about one vertebral body height below the roof of the left atrium, and midway between the aorta (identified fluoroscopically by a pigtail catheter introduced from the right radial artery) and the anterior border of the spine (Fig. 4.88D–E). (Note that contrast injection through the needle delineates the floor of the left atrium.) A 14F J-shaped sheath was advanced into the left atrium over a 0.025-inch curved left atrial wire. A stiff 0.035-inch wire with a large, soft J-tip was then placed at the left ventricular apex and the mitral valve was dilated using an over-the-wire cylindrical single balloon (Fig. 4.88F). (Note the almost straight-line access to the mitral valve afforded by the jugular approach.) The planimetric mitral valve area increased from 1.0 to 1.72 cm^2. The entire procedure took 45 minutes and was performed without echocardiographic guidance. There were no complications. The transjugular approach to transseptal BMV is a useful alternative in patients with venous anomalies that preclude the conventional femoral venous approach.

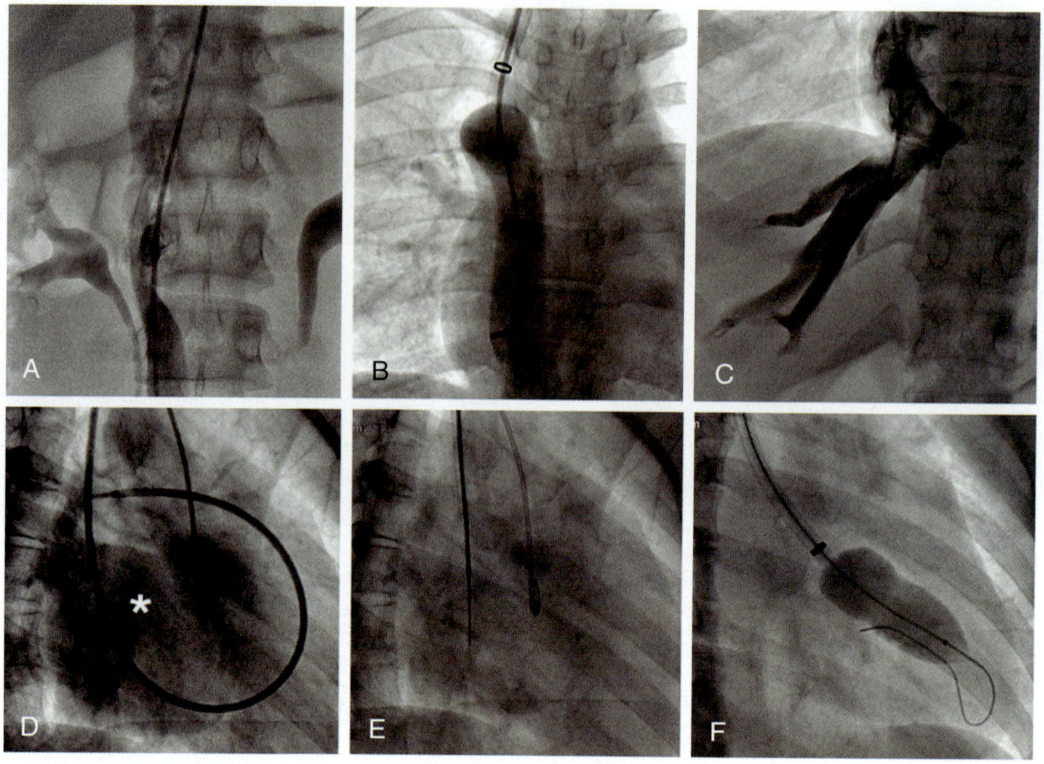

FIG. 4.88 Cine Images Demonstrating Inferior Vena Cava Interruption and Transjugular Balloon Mitral Valvotomy. *Asterisk* in (D) demarcates intended site of interatrial septal puncture.

Transseptal Anchored Vascular Plug Closure of Mitral Valve Perforation

Elena K. Grant, MBChB, Dennis W. Kim, MD, William L. Border, MBChB, MPH, Stamatios Lerakis, MD, Vasilis Babaliaros, MD, Robert N. Vincent, MD

A 15-year-old patient who had undergone neonatal repair of truncus arteriosus sustained an anterior leaflet mitral valve injury during elective aortic root replacement and aortic valve repair, resulting in severe mitral regurgitation (Fig. 4.89, Online Video 4.99). He was deemed not to be a surgical candidate in the setting of multiorgan failure on extracorporeal membrane oxygenation 1 month after valve injury. Amplatzer septal occluders (10 mm, then 12 mm) (St. Jude Medical, Minneapolis, Minnesota), a 25-mm Gore Cardioform septal occluder (Gore Medical, Flagstaff, Arizona) and a 22-mm Amplatzer vascular plug type II (St. Jude Medical) pulled through the defect during attempted device deployment. A 22-mm Amplatzer vascular plug type II was successfully deployed across both the atrial septum and the mitral valve defect, thus slightly suspending the anterior mitral valve leaflet and reducing tension on the defect rims (Figs. 4.90 and 4.91, Online Video 4.99). Mitral regurgitation (Fig. 4.91, Online Video 4.99) and clinical status improved, including successful extracorporeal membrane oxygenation decannulation. Sadly, the patient suffered a cerebral hemorrhage, and care was withdrawn 8 days after intervention. Although the length of device follow-up in this case is too limited to assess this strategy for long-term management, transcatheter closure using a transseptal anchor technique for challenging defects may at least provide acute hemodynamic improvement as a bridge to surgery for high-risk patients.

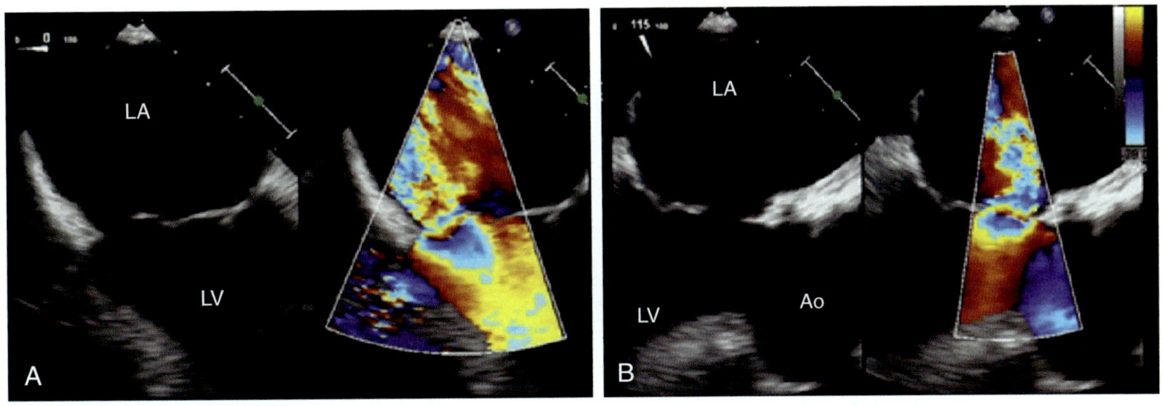

FIG. 4.89 Baseline Transesophageal Echocardiogram. Baseline transesophageal echocardiogram demonstrating anterior mitral valve leaflet defect (Online Video 4.99). *Ao*, aorta; *LA*, left atrium; *LV*, left ventricle.

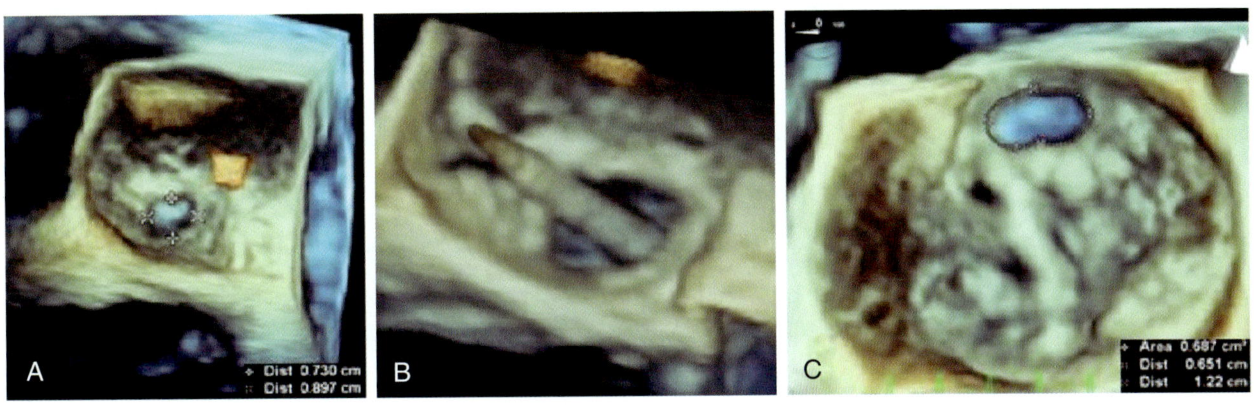

FIG. 4.90 Three-Dimensional Transesophageal Echocardiographic Guidance. (A) Three-dimensional transesophageal echocardiogram baseline mitral valve defect measurement. (B) Defect crossing guidance. (C) Repeat defect measurement after large device pull-through (Online Video 4.99).

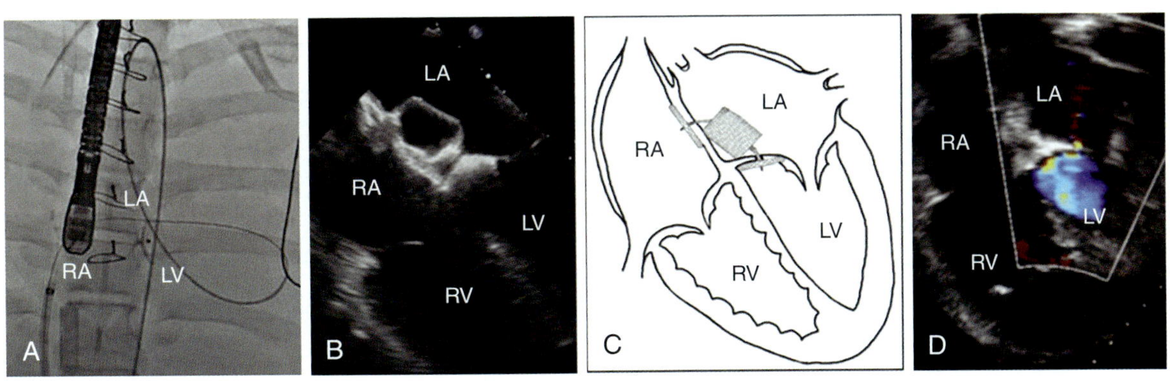

FIG. 4.91 Transseptal Anchored Vascular Plug Closure of Mitral Valve Perforation. (A) Fluoroscopy and (B) transesophageal echocardiogram of successful 22-mm Amplatzer vascular plug type II (St. Jude Medical, Minneapolis, Minnesota) placement with distal disk in the left ventricle (*LV*), mid portion in the left atrium (*LA*), and proximal disk in the right atrium (*RA*), as illustrated in (C), with mild mitral regurgitation by transthoracic echocardiogram (D) 5 days after the procedure (Online Video 4.99). *RV*, right ventricle.

Atrial Interventions (Left Atrial Appendage, Atrial Septal Defect, and Patent Foramen Ovale)

Thromboembolic Risk Reduction via Transseptal Thrombus Aspiration in a Patient With Spontaneous Left Atrial Thrombus and Stroke

Fabian Stimpfle, MD, Karin Müller, MD, Tobias Geisler, MD, Jürgen Schreieck, MD, Dennis Schlak, MD, Ulf Ziemann, MD, Meinrad Gawaz, MD, Peter Seizer, MD

We report the case of a 73-year-old male patient who first presented for cardiology consultation after transient ischemic attack. No preexisting conditions, other than hypertension, were known. Long-term electrocardiography did not reveal atrial fibrillation. Transesophageal echocardiography (TEE) showed a hyperechogenic structure in the left atrial appendage suspicious for an older thrombus. Thus, phenprocoumon therapy was initiated (target international normalized ratio: 2–3). However, 9 months later, the patient presented again after retinal embolism. Despite sufficient phenprocoumon therapy, TEE revealed a big thrombus in the left atrium (LA) adherent to the anterior wall. Therapeutic heparinization (activated partial thromboplastin time ratio: 1.5–2.5) was initiated to await spontaneous international normalized ratio drop to 1.7 before intended thrombolysis or surgery.[1] Unfortunately, a cerebral infarction in the right medial cerebral artery territory (National Institutes of Health Stroke Scale score:18) occurred instantly, and systemic thrombolysis (recombinant tissue plasminogen activator 0.9 mg/kg) was performed after administration of protamine. However, TEE showed an unaltered thrombus (Fig. 4.92A, Online Video 4.100). Because on-pump surgery or a repeated thrombolysis was impossible because of increased intracerebral bleeding risk, interventional thrombus aspiration was planned as a bail-out strategy to reduce thrombus burden and systemic thromboembolic risk. Thus, the Sentinel Cerebral Protection System (Claret Medical, Santa Rosa, California) was placed to protect the patient from further embolism (Fig. 4.93). After TEE-guided transseptal puncture,

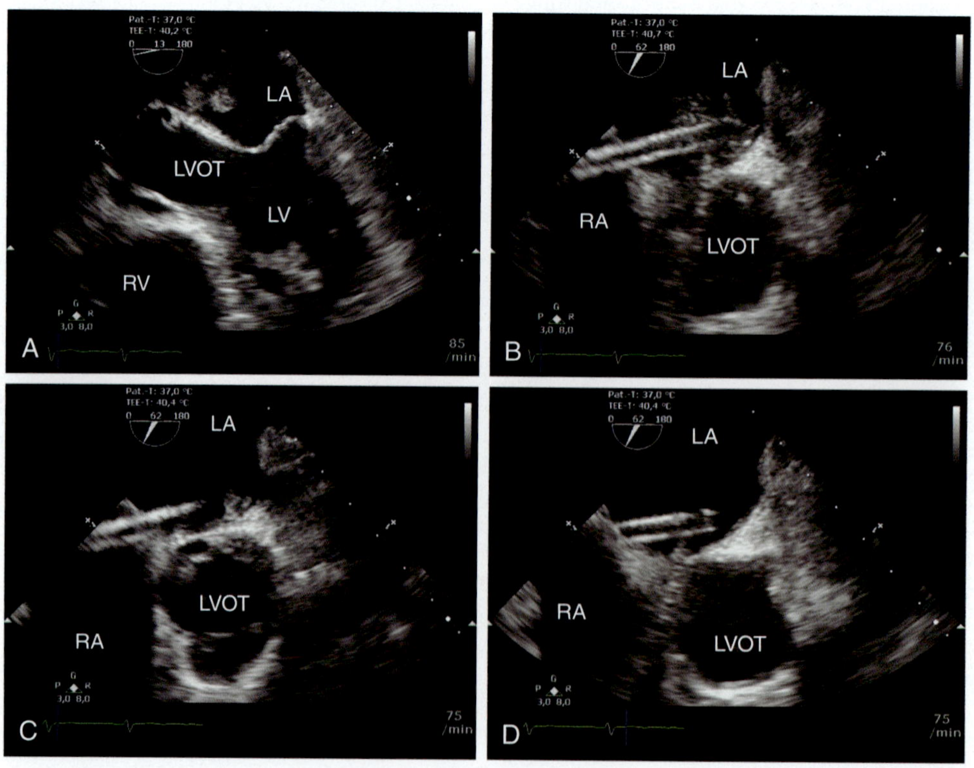

FIG. 4.92 Thrombus Aspiration: Transesophageal Echocardiography Imaging of Thrombus Aspiration from the Left Atrium. (A) Thrombus before transseptal puncture. (B) The 12F FlexCath Advance Steerable Sheath (Medtronic, Minneapolis, Minnesota) advanced into the left atrium (*LA*). (C) Most of the thrombotic material aspirated. (D) Thrombotic material almost completely aspirated (Online Video 4.100). *LV*, left ventricle; *LVOT*, left ventricular outflow tract; *RA*, right atrium; *RV*, right ventricle.

a 12F FlexCath Advance Steerable Sheath (Medtronic, Minneapolis, Minnesota) was advanced into the LA (Fig 4.92B, Online Video 4.100). Guided by TEE, the thrombotic material could be almost completely aspirated using a 50-mL syringe (Fig. 4.92C–D, Online Video 4.100). Only a minimal residue, adhesive to the anterior wall, remained in the LA (Fig. 4.92D, Online Video 4.100). Histologic investigation of the aspirated clot confirmed thrombotic origin.

Our case reports for the first time that interventional thrombus aspiration can be an alternative strategy to remove LA thrombotic material if surgery or thrombolysis is impossible.

Reference

1. Xian Y, Liang L, Smith EE, et al. Risks of intracranial hemorrhage among patients with acute ischemic stroke receiving warfarin and treated with intravenous tissue plasminogen activator. *JAMA*. 2012;307:2600-2608.

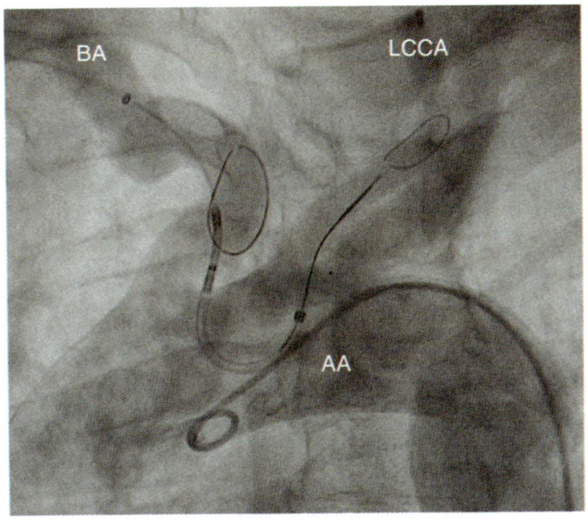

FIG. 4.93 Protection From Cerebral Embolism: Fluoroscopy of Cerebral Protection System. A Sentinel Cerebral Protection System (Claret Medical, Santa Rosa, California) is placed into the left common carotid artery (*LCCA*) and the brachiocephalic artery (*BA*). *AA*, aortic arch.

A Marble in the Heart

Juan Caro-Codón, MD, Guillermo Galeote, MD, Carlos Álvarez-Ortega, MD, Raul Moreno, MD, PhD, Jose-Luis López-Sendón, MD, PhD

An 83-year-old woman with chronic atrial fibrillation and hypertension underwent left atrial appendage occlusion at another center with a 22-mm Amplatzer cardiac plug (St. Jude Medical, Minneapolis, Minnesota) after embolic central retinal artery occlusion while receiving treatment with dabigatran. Dual-antiplatelet therapy with aspirin and clopidogrel was initiated, but both drugs were stopped after 3 months of follow-up with transthoracic echocardiography. Two years later, she was admitted to our hospital with acute cholecystitis. A computed tomography scan requested during admission to rule out pulmonary embolus showed a large filling defect in the left atrium, next to the left atrial appendage occluder, which was suggestive of atrial thrombus (Fig. 4.94A). Subsequent transesophageal echocardiography confirmed the presence of a giant ball-shaped thrombus on the atrial aspect of the occluder disk (Fig. 4.94B–C, Online Videos 4.101 and 4.102). The patient was discharged against medical advice. On follow-up, she experienced a second episode of embolic central retinal artery occlusion despite treatment with low-molecular-weight heparin.

Device-related thrombus after percutaneous left atrial appendage closure occurs in a significant proportion of patients in real-life

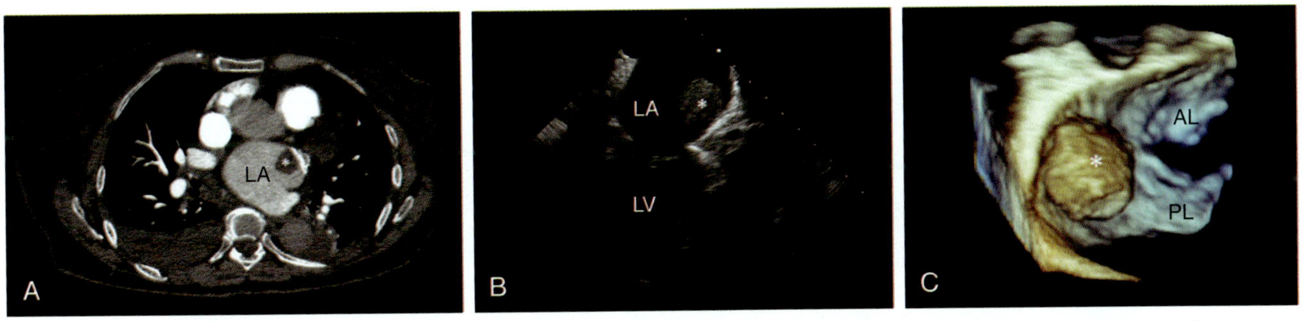

FIG. 4.94 Imaging Studies. (A) Axial contrast-enhanced computed tomography showing a large filling defect *(asterisk)* in the left atrium (*LA*) next to the occluder device. (B) Two-chamber view with transesophageal echocardiography demonstrates a giant ball-shaped thrombus *(asterisk)* next to the Amplatzer cardiac plug (Online Video 4.101). (C) Transesophageal three-dimensional en face view of the mitral valve from the left atrium with the giant thrombus *(asterisk)* covering the atrial aspect of the occluder disk (Online Video 4.102). *AL*, anterior leaflet; *LV*, left ventricle; *PL*, posterior leaflet.

registries.[1] Evidence regarding postprocedural antithrombotic management is lacking, but dual-antiplatelet therapy is usually used after Amplatzer cardiac plug implantation, followed by single-antiplatelet treatment. This case illustrates that even in patients without known risk factors for device-related thrombus,[2] changes in the antithrombotic regimen should be guided by follow-up transesophageal echocardiography. It also confirms the useful role of computed tomography scan as a noninvasive technique for device surveillance.[3]

References

1. López-Mínguez JR, Eldoayen-Gragera J, González-Fernández R, et al. Immediate and one-year results in 35 consecutive patients after closure of left atrial appendage with the Amplatzer Cardiac Plug. *Rev Española Cardiol.* 2013;66:90-97.
2. Plicht B, Konorza TFM, Kahlert P, et al. Risk factors for thrombus formation on the Amplatzer cardiac plug after left atrial appendage occlusion. *J Am Coll Cardiol Intv.* 2013;6:606-613.
3. Saw J, Fahmy P, DeJong P, et al. Cardiac CT angiography for device surveillance after endovascular left atrial appendage closure. *Eur Heart J Cardiovasc Imaging.* 2015;16: 1198-1206.

A Novel Mechanism of Atrioventricular Block After Transcatheter Closure of an Atrial Septal Defect

Tsunehisa Yamamoto, MD, Hideaki Kanazawa, MD, PhD, Sho Tanosaki, MD, Shinichi Goto, MD, Mai Kimura, MD, Hikaru Tsuruta, MD, Yuji Itabashi, MD, PhD, Mitsushige Murata, MD, PhD, Akira Kunitomi, MD, Yoshiyasu Aizawa, MD, PhD, Takahiko Nishiyama, MD, PhD, Takashi Kohno, MD, PhD, Yuichiro Maekawa, MD, PhD, Seiji Takatsuki, MD, PhD, Motoaki Sano, MD, PhD, Osamu Igawa, MD, PhD, Keiichi Fukuda, MD, PhD

A 58-year-old woman visited the emergency room for faintness on exertion 1 month after treatment of an atrial septal defect (ASD) by transcatheter closure (Amplatzer septal occluder [ASO], St. Jude Medical, St. Paul, Minnesota). An electrocardiogram showed advanced atrioventricular (AV) block (Fig. 4.95A). Transesophageal echocardiography and three-dimensional computed tomography revealed no compression of the Valsalva sinus by ASO, and there was a sufficient margin from the edge to the ASO to the AV node (Fig. 4.95B–C, Online Video 4.103), which are major risk factors of AV block after device closure of ASD. The AV block with reproducible presyncope occurred during the treadmill exercise test. Based on these findings, we reevaluated the impact of blood supply impairment to the conduction system. The coronary angiography of right coronary artery obtained before device deployment showed a small branch arising from the sinoatrial nodal artery (Fig. 4.96A–B, Online Video 4.104). Three-dimensional computed tomography demonstrated that this branch, named the right superior descending artery, provided an alternative blood supply to the AV node from the proximal right coronary artery, extending toward the AV node (Fig. 4.96C, Online Video 4.105), which was compressed by the ASO proximal to the bifurcation (Fig. 4.96D, Online Video 4.106). We concluded that compression by ASO caused exercise-induced ischemia of the AV node.

This is the first reported case of an adult patient with symptomatic AV block caused by involvement of the right superior descending artery with an ASD closure device.

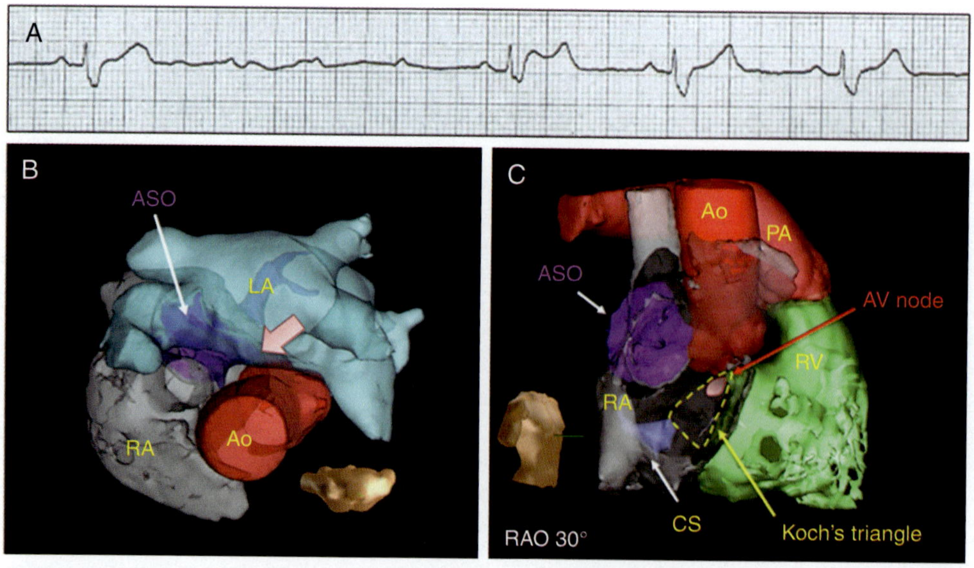

FIG. 4.95 Anatomic Relationship Between Amplatzer Septal Occluder and Atrioventricular Node. (A) Electrocardiogram recorded in the emergency department. (B and C) Reconstructed three-dimensional computed tomography (EnSite Verismo Segmentation Tool, St. Jude Medical, St. Paul, Minnesota) indicates that the Amplatzer septal occluder (*ASO*) was implanted far from the Valsalva sinus (*red arrow*) and the atrioventricular (*AV*) node located in Koch's triangle (Online Video 4.103). *Ao*, aorta; *CS*, coronary sinus; *LA*, left atrium; *PA*, pulmonary artery; *RA*, right atrium; *RAO*, right anterior oblique; *RV*, right ventricle.

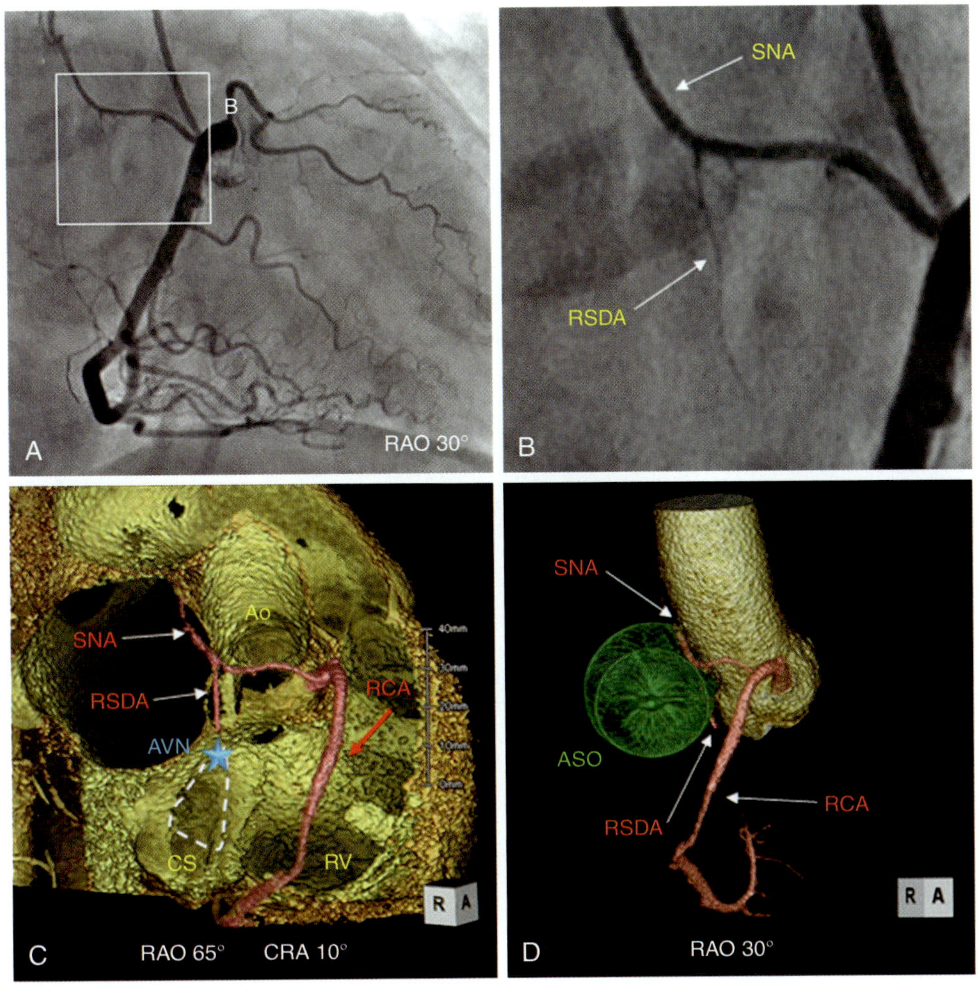

FIG. 4.96 Amplatzer Septal Occluder Impairs Alternative Blood Supply to the Atrioventricular Node. (A) Coronary angiography of the right coronary artery (*RCA*) obtained before device deployment. (B) The right superior descending artery (*RSDA*) arose from the sinoatrial nodal artery (*SNA*) (Online Video 4.104). (C and D) Anatomic evaluation of the relationship between the Amplatzer septal occluder (*ASO*) and RSDA by reconstructed three-dimensional computed tomography (Ziostation2, Ziosoft Inc., Tokyo, Japan) (Online Videos 4.105 and 4.106). *Ao*, aorta; *AVN*, atrioventricular node; *CRA*, cranial; *CS*, coronary sinus; *LA*, left atrium; *PA*, pulmonary artery; *RA*, right atrium; *RAO*, right anterior oblique; *RV*, right ventricle.

A Double-Snare Technique for Safe Retrieval of Embolized Left Atrial Appendage Occluders

Mohamad Alkhouli, MD, Sami Aljohani, MD, Ryan Kucera, RT, Naser Moiduddin, MD, Robert Hull, MD

A 71-year-old patient with hypertension, hyperlipidemia, diabetes, and atrial fibrillation, CHA_2DS_2-VASc (congestive heart failure, hypertension, age ≥75 years, diabetes mellitus, prior stroke or transient ischemic attack or thromboembolism, vascular disease, age 65–74 years, sex category) score of 3, and HAS-BLED (hypertension, abnormal renal and liver function, stroke, bleeding, labile international normalized ratios, elderly, drugs or alcohol) score of 4, was referred for a left atrial appendage occluder (LAAO) implantation. He has been intolerant to oral anticoagulation because of recurrent epistaxis. After a multidisciplinary team evaluation, the patient underwent an implantation of a 20-mm Amplatzer Amulet LAAO (St. Jude Medical, St. Paul, Minnesota). Postimplant day 1, the patient developed a short run of asymptomatic nonsustained ventricular tachycardia. Chest radiograph suggested migration of the LAAO from the appendage. Fluoroscopy revealed the lodging of the embolized device in the midabdominal aorta at the level of the renal arteries (Fig. 4.97A, Online Video 4.107).

Concerns about percutaneous retrieval were raised because the barbs of the device were pointing caudally (Fig. 4.97A, *inset*). A novel method was used to ensure safe percutaneous retrieval of the device. The button of the cephalic disk was snared with a 12- to 20-mm EN Snare device (Merit Medical Systems, South Jordan, Utah) advanced inside a 7F catheter right coronary guiding catheter via a right radial artery approach. The caudal disk of the device was snared with an 18- to 30-mm EN Snare device advanced inside a 20F catheter Check-Flo sheath (Cook Medical, Bloomington, Indiana) via a right

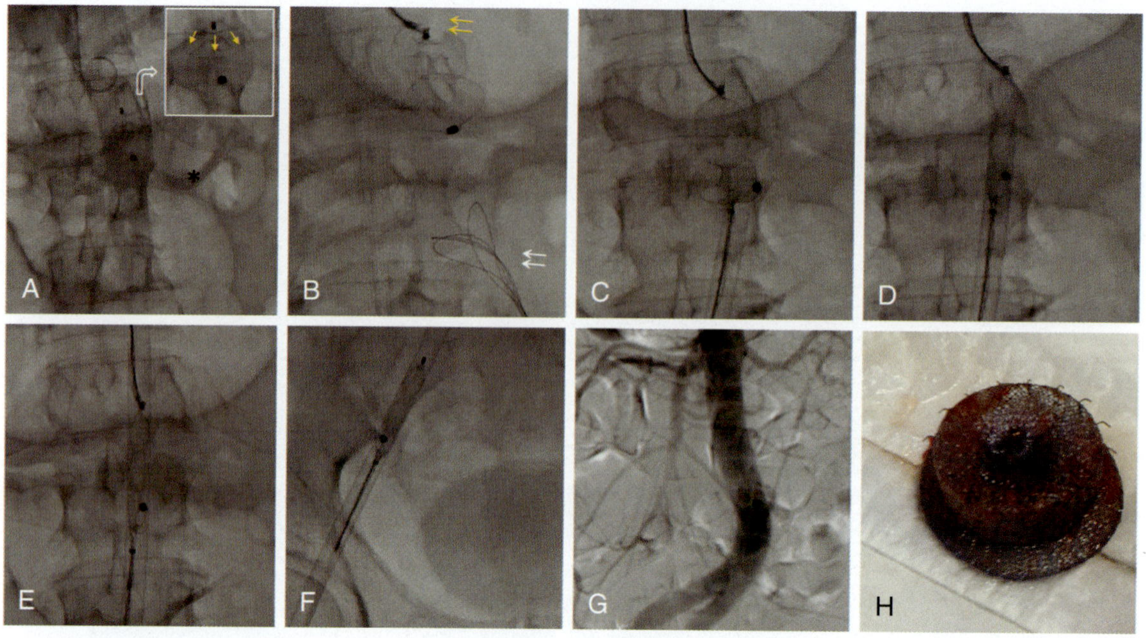

FIG. 4.97 Percutaneous Retrieval of the Embolized Left Atrial Appendage Occluder. (A) The embolized Amulet device is seen in the midabdominal aorta at the level of the renal arteries (*asterisk*). The down-pointing direction of the device's barbs is depicted by the *yellow arrows* in the *inset* (Online Video 4.107). (B) Snaring the cephalic disk (*yellow arrows*) and the caudal disk (*white arrows*) (Online Video 4.108). (C) Engulfing the stabilized and slenderized device with the 20F catheter sheath (Online Video 4.109). (D) Removing the device from the body. (E) to (G) Postremoval aortogram confirming no vascular complications (Online Video 1.110). (H) The retrieved Amulet device.

common femoral artery approach (Fig. 4.97B, Online Video 4.108). Bidirectional tugging was applied on both of the snares to stabilize the cranial disk in place and prevent distal migration and possible damage to the aorta with the barbs, and elongate the device and facilitate its retrieval (Fig. 4.97C). The Check-Flo sheath was then advanced into the slenderized device, and the device was removed from the body (Fig. 4.97D–E, Online Video 4.109). A second abdominal aortic angiography showed no vascular complications (Fig. 4.97G–H, Online Video 4.110). A 25-mm Amulet LAAO was implanted on day 4, and the patient was discharged home on day 5 without further complications.

Device embolization into the aorta is an uncommon complication of LAAO implantation.[1-3] Percutaneous retrieval can be challenging because of the potential risk of vascular wall damage with the device's barbs. A double-snare technique can be used to avoid this risk and ensure safe percutaneous retrieval.

References

1. Mester P, Dompnier A, Belle L. Asymptomatic migration of an AMPLATZER™ Amulet™ left atrial appendage occluder through the mitral valve. *Catheter Cardiovasc Interv.* 2017;90(2):346-349. doi:10.1002/ccd.26557. [Epub 2016 May 3.]
2. Fahmy P, Eng L, Saw J. Retrieval of embolized left atrial appendage devices. *Catheter Cardiovasc Interv.* 2018;91(7):E75-E80. doi:10.1002/ccd.26800. [Epub 2016 Sep 28.].
3. Aminian A, Lalmand J, Tzikas A, Budts W, Benit E, Kefer J. Embolization of left atrial appendage closure devices: a systematic review of cases reported with the watchman device and the Amplatzer cardiac plug. *Catheter Cardiovasc Interv.* 2015;86:128-135.

Acute Heart Failure Caused by Dislocation of a Watchman Left Atrial Appendage Occluder

Hai Deng, MD, Hongtao Liao, MD, Yang Liu, MD, PhD, Shuo Chen, MD, Yumei Xue, MD, Xianzhang Zhan, MD, Xianhong Fang, MD, Yigao Huang, MD, Jianfang Luo, MD, Hongwen Fei, MD, Zhiwei Zhang, MD, Shulin Wu, MD

A 75-year-old man with permanent atrial fibrillation was referred to our hospital. Because of a high risk of cardioembolic stroke with a CHA_2DS_2-VASc (congestive heart failure, hypertension, age ≥75 years, diabetes mellitus, prior stroke or transient ischemic attack or thromboembolism, vascular disease, age 65–74 years, sex category) score of 4 points and a strong contraindication for anticoagulants with a HAS-BLED (hypertension, abnormal renal and liver function, stroke, bleeding, labile international normalized ratios, elderly, drugs or alcohol) score of 4 points, he was a good candidate for percutaneous left atrial appendage (LAA) occlusion. A standard implant procedure was performed with the patient under general anesthesia. The procedure protocol has been described previously.[1] A Watchman LAA occluder (Boston Scientific, Marlborough, Massachusetts) (diameter, 30 mm) was successfully released at the LAA ostium under fluoroscopic guidance and continuous transesophageal echocardiographic monitoring (Fig. 4.98A). The patient was asymptomatic and hemodynamically stable at discharge. However, he experienced acute left-sided heart failure with dyspnea on exertion 30 days after the procedure. His symptoms were suddenly relieved with oral administration of digoxin and diuretic drugs. Echocardiographic

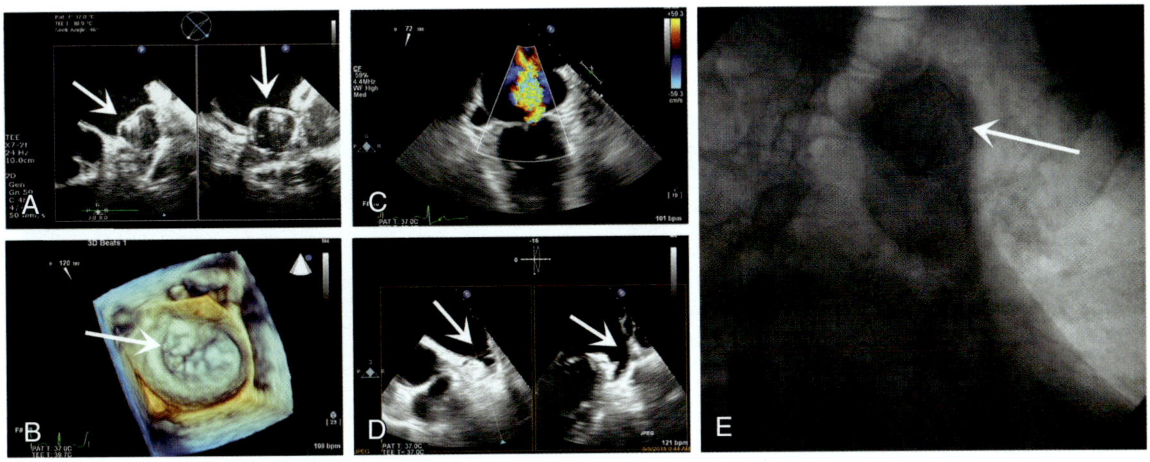

FIG. 4.98 Dislocated Watchman Device Causing Severe Mitral Regurgitation. (A) The final position of the device deployed at the left atrial appendage (LAA) ostium under transesophageal echocardiographic monitoring (*arrows*). (B) Three-dimensional transesophageal echocardiography showing the anterior mitral leaflet prolapse (*arrow*). (C) Transesophageal echocardiography showing severe mitral regurgitation. (D) Transesophageal echocardiography showing the absence of the device in the LAA (*arrows*). (E) Fluoroscopic imaging showing the LAA device dislocated in the aortic arch (*arrow*).

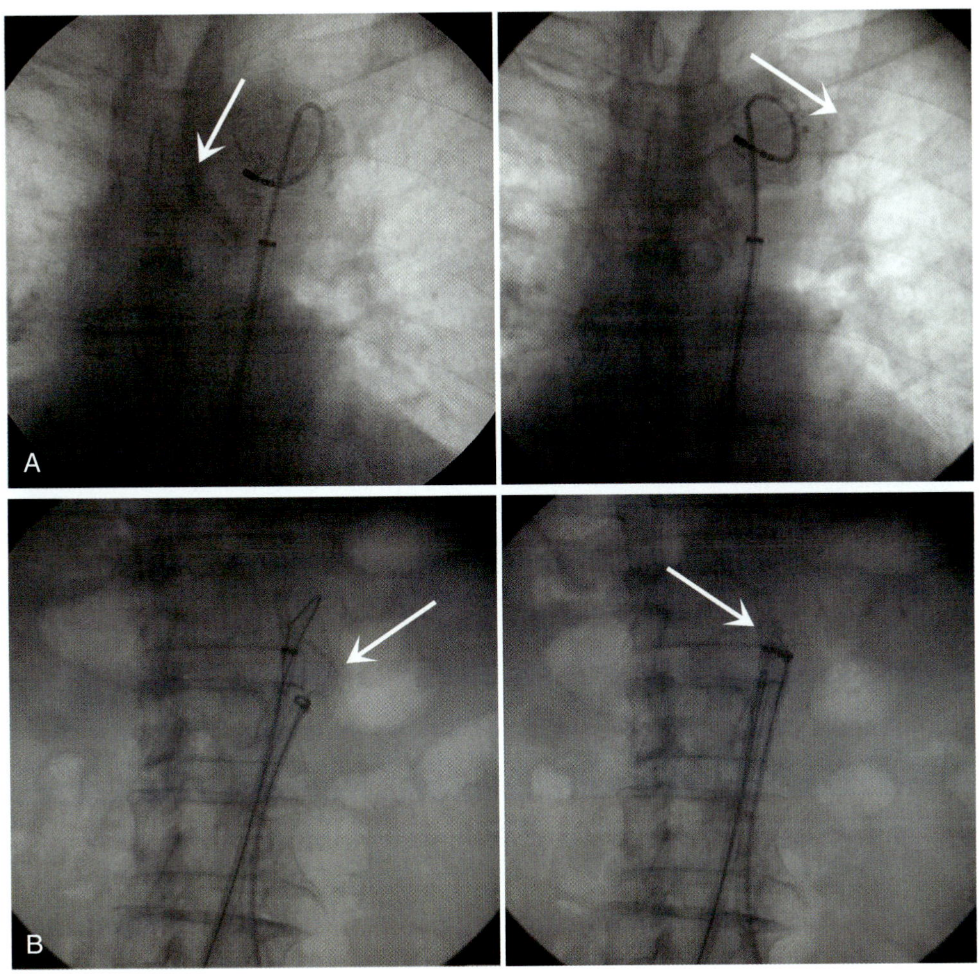

FIG. 4.99 Percutaneous Retrieval of the Device by Combined Deflectable Ablation Catheter and Double Gooseneck Snare. (A) Reversing direction (*arrows*) of the device with a deflectable ablation catheter. (B) The device (*arrows*) being pulled out by double gooseneck snares.

assessment at the 45-day follow-up visit demonstrated ruptured mitral chordae tendineae (Fig. 4.98B), severe mitral regurgitation (Fig 4.98C), and the absence of the implant either in the LAA or in any of the heart cavities (Fig. 4.98D). Fluoroscopic imaging confirmed that the LAA device was located in the aortic arch (Fig. 4.98E). After changing the direction of the device hub to the descending aorta by a deflectable ablation catheter (Fig. 4.99A), the device was retrieved successfully using double gooseneck snares (10 and 15 mm in diameter) via bilateral femoral artery access with 14F sheaths (Fig. 4.99B). A completely endothelialized disk was observed (Fig. 4.100).

This case shows that acute heart failure after successful LAA occlusion may imply acute mitral dysfunction caused by mechanical damage of the mitral valve because of an LAA occluder dislocation. The unexpected symptom relief would most likely be due to the dislocated device running into aorta, which relieves obstruction of the left ventricular outflow tract. Percutaneous retrieval of the device is feasible, obviating further surgical intervention.

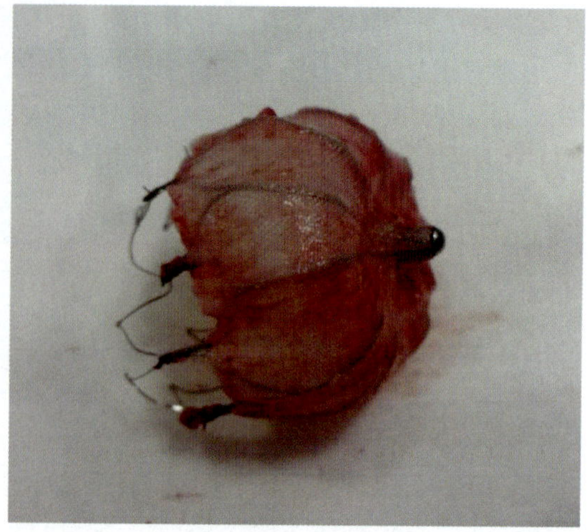

FIG. 4.100 Retrieved Device With a Completely Endothelialized Disk. The retrieved Watchman device with a completely endothelialized disk.

Reference

1. Fountain RB, Holmes DR, Chandrasekaran K, et al. The PROTECT AF (WATCHMAN Left Atrial Appendage System for Embolic PROTECTion in Patients with Atrial Fibrillation) trial. *Am Heart J.* 2006;151:956-961.

Amplatzer Septal Occluder Sealed the Complicating Aortic Root Perforation During Transseptal Procedure

Beny Hartono, MD, Omar Abdul Razakjr, MD, Muhammad Munawar, MD, PhD

An octogenarian man with severe rheumatic mitral stenosis underwent percutaneous transvenous mitral commissurotomy. The procedure was complicated by accidental unrecognized aortic root puncture by Brockenbrough needle followed by the delivery of the 8F Mullins sheath (Medtronic, Minneapolis, Minnesota). Subsequent contrast injection demonstrated the left coronary artery (Fig. 4.101A). The complication could be avoided if some cautious procedure were performed, such as measuring the pressure from the Brockenbrough needle to differentiate the left atrial and aortic pressure before advancing the Mullins sheath. We decided to seal the hole with a 4-mm Amplatzer Septal Occluder (ASO) device (St. Jude Medical, St. Paul, Minnesota) instead of surgical intervention. A coiled guidewire (Fig. 4.101B, *arrows*) was advanced to the aorta to facilitate the exchange of the Mullins sheath with an 8F ASO delivery sheath. A test injection of contrast medium confirmed position within aortic root. The loader with the collapsed device was then advanced into the delivery catheter by pushing the delivery cable. Under fluoroscopic and ultrasonic guidance, the ASO device (Fig. 4.101C, *arrow*) was deployed and the left atrial disk and pulled gently against the aortic wall, which was both felt and observed by two-dimensional echocardiography. Using gentle tension on the delivery cable, the sheath (Fig. 4.101C, *arrowhead*) was pulled back and the right atrial disk was deployed. Echocardiography and contrast fluoroscopy confirmed optimal position across the communication and the position of the right coronary artery. After release of the ASO (Fig. 4.101D), both color Doppler echocardiography and angiography showed the absence of the residual shunt. During 6-month echocardiographic follow-up, the ASO device remained in place without any residual flow observed. This is the first usage of such a device for a complication that always requires an open-heart surgery (Online Video 4.111).

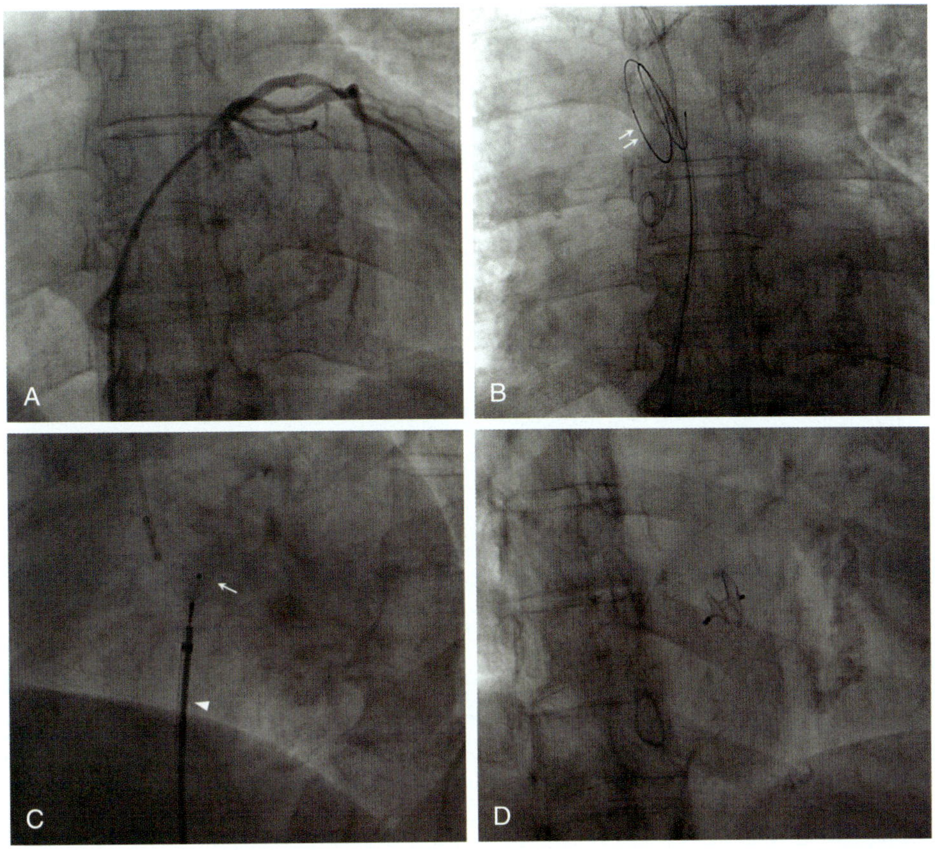

FIG. 4.101 Aortic Root Perforation Closed With Amplatzer Septal Occluder. (A) Transseptal procedure perforated the aortic root. The left coronary artery was noted with injection of contrast. (B) A coiled guidewire (*arrow*) was used to facilitate the exchange of the Mullins sheath (Medtronic, Minneapolis, Minnesota) for an Amplatzer Septal Occluder (ASO) delivery sheath. Panel (C) shows the deployment of the ASO (*arrow*) from the delivery sheath (*arrowhead*) by gentle tension of the delivery cable. Panel (D) shows the final ASO position after being released from the delivery sheath.

Early Anterior Mitral Valve Leaflet Mechanical Erosion After Left Atrial Appendage Occluder Implantation

Alain Berrebi, MD, Frederic A. Sebag, MD, Christelle Diakov, MD, Nicolas Amabile, MD, PhD

An 84-year-old woman was referred to our center for a left atrial appendage (LAA) occlusion (LAAO) procedure. Her medical history included alcoholic cirrhosis, permanent atrial fibrillation, and recent hemorrhagic shock related to gastrointestinal bleeding under oral anticoagulation. CHA_2DS_2-VASc (congestive heart failure, hypertension, age ≥75 years, diabetes mellitus, prior stroke or transient ischemic attack or thromboembolism, vascular disease, age 65–74 years, sex category) and HAS-BLED (hypertension, abnormal renal and liver function, stroke, bleeding, labile international normalized ratios, elderly, drugs or alcohol) scores were both equal to 5. LAA ostium and neck dimensions were 31 mm and 26 mm, respectively, by computed tomography scan (Fig. 4.102A).

The procedure was performed under general anesthesia and transesophageal echocardiography guidance that confirmed LAA dimensions. A 28-mm Amplatzer Amulet occluder (St. Jude Medical, St. Paul, Minnesota) was thus implanted. Postprocedural results showed device correct position and compression (Fig. 4.102B), and absence of residual peridevice atrial leakage and filling. Mitral valve kinetics was normal, although the device was in contact with the anterior leaflet, but no additional valvular regurgitation was noticed (Fig. 4.102C, Online Videos 4.112 and 4.113).

The patient was discharged under single-antiplatelet therapy (aspirin) and had an uneventful clinical evolution. Routine transesophageal echocardiography control was performed 6 weeks after procedure and revealed neither residual peridevice leakage nor thrombus. However, a de novo mild mitral regurgitation was identified (Fig. 4.102D, Online Video 4.114), which was related to a device-induced tear of the A1 portion of the anterior leaflet.

To our best knowledge, this is the first case of a mitral valve perforation after an LAAO procedure. The most plausible mechanism here is the progressive leaflet erosion by the 35-mm-diameter device outer disk. Hemolysis and endocarditis might represent theoretic complications and thus require close patient follow-up. This case advocates for the need to anticipate the anatomic relationships between device and native heart structure during LAAO procedures to avoid unexpected complications.

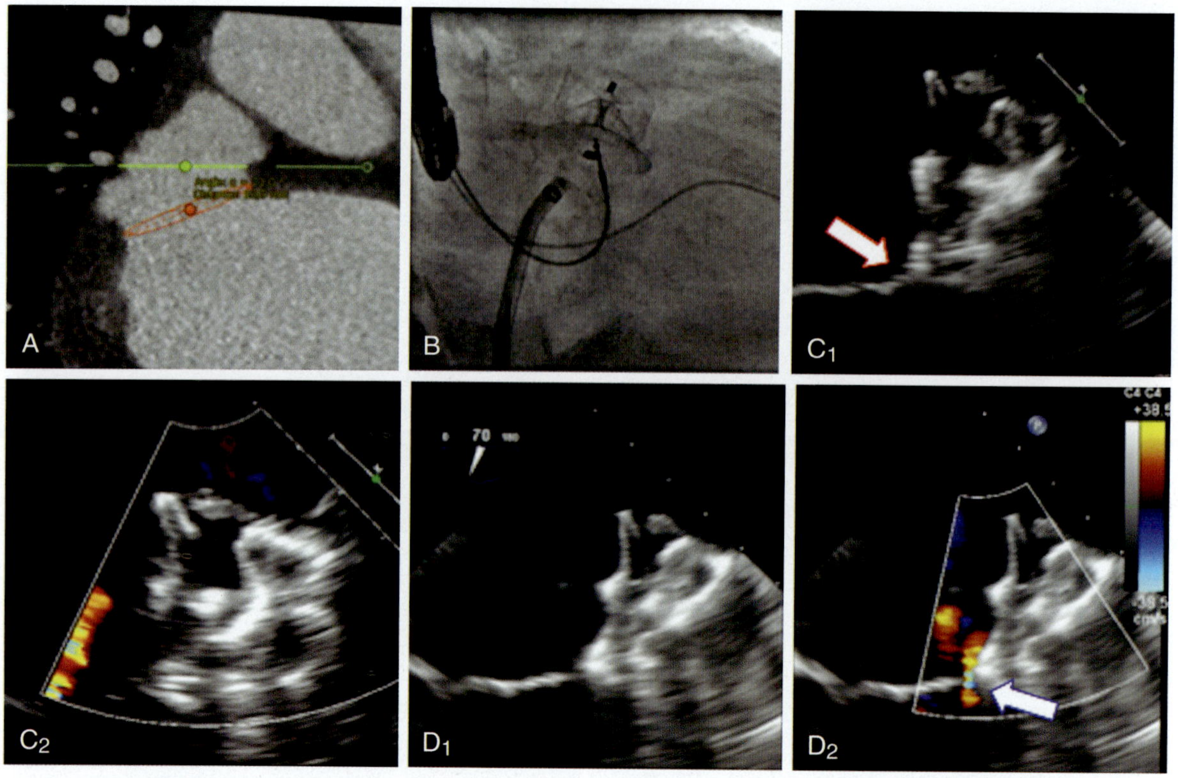

FIG. 4.102 Left Atrial Appendage Occlusion: Preparation, Procedure, and Follow-Up. (A) Left atrial appendage dimensions as assessed by preintervention computed tomography scan. Ostium diameter was measured to 31 mm and the device's lobe landing zone (neck) was measured to 26 mm. (B) Final angiographic view after the 28-mm Amplatzer Amulet occluder (St. Jude Medical, St. Paul, Minnesota) implantation. (C) Immediate postimplantation transesophageal echocardiography (TEE) view (Online Videos 4.112 and 4.113). (C_1) The device outer disk was in contact with anterior leaflet (*arrow*), but no valvular regurgitation was identified (C_2). (D) Six-week control TEE. An erosion was identified in the anterior mitral leaflet (D_1) related a shearing process by the outer disk and (D_2) creating a mild regurgitation (*arrow*) (Online Video 4.114).

Embolization of Left Atrial Appendage Thrombus During Transcatheter Aortic Valve Replacement: A Potential Mechanism of Periprocedural Stroke

Paul D. Williams, BM, BCh, MA, MD, Mark A. de Belder, MA, MD, Neil Maredia, MB ChB, MD, Douglas F. Muir, MB ChB

An 81-year-old man with severe symptomatic aortic stenosis, permanent atrial fibrillation, and a previous stroke underwent transcatheter aortic valve replacement (TAVR). His long-term warfarin therapy was stopped 5 days before admission.

At the beginning of the procedure, transesophageal echocardiography (TEE) identified thrombus within the left atrial appendage (LAA) (Fig. 4.106A, Online Video 4.115). It initially proved difficult to position a preshaped guidewire within the left ventricle, and there was frequent wire prolapse through the mitral valve into the left atrium. After balloon aortic valvuloplasty, a large mobile filling defect was seen within the left ventricle (Fig. 4.106B, Online Video 4.116), and the LAA was now empty (Fig. 4.103C, Online Video 4.117). The activated clotting time was >300 s. Aspiration was performed via an 8-F guide catheter, which caused the filling defect to migrate distally to straddle the aortic valve (Fig. 4.103D, Online Video 4.118).

A 16F snare delivery sheath was advanced over the wire to the aortic root, and the wire was withdrawn across the aortic valve and into the sheath during continuous aspiration. A large thrombus with the appearance of an appendage "cast" was retrieved (Fig. 4.103E).

Subsequent implantation of a 29-mm SAPIEN XT valve (Edwards Lifesciences, Inc., Irvine, California) was uncomplicated. The patient made a good recovery with no clinical evidence of an embolic event.

Atrial fibrillation is common in patients undergoing TAVR, and this case demonstrates that LAA thrombus embolization is a potential mechanism of periprocedural stroke. Investigation for LAA thrombus should be performed in all patients with atrial fibrillation as part of their workup for TAVR. This is of particular importance for cases performed under conscious sedation in which intraprocedural TEE is not available. There may be a role for embolic protection devices in patients with persistent LAA thrombus despite adequate anticoagulation.

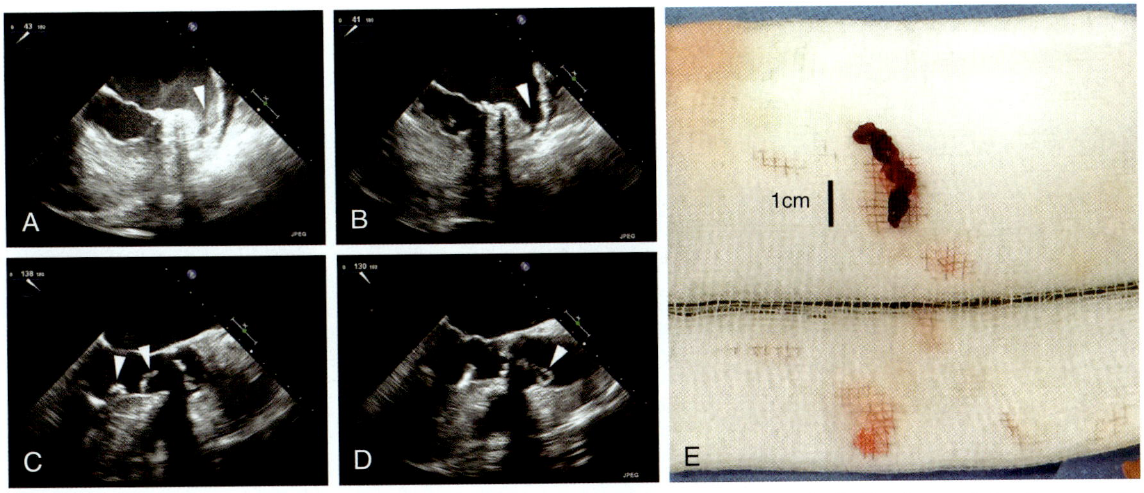

FIG. 4.103 Transesophageal Echocardiography Images of Left Atrial Appendage Thrombus Embolization and the Extracted Thrombus. (A) Transesophageal echocardiography showing thrombus within the left atrial appendage (Online Video 4.115). (B) After wire positioning in the left ventricle and aortic valvuloplasty, a mobile filling defect is noted within the left ventricle and outflow tract (Online Video 4.116). (C) The appendage is now empty (Online Video 4.117). (D) After aspiration, the filling defect has migrated to straddle the aortic valve into the sinus of Valsalva (Online Video 4.118). (E) The retrieved thrombus with the appearance of an appendage "cast."

Run With the Hare and Hunt With the Hounds: Watchman Device Surgical Resection in the Setting of Recurrent Device–Related Thrombi in a Patient With Bleeding Diathesis

Catherine O'Hara, MD, Gilles E. O'Hara, MD, Frédéric Jacques, MD, Jean Champagne, MD, Maryse Lemyre, NP, Lyne Charbonneau, NP, Kim O'Connor, MD, Mathieu Bernier, MD, Jonathan Beaudoin, MD, Josep Rodés-Cabau, MD, Jean-Michel Paradis, MD

A 63-year-old man with a medical history of hypertension, dyslipidemia, coronary disease, and left ventricular dysfunction (left ventricular ejection fraction, 45%), received anticoagulant therapy for atrial fibrillation because of high thromboembolic risk (CHA_2DS_2-VASc [congestive heart failure, hypertension, age ≥75 years, diabetes mellitus, prior stroke or transient ischemic attack or thromboembolism, vascular disease, age 65–74 years, sex category] score, 3). Under rivaroxaban, the patient experienced recurrent episodes of lower gastrointestinal bleeding caused by hemorrhoids. Despite rubber band ligation and argon laser therapy, major bleeding returned every time anticoagulation was resumed.

Because of this contraindication for anticoagulation therapy, the patient was referred to our institution to undergo a percutaneous closure of the left atrial appendage (LAA). Under general anesthesia, with transesophageal echocardiography (TEE) and fluoroscopic guidance (Fig. 4.104A), a 24-mm Watchman device (Boston Scientific, St. Paul, Minnesota) (Fig. 4.105) was successfully implanted (Fig. 4.104B). Treatment at discharge consisted of aspirin 80 mg, clopidogrel 75 mg, and rivaroxaban 15 mg daily. However, the latter agent had to be stopped 18 days after the procedure because of significant lower gastrointestinal bleeding and epistaxis.

During routine TEE performed 45 days after the procedure, the device was well positioned and there was no residual peridevice leak. Nonetheless, a thrombus was now visualized on the face of the LAA occluder, probably attached to the central threaded insert (Fig. 4.104C–D). Dalteparin (200 U/kg) was initiated rapidly but had to be discontinued because of another episode of life-threatening epistaxis. Because the thrombus was still progressing under double-antiplatelet therapy, warfarin was initiated. A consultation with the hematologist revealed no specific clotting disorders.

After 5 months of antithrombotic therapy (aspirin, clopidogrel, and warfarin), the thrombus finally disappeared (Fig. 4.104E–F). Thus, the patient was empirically placed on apixaban 2.5 mg twice a day alone. However, because of persistent disabling rectal bleeding, apixaban was switched to aspirin 80 mg daily.

Unfortunately, routine 1-year TEE revealed a pedunculated thrombus recurrence on the Watchman device (Fig. 4.104G–H). Because the patient refused to take any form of oral anticoagulation ever again, the heart team elected to proceed with a surgical excision of the Watchman device combined with an LAA ligature (Fig. 4.106). The postoperative course was uneventful. The patient was to be treated with warfarin for 3 months and lifelong aspirin afterward.

To our knowledge, this is one of the first worldwide reports of Watchman device surgical excision. LAA device thrombosis is one of the most dreaded complications. Most of the published cases resolved after oral anticoagulation therapy.[2–4] Current postprocedural antithrombotic regimens are empirical. Considering the complexity of patients undergoing LAA closure, further studies are needed not only to define evidence-based antithrombotic strategies to prevent device thrombosis but also to better determine predisposing factors of this feared complication.

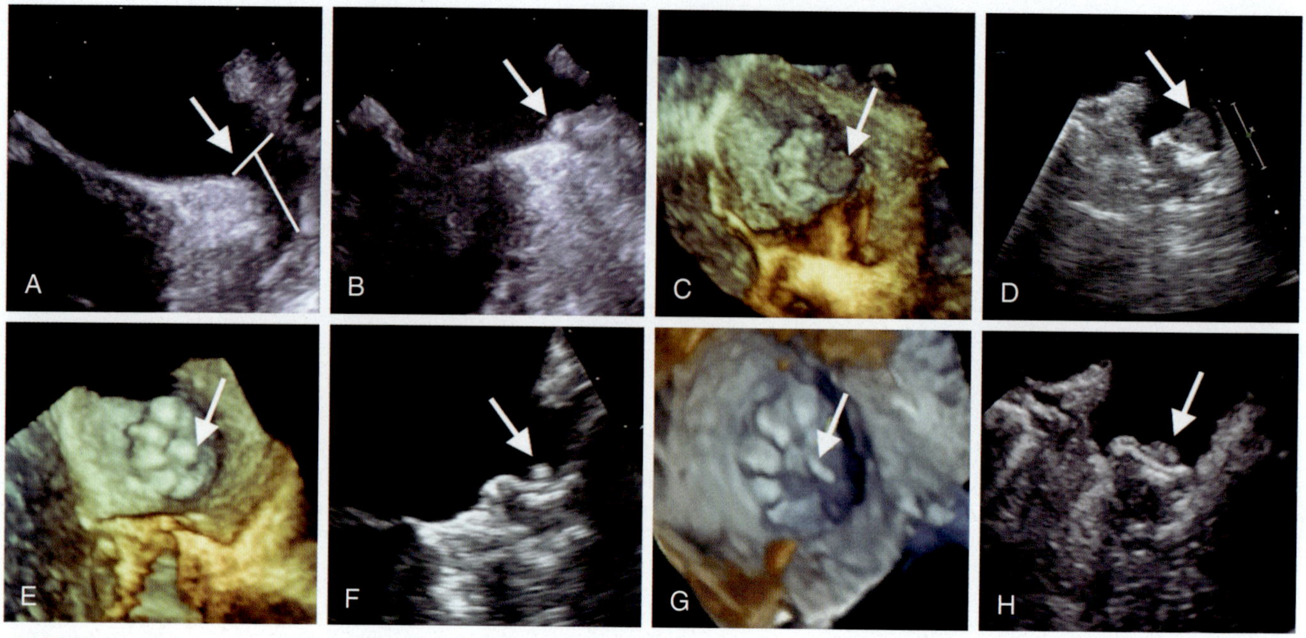

FIG. 4.104 Transesophageal Echocardiography Images of the Left Atrial Appendage. (A) Preprocedural maximal left atrial appendage ostial diameter measured 19 mm (with a depth of 24 mm) (*arrow*), 90° two-dimensional [2D] transesophageal echocardiography [TEE]. (B) LAA immediately after Watchman device implantation (*arrow*) (90°2D TEE). (C and D) Thrombus visualized 45 days postprocedure, probably attached to the central threaded insert (*arrow*). (C) 3D TEE and (D) 120° 2D TEE. (E and F) Resolution of the thrombus after 5 months of antithrombotic therapy with thrombus-free threaded insert (*arrow*) (E) 3D TEE and (F) 90° 2D TEE. (G and H) Pedunculated device-related thrombus recurrence (*arrow*) at the routine 1-year follow-up TEE. (G) 3D TEE and (H) 120° 2D TEE.

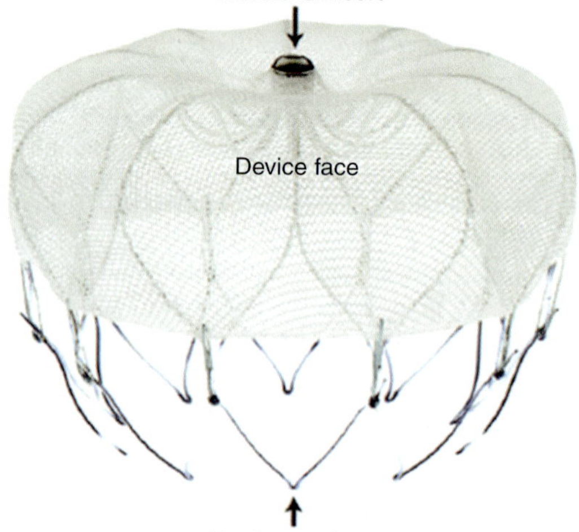

FIG. 4.105 Watchman Device. Watchman (Boston Scientific, St. Paul, Minnesota) left atrial appendage closure device.[1]

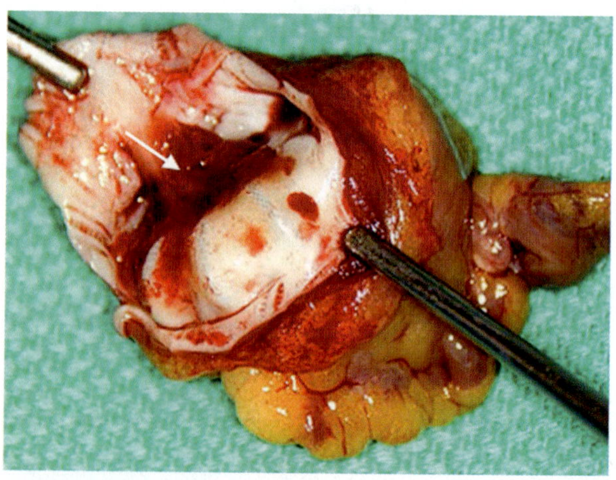

FIG. 4.106 Resected Atrial Appendage. Resected atrial appendage and device-related thrombus (*arrow*) probably attached to the central threaded insert. The Watchman device was completely endothelialized.

References

1. Main ML, Fan D, Reddy VY, et al. Assessment of device-related thrombus and associated clinical outcomes with the WATCHMAN Left Atrial Appendage Closure Device for Embolic Protection in Patients With Atrial Fibrillation (from the PROTECT-AF trial). *Am J Cardiol.* 2016;117:1127-1134.
2. Viles-Gonzalez JF, Kar S, Douglas P, et al. The clinical impact of incomplete left atrial appendage closure with the Watchman device in patients with atrial fibrillation: a PROTECT AF (Percutaneous Closure of the Left Atrial Appendage Versus Warfarin Therapy for Prevention of Stroke in Patients With Atrial Fibrillation) substudy. *J Am Coll Cardiol.* 2012;59:923-929.
3. Reddy VY, Möbius-Winkler S, Miller MA, et al. Left atrial appendage closure with the Watchman device in patients with a contraindication for oral anticoagulation: the ASAP study (ASA Plavix Feasibility Study With Watchman Left Atrial Appendage Closure Technology). *J Am Coll Cardiol.* 2013;61:2551-2556.
4. Reddy VY, Holmes D, Doshi SK, Neuzil P, Kar S. Safety of percutaneous left atrial appendage closure: results from the Watchman Left Atrial Appendage System for Embolic Protection in Patients with AF (PROTECT AF) clinical trial and the Continued Access Registry. *Circulation.* 2011;123:417-424.

A Novel Wire-Assisted Technique for Closing Large Atrial Septal Defects: New Concepts of Closure Mechanism

Hideaki Kanazawa, MD, PhD, Akio Kawamura, MD, PhD, Mai Kimura, MD, Keitaro Akita, MD, Fumiaki Yashima, MD, Takahide Arai, MD, Takashi Kawakami, MD, PhD, Kentaro Hayashida, MD, PhD, Hikaru Tsuruta, MD, Shinsuke Yuasa, MD, PhD, Yuji Itabashi, MD, PhD, Mitsushige Murata, MD, PhD, Yuichiro Maekawa, MD, PhD, Keiichi Fukuda, MD, PhD

Transcatheter closure of an atrial septal defect (ASD) with the Amplatzer Septal Occluder (ASO) (St. Jude Medical, St. Paul, Minnesota) is a well-established treatment strategy. Although most ASDs are easy to close percutaneously, large ASDs or those with deficient aortic/superior rims are challenging to close with conventional techniques.

Case 1 shows a large ASD with deficient aortic and superior rims (Fig. 4.107A–C, Online Video 4.119). After several attempts using conventional techniques failed, an Amplatz stiff guidewire was placed into the left upper pulmonary vein (LUPV). The ASO (26 mm) was deployed successfully via the LUPV approach. Theoretically, the wire helps keep the left atrial disk parallel to the septum and prevents prolapse into the right atrium (Fig. 4.107C, *yellow arrow*).

Case 2 shows a large elliptical ASD (26 × 16 mm) (Fig. 4.108A, Online Video 4.120). It was difficult to deploy the ASO using several techniques. Therefore, the wire (with a multipurpose catheter to avoid tearing the posterior septum) was placed into the right upper pulmonary vein (Fig. 4.108B). The ASO was successfully implanted in the appropriate position (Online Video 4.120). The wire likely causes the deformity in the defect (Fig. 4.108C). This deformity brings down the superior rim (Fig. 4.108C, *yellow arrows*) and provides adequate tension at the superior rim (Fig. 4.108C, *red arrow*) to maintain the top edge of the left atrial disc in position.

This technique is a novel, simple, and less invasive maneuver that shows promise in challenging ASDs. It is called the wire-assisted technique.

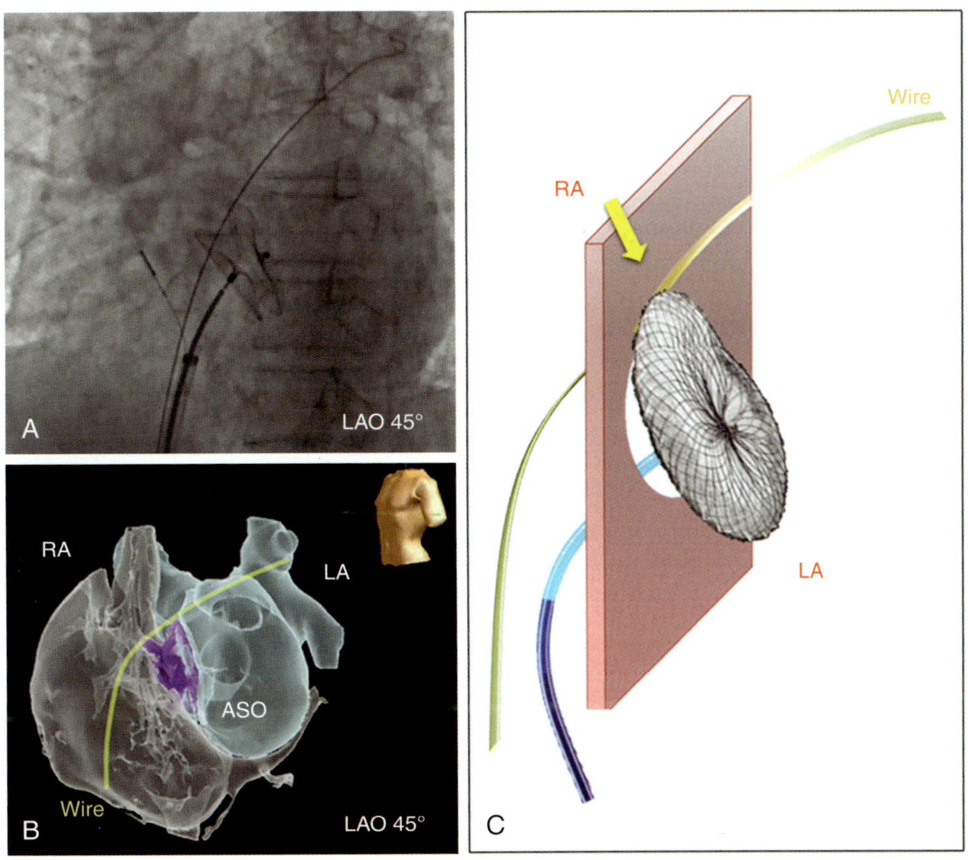

FIG. 4.107 Wire-Assisted Technique 1. (A) Fluoroscopic image of the wire-assisted technique 1 (Online Video 4.119). (B) A three-dimensional computed tomography image (using EnSite Verismo Segmentation Tool [St. Jude Medical, St. Paul, Minnesota]) of the relationship between the wire position and the Amplatzer device. (C) Illustration of the mechanism of wire-assisted technique 1. *Yellow arrow* indicates prevention of left atrial disk prolapse into the right atrium. *ASO*, Amplatzer Septal Occluder; *LA*, left atrium; *LAO*, left anterior oblique; *RA*, right atrium.

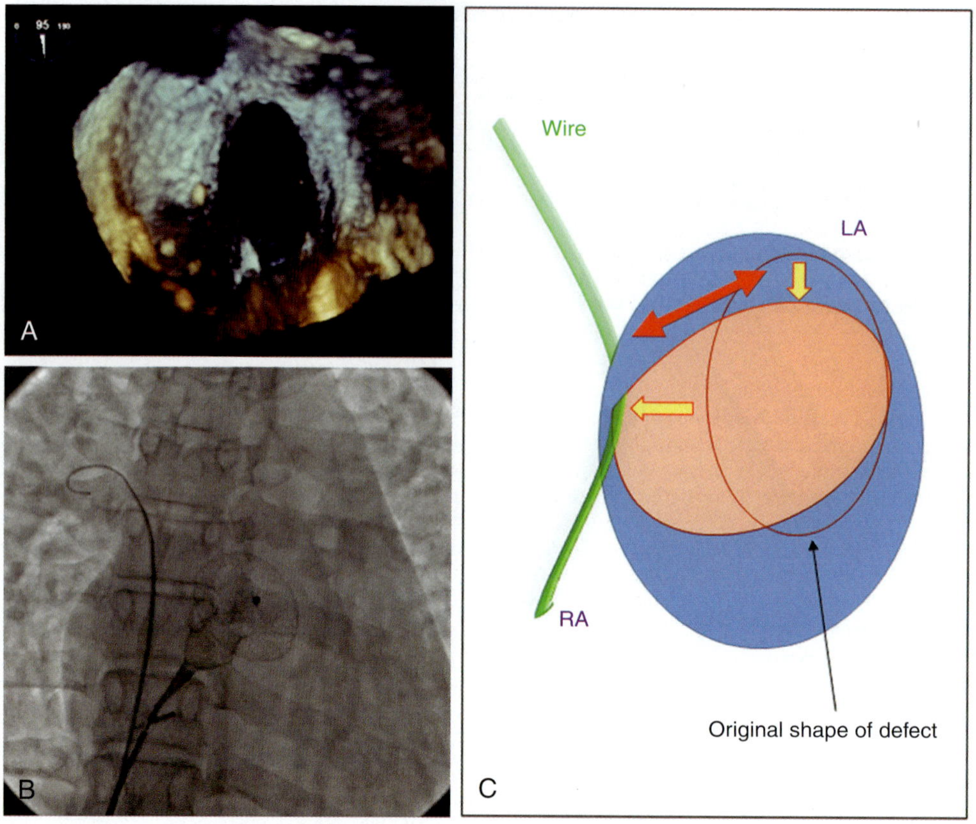

FIG. 4.108 Wire-Assisted Technique 2. (A) Three-dimensional transesophageal echocardiography of a large elliptical atrial septal defect. (B) Fluoroscopic image of wire-assisted technique 2 (Online Video 4.120). (C) Illustration of the mechanism of wire-assisted technique 2. *ASO*, Amplatzer Septal Occluder; *LA*, left atrium; *LAO*, left anterior oblique; *RA*, right atrium.

Integrated Three-Dimensional Echo-X-Ray Navigation-Guided Transcatheter Closure of Complex Multiple Atrial Septal Defects

Yoichi Takaya, MD, Teiji Akagi, MD, Koji Nakagawa, MD, Hiroshi Ito, MD

A 73-year-old woman was referred to our institution for transcatheter closure of an atrial septal defect (ASD). Three-dimensional transesophageal echocardiography (3D TEE) showed complex multiple ASDs of 26 mm (ASD1), 10 mm (ASD2), 8 mm (ASD3), and 15 mm (ASD4) (Fig. 4.109A). We planned to close relatively large ASDs (ASD1 and ASD4) using two devices. The 3D echo-x-ray navigation system (EchoNavigator, Philips Medical Systems, Andover, Massachusetts) was used to guide the accurate delivery of the Amplatzer delivery sheaths, marking the shape and location of ASD1 and ASD4 during the procedure (Fig. 4.109B–C). Catheters were then advanced to the identified location (Fig. 4.109D, Online Video 4.121A–B). After balloon sizing, 28-mm and 20-mm Amplatzer Septal Occluders (St. Jude Medical, St. Paul, Minnesota) were deployed at the appropriate sites (Fig. 4.109E–F).

This is the first report of successful transcatheter closure of complex multiple ASDs under 3D echo-x-ray navigation guidance. Transcatheter closure of multiple ASDs remains challenging because of complicated techniques, including the risk of incorrect device delivery into unexpected defects. The 3D echo-x-ray navigation system integrates TEE and fluoroscopy images,[1] identifying the shape and location of ASDs evaluated by 3D TEE on fluoroscopy. This system provides a more comprehensible image, and contributes to valuable guidance in the approach to complex multiple ASDs.

Reference

1. Clegg SD, Chen SJ, Nijhof N, et al. Integrated 3D echo-x-ray to optimize image guidance for structural heart intervention. *J Am Coll Cardiol Img*. 2015;8:371-374.

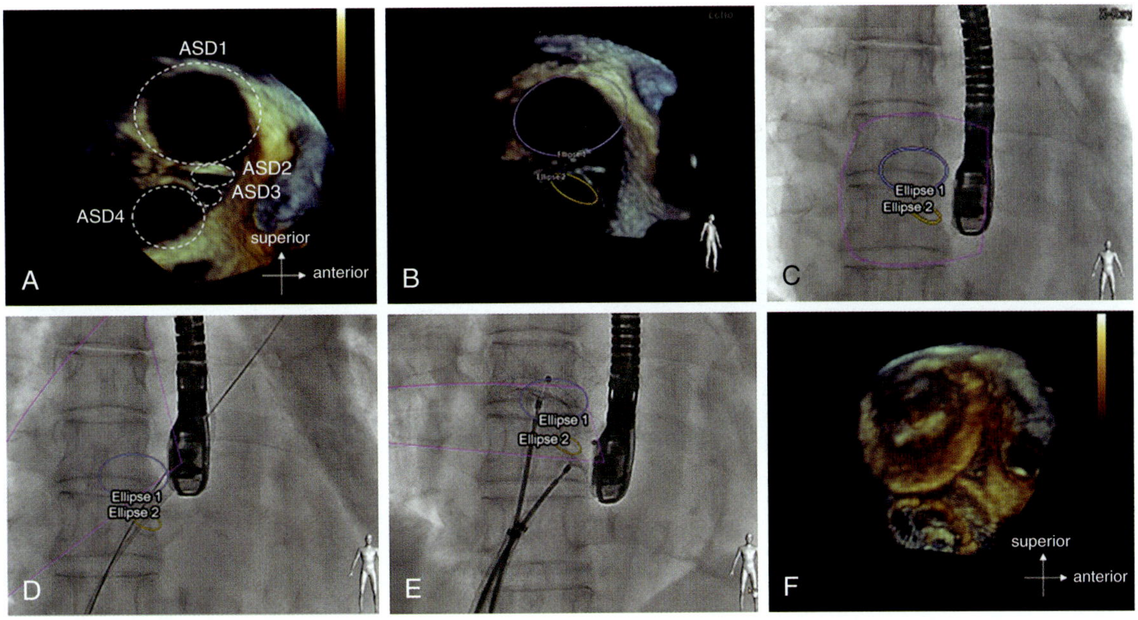

FIG. 4.109 Three-Dimensional Echo-X-Ray Navigation Guidance. (A) Three-dimensional transesophageal echocardiography (3D TEE) showed complex atrial septal defects (ASDs). 3D echo-x-ray navigation system marked (B) the shape and location of ASDs on TEE, and (C) integrated on fluoroscopy. Catheters were advanced to (D) the identified location (Online Video 4.121A–B), and (E) devices were deployed. (F) 3D TEE showed suitable device deployment.

Transcatheter Closure of Aorta-to-Right Atrium Fistula Caused by Erosion of an Amplatzer Septal Occluder

Jun-Yi Wan, MD, Ge-Jun Zhang, MD, Shi-Liang Jiang, MD, Yun-Ching Fu, MD

Cardiac perforation or erosion is a rare but potentially lethal complication of transcatheter closure of an atrial septal defect (ASD). The usual solution would be surgical repair.[1] We present a patient who underwent device closure of an ASD with an Amplatzer Septal Occluder (ASO) (AGA Medical, Golden Valley, Minnesota) and later developed an aorta-to-right atrium fistula. The fistula was successfully closed using a transcatheter technique.

A 7-year-old girl with a 12-mm secundum-type ASD and a deficient aortic rim underwent successful ASD closure using a 16-mm ASO. Follow-up echocardiography 1 month later showed a small aorta-to-right atrium fistula (Fig. 4.110). The patient was asymptomatic initially but developed hematuria and fatigue 3 weeks later. Hemoglobin dropped to 9.8 g/dL from 13.4 g/dL. After informed consent was obtained from the patient's parents, cardiac catheterization was performed under general anesthesia with fluoroscopic and transthoracic echocardiographic guidance. Aortography showed that the diameter of the fistula was 3 mm (Fig. 4.111). The fistula was crossed in a retrograde fashion from the aorta using a 5F Judkins right coronary catheter. A 0.035-inch Glidewire was advanced into the superior vena cava and exteriorized out of the femoral vein. A 6F patent ductus arteriosus delivery sheath (Lifetech Scientific, Shenzhen, China) was advanced in an antegrade manner into the ascending aorta. A 6/4-mm patent ductus arteriosus device (Lifetech Scientific) was deployed to close the fistula (Fig. 4.112). The patient is doing well with good device position and no residual leak on echocardiography through 3-year follow-up (Fig. 4.113).

Transcatheter closure of ASDs has been proved to be safe and effective. The complication of cardiac perforation or erosion is very rare (0.1%) but potentially lethal.[1–3]

Suggested risk factors for erosion include: (1) an atrial rim size of <5 mm, (2) excessive mobility of the device, (3) excessive oversizing of the ASO (≥1.5 times the size of the ASD), (4) splaying of the atrial disks across the aortic root, and (5) extreme movement of the deployed device before release.[1,4] In our patient, there was a deficient aortic rim. The edge of the right atrial disk likely moved with the cardiac cycle and eroded the atrial wall.

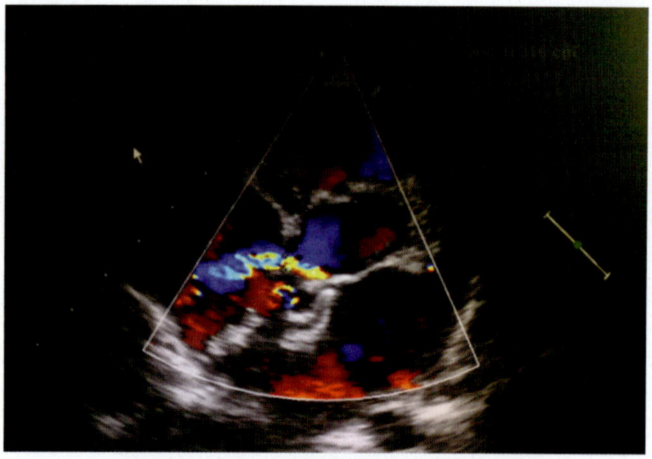

FIG. 4.110 **Transthoracic Echocardiogram Showing the Aorta-to-Right Atrium Fistula.**

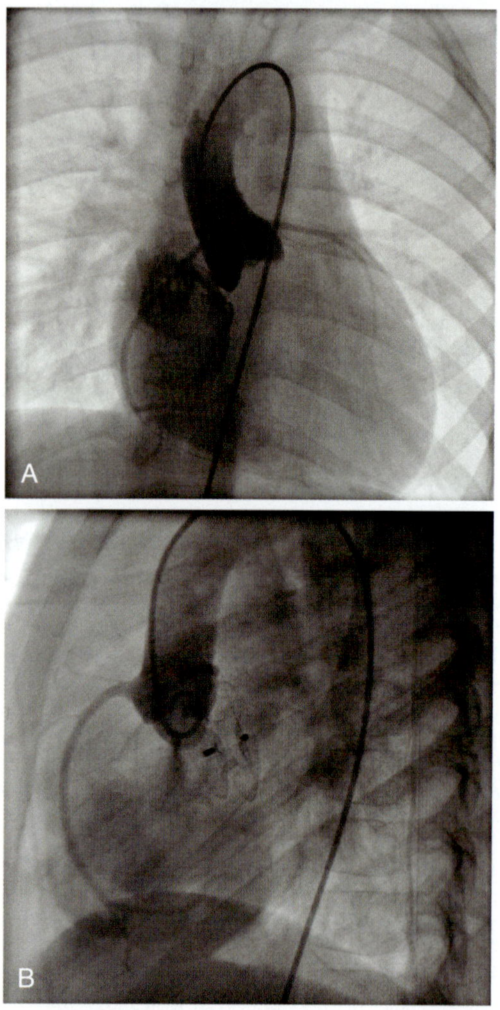

FIG. 4.111 **Aortogram Showing a Fistula From the Noncoronary Sinus to the Right Atrium.**

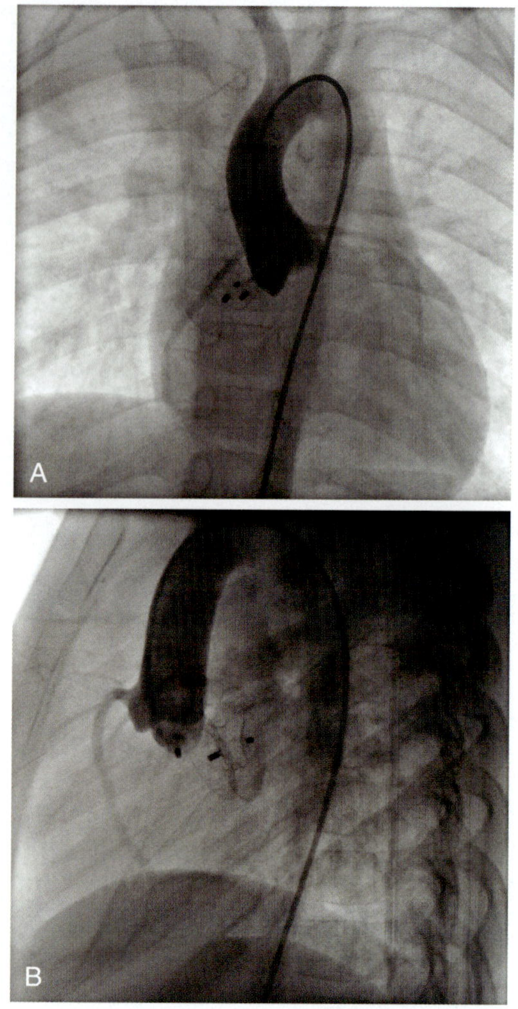

FIG. 4.112 **Postprocedural Aortogram Showing Good Device Position and Absence of Aortic Regurgitation.**

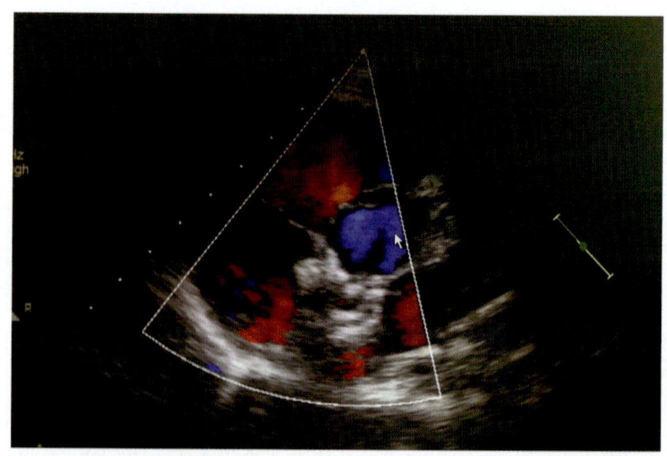

FIG. 4.113 **Follow-Up Transthoracic Echocardiogram Showing Complete Closure of the Fistula.**

This is the first reported case, to the best of our knowledge, of device closure of an aorta–to–right atrium fistula caused by an ASO device. After 3 years of follow-up, the patient is doing well without additional problems.

In conclusion, our limited experience demonstrates that device closure of an ASO-related fistula is feasible, safe, and effective.

References

1. Amin Z, Hijazi ZM, Bass JL, Cheatham JP, Hellenbrand WE, Kleinman CS. Erosion of Amplatzer septal occluder device after closure of secundum atrial septal defects: review of registry of complications and recommendations to minimize future risk. *Catheter Cardiovasc Interv.* 2004;63:496-502.
2. Delaney JW, Li JS, Rhodes JF. Major complications associated with transcatheter atrial septal occluder implantation: a review of the medical literature and the Manufacturer and User Facility Device Experience (MAUDE) database. *Congenit Heart Dis.* 2007;2:256-264.
3. DiBardino D, McElhinney D, Kaza A, Mayer J Jr. Analysis of the US Food and Drug Administration Manufacturer and User Facility Device Experience database for adverse events involving Amplatzer septal occluder devices and comparison with the Society of Thoracic Surgery congenital cardiac surgery database. *J Thorac Cardiovasc Surg.* 2009;137:1334-1341.
4. Yared K, Baggish AL, Solis J, et al. Echocardiographic assessment of percutaneous patent foramen ovale and atrial septal defect closure complications. *Circ Cardiovasc Imaging.* 2009;2:141-149.

Transcatheter Left Atrial Appendage Closure After Incomplete Surgical Ligation

Takashi Matsumoto, MD, Mamoo Nakamura, MD, Wen-Loong Yeow, MD, Robert J. Siegel, MD, Saibal Kar, MD

An 82-year-old woman with chronic atrial fibrillation on full anticoagulation with warfarin was referred for a repeat attempt to close the left atrial appendage (LAA) with a transcatheter, transseptal approach. The patient underwent surgical mitral and tricuspid repair, ligation of the LAA, and unsuccessful maze procedure. A subsequent transesophageal echocardiogram (TEE) demonstrated residual communication between the left atrium and LAA by pulsed and color flow Doppler (Fig. 4.114A–B, *asterisk* and *white arrow*).

After successful transseptal puncture under general anesthesia and TEE guidance, the baseline LAA angiogram was performed (Fig. 4.115A). Given its nonthrombogenic property and the sufficient LAA ostium rim, the Gore Helex Septal Occluder (W. L. Gore & Associates, Newark, Delaware) was used. The 15-mm occluder device was selected because the diameter of residual LAA ostium communication was 7 mm.

After dilation of the septal puncture site using an 8.0- × 20-mm balloon catheter, the 10F Arrow sheath (Arrow International, Reading, Pennsylvania) was introduced into the left atrium. To place the 8F occluder deployment system, the 10F sheath was further advanced into the LAA over the deflating balloon catheter that was positioned in the LAA (Fig. 4.115B). The deployment system was then advanced into the LAA through the 10F sheath. The occluder device was deployed successfully (Fig. 4.115C). The final angiogram and TEE showed a well-seated occluder device, with no residual flow, that completely closed the LAA ostium (Fig. 4.114C–D).

This is the first report of LAA closure using the Gore Helex Septal Occluder. Unfortunately, surgical LAA ligation is frequently incomplete (77%). Moreover, 41% of patients with unsuccessful surgical closure have LAA thrombus, which puts patients at an increased risk for systemic embolism and stroke.[1] Our case demonstrates that the residual communication secondary to incomplete surgical ligation can be closed percutaneously to reduce the risk of thromboembolism and stroke.

Reference

1. Kanderian AS, Gillinov AM, Pettersson GB, Blackstone E, Klein AL. Success of surgical left atrial appendage closure: assessment by transesophageal echocardiography. *J Am Coll Cardiol.* 2008;52:924-929.

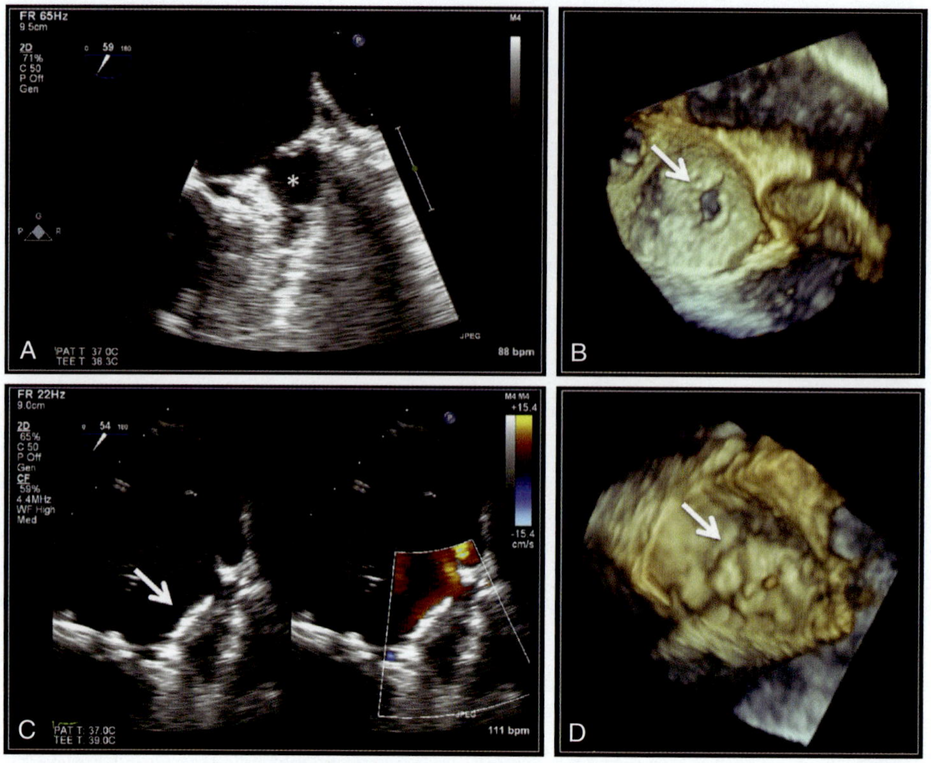

FIG. 4.114 Two- and Three-Dimensional- Transesophageal Echocardiography Images of the Left Atrial Appendage and the Gore Helex Septal Occluder. (A and B) Baseline study showed the residual communication between the left atrial appendage (*LAA*) and left atrium (*asterisk*, *white arrow*). (C and D) After device deployment no residual flow was seen across the device (*arrow*) and the device was well seated (*arrow*).

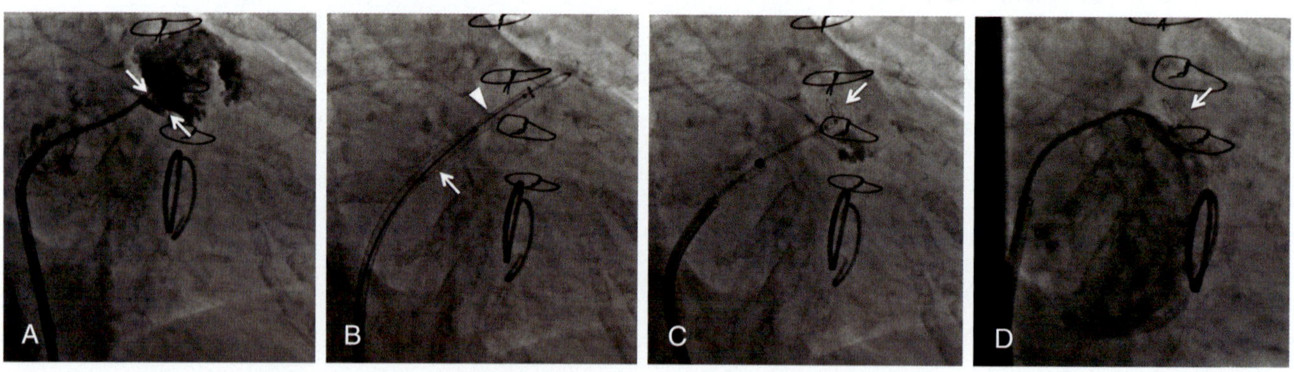

FIG. 4.115 Cineangiogram of Left Atrial Appendage Closure. (A) The left atrial appendage (LAA) with rim (*arrow*). (B) The 10F sheath (*arrow*) advanced into the LAA with support of the balloon (*arrowhead*). (C) The 15-mm Gore Helex Septal Occluder deployed across the LAA ostium (*arrow*). (D) Final angiogram showing no residual flow across the device (*arrow*).

Transseptal Puncture Through Amplatzer Atrial Septal Occluder for Left Atrial Appendage Closure

Steffen Gloekler, MD, Samera Shakir, MD, Bernhard Meier, MD

A 54-year-old woman with persistent atrial flutter or fibrillation requested left atrial appendage (LAA) closure because of poor dabigatran tolerance at a tertiary center in the United States. She had undergone atrial septal defect device closure there 9 years earlier. The 24-mm Amplatzer Septal Occluder (ASO) (Abbott, Plymouth, Minnesota) with a 36-mm disk diameter was deemed prohibitive for transseptal passage based on transesophageal echocardiography (TEE) and computed tomography.[1] She traveled to Switzerland for treatment.

Under local anesthesia with exclusively fluoroscopic guidance (TEE not repeated), an 8F transseptal sheath–needle set (Medtronic,

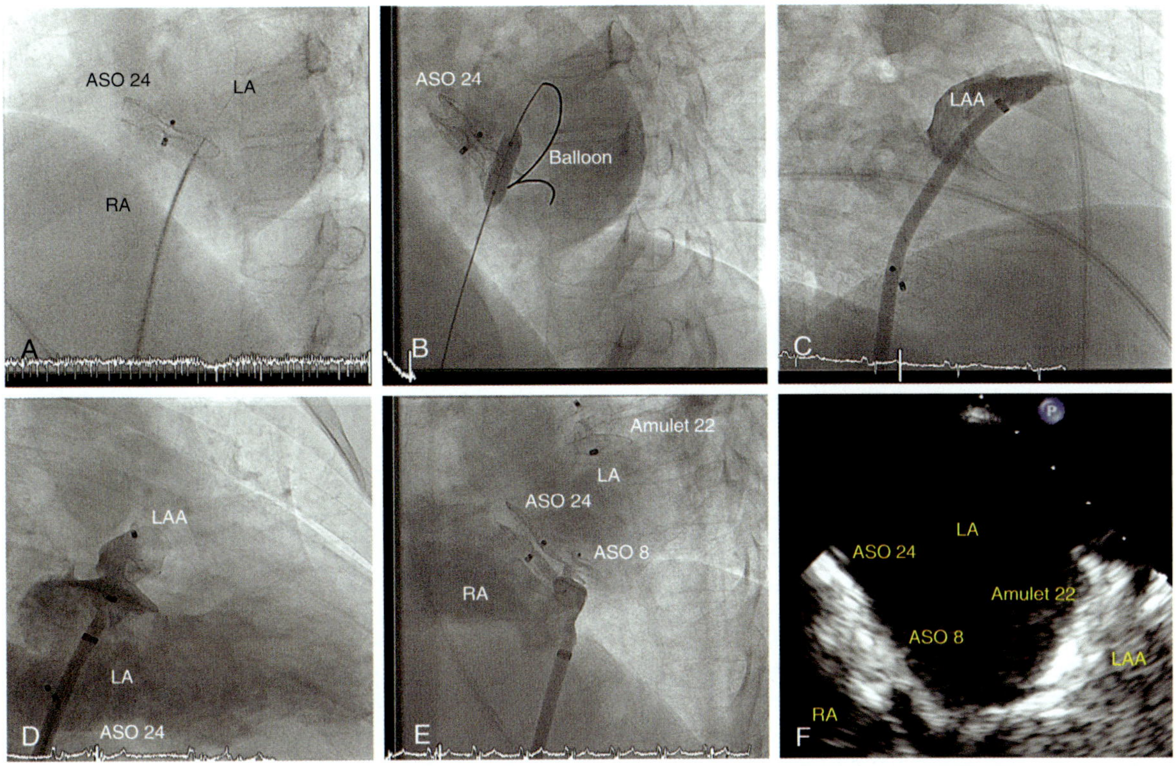

FIG. 4.116 Transseptal Puncture Through Atrial Septal Defect Occluder for Left Atrial Appendage Closure. (A) Puncture of the 38-mm left disk of the 24-mm Amplatzer Septal Occluder occluder (Abbott, Plymouth, Minnesota) (*ASO 24*) with the stiff end of a coronary 0.014-inch guidewire through a Brockenbrough needle (Medtronic, Minneapolis, Minnesota) in a left anterior oblique (LAO) projection. (B) Passage of 12F TorqVue sheath (Abbott) was only possible after predilation with a 7-mm balloon over a 0.035-inch backup wire (Boston Scientific, Marlborough, Massachusetts) (LAO projection) (Online Video 4.122). (C) Contrast medium injection into the left atrial appendage (*LAA*) in a right anterior oblique cranial projection. (D) Implantation of an Amulet 22-mm LAA occluder (Abbott) (*Amulet 22*) in a right anterior oblique cranial projection. (E) Closure of the hole in the left disk of the ASO 24 with an ASO 8-mm occluder (Abbott) (*ASO 8*) in an LAO projection. (F) Transesophageal echocardiography at 6 months showing a perfect result. *LA*, left atrium; *RA*, right atrium.

Minneapolis, Minnesota) was selected to perforate the lower part of the left disk of the ASO (Fig. 4.116A). After preperforation with the stiff end of a 0.014-inch coronary guidewire, the needle and the dilator of the transseptal sheath could be passed. During predilation with a 7-mm angioplasty balloon catheter over a 0.035-inch Backup wire (Boston Scientific, Marlborough, Massachusetts), the patient surprisingly converted into sinus rhythm (Fig. 4.116B, Online Video 4.122). Through a 12F TorqVue sheath (Abbott), LAA angiography (Fig. 4.116C) and closure with an Amplatzer Amulet 22-mm device (Abbott) (Fig. 4.116D) were performed. On the way out, the trans-ASO access hole was closed with an 8-mm ASO (Fig. 4.116E). Dabigatran was immediately discontinued. Clopidogrel (75 mg) for 1 month and acetylsalicylic acid (100 mg) for 5 months were prescribed. The patient left the hospital the next morning after transthoracic echocardiography had verified correct positions of the three devices.

TEE follow-up at 6 months (patient had remained in sinus rhythm and well) showed complete closure of the LAA and the atrial septum with all three devices free of thrombus and in correct positions (Fig. 4.116F).

This is the first report on catheter-based transdevice transseptal LAA closure expanding on reports on transdevice[2] and paradevice[3] transseptal left atrial ablation procedures.

References

1. Wagdi P, Alkadhi H. Can computer tomography help predict feasibility of transseptal puncture after percutaneous closure of an interatrial septal communication? *J Interv Card Electrophysiol.* 2012;34:167-172.
2. Li X, Wissner E, Kamioka M, et al. Safety and feasibility of transseptal puncture for atrial fibrillation ablation in patients with atrial septal defect closure devices. *Heart Rhythm.* 2014;11:330-335.
3. Zaker-Shahrak R, Fuhrer J, Meier B. Transseptal puncture for catheter ablation of atrial fibrillation after device closure of patent foramen ovale. *Catheter Cardiovasc Interv.* 2008;71:551-552.

Ventricles (Left Ventricle, Right Ventricle, Ventricular Septal Defects)

A Man With Three Lives: Long-Term Follow-Up After Percutaneous Closure of Left Ventricular Pseudoaneurysm Neck

Jonathon M. White, MB ChB, Boris S. Lowe, MB ChB, Peter N. Ruygrok, MB ChB, MD

An 81-year-old man presented with fever and weight loss 5 years after coronary artery bypass surgery and open repair of a ventricular septal defect (VSD) with a Dacron patch after an anterior myocardial infarction. He had remained under clinical and echocardiographic surveillance with moderate left ventricular (LV) systolic dysfunction and a stable VSD repair. He was febrile and multiple blood cultures grew *Staphylococcus warneri*. Transthoracic echocardiography showed a large LV apical pseudoaneurysm with a stable VSD repair and moderate LV impairment. Transesophageal echocardiography documented a large vegetation attached to the right ventricular side of the VSD patch. Computed tomography (CT) confirmed a 5- × 7-cm thin-walled saccular apical aneurysm (Fig. 4.117). He responded promptly to treatment for endocarditis with 2 weeks of intravenous vancomycin followed by oral clindamycin. Surgical debridement and aneurysm repair were considered an unacceptable risk, so, after 4 weeks of treatment, he underwent percutaneous closure of the apical aneurysm neck with a 16-mm Amplatzer muscular VSD occluder (Fig. 4.118, Online Video 4.123). He continued

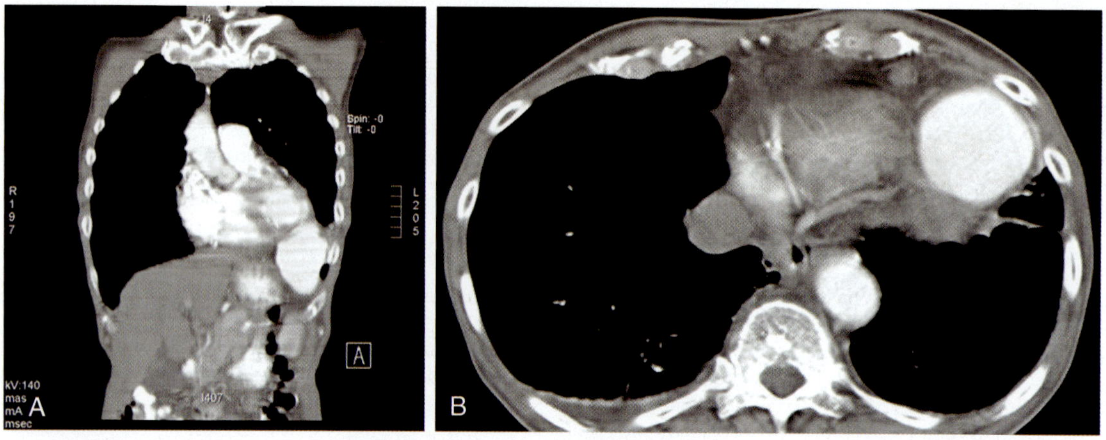

FIG. 4.117 Saccular Left Ventricular Aneurysm 5 Years After Myocardial Infarction. Computed tomography 5 years after myocardial infarction and coronary artery bypass surgery demonstrates a 5- × 7-cm saccular left ventricular aneurysm. (A) Coronal view. (B) Transverse view.

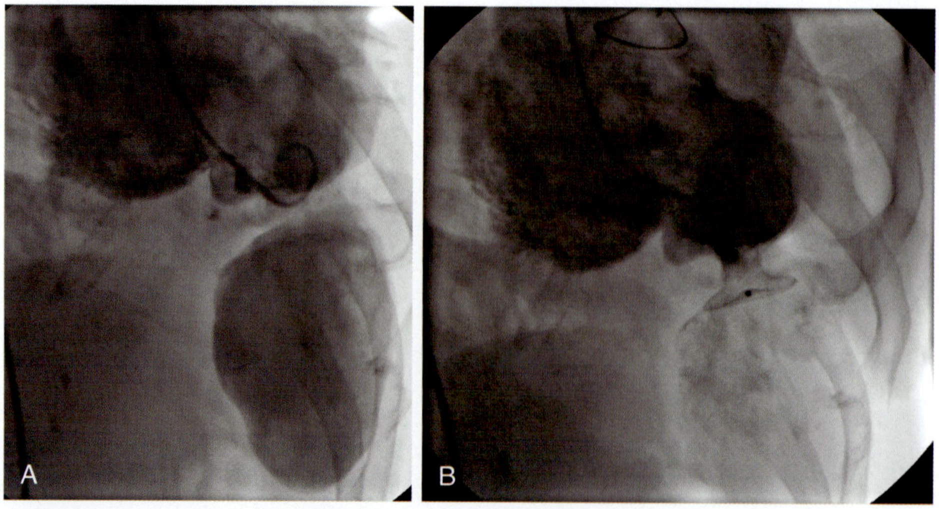

FIG. 4.118 Angiography Before and After Closure. Angiography before (A) (Online Video 4.123) and after (B) closure with a 16-mm Amplatzer muscular ventricular septal defect occluder (St. Jude Medical, St. Paul, Minnesota).

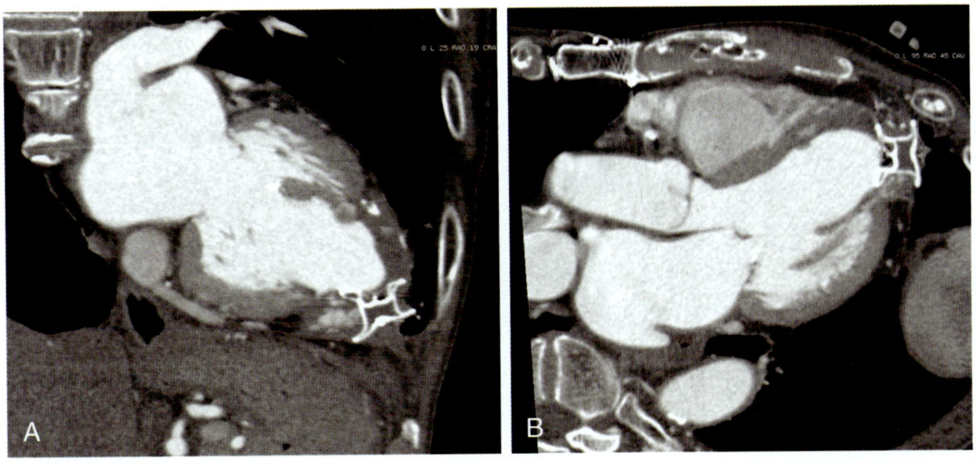

FIG. 4.119 Exclusion and Contraction of Apical Left Ventricular Aneurysm. Computed tomography 5 years after percutaneous closure demonstrating exclusion (A) and contraction (B) of apical left ventricular aneurysm.

lifelong clindamycin and remained well at 5-year follow-up (age 86 years), a follow-up CT documented continued stable appearances of the VSD occluder, contraction of the pseudoaneurysm, and no evidence of right ventricular vegetation (Fig. 4.119). This case demonstrates the very good long-term result that can be achieved by percutaneous LV pseudoaneurysm closure of even very large defects in inoperable patients.

Complete Percutaneous Obliteration of a Postinfarction Left Ventricular Inferior Wall Pseudoaneurysm

Grzegorz Smolka, MD, Ewa Peszek-Przybyla, MD, Maciej Sosnowski, MD, Andrzej Ochala, MD

A 67-year-old woman with a history of inferior wall myocardial infarction presented at a general hospital with a 4-week history of sudden-onset heart failure in New York Heart Association functional class III. Echocardiography revealed inferior wall pseudoaneurysm formation, probably because of recent myocardial infarction (Fig. 4.120A). Because the patient refused the proposal of immediate surgical treatment, we planned a percutaneous procedure. Coronary angiography revealed occlusion of the peripheral segment of the right coronary artery, multilevel critical stenoses in the left anterior descending coronary artery (LAD), and rupture of the left ventricular inferior wall with opacification of a pseudoaneurysm cavity (Fig. 4.120B). Cardiac imaging was supplemented by multidetector computed tomography, which visualized the pseudoaneurysm cavity (Fig. 4.120C) and noticeably thinned necrotic tissue within the inferior wall and allowed us to precisely determine the relation between rupture site and papillary muscle (Fig. 4.120D). Therefore, we decided that a staged procedure should be performed: a percutaneous closure of the pseudoaneurysm and, afterward, elective LAD angioplasty. A pigtail catheter was introduced transfemorally into the left ventricle, and another one—via transbrachial access with a 7-F sheath—served as a gateway for the closing device delivery system. The procedure was performed under fluoroscopic and transthoracic echocardiographic guidance. During the implantation, the pigtail catheter was used to temporarily move the papillary muscle body away from the lesion (Fig. 4.121A). This technique facilitated accurate placement and full expansion of an 8-mm Amplatzer Septal Occluder. As a result, complete sealing of the pseudoaneurysm orifice was achieved. Moreover, originally moderate ischemic mitral regurgitation diminished to trivial instantaneously (probably due to ventricle geometry improvement promoted by inferior wall stabilization). No early complications occurred, and after 2 days, the patient, in New York Heart Association functional class I, was discharged from the hospital. Three weeks later complete pseudoaneurysm closure was confirmed by echocardiography (Fig. 4.121B), multislice computed tomography (Fig. 4.121C), and ventriculography (Fig. 4.121D), and elective LAD angioplasty with implantation of two drug-eluting stents was performed. At 6-month follow-up, the result of the aforementioned staged procedure was satisfactory, and our patient was asymptomatic.

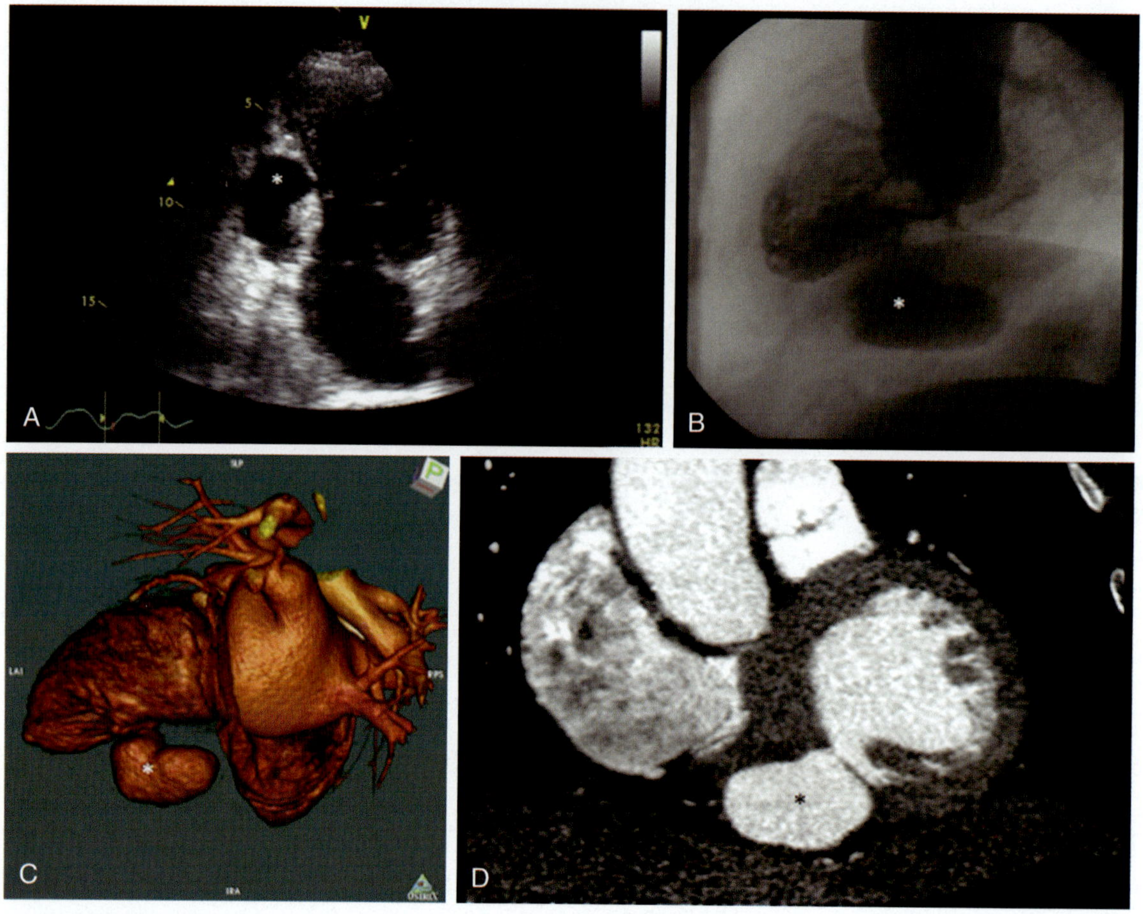

FIG. 4.120 Inferior Wall Pseudoaneurysm Formation. (A) Echocardiography (apical two-chamber view) showing inferior wall pseudoaneurysm cavity (*asterisk*). (B) Left ventriculography view shows rupture in the left ventricular inferior wall and opacification of pseudoaneurysm cavity (*asterisk*). (C) Multislice computed tomography reconstruction. For optimal visualization of pseudoaneurysm cavity (*asterisk*), the right ventricle was removed. (D) Left ventricle and pseudoaneurysm cavity (*asterisk*), largest dimension cross section. Note noticeably thinned myocardium within postinfarction necrotic tissue in the region of inferior wall and myocardial discontinuity visible. Posteromedial papillary muscle is localized superior to the pseudoaneurysm orifice.

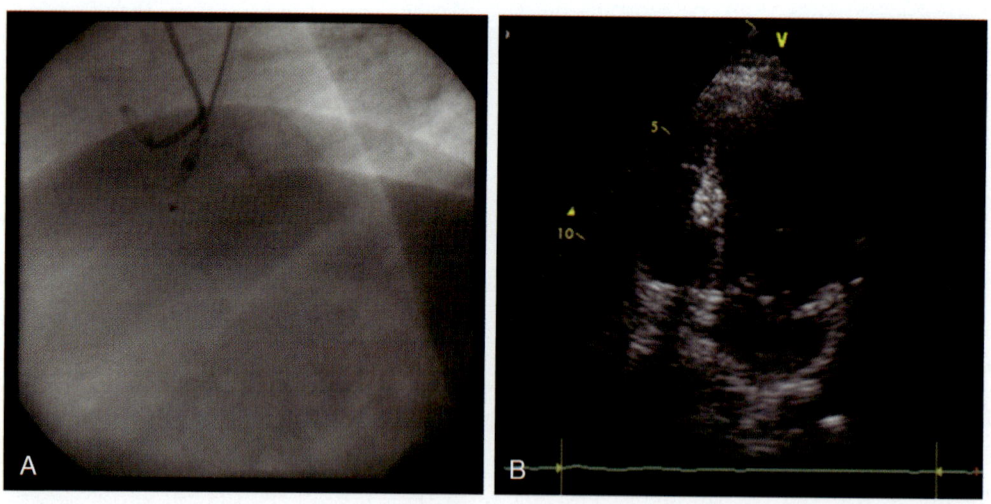

FIG. 4.121 Procedure Views. (A) Pseudoaneurysm closure with occluder: distal disk placed in the pseudoaneurysm cavity. Proximal disk placement was preceded by pigtail catheter maneuver to temporarily "displace" the posteromedial papillary muscle body. (B) Transthoracic echocardiography 3 weeks after pseudoaneurysm closure: 8-mm atrial septal occluder tightly covers the tear of the inferior wall of the left ventricle.

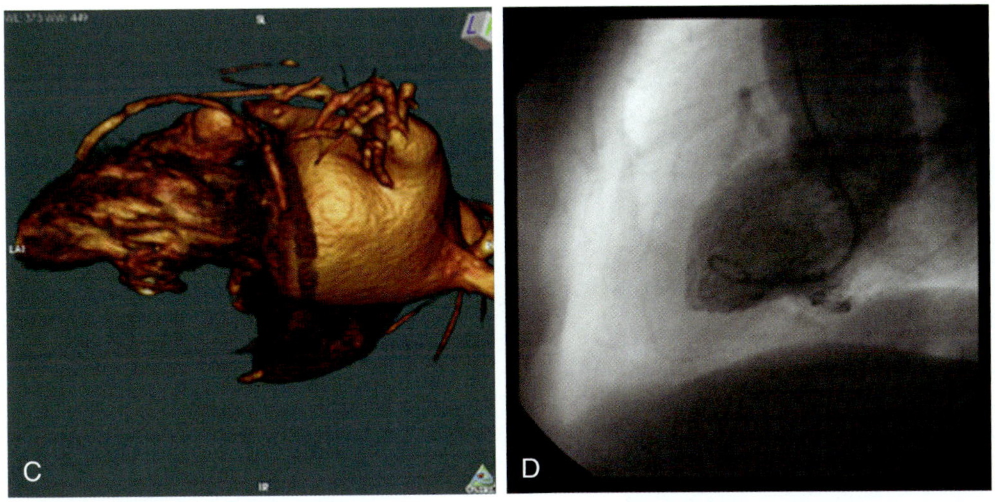

FIG. 4.121, cont'd (C) Multislice computed tomography reconstruction 3 weeks after pseudoaneurysm closure: the occluder is localized in the former rupture site. (D) Left ventricle ventriculography 3 weeks after pseudoaneurysm closure: pseudoaneurysm cavity is not opacified.

Percutaneous Angioplasty of Stenotic Outflow Graft Anastomosis of HeartMate II

Richard K. Cheng, MD, Jamil Aboulhosn, MD, Ali Nsair, MD

A 55-year-old man with nonischemic dilated cardiomyopathy who had undergone HeartMate II (HM2) (Thoratec, Pleasanton, California) implantation for destination therapy was readmitted 1.5 years later because of low-flow alarms with dizziness. Transesophageal echocardiogram showed decreased velocity proximal to the HM2 outflow–aortic anastomosis, raising concerns for obstruction, and flow acceleration distal to the anastomosis (Fig. 4.122). His left ventricular end-diastolic diameter (LVEDD) was 59 mm. Inflows were estimated at 0.6 m/s (Fig. 4.123), velocity within the outflow cannula was 0.5 m/s, and outflow–aortic anastomosis velocity was 1.9 m/s. Computed tomography angiograms confirmed the outflow cannula was stenotic near the aortic insertion (Fig. 4.124), with a reference diameter in the Dacron graft of 16 mm and narrowing to 8 mm × 12 mm near the anastomosis.

He was believed to be too high a risk for surgery, and it was decided to attempt percutaneous angioplasty. A 4F cut pigtail catheter

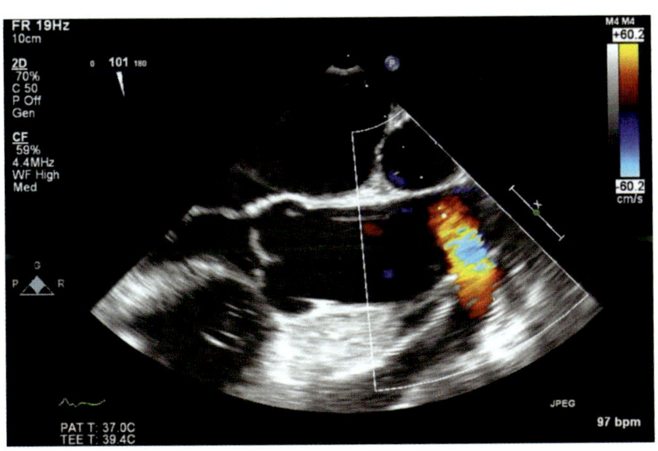

FIG. 4.122 Narrowing of HeartMate II Outflow Graft-Aortic Anastomosis. Color Doppler echocardiography demonstrates turbulent flow with flow acceleration in this region.

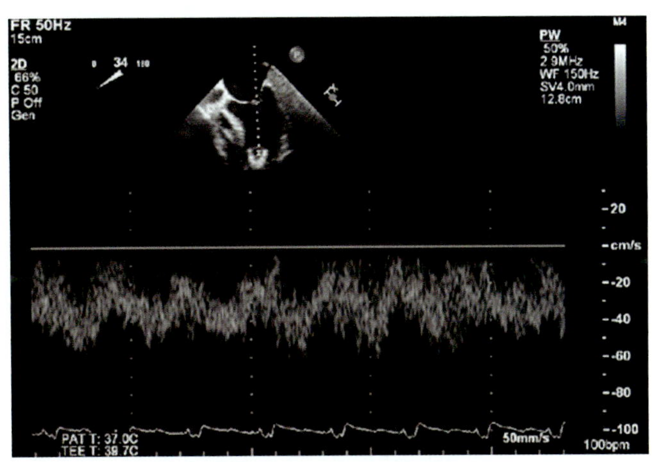

FIG. 4.123 Pulsed Doppler Echocardiography of HeartMate II Inflow Cannula by Transesophageal Echocardiography. There is low velocity of 0.5 to 0.6 m/s, raising concerns for obstruction or thrombus along the inflow-to-outflow graft.

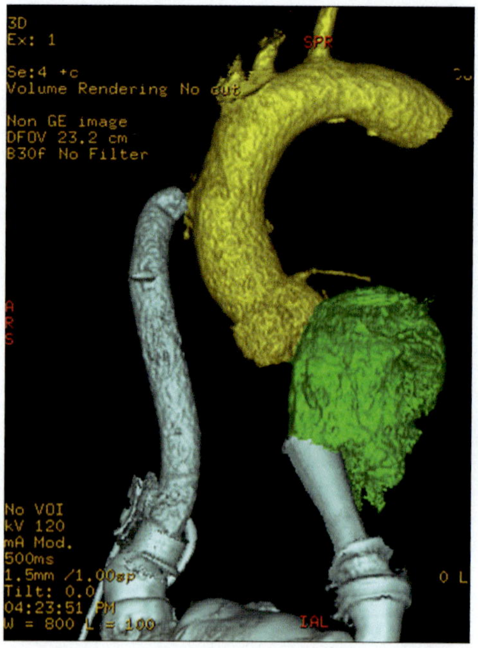

FIG. 4.124 Three-Dimensional Cardiac Computed Tomography Scan Reconstruction of HeartMate II Outflow Graft–Aortic Anastomosis. There is a stenotic narrowing at the outflow graft insertion site.

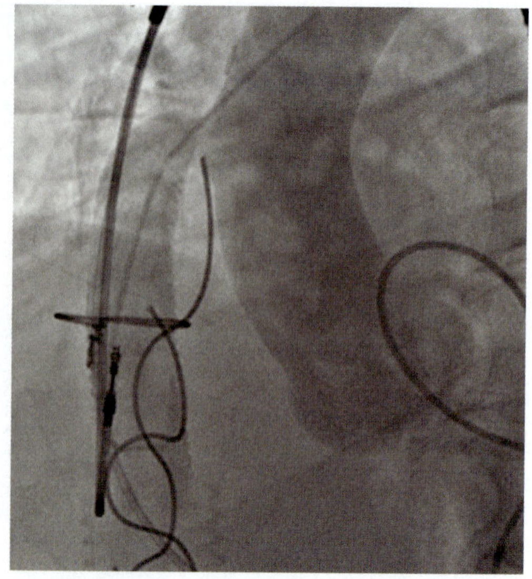

FIG. 4.125 Preangioplasty Aortogram of the HeartMate II Outflow Graft–Aortic Anastomosis. The narrowing at the outflow graft insertion site was confirmed.

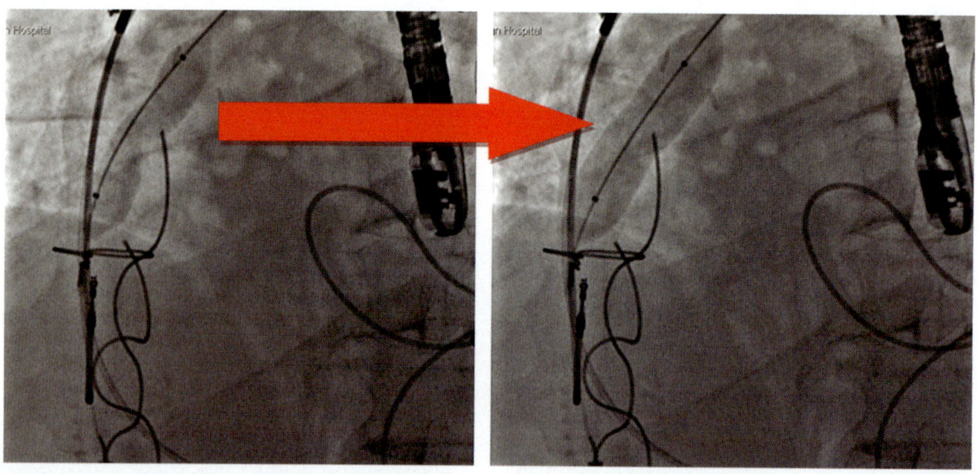

FIG. 4.126 Balloon Angioplasty of the Narrowing at the Anastomosis Site. There was notable narrowing preangioplasty (*left*) (Online Video 4.124). After balloon inflation twice at this region, there is minimal residual narrowing with full expansion of the balloon (*right*). The *red arrow* points to the area of anastomosis between the outflow graft and the aorta.

and straight 0.035-inch wire was used to access the outflow cannula. Reference vessel diameter was 14 to 15 mm, and the region of stenosis was 8 to 9 mm in diameter (Fig. 4.125). An Amplatz 0.035-inch Super Stiff guidewire (St. Jude Medical, Golden Valley, Minnesota) was placed in the midcannula retrograde through the outflow graft, and a 14 mm × 4-cm Cordis Opta Pro balloon angioplasty balloon (Cordis Corp., Miami, Florida) was inflated twice at the anastomosis to a maximal pressure of 4 atm. There was resolution of the waist narrowing with the second inflation (Figs. 4.126 and 4.127, Online Videos 4.124 and 4.125). During each inflation, HM2 flow was decreased transiently to 1 L/min for 3 to 4 seconds at a time. Postangioplasty, Doppler flow velocity at the anastomosis improved from 1.9 m/s to 1 m/s. LVEDD decreased from 59 mm to 39 mm. The patient was discharged 4 days later, and HM2 function has remained stable 6 months postangioplasty.

The incidence of outflow graft stenosis in the intermediate to long-term setting after left ventricular assist device implantation is not well documented. It is likely that even though the occurrence is low, it remains underdiagnosed except in the most severe cases. Percutaneous approaches offer an attractive alternative to surgical intervention in this high-risk group by avoiding redo sternotomy.

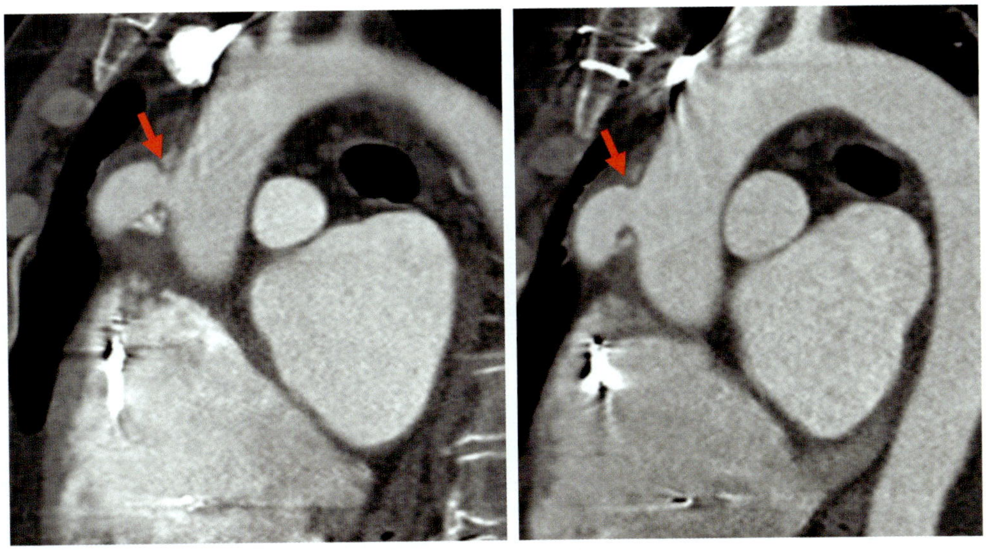

FIG. 4.127 Pre- and Postangioplasty Computed Tomography Angiograms of the HeartMate II Outflow Graft-Aortic Anastomosis. Pre- (*left*) and postangioplasty (*right*) computed tomography (CT) angiograms of the HeartMate II outflow graft–aortic anastomosis (Online Video 4.125). Before angioplasty, there was significant narrowing, which remains much improved on follow-up CT angiogram several months after the intervention. The *red arrows* point to the area of anastomosis between the outflow graft and the aorta before (*left*) and after (*right*) the procedure.

Percutaneous Closure of Left Ventricular Pseudoaneurysm With Septal Occluder Device and Coils: A Multimodality Imaging Approach

Matias B. Yudi, MBBS, Barry Love, MD, Adnan Nadir, MBBS, Annapoorna Kini, MD, Samin K. Sharma, MD

A 79-year-old man presented to our institution for follow-up 2 weeks after delayed presentation of anterior ST-segment elevation myocardial infarction and consequent successful percutaneous coronary intervention to the occluded saphenous vein to left anterior coronary artery graft. He has a medical history of coronary artery bypass surgery, hypertension, hyperlipidemia, and peripheral vascular disease. Echocardiogram (Fig. 4.128A) showed akinetic anteroseptal, inferoseptal, and apical walls with color flow demonstrating a left ventricular pseudoaneurysm. Cardiac magnetic resonance imaging (Fig. 4.128B) and computed tomography angiogram (Fig. 4.128C) confirmed a 34- × 10-mm bilobed left ventricular pseudoaneurysm with a 4-mm neck. A multidisciplinary heart team evaluation deemed the patient to be high risk for surgery, and the decision was made to undertake percutaneous closure. Under fluoroscopic guidance, an 8F multipurpose guide was placed in the pseudoaneurysm and a 10-mm Amplatzer muscular ventricular septal defect occluder (Abbott Vascular, Santa Clara, California) was successfully deployed via a retrograde transaortic approach (Fig. 4.129B). A follow-up contrast echocardiogram showed continued flow into the pseudoaneurysm (Fig. 4.128D). The patient was brought back to the catheterization laboratory 3 days later for direct chest wall entry into the pseudoaneurysm using a micropuncture needle (Fig. 4.129C) with deployment of 14-mm, 10-mm, and 6-mm 0.018-inch Interlock two-dimensional coils (Boston Scientific, Natick, Massachusetts) (Fig. 4.129D). After coil deployment, left ventriculography and echocardiography did not reveal any residual flow into the pseudoaneurysm. The patient was successfully discharged home.

Left ventricular pseudoaneurysms are most commonly sequelae of myocardial infarction and are associated with an unacceptable risk of sudden cardiac death.[1] Although surgery is the preferred treatment strategy, a percutaneous approach is emerging as an appropriate option in high-risk surgical candidates.[2,3] Multimodality imaging is essential for diagnosis, to completely understand the pseudoaneurysm anatomy, for procedural planning, and ultimately to guide the intervention. This was particularly highlighted in our case because we initially used a retrograde transaortic approach and then completed the occlusion with a second procedure through an apical approach.

References

1. Frances C, Romero A, Grady D. Left ventricular pseudoaneurysm. *J Am Coll Cardiol.* 1998;32:557-561.
2. Acharya D, Nagaraj H, Misra VK. Transcatheter closure of left ventricular pseudoaneurysm. *J Invasive Cardiol.* 2012;24:E111-E114
3. Singh A, Kliger C, Ruiz CE. Novel approach for the percutaneous treatment of left ventricular pseudoaneurysms. *Catheter Cardiovasc Interv.* 2015;85:1092-1096.

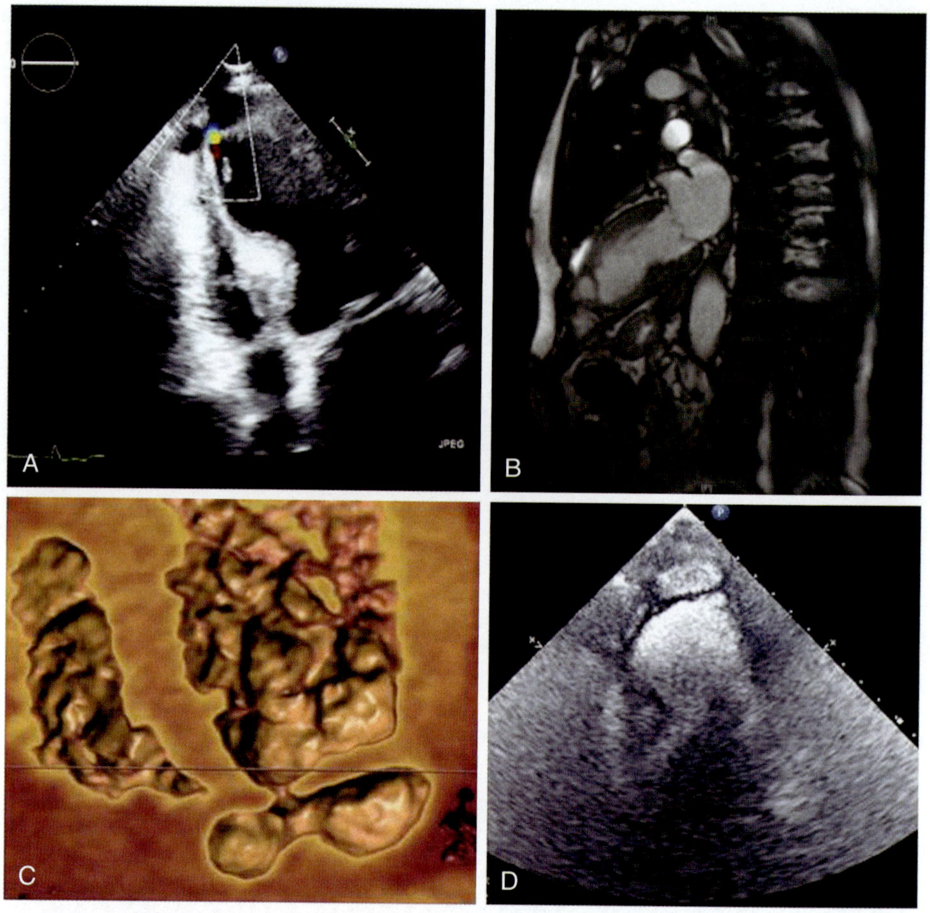

FIG. 4.128 Multimodality Assessment of Left Ventricular Pseudoaneurysm. (A) Echocardiogram initially diagnosed flow into an apical pseudoaneurysm. (B) Cardiac magnetic resonance imaging showed the size of pseudoaneurysm but could not identify the ostium. (C) Computed tomography angiogram reconstruction revealed the ostium of the bilobed pseudoaneurysm. (D) Contrast echocardiogram highlighted ongoing flow into the pseudoaneurysm after deployment of the vascular occlusion device.

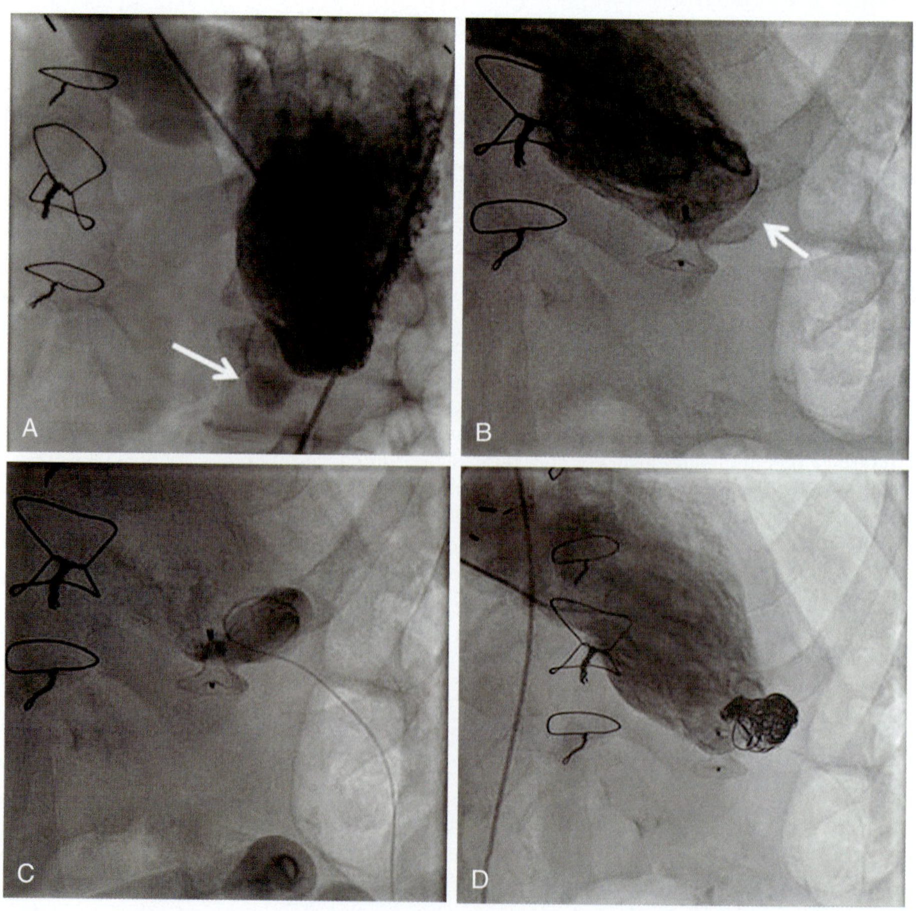

FIG. 4.129 Left Ventriculogram Before, During, and After Percutaneous Closure. (A) Left ventriculography showing the neck of the pseudoaneurysm (*arrow*). (B) Imaging after deployment of the vascular occlusion device shows residual flow into the pseudoaneurysm (*arrow*). (C) Injection into the pseudoaneurysm from a transapical approach. (D) No residual flow into the pseudoaneurysm after coiling.

Transseptal Closure of Left Ventricular Pseudoaneurysm After Transapical Transcatheter Aortic Valve Replacement

Takashi Matsumoto, MD, Kazuaki Okuyama, MD, Wen Cheng, MD, Raj R. Makkar, MD, Saibal Kar, MD

An 81-year-old woman presented for a scheduled 1-month follow-up after an uneventful valve-in-valve transapical transcatheter aortic valve replacement (TA-TAVR) using a 23-mm SAPIEN XT prosthesis (Edwards Lifesciences, Irvine, California). Although the patient remained asymptomatic after discharge, a transthoracic echocardiogram revealed a left ventricular (LV) pseudoaneurysm, with a 10-mm neck, at the location of the transapical access site (Fig. 4.130A, Online Video 4.126). Subsequent heart team discussion led to the decision to proceed with percutaneous closure via an antegrade transseptal approach. The procedure was performed under general anesthesia and transesophageal echocardiographic guidance. After transseptal puncture, an 8F Mullins sheath was further advanced into the LV through the mitral valve with support of a 6F balloon floating catheter, and then an initial LV angiogram was performed (Fig. 4.131A). A 6F multipurpose catheter was manipulated into the pseudoaneurysm; the catheter was then exchanged for an 80-cm 8F Amplatzer TorqVue sheath (St. Jude Medical, Minneapolis, Minnesota). On the basis of echocardiographic and balloon-sizing measurement, a 12-mm muscular ventricular septal defect occluder (St. Jude Medical) was prepared in standard fashion and deployed successfully (Fig. 4.131B–C). The final angiogram showed a well-seated device without significant shunt (Fig. 4.131D). At discharge (postoperative day 2), a transthoracic echocardiogram showed the occluder device completely sealing the pseudoaneurysm (Fig. 4.130B, Online Video 4.127).

LV pseudoaneurysm is a rare but serious complication after TA-TAVR.[1] Percutaneous pseudoaneurysm closure after TA-TAVR via a retrograde transfemoral approach was previously reported,[2] but this technique has some concerns, including the long access route to the LV apex and potential risk of valve injury. By contrast, the antegrade transseptal approach provides an appropriate access route, allowing the usage of a standard delivery system for the occluder device, and eliminates the risk of damaging the implanted valve. Therefore, it is suggested that the present technique be considered the first-line option for LV pseudoaneurysm closure after TA-TAVR.

References

1. Pasic M, Unbehaun A, Dreysse S, et al. Transapical aortic valve implantation in 175 consecutive patients: excellent outcome in very high-risk patients. *J Am Coll Cardiol.* 2010;56:813-820.
2. Bortnick AE, Gordon E, Gutsche J, et al. Percutaneous closure of a left ventricular pseudoaneurysm after Sapien XT transapical transcatheter aortic valve replacement. *J Am Coll Cardiol Intv.* 2012;5:e37-e38.

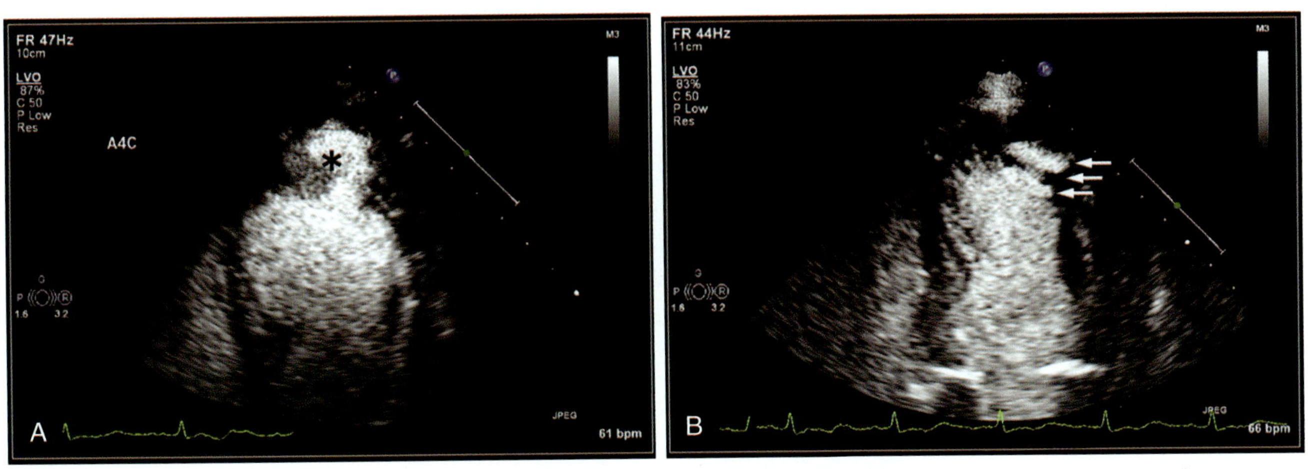

FIG. 4.130 Transthoracic Echocardiogram With Contrast (Apical Four-Chamber View). (A) Transthoracic echocardiogram with contrast at 1-month follow-up post-transapical transcatheter aortic valve replacement revealed a left ventricular (LV) pseudoaneurysm (*asterisk*) with a neck (Online Video 4.126). (B) Transthoracic echocardiogram with contrast after pseudoaneurysm closure showed a well-seated 12-mm Amplatzer muscular ventricular septal defect occluder (*white arrows*) across the neck of the LV pseudoaneurysm without significant shunt (Online Video 4.127).

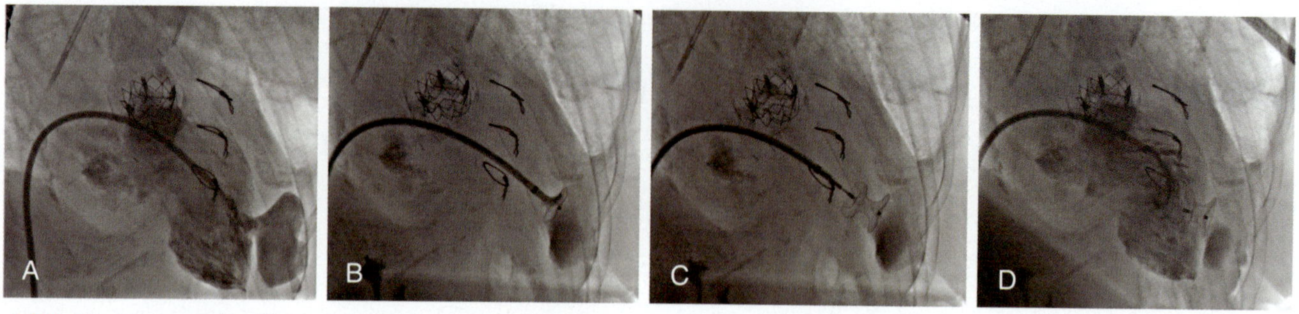

FIG. 4.131 Cineangiography. (A) Initial left ventriculogram demonstrated left ventricular (LV) pseudoaneurysm with a neck. (B) A distal disk of the occluder device was deployed. (C) A proximal disk of the occluder device was deployed. (D) The final left ventriculogram showed occlusion of the pseudoaneurysm with the 12-mm Amplatzer muscular ventricular septal defect occluder.

Transcatheter Closure of a Postmyocardial Infarction Ventricular Septal Rupture Using a Parachute Device

Daxin Zhou, MB, Wenzhi Pan, MD, Lihua Guan, MB, Cuizhen Pan, MB, Junbo Ge, MD

A 58-year-old man with exertional dyspnea (New York Heart Association functional class II) was admitted to our hospital. He suffered from acute anterior myocardial infarction 1 year earlier and had undergone percutaneous coronary intervention and closure of ventricular septal rupture (VSR) with an Amplatzer Septal Occluder (St. Jude Medical, St. Paul, Minnesota) 9 months before admission. Echocardiography taken on admission showed large residual apical ventricular septal shunts near the occluder (Fig. 4.132A, Online Video 4.128) and left ventricular aneurysm, with left ventricular ejection fraction of 49%. An 85-mm Parachute device (CardioKinetix, Inc., Menlo Park, California) was used to restore the left ventricle and close the apical VSR simultaneously, with the method reported previously.[1] After the procedure, the Qp/Qs ratio decreased from 1.8 to 1.2. An x-ray showed that the Parachute device was located at the left ventricular apex and the Amplatzer occluder intruded into the device (Fig. 4.133). At 3-month follow-up, the patient's symptom was relieved, and New York Heart Association functional class was improved to class I. Echocardiography demonstrated that apical ventricular septal shunts decreased significantly (Fig. 4.132B, Online Video 4.129). The Amplatzer occluder intruded into the Parachute device, causing incomplete apposition of the device and blood flow into the portioned apical cavity from the left ventricular chamber (Fig. 4.134), and then went through the apical ventricular septal rupture (Fig. 4.132B).

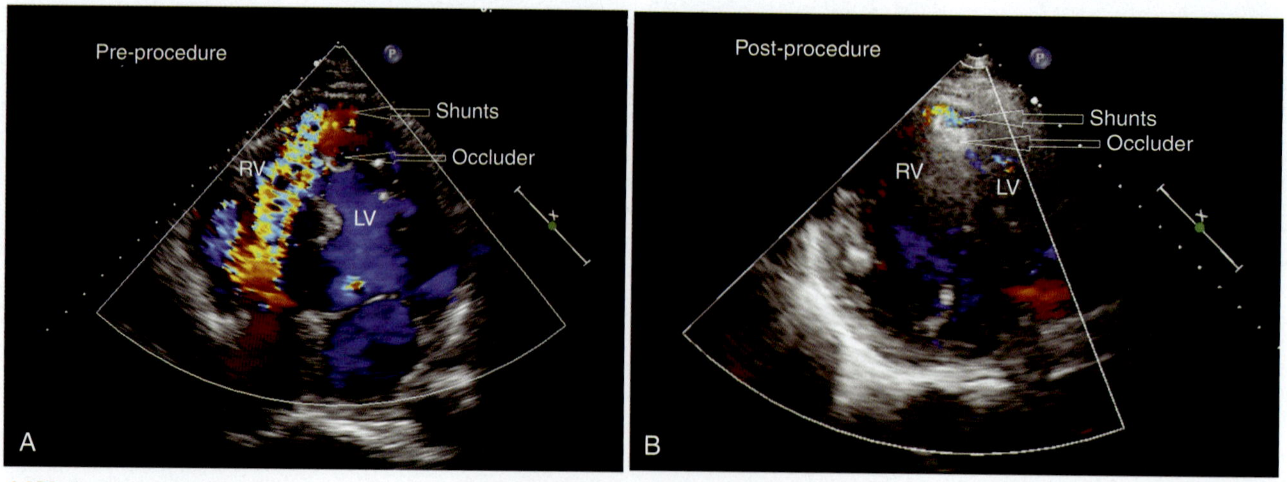

FIG. 4.132 Preprocedure and Postprocedure Color Doppler Flow Images. (A) Before the procedure, large residual ventricular septal shunts could be seen between the occluder and the peak of apex (Online Video 4.128). (B) After the procedure, the shunts decreased significantly (Online Video 4.129). *LV*, left ventricle; *RV*, right ventricle.

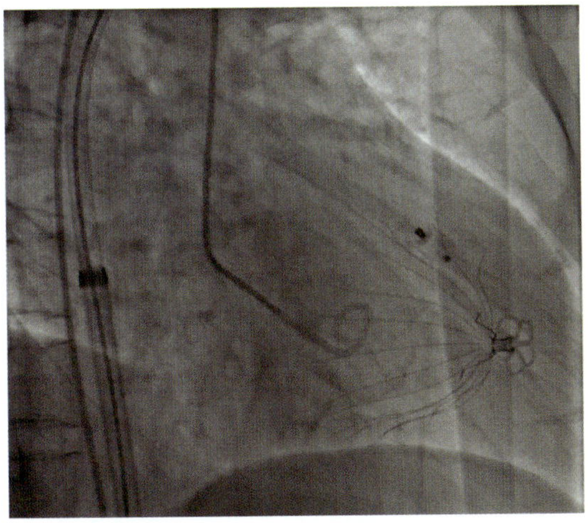

FIG. 4.133 X-Ray Taken During the Procedure. The Parachute device was located at the left ventricular apex and the Amplatzer occluder intruded into the device.

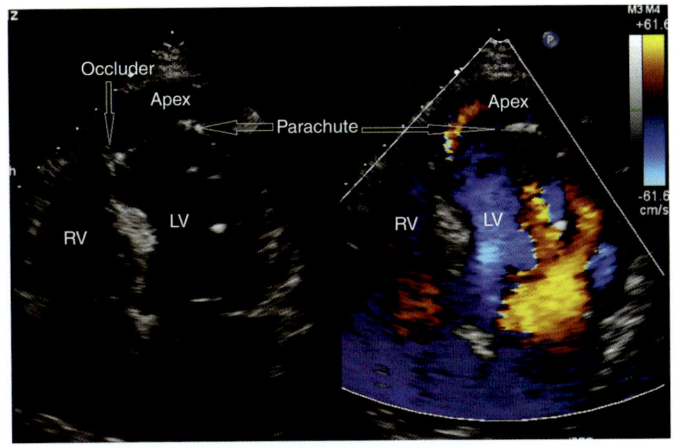

FIG. 4.134 Echocardiographic View. The Amplatzer occluder intruded into the Parachute device, causing incomplete apposition of the device and blood flow into the portioned apical cavity from the left ventricular chamber. *LV*, left ventricle; *RV*, right ventricle.

Postmyocardial infarction VSR is a serious disease. Even if treated with surgery or percutaneous intervention, it is still associated with high mortality. Previously, VSR was percutaneously closed using double-umbrella devices,[2] which were not effective for multihole VSRs. This is the first time we have explored the feasibly of transcatheter closure of apical VSR using a Parachute device (the schematic diagram appears in Fig. 4.135). Because the Amplatzer occluder affected the partitioning effect of the Parachute device, residual shunts still existed. If the case had not been treated by an Amplatzer occluder previously, the result might be better.

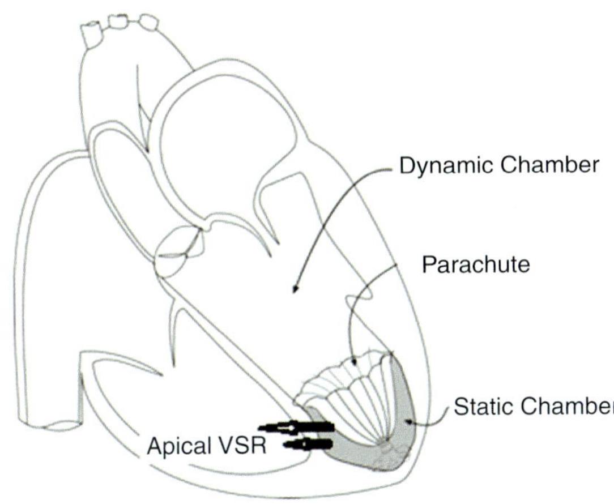

FIG. 4.135 Schematic Diagram of Transcatheter Closure of Apical Ventricular Septal Rupture Using a Parachute Device. The Parachute device partitions the apical cavity, as well as the apical ventricular septal rupture.

References

1. Mazzaferri EL Jr., Gradinac S, Sagic D, et al. Percutaneous left ventricular partitioning in patients with chronic heart failure and a prior anterior myocardial infarction: results of the PercutAneous Ventricular Restor Ation in Chronic Heart failUre PaTiEnts Trial. *Am Heart J.* 2012;163: 812-820.e1.
2. Assenza GE, McElhinney DB, Valente AM, et al. Transcatheter closure of post myocardial infarction ventricular septal rupture. *Circ Cardiovasc Interv.* 2013;6:59-67.

Transapical Transcatheter Closure of Pseudoaneurysm in the Left Ventricular Outflow Tract After Aortic Valve Replacement

Yoshiaki Katada, MD, PhD, Joji Ito, MD, Kentaro Shibayama, MD, Daisuke Nakatsuka, MD, Yuji Kawano, MD, Hiroyuki Watanabe, MD, Minoru Tabata, MD, PhD, MPH

A 74-year-old woman underwent reconstruction of the infected annulus and redo aortic valve replacement with a bioprosthetic valve for prosthetic valve endocarditis. Postoperative computed tomography revealed a pseudoaneurysm of the posterior left ventricular outflow tract (LVOT) (Fig. 4.136).

The ventricular apex was exposed with a left minithoracotomy. A 9F, 10-cm sheath was inserted into the left ventricle, and a 6F, 45-cm guiding sheath was inserted into the pseudoaneurysm. Under the guidance of transesophageal echocardiography (Fig. 4.137), a 10-mm Amplatzer vascular plug II (St. Jude Medical, St. Paul, Minnesota) was deployed by placing the first disk in the LVOT and the other two disks in the pseudoaneurysm. No blood flow and clot formation inside the pseudoaneurysm were confirmed intraoperatively (Figs. 4.137 and 4.138). Preoperative computed

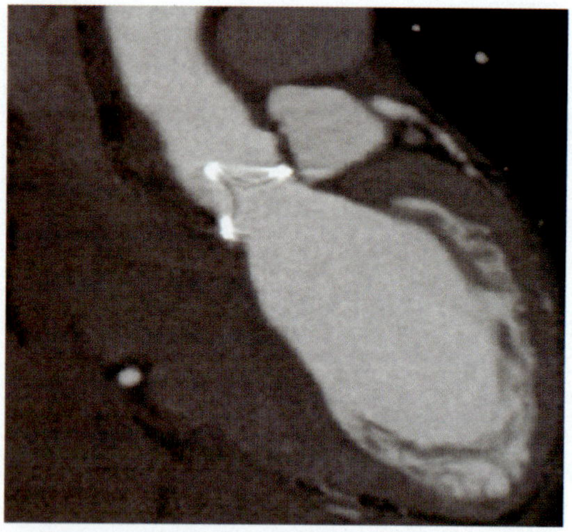

FIG. 4.136 Preoperative Contrast-Enhanced Computed Tomography. A pseudoaneurysm is found in the left ventricular outflow tract.

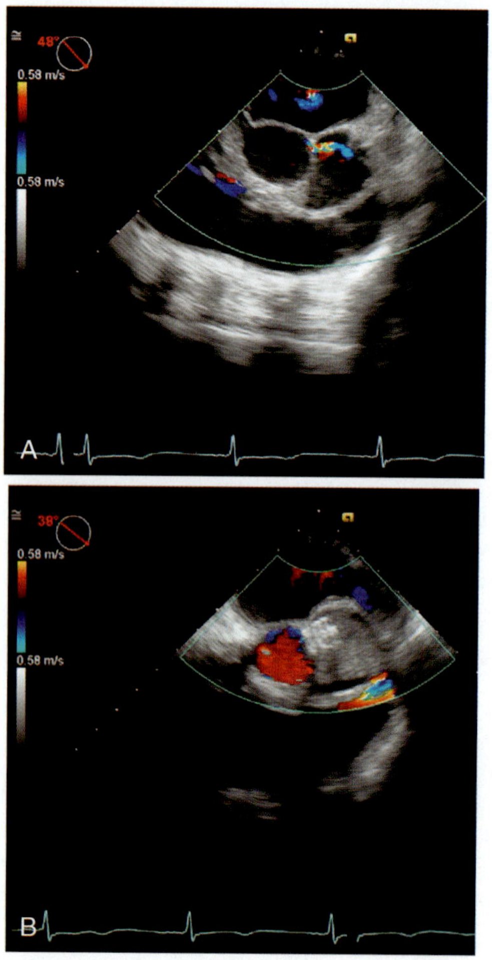

FIG. 4.137 Intraoperative Transesophageal Echocardiography. Intraoperative transesophageal echocardiography showed pseudoaneurysm entry (A) and clot formation inside the pseudoaneurysm immediately after device deployment (B).

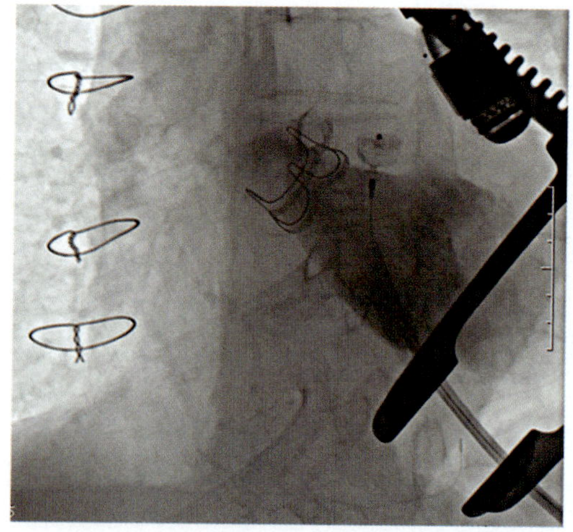

FIG. 4.138 Intraoperative Fluoroscopy After Deployment. The closure device is positioned at the entry of the pseudoaneurysm and there is no contrast flow into the pseudoaneurysm.

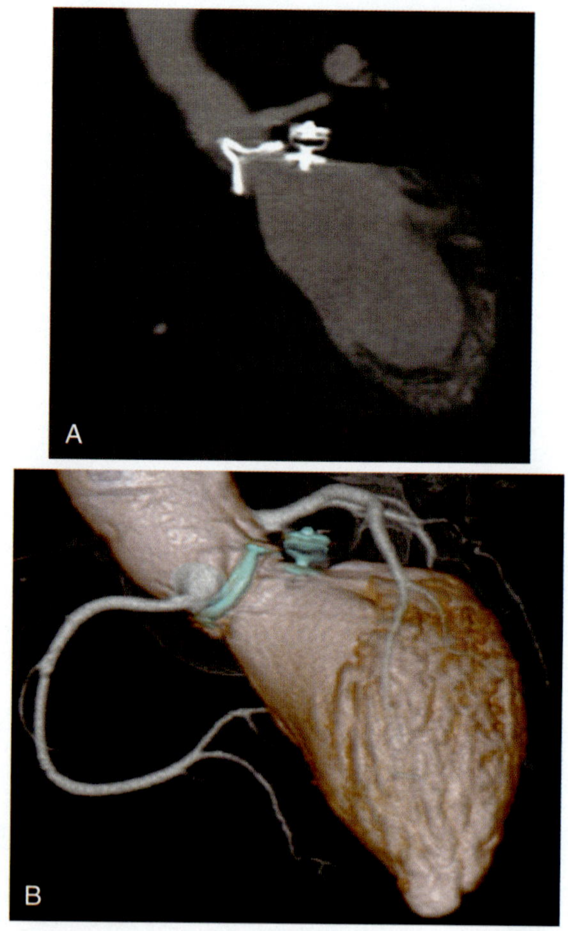

FIG. 4.139 Postoperative Contrast-Enhanced Computed Tomography. Two-dimensional (A) and three-dimensional (B) images of postoperative computed tomography revealed complete thrombosis of the pseudoaneurysm cavity.

tomography confirmed complete occlusion of the pseudoaneurysm cavity (Fig. 4.139).

Compared with the percutaneous transseptal approach,[1] the transapical approach provides shorter and more linear access to the LVOT.[2] Heart team transapical closure is an efficient and safe option for LVOT pseudoaneurysm.

References

1. Romaguera R, Slack MC, Waksman R, et al. Percutaneous closure of a left ventricular outflow tract pseudoaneurysm causing extrinsic left coronary artery compression by transseptal approach. *Circulation.* 2010;121:e20-e22.
2. Babaliaros VC, Lerakis S, Thourani VH, et al. Transapical closure of a pseudoaneurysm of the mitral-aortic intervalvular fibrosa. *Tex Heart Inst J.* 2015;42:285-288.

Alcohol Ablation of Right Ventricular Outflow Tract Obstruction

Sivasubramanian Ramakrishnan, DM, Balram Bhargava, DM, Sandeep Seth, DM, Balram Airan, MCh

A 28-year-old woman with valvular and infundibular pulmonary narrowing (peak Doppler gradients of 120 mm Hg) had presented to us in the last trimester of pregnancy. She had an uneventful delivery, and subsequently underwent elective pulmonary valve balloon dilation (Fig. 4.140A–B). After the valvuloplasty, the right ventricular (RV) pressures rose markedly despite adequate dilation of the pulmonary valve, and the gradients across the valve and at the infundibulum level were 30 and 100 mm Hg, respectively. She remained stable and was started on oral metoprolol (sustained release) 50 mg twice daily. Follow-up echocardiogram after 6 months of therapy with metoprolol showed persistent right ventricular outflow track (RVOT) gradients (150 mm Hg) at the infundibular level. The pulmonary valve was opening well, with mild pulmonary regurgitation. A computed tomography coronary angiogram delineated the anomalous infundibular bundle with a large conal artery supply. After a detailed conversation and providing informed consent, percutaneous alcohol ablation of the conal artery was planned in view of the patient's reluctance to undergo open-heart surgery.

The RV pressure was systemic, with a gradient of 90 mm Hg across the infundibulum (Fig. 4.141). A simultaneous RV and conal artery angiogram clearly delineated the conal artery supply to the large, anomalous infundibular muscle bundle (Online Video 4.130). A temporary transvenous pacemaker lead was inserted. The conal artery had a separate origin from the right coronary artery (Fig. 4.140C), and selective engagement of the conal artery was done with difficulty. A 0.014-inch exchange-length BMW guidewire (Abbott Laboratories, Abbott Park, Illinois) was placed distally in the conal artery. A 2.5- × 12-mm over-the-wire Fire Star balloon (Cordis Corporation, Asia Pacific, Singapore) was inflated in the conal artery. After guidewire removal, 1 mL of contrast was injected distally (Fig. 4.140D). This showed marked staining of the infundibular muscle on fluoroscopy (Online Video 4.131), which was confirmed by echocardiography. Sustained balloon inflation (10 minutes) demonstrated clear reduction in gradients across the RVOT. On confirming assured target and success, both radiographically and hemodynamically, 1 mL of absolute alcohol was injected distally into the

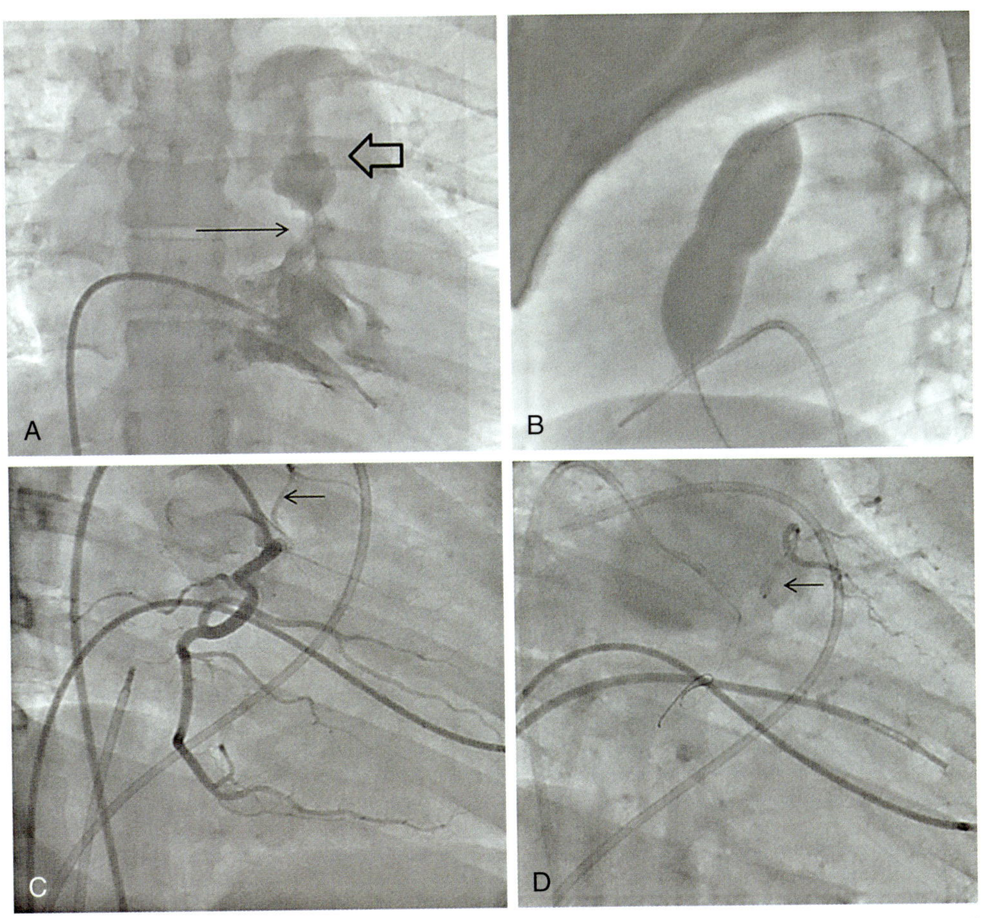

FIG. 4.140 Angiographics Details of the Procedure. (A) Right ventricular angiogram in anteroposterior view showing tight infundibular (*large, open arrow*) and valvular (*thin arrow*) pulmonary stenosis. (B) Fluoroscopic image in lateral view showing pulmonary valve balloon dilation with an appropriately sized balloon. (C) Right coronary injection in the right anterior oblique (RAO) view showing the right coronary artery and the separate origin of the conal artery (*arrow*). (D) Fluoroscopic image in RAO view with injection made through an over-the-wire coronary balloon (*arrow*) showing selective opacification of the conal artery (Online Videos 4.130 and 4.131). The guidewire placed in the native right coronary artery for stability can also be seen.

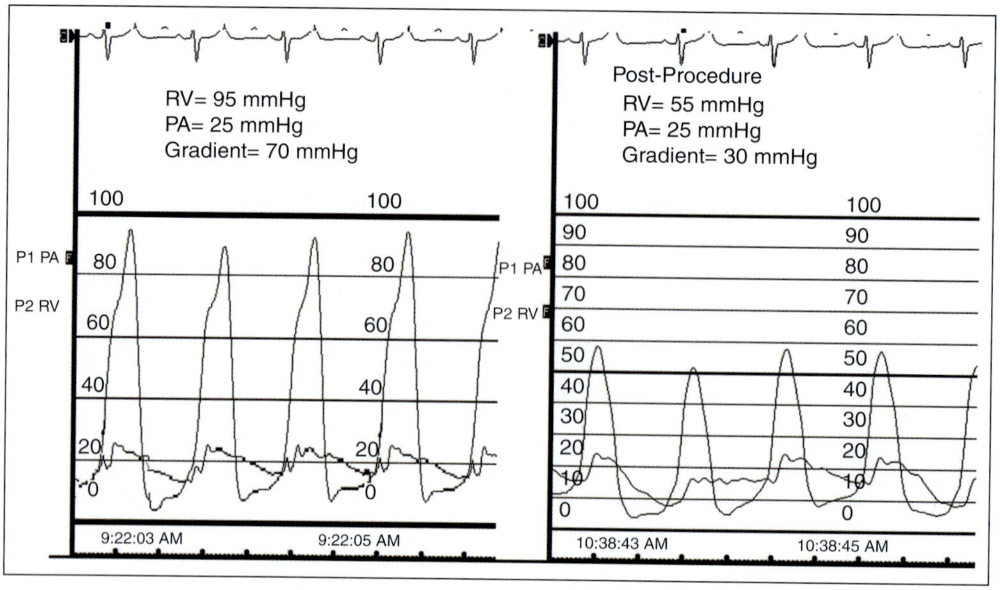

FIG. 4.141 Pressure Gradients Preprocedure and Postprocedure. Simultaneous right ventricle (*RV*) and pulmonary artery (*PA*) traces showing the gradients across the right ventricular outflow track before (*left*) and after (*right*) the procedure.

conal artery through the lumen of the inflated balloon catheter. The patient complained of mild chest pain. Ten minutes later, the balloon was flushed and then deflated. The suprasystemic RV pressures dropped dramatically, with significant reductions of the RVOT gradients from 90 mm Hg preprocedure to 40 mm Hg (Fig. 4.141). The creatine kinase-myocardial band isoform increased progressively over the next 12 hours and peaked at 546 IU/mL. The patient had an uneventful intensive care unit stay and was electively discharged on day 3. On follow-up at 3 months, the patient was well, and the routine echocardiogram showed further reduction in gradients to 30 mm Hg across the RVOT.

Brock,[1] in his historic paper in 1948, first described closed RVOT dilation that paved the way for several intracardiac corrective surgeries. Open-heart surgery is currently the established treatment for muscular RVOT obstruction. Several percutaneous palliative procedures have been tried with limited success for relieving RVOT obstruction. Balloon dilation, cutting balloons, stents, and even atherectomy have been used in the past.[2,3] Alcohol ablation for hypertrophic cardiomyopathy is now an established procedure.[4] Procedural complications of septal alcohol ablation, including dissection, alcohol spillage, dreaded complications of complete heart block, and cardiac perforations, are likely to be lower in alcohol ablation of RVOT as compared with the left side. The long-term risk of ventricular arrhythmias as a result of scarring is a remote, albeit real, risk. The lack of mid- to long-term data on the safety and efficacy of this procedure is a major limitation.

Alcohol ablation for RVOT obstruction is novel, and may prove to be an elegant cure for RVOT obstruction in selected patients.

References

1. Brock RC. Pulmonary valvulotomy for the relief of congenital pulmonary stenosis: report of three cases. *Br Med J.* 1948;1:1121-1126.
2. Dryzek P, Mazurek-Kula A, Moszura T, Sysa A. Right ventricle outflow tract stenting as a method of palliative treatment of severe tetralogy of Fallot. *Cardiol J.* 2008;15:376-379.
3. Qureshi SA, Parsons JM, Tynan M. Percutaneous transcatheter myectomy of subvalvar pulmonary stenosis in tetralogy of Fallot: a new palliative technique with an atherectomy catheter. *Br Heart J.* 1990;64: 163-165.
4. Maron BJ, Maron MS. Hypertrophic cardiomyopathy. *Lancet.* 2013;381: 242-255.

Percutaneous Closure of Right Ventricular Pseudoaneurysm

Mohamad Alkhouli, MD, Bryan Waits, MD, Abhishek Chaturvedi, MBBS, Frederick S. Ling, MD

Ventricular pseudoaneurysm is a contained rupture of the ventricular wall that may occur after myocardial infarction, trauma, infection, transcatheter valve replacement, or cardiac surgery.[1–4] It usually occurs in the left ventricle, with very few reports of right ventricular (RV) pseudoaneurysm.[3] Left untreated, this serious complication is associated with a 40% incidence of rupture at 1 year.[1] Surgical repair is generally considered the standard treatment, but is associated with high morbidity and mortality.[2] Percutaneous pseudoaneurysm closure has emerged as a new alternative for high-risk surgical patients. This technique has been described in small case series of patients with left ventricular pseudoaneurysm.[1,3,4] We describe a case of an acquired RV pseudoaneurysm after pericardiocentesis that was successfully treated with percutaneous closure.

A 71-year-old man with hypertension, diabetes, atrial fibrillation, morbid obesity, and oxygen-dependent obstructive pulmonary disease presented with worsening dyspnea and was found to have a large pericardial tamponade. Pericardiocentesis was attempted via the apical route under ultrasound guidance, but images were very limited by body habitus. The attempt was complicated with RV puncture, severe tamponade, and shock requiring intubation, and emergent pericardial window. Two days later, an abdominal computed tomography was done after an episode of hematemesis and incidentally revealed an RV pseudoaneurysm. This was further confirmed on transthoracic echocardiogram (Online Video 4.132). He was at an excessive risk for open repair and was therefore referred for a percutaneous closure of the pseudoaneurysm. A planning cardiac computed tomography revealed a pseudoaneurysm sac size of 3.6 × 3.2 cm, and a tortuous neck that measured 15.3 × 7.9 mm in diameter and 5.1 to 7.2 mm in length (Figs. 4.142 and 4.143, Online Videos 4.132 and 4.133).

Right ventriculography was performed revealing the RV pseudoaneurysm (Fig. 4.144A, Online Videos 4.134 and 4.135). The position of the RV pseudoaneurysm relative to the chest wall was confirmed with angiography and transthoracic echocardiography. An intracardiac echocardiography catheter was positioned in the RV for further guidance, but was technically limited. The pseudoaneurysm sac was

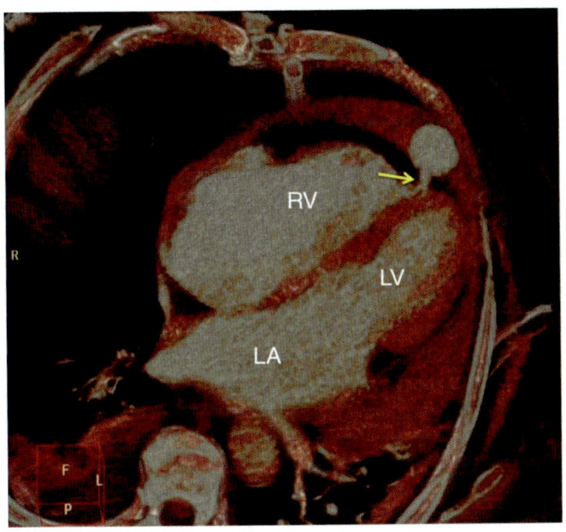

FIG. 4.142 Three-Dimensional Computed Tomography Long-Axis View of Right Ventricular Pseudoaneurysm. Cardiac computed tomography three-dimensional reconstruction showing the right ventricular (*RV*) pseudoaneurysm in long-axis view (*yellow arrow*) (Online Videos 4.132 and 4.133). *LA*, left atrium; *LV*, left ventricle.

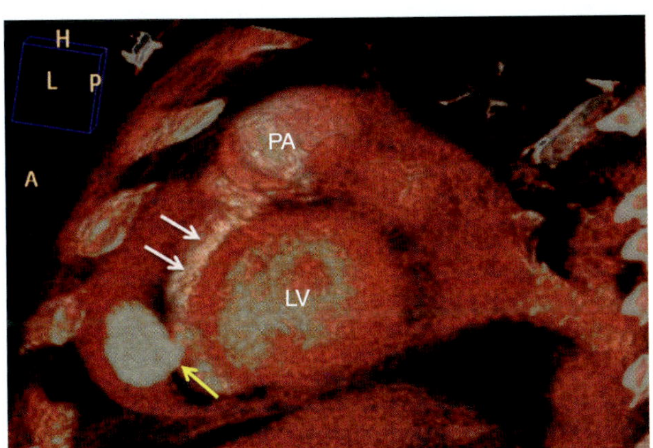

FIG. 4.143 Three-Dimensional Computed Tomography Sagittal View of Right Ventricular Pseudoaneurysm. Cardiac three-dimensional reconstruction showing the right ventricular pseudoaneurysm in a sagittal view (*yellow arrow*). The *white arrows* point to the right ventricle (Online Video 4.133). *LV*, left ventricle; *PA*, main pulmonary artery.

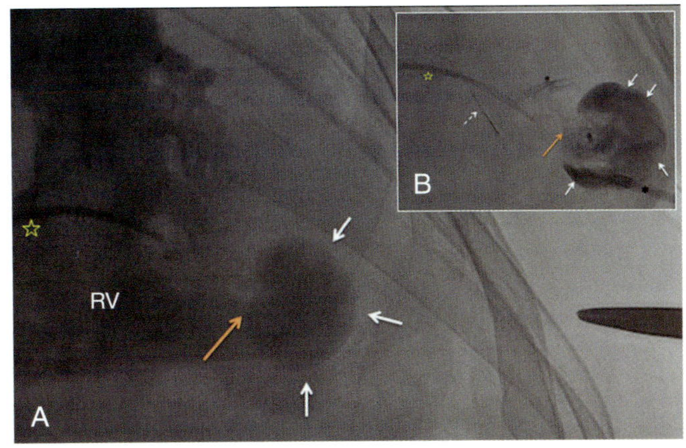

FIG. 4.144 Cineangiography Before and After Vascular Plug Deployment. Still frames of cineangiography showing the right ventricular (*RV*) pseudoaneurysm before (A) (Online Videos 4.134 and 4.135) and after (B) (Online Videos 4.136–4.138) the vascular plug deployment. *Orange arrow* indicates the neck of the pseudoaneurysm; *white arrows* indicate the sac of the pseudoaneurysm; *dashed arrow* in (B) shows the intravascular ultrasound catheter; *star* indicates the angiographic catheter in the RV; *asterisks* indicate the 8F Bright Tip sheath.

entered with a micropuncture needle, and a 0.014-inch Choice PT Extra Support wire (Boston Scientific, Marlborough, Massachusetts) was manipulated across the pseudoaneurysm neck into the right atrium. The tract was dilated with a 5F micropuncture dilator, and a 4F sheath was advanced into the pseudoaneurysm. A 4F angled glide catheter (Terumo, Tokyo, Japan) was then advanced into the inferior vena cava to allow exchange for a 0.035-inch Amplatz Extra Support wire (Boston Scientific). The 4F sheath was then exchanged for an 8F Brite Tip sheath (Cordis, Bridgewater, New Jersey), which was advanced into the right atrium. A 0.018-inch SV-5 wire (Cordis) was advanced alongside the Amplatz Extra-Stiff wire into the superior vena cava for support during device deployment and to act as a safety wire. The Amplatz Extra-Stiff wire was removed and the sheath was retracted into the RV. A 16-mm Amplatzer vascular plug II device (AGA Medical, Golden Valley, Minnesota) was deployed across the defect using RV injections for guidance (Online Videos 4.135 and 4.136). Subsequent RV angiography showed no significant flow into the pseudoaneurysm sac (Online Video 4.137). With the sheath's tip still in the pseudoaneurysm, thrombin was injected into the sac to ensure complete thrombosis of the sac (Fig. 4.144B, Online Videos 4.136–4.138). The sheath was then removed and the chest wall tissue tract was filled with Tisseel fibrin sealant (Baxter, Deerfield, Illinois). A follow-up echocardiogram showed complete cessation of flow into the pseudoaneurysm sac (Online Video 4.137), and the patient was discharged to a rehabilitation facility 1 week later.

References

1. Dudiy Y, Jelnin V, Einhorn BN, Kronzon I, Cohen HA, Ruiz CE. Percutaneous closure of left ventricular pseudoaneurysm. *Circ Cardiovasc Interv.* 2011;4:322-326.
2. Prêtre R, Linka A, Jenni R, Turina MI. Surgical treatment of acquired left ventricular pseudo-aneurysms. *Ann Thorac Surg.* 2000;70:553-537.
3. Bortnick AE, Gordon E, Gutsche J, et al. Percutaneous closure of a left ventricular pseudoaneurysm after Sapien XT transapical transcatheter aortic valve replacement. *J Am Coll Cardiol Intv.* 2012;5:e37-e38.
4. Kumar PV, Alli O, Bjarnason H, Hagler DJ, Sundt TM, Rihal CS. Percutaneous therapeutic approaches to closure of cardiac pseudoaneurysms. *Catheter Cardiovasc Intv.* 2012;80:687-699.

Percutaneous Pulmonary Valve Implantation in a Native Outflow Tract: Three-Dimensional DynaCT Rotational Angiographic Reconstruction and Three-Dimensional Printed Model

Joseph T. Poterucha, DO, Thomas A. Foley, MD, Nathaniel W. Taggart, MD

A 15-year-old girl with dextro-transposition of the great arteries presented with combined neopulmonary stenosis and regurgitation after an arterial switch operation as a neonate and neopulmonary valvectomy at 6 years of age. Echocardiography revealed right ventricular enlargement and severe neopulmonary regurgitation and stenosis with a mean Doppler gradient of 47 mm Hg. Right ventricular end-diastolic volume by cardiac magnetic resonance was 201 mL/m^2. She underwent cardiac catheterization with three-dimensional (3D) DynaCT rotational angiography and 3D reconstruction (Siemens, Munich, Germany) (Fig. 4.145A, Online Videos 4.139 and 4.140). Catheterization demonstrated a peak-to-peak pulmonary gradient of 38 mm Hg. The right ventricular outflow tract (RVOT) measured 16 mm angiographically. Sequential placement of a 26-mm ev3 IntraStent LD Max (ev3-Endovascular, Plymouth, Minnesota) and a Palmaz XL 3110 stent (Cordis, Johnson & Johnson, Bridgewater Township, New Jersey), both delivered over a 22 mm × 4-cm Z-Med balloon (PFM Medical, Cologne, Germany), established a satisfactory landing zone for percutaneous pulmonary valve implantation. A Medtronic Melody valve (Medtronic, Fridley, Minnesota) was successfully placed in the RVOT using a 22F Ensemble delivery system (Medtronic), resulting in resolution of neopulmonary regurgitation and improvement in peak-to-peak gradient to 15 mm Hg. DynaCT rotational angiography and reconstruction was again performed (Fig. 4.145B, Online Videos 4.141 and 4.142). The 3D rotational angiogram DICOM (Digital Imaging and Communications in Medicine) data was then processed offline using dedicated software (Materialize, Leuven, Belgium) to create STL (stereolithography) files for 3D printing. Life-size 3D printing was performed using an Objet Connex350 3D Printer (Stratasys Ltd., Eden Prairie, Minnesota) (Fig. 4.145C–D).

Off-label percutaneous pulmonary valve implantation has been safely demonstrated in patients with unfavorable anatomy including patients with conduit-free RVOT, native pulmonary valves, and small conduits. Creation of an adequate landing zone with prestenting of the RVOT is critical to successful placement.[1] This is the first reported case of percutaneous pulmonary valve implantation into a native RVOT using 3D rotational angiography for guidance of stent and valve implantation. 3D printed models provide a novel and valuable tool for patient and trainee education.

Reference

1. Thanopoulos BV, Giannakoulas G, Arampatzis CA. Percutaneous pulmonary valve implantation in the native right ventricular outflow tract. *Catheter Cardiovasc Interv.* 2012;79:427-429.

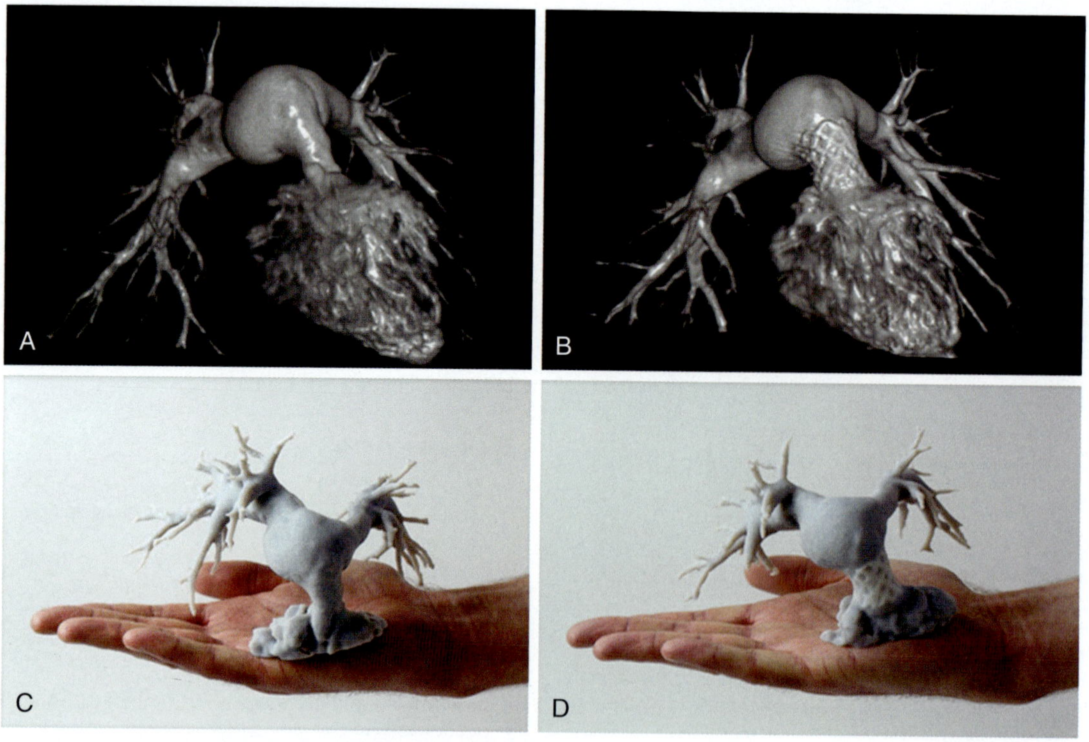

FIG. 4.145 Three-Dimensional Reconstruction and Printed Model Before and After Percutaneous Pulmonary Valve Implantation. (A and C) Before implantation with Melody valve (Medtronic, Fridley, Minnesota) (Online Videos 4.139 and 4.140). (B and D) After implantation (Online Videos 4.141 and 4.142). (A and B) Three-dimensional DynaCT reconstruction. (C and D) Printed models.

Not Your Typical Hole-in-the-Wall: Percutaneous Closure of an Acquired Postmyocardial Infarction Ventriculoatrial Gerbode Defect

Richard Cheng, MD, Reza Arsanjani, MD, Emily Tat, BA, Justin Cox, MD, Abhimanyu Uberoi, MD, MS, Rebecca Aron, MD, Saibal Kar, MD

A 58-year-old male patient presented with an inferior ST-segment elevation myocardial infarction complicated by a ventricular septal defect (VSD). The VSD was surgically repaired, but basal extension of necrotic tissue obligated a second repair 2 weeks later. Subsequently, he again presented in cardiogenic shock and was found to have a significant residual VSD; he was referred to our institution for cardiac transplantation.

Transthoracic echocardiogram showed further basal extension of the VSD (Fig. 4.146A) with left ventricular (LV) to right ventricular shunting. However, transesophageal echocardiogram instead revealed LV to right atrial (RA) shunting through an 11-mm Gerbode defect with direct extension through the atrioventricular portion of the septum, which was thought to be from further basal extension of infarct necrosis (Fig. 4.146B). Percutaneous closure was planned because a third sternotomy could preclude future transplantation listing.

Shunt run demonstrated elevated RA pressures, with the a wave at 24 mm Hg and the v wave at 28 mm Hg. Shunt size was estimated at 4.57 L/min (Qp/Qs ratio, 1.72). With a retrograde transfemoral approach and directed by an internal mammary catheter, a coated guidewire was advanced through the defect into the RA, where it was snared and externalized through the internal jugular vein (Fig. 4.146C). A delivery sheath was advanced over the guidewire from the neck into the LV and ascending aorta (Fig. 4.146D), and a 14-mm Amplatzer atrial septal occluder (St. Jude Medical, St. Paul, Minnesota) was successfully deployed with minimal residual shunting (Figs. 4.146E–G) and an immediate 4-mm Hg improvement in mean RA and right ventricular pressures. Shunt size was reduced to 2.18 L/min (Qp/Qs ratio, 1.37) with residual shunting through the device itself, which was expected to improve with endothelialization. Tricuspid valve leaflets were free from impingement after device deployment as assessed by transesophageal echocardiogram with no significant regurgitation. The patient was successfully discharged and was stable at 2-month follow-up.

Acquired Gerbode defects are rare, and percutaneous closure has only previously been described in three cases of surgically acquired defects[1–3] but not after myocardial infarction. In this case, successful percutaneous closure allowed for immediate hemodynamic and clinical stabilization and the avoidance of a third sternotomy, which may have excluded the option of cardiac transplantation in the future.

References

1. Fanari Z, Barekatain A, Abraham N, Hopkins JT. Percutaneous closure of acquired Gerbode defect: management of a rare complication of cardiac surgery. *Interact Cardiovasc Thorac Surg.* 2015;21:127-128.
2. Rothman A, Galindo A, Channick R, Blanchard D. Amplatzer device closure of a tortuous Gerbode (left ventricle-to-right atrium) defect complicated by transient hemolysis in an octogenarian. *J Invasive Cardiol.* 2008;20: E273-E276.
3. Trehan V, Ramakrishnan S, Goyal NK. Successful device closure of an acquired Gerbode defect. *Catheter Cardiovasc Interv.* 2006;68:942-945.

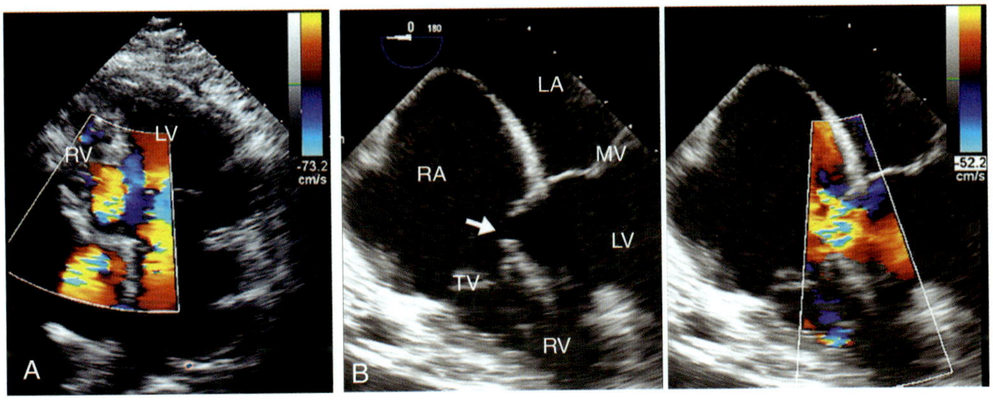

FIG. 4.146 Echocardiography- and Fluoroscopy-Guided Percutaneous Closure of a Gerbode Defect. (A) Apical four-chamber view on transthoracic echocardiogram of shunting from the left ventricle (*LV*) to what appears to be the right ventricle (*RV*). (B) Midesophageal four-chamber view on transesophageal echocardiogram instead reveals a Gerbode defect (*arrow*) to the right atrium (*RA*). The left atrium (*LA*), mitral valve (*MV*), and tricuspid valve (*TV*) are also shown. (C) Cranial left anterior oblique view on angiogram shows a guidewire being snared (*arrow*).

Continued

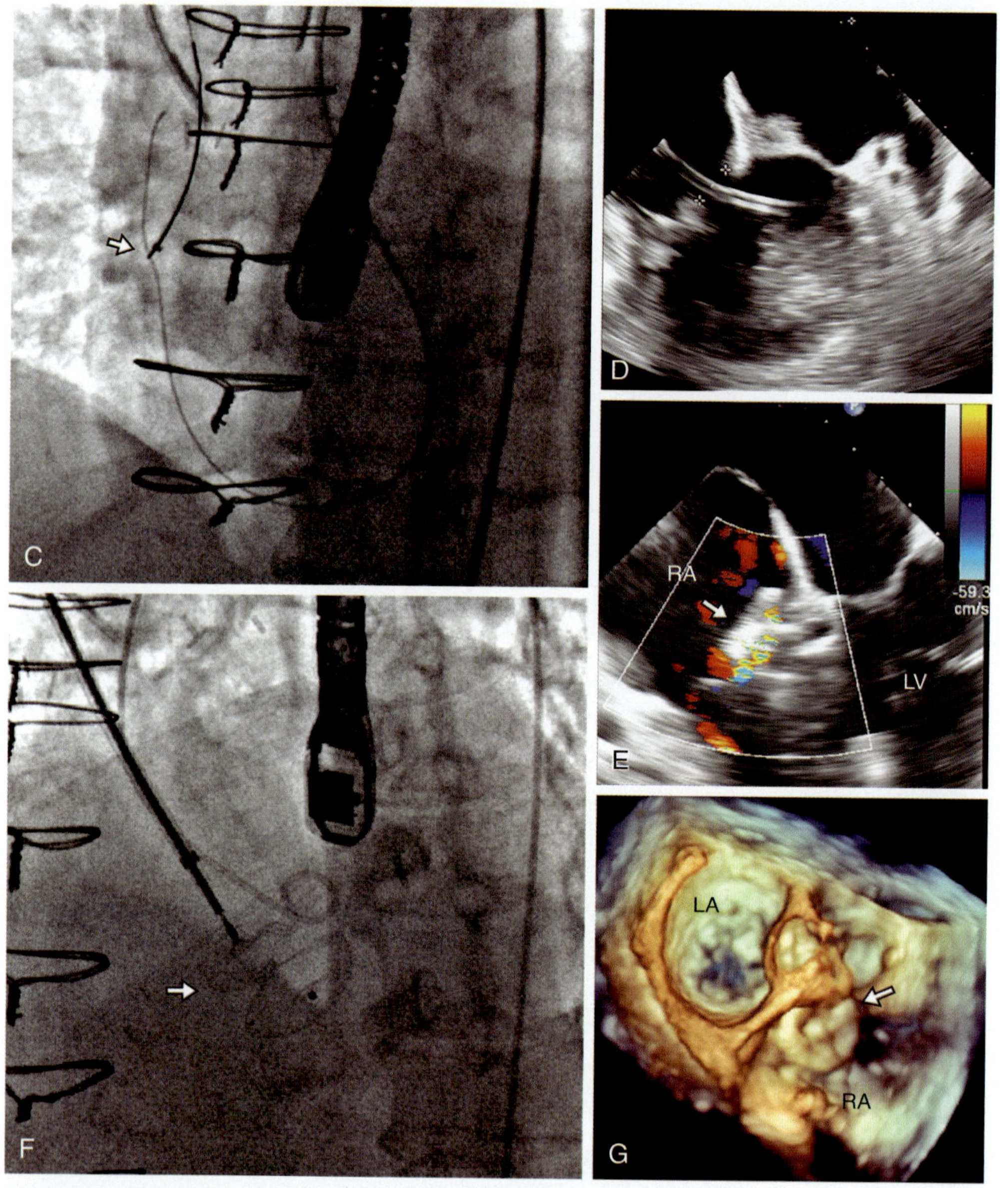

FIG. 4.146, cont'd (D) An Amplatzer delivery sheath across the 11-mm defect. (E and F) An Amplatzer 14-mm atrial septal occluder (*arrow*) is deployed with minimal residual shunting. (G) Three-dimensional transesophageal echocardiogram shows no residual defect and a well-situated device (*arrow*).

Utility of the Gore Septal Occluder in Transcatheter Closure of Postmyocardial Infarction Ventricular Septal Defect: Initial Experience

Eduardo A. Arias, MD, Amit Bhan, MD, Zhan Y. Lim, MD, Michael Mullen, MD

We present two examples of postmyocardial infarction ventricular septal defect (PMIVSD) successfully treated by percutaneous closure using the Gore septal occluder (GSO) (W. L. Gore & Associates, Flagstaff, Arizona).

A 71-year-old woman was transferred to our institution after elective percutaneous intervention to the left anterior descending artery, complicated by coronary dissection and a periprocedural myocardial infarction. Two days later, a new pansystolic murmur was detected and echocardiography confirmed an apical PMIVSD. With incipient multiorgan failure, she underwent successful percutaneous closure of the defect using a 30-mm GSO on day 10 after the myocardial infarction.

A 79-year-old woman with a late presentation anterior myocardial infarction and PMIVSD underwent surgical repair with a bovine pericardial patch and bypass grafting. Postoperative echocardiography revealed two large separate residual PMIVSDs. Twenty-two days after surgery, she underwent percutaneous closure.

In both examples, procedural access was via the right internal jugular vein and right femoral artery. Left ventriculography showed severe left-to-right shunt. Standard percutaneous techniques, including crossing of the defect retrogradely and arteriovenous circuit formation, were performed.[1] Transesophageal echocardiography and fluoroscopy were used for guidance.

In the first example, a 30-mm GSO was deployed and control angiogram showed a second separate apical defect with a mild to moderate shunt. After the procedure, liver and renal function normalized and the patient was discharged with a plan for elective surgery (Fig. 4.147, Online Video 4.143). In the second example two 30-mm GSO devices were deployed in the inferior and posterior aspects of the septum surrounding the bovine pericardial patch. A control angiogram showed no residual shunt and the patient was discharged 5 days later (Fig. 4.148, Online Video 4.144). After the procedure, a gated computed tomography scan showed devices in situ with excellent conformation to the ventricular chambers (Figs. 4.149 and 4.150). In both examples, an immediate hemodynamic improvement was noted.

Closure by PMIVSD is a complex procedure and technical challenges include unstable septal anatomy and a huge variation in size and shape of the defects. Early after the insult, the myocardium remains friable and in some cases stiffer devices could potentially extend the defect. In addition, we decided to use this device for the following reasons: (1) the presence of slitlike defect at the infarct borders, (2) soft and compliant disks that could mold to the shape of the LV, and (3) a small waist so there was less chance of stretching the defect further. To the best of our knowledge, the information presented herein demonstrates the first successful use of the GSO to close PMIVSDs.[2]

REFERENCES

1. Al-Kashkari W, Balan P, Kavinsky CJ, Cao QL, Hijazi ZM. Percutaneous device closure of congenital and iatrogenic ventricular septal defects in adult patients. *Catheter Cardiovasc Interv.* 2011;77:260-267.
2. Hagler DJ, Latson LA, Goble J, Mathewson JW, Cutright W. Failure of the GORE HELEX atrial septal defect occluder to treat membranous VSDs in swine. *Catheter Cardiovasc Interv.* 2010;76:874-877.

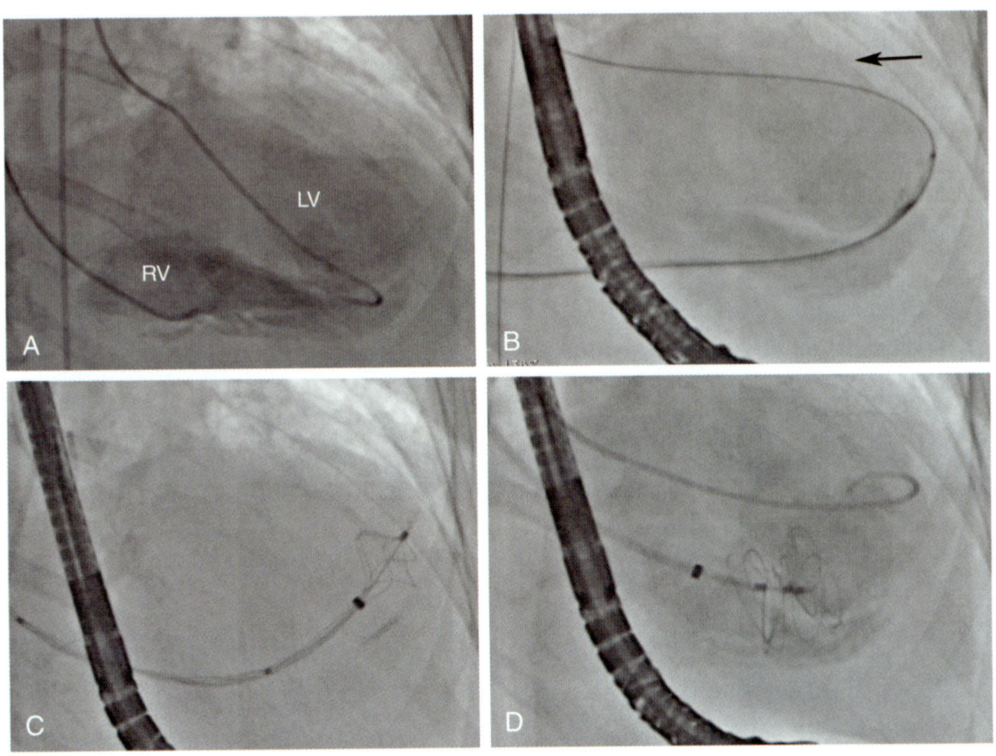

FIG. 4.147 Deployment of the Gore Septal Occluder Device. (A) An angiogram is undertaken using a pigtail catheter in the left ventricle (*LV*) to delineate the defect (Online Video 4.143). The catheter in the right ventricle (*RV*) is a JR4. (B) The defect has been crossed from the LV side with a Terumo wire and an arteriovenous loop has been created. A multitrack catheter has been advanced on the wire. The *black arrow* points to the previously implanted left anterior descending artery stents. (C) The device has been advanced from the venous sheath and the left-sided disk has been deployed. (D) The device has been pulled back on to the ventricular septum and the right-sided disk deployed in the RV.

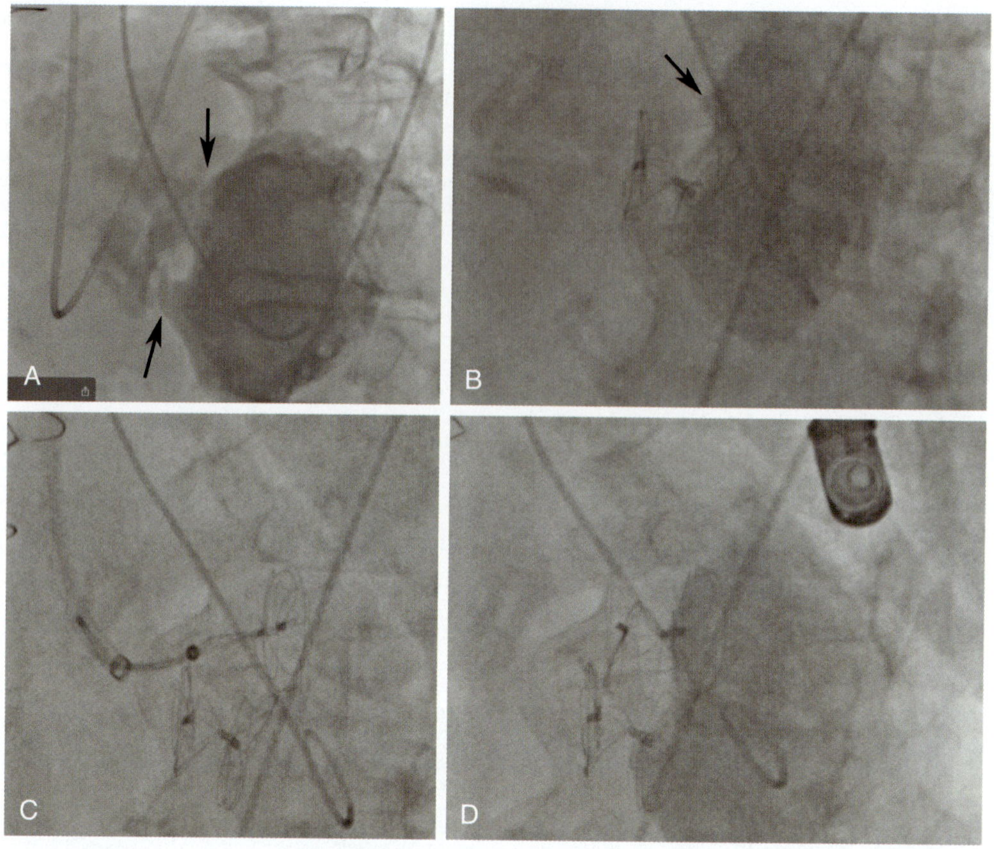

FIG. 4.148 Deployment of Two Gore Septal Occluder Devices. (A) Initial left ventriculography (Online Video 4.144) demonstrates two separate shunts on either side of the surgical patch (*black arrows*). (B) The first device has been deployed across the more apical defect, but a shunt is still seen from the other defect (*black arrow*). (C) A second device being deployed in the second defect. (D) Final result demonstrating no residual shunt.

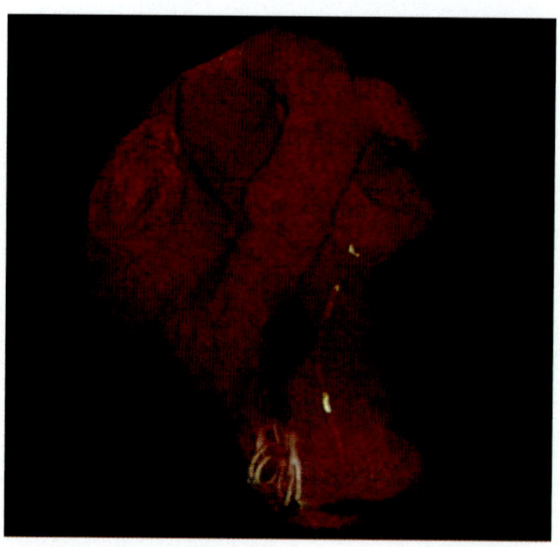

FIG. 4.149 Computed Tomography Reconstruction. Computed tomography reconstruction demonstrating the apical position of the Gore septal occluder device in the first example. Artifact from the left anterior descending arterial stents is clearly seen.

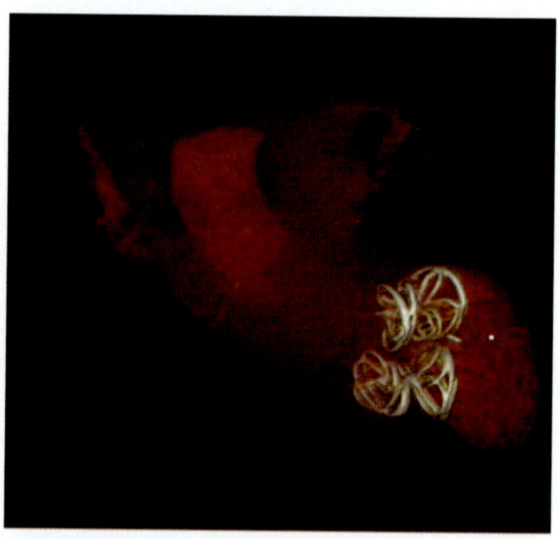

FIG. 4.150 Computed Tomography Reconstruction. Computed tomography reconstruction demonstrating the two Gore septal occluder devices sited in the second example.

Tricuspid Valve

Sustained Reduction of Tricuspid Regurgitation After Percutaneous Repair With the MitraClip System in a Patient With a Dual-Chamber Pacemaker

Damiano Regazzoli, MD, Alfonso Ielasi, MD, Giuseppe Lanzillo, MD, Marco Bruno Ancona, MD, Eustachio Agricola, MD, Francesco Giannini, MD, Antonio Mangieri, MD, Francesco Ancona, MD, Jorg Hausleiter, MD, Michael Nabauer, MD, Antonio Colombo, MD, Azeem Latib, MD

A 73-year-old woman presented with heart failure, systemic congestion, and fatigue despite optimal medical therapy. Her medical history included stage IV kidney disease and previous hepatitis B virus infection.

In 2014, she experienced a non–ST-segment elevation myocardial infarction. Coronary angiography was performed and showed two-vessel disease with stenosis of the left anterior descending artery that was treated with drug-eluting stent implantation; chronic total occlusion of right coronary artery was also found and left to medical therapy. She underwent dual-chamber permanent pacemaker (PM) implantation for third-degree atrioventricular block a year later. After this last procedure, progressive tricuspid regurgitation (TR) developed. This finding was confirmed at echocardiography performed at admission (Fig. 4.151, Online Video 4.145); TR was secondary to annular dilatation and PM lead interference with the septal leaflet. Both right and left ventricular function, as well as pulmonary pressure, were normal.

Pacing leads in the right ventricle (RV) are present in 40% to 50% of patients with severe TR, and an increased mortality rate has been observed in this population, compared with those with TR but no PM.[1] In the present case, the pacing lead may have actively contributed to the mechanism of TR by displacing the septal leaflet and by causing asynchrony in RV contraction.[2] Furthermore, the presence of this foreign body across the valve may interfere with potential surgical or percutaneous treatment for TR.[3]

After heart team discussion, the patient was deemed inoperable and was then evaluated for percutaneous transcatheter tricuspid repair with the MitraClip system (Abbott Vascular, Santa Clara, California). The procedure was performed under general anesthesia with fluoroscopic and transesophageal echocardiographic guidance via percutaneous right transfemoral venous access. The guiding catheter was placed into the right atrium, and a clip was then advanced through the transcatheter valve and oriented in order to reach the anteroseptal commissure (Fig. 4.152A–B). A second clip was advanced near the first one, toward the posteroseptal commissure (Fig. 4.152C–D), thus effectively excluding the lead into the commissure and substantially reducing TR (Fig. 4.152E–F, Online Video 4.146). The patient was discharged on postoperative day 2 with mild residual TR (Fig. 4.153A, Online Video 4.147). At 6-month

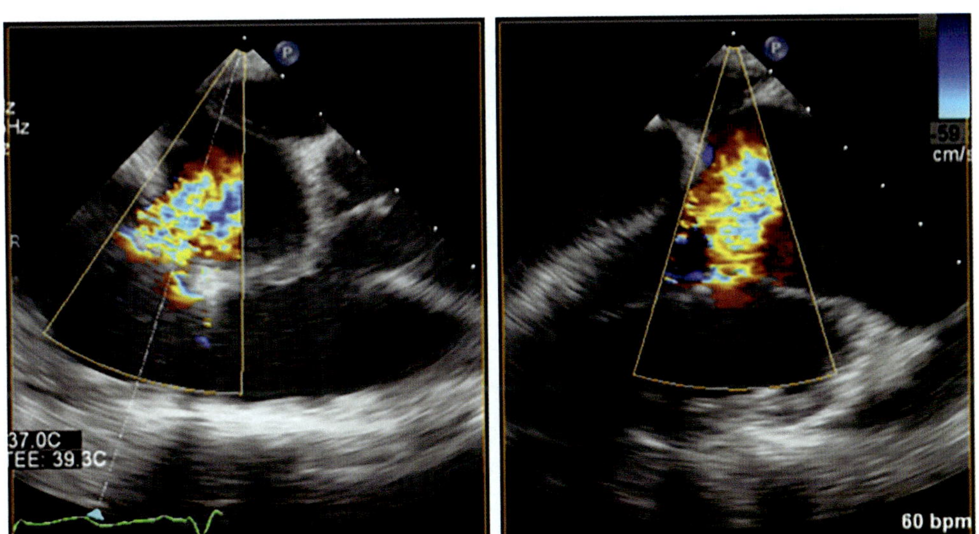

FIG. 4.151 Baseline Transesophageal Echocardiography. The images show severe tricuspid regurgitation secondary to annular dilatation and pacemaker lead interference with the septal leaflet (Online Video 4.145).

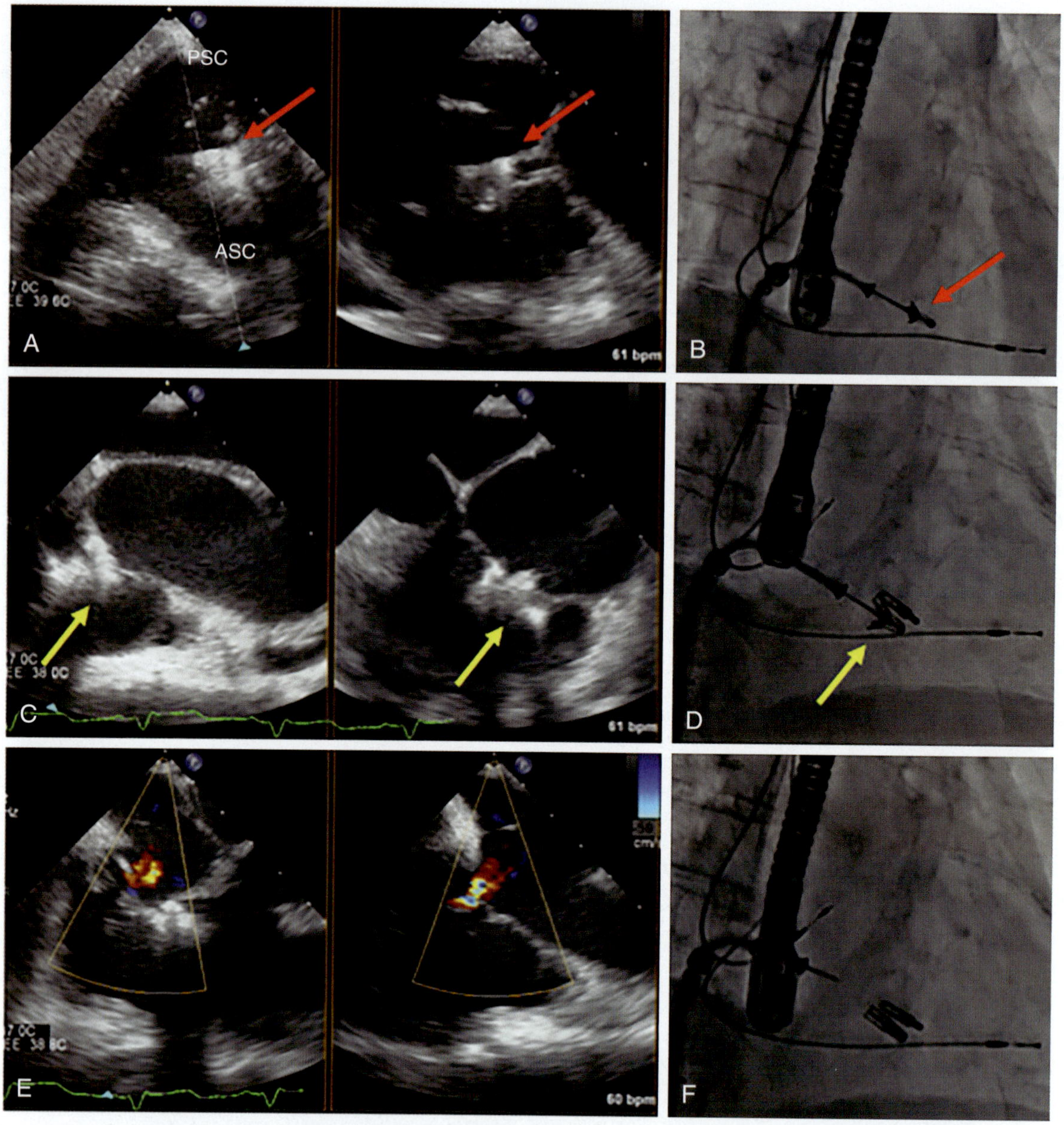

FIG. 4.152 Procedural Imaging. (A and B) The first clip (*red arrow*) implanted near the anteroseptal commissure (*ASC*). *PSC*, posteroseptal commissure. (C and D) The *yellow arrow* indicates the second clip, implanted toward the PSC. (E and F) Good final result (Online Video 4.146).

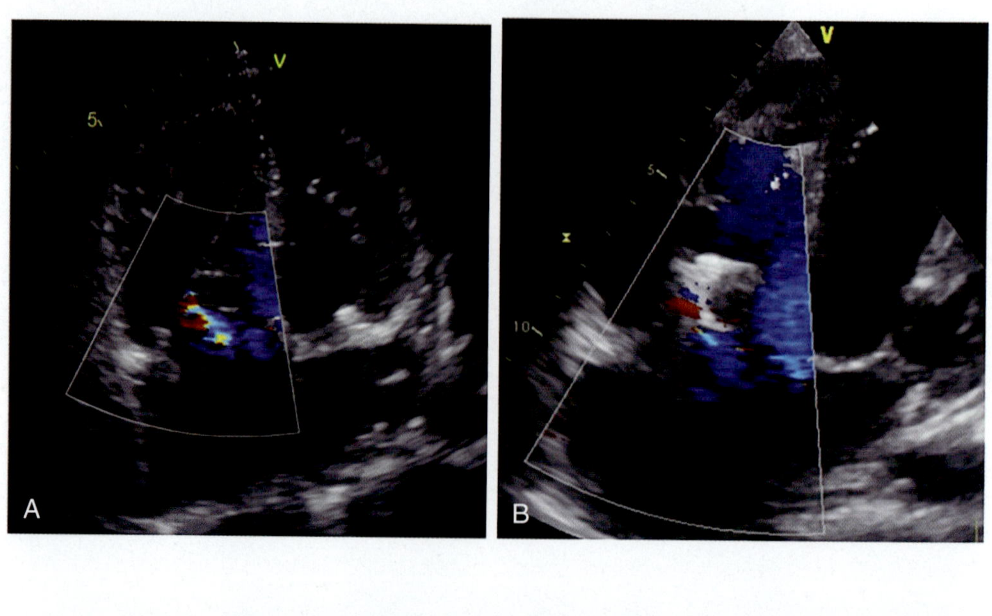

FIG. 4.153 Discharge and Follow-Up Echocardiograms. Echocardiograms show consistent reduction of tricuspid regurgitation (A), confirmed also after 6 months (B), as well as positive right ventricular remodeling (Online Video 4.147).

follow-up, she reported clinical improvement with reduction in lower limb edema and fatigue; echocardiography confirmed the consistent reduction of TR (Fig. 4.153B).

In this specific setting, percutaneous transcatheter valve repair with the MitraClip system seems to be a promising option with minimal procedural risk as well as good and sustained clinical and echocardiographic results.

References

1. Delling FN, Hassan ZK, Piatkowski G, et al. Tricuspid regurgitation and mortality in patients with transvenous permanent pacemaker leads. *Am J Cardiol.* 2016;117:988-992.
2. Stryjewski PJ, Osika A, Kuczaj A, et al. Pathogenesis of tricuspid valve regurgitation in patients with implanted of right-ventricular electrode. *Przegl Lek.* 2015;72:71-73.
3. Pfannmueller B, Hirnle G, Seeburger J, et al. Tricuspid valve repair in the presence of a permanent ventricular pacemaker lead. *Eur J Cardiothorac Surg.* 2011;39:657-661.

Tricuspid Valve Replacement: A Percutaneous Transfemoral Valve-in-Ring Approach

Alduz S. Cabasa, MD, Mackram F. Eleid, MD, Charanjit S. Rihal, MD, Hector R. Villarraga, MD, Thomas A. Foley, MD, Rakesh M. Suri, MD, DPhil

We describe a percutaneous transcatheter tricuspid valve-in-ring implantation using the SAPIEN XT prosthesis (Edward Lifesciences, Irvine, California).[1,2] A 68-year-old woman with rheumatic heart disease and two previous sternotomies including tricuspid valve repair with a 32-mm Carpentier-Edwards (Irvine, California) annuloplasty ring presented 2 years prior with severe tricuspid valve regurgitation (annulus dilatation and tenting of the leaflet) and pulmonary hypertension (right ventricular systolic pressure of 46 mm Hg) related to left ventricular diastolic dysfunction. After multidisciplinary evaluation, a percutaneous approach was recommended to avoid increased risk of third-time redo sternotomy. The procedure was planned using a cardiac computed tomography–derived three-dimensional printed model created using an Objet Connex 350 printer (Stratasys, Eden Prairie, Minnesota) (Fig. 4.154). Using this model, the prosthesis size was selected and "test deployed" to verify adequacy (Online Video 4.148). The actual transcatheter tricuspid valve-in-ring implantation was performed in the hybrid operating suite under general anesthesia. The right common femoral vein was accessed percutaneously. With an Amplatz Super Stiff guidewire (Boston Scientific, Marlborough, Massachusetts) acting as a rail, a 29-mm SAPIEN XT valve was advanced across the tricuspid valve annulus. The stented valve was balloon-inflated with an additional 1 mL of contrast saline solution to achieve optimal conical deployment (Fig. 4.155, Online Video 4.149). Transesophageal echocardiography showed only mild perivalvular regurgitation in the septal region, as predicted in the printed model. Postprocedural two-dimensional echocardiography showed mild tricuspid valve regurgitation with a transvalvular gradient of 3 mm Hg (Fig. 4.156, Online Video 4.150). The patient's dyspnea improved before discharge from hospital 4 days later. The long-term effectiveness of this off-label procedure is still unknown and warrants further studies.

References

1. Hoendermis ES, Douglas YL, van den Heuvel AF. Percutaneous Edwards Sapien valve implantation in the tricuspid position: case report and review of literature. *EuroIntervention.* 2012;8:628-633.
2. Raval J, Nagaraja V, Eslick GD, Denniss AR. Transcatheter valve-in-valve implantation: a systemic review of literature. *Heart Lung Circ.* 2014;23:1020-1028.

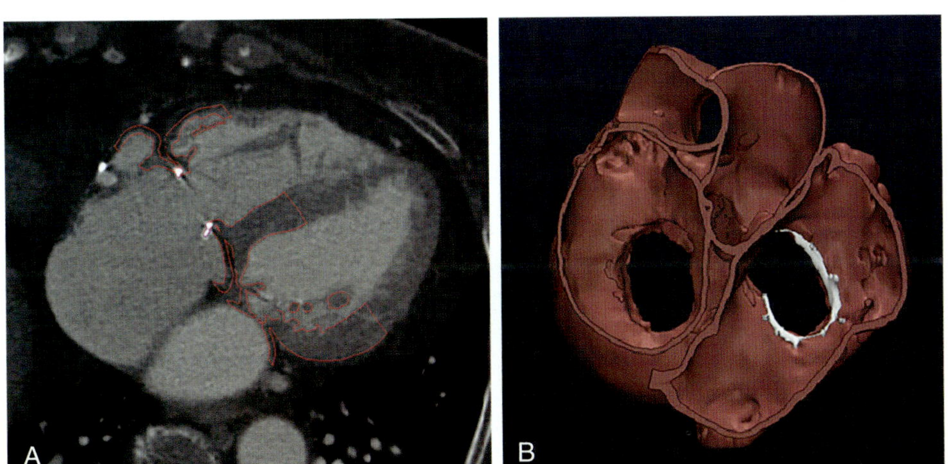

FIG. 4.154 Preprocedure and Postprocedure Computed Tomography Imaging and Three-Dimensional Printed Model. (A) Preprocedure electrocardiography-gated cardiac computed tomography (CT) scan with the outline of the standard template library files (*red and purple outlines*) used for printing of the three-dimensional (3D) model projected on the CT image. (B) The 3D reconstruction of the standard template library files showing the anatomy included in the printed model.

Continued

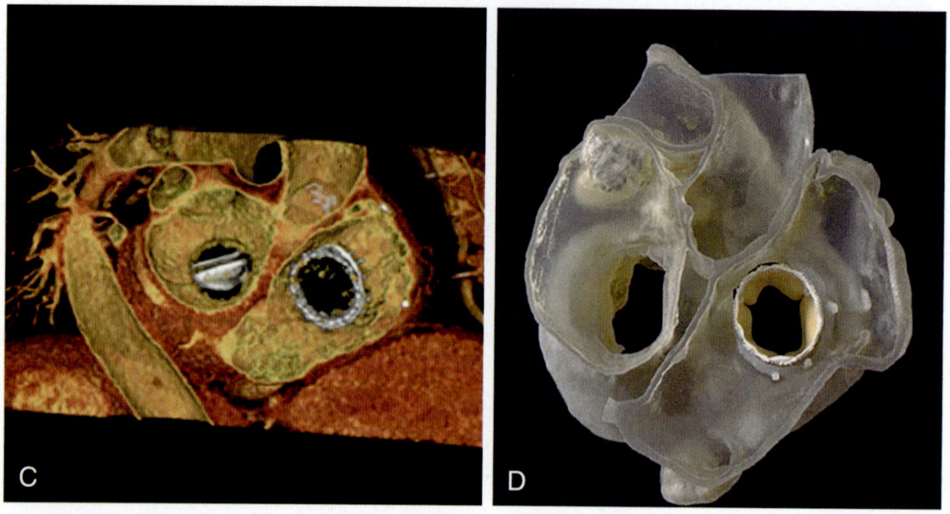

FIG. 4.154, cont'd (C) Postoperative volume-rendered 3D image showing the implanted SAPIEN XT valve within the annulus. (D) The 3D printed model, which is made up of acrylic-based photopolymer resins of differing stiffness for the annuloplasty band and myocardium. The appropriate size of the SAPIEN XT valve was preoperatively determined using the model. See Online Video 4.148.

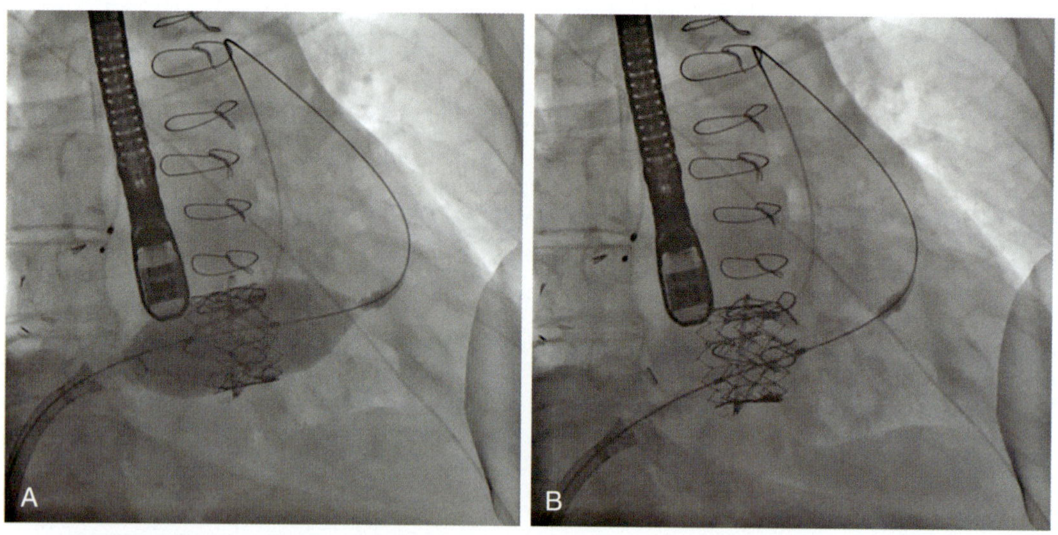

FIG. 4.155 Fluoroscopy Images of the Procedure. (A) Additional 1 mL of contrast saline solution was used to achieve optimal conical deployment. (B) Postballoon expansion of the SAPIEN XT valve image showing a well-seated valve with most of the stent on the right atrial side of the annulus. See Online Video 4.149.

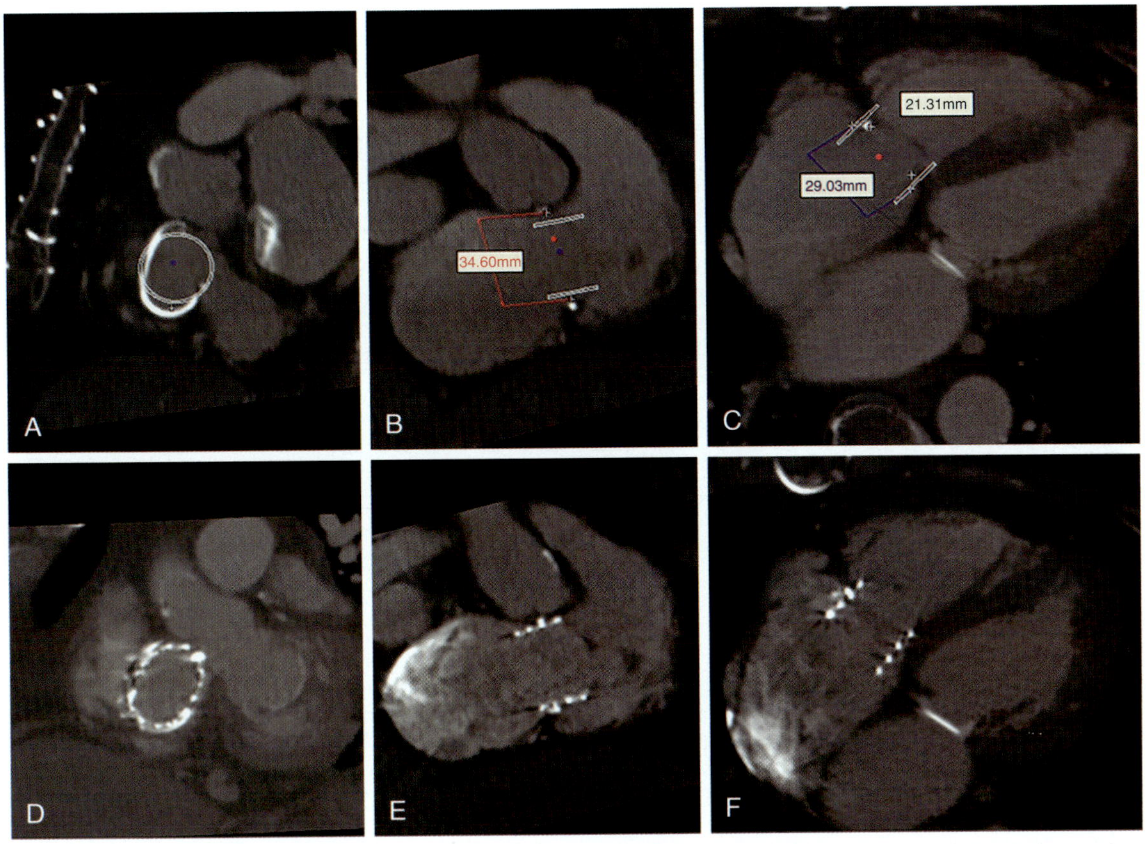

FIG. 4.156 Virtual Model of SAPIEN XT Projected on Computed Tomography Image. (A)–(C) Reformatted preprocedure cardiac computed tomography (CT) images with "virtual" model of the 29-mm SAPIEN XT valve projected on the CT image in the tricuspid position. (D)–(F) Reformatted postprocedure implantation cardiac CT images showing the position of the SAPIEN valve after implantation. The valve stent appears well opposed to the annulus and annuloplasty band. See Online Video 4.150.

Chapter 5
Vascular, Congenital, and Other Anatomy and Pathophysiology

Hemodynamic Findings of Effusive-Constrictive Pericarditis

Anand D. Shah, MD, Daniel L. Molloy, MD, John E.A. Blair, MD

A 64-year-old man with rheumatoid arthritis presented with progressive abdominal and leg swelling, anorexia, and dyspnea for several years. Physical examination was notable for a pericardial knock, pulsatile hepatomegaly, and lower extremity edema. The jugular vein was distended past the angle of the jaw and did not decrease with inspiration (Kussmaul sign). Transthoracic echocardiography demonstrated normal left ventricular function, a thickened pericardium, and a large pericardial effusion. Computed tomography showed the pericardium to measure 8 mm (normal, <3 mm). To clarify a diagnosis of symptomatic pericardial effusion versus constrictive pericarditis, the patient was referred for left-side and right-side heart catheterization and pericardiocentesis.

Left and right ventricular pressures were transduced simultaneously with right atrial pressure (RAP) at baseline; interventricular dependence of left and right ventricular filling was noted (Fig. 5.1A, *arrowheads*, scales optimized), along with a dip-and-plateau pattern

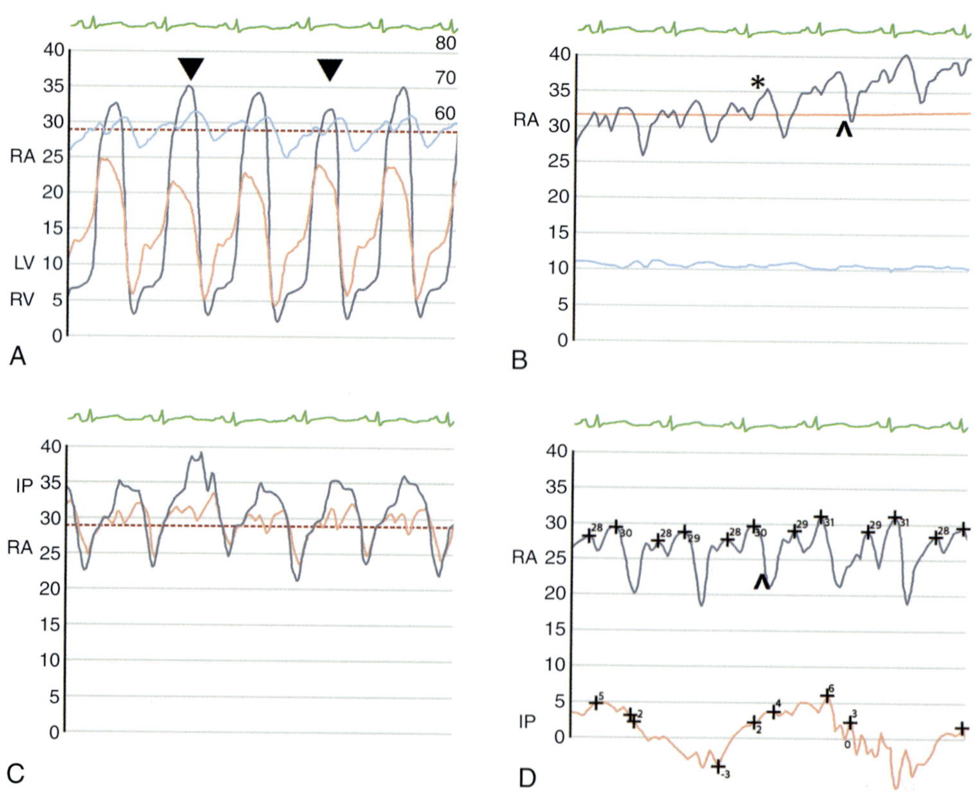

FIG. 5.1 Hemodynamic Findings in Effusive-Constructive Pericarditis. (A) Simultaneous left ventricular and right ventricular pressure tracings show ventricular interdependence and dip-and-plateau filling pattern during diastole. (B) Right atrial pressure (RAP) rises with inspiration, demonstrating Kussmaul sign; prominent *y* descents are noted. (C) Before pericardiocentesis, intrapericardial (*IP*) pressure and RAP are superimposed. (D) After pericardiocentesis, IP pressure is normalized but remains unchanged in the right atrium, demonstrating the visceral pericardial contribution to constriction. *LV*, left ventricle; *RA*, right atrium; *RV*, right ventricle.

of ventricular filling. RAP was severely elevated and failed to decrease with inspiration (Fig. 5.1B, *asterisk*). The preserved *y* descent in RAP was not consistent with tamponade. Intrapericardial pressure was measured with RAP at baseline (Fig. 5.1C) and after complete drainage of pericardial fluid (Fig. 5.1D). RAP was dissociated from intrapericardial pressure, remaining elevated at 25 mm Hg, despite normalization of intrapericardial pressure to 0 mm Hg. The typical, exaggerated *y* descent of pericardial constriction was more apparent after pericardiocentesis because the holodiastolic four-chamber impediment to filling associated with tamponade was eliminated, leaving only the limitation to filling in mid- and end-diastole, characteristic of constrictive pericarditis. Thus the findings demonstrated that the patient's elevated filling pressures were related to constrictive pericarditis. Despite adjustment of the patient's immunosuppressive regimen, severe congestive symptoms persisted. The patient underwent successful pericardiectomy, at which time the diagnosis was confirmed. Pericardial involvement is noted in 50% of patients with rheumatoid arthritis, although ≥90% are asymptomatic.[1]

Reference

1. Prasad M, Hermann J, Gabriel SE, et al. Cardiorheumatology: cardiac involvement in systemic rheumatic disease. *Nat Rev Cardiol.* 2015;12: 168-176.

Hypoxemia Due to Patent Foramen Ovale in the Setting of New Right Hemidiaphragmatic Paralysis

Cory R. Trankle, MD, Hem L. Bhardwaj, MD, Walter H.J. Paulsen, MD, John D. Grizzard, MD, Rachit D. Shah, MD, Zachary M. Gertz, MD, MBE

A 58-year old man with no history of cardiac pathology presented with dyspnea and was found to be hypoxemic (oxygen saturation, 88% on room air) with platypnea-orthodeoxia. The symptoms had started soon after a laparoscopic cholecystectomy 3 weeks before.

Imaging revealed new right hemidiaphragmatic paralysis (confirmed with sniff testing showing paradoxic motion) and no pulmonary embolism (Fig. 5.2A–B). Transthoracic echocardiography with agitated saline demonstrated the early appearance of a large number of microbubbles in the left side of the heart, consistent with a right-to-left interatrial shunt (Fig. 5.2C, Online Video 5.1). Transesophageal echocardiography confirmed a patent foramen ovale (PFO) with near continuous right-to-left flow (Fig. 5.2D–E).

The patient was referred for percutaneous PFO closure. Pulmonary vein oxygen saturation was 96% (arterial room air saturation, 87%). A 25-mm Amplatzer cribriform Septal Occluder device (St. Jude Medical, St. Paul, Minnesota) was deployed, and the patient's arterial saturation immediately improved to 96% (Fig. 5.2F). His symptomatic shortness of breath was improved but not completely resolved, so he was referred for diaphragmatic plication. After successful plication, the patient's dyspnea nearly completely resolved (Fig. 5.2F–H, Online Videos 5.2 and 5.3).

Platypnea-orthodeoxia syndrome is a rare phenomenon that can be caused by a hemodynamically significant PFO. It has been reported several times as a complication after right pneumonectomy[1,2] and less frequently as a result of right hemidiaphragmatic elevation.[3,4] Timely diagnosis and closure of the PFO can lead to rapid correction of hypoxemia.

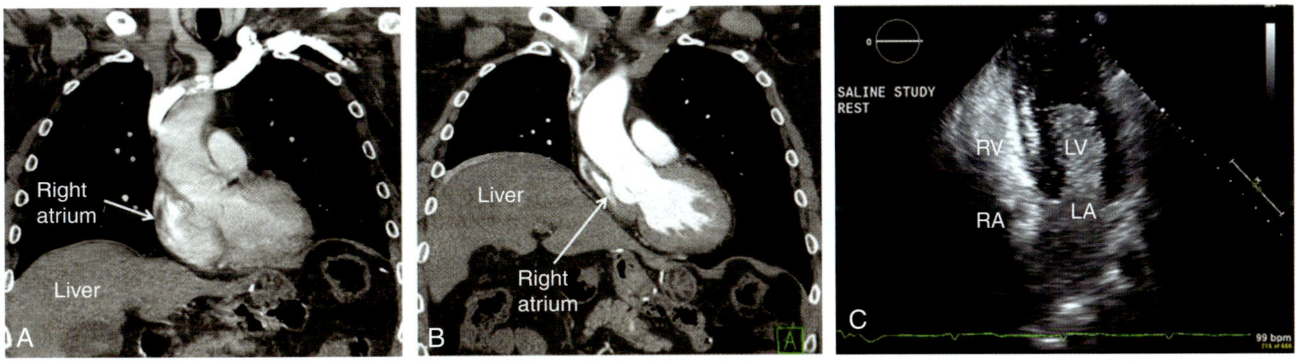

FIG. 5.2 Patent Foramen Ovale With Hypoxemia After Diaphragmatic Paralysis. (A) Chest computed tomography (CT) from 18 months before, without hemidiaphragmatic elevation. (B) Chest CT showing elevated right hemidiaphragm with compression of the right atrium. (C) Resting transthoracic echocardiography with bubble study showing the early appearance of a large amount of microbubbles in the left side of the heart (Online Video 5.1).

Continued

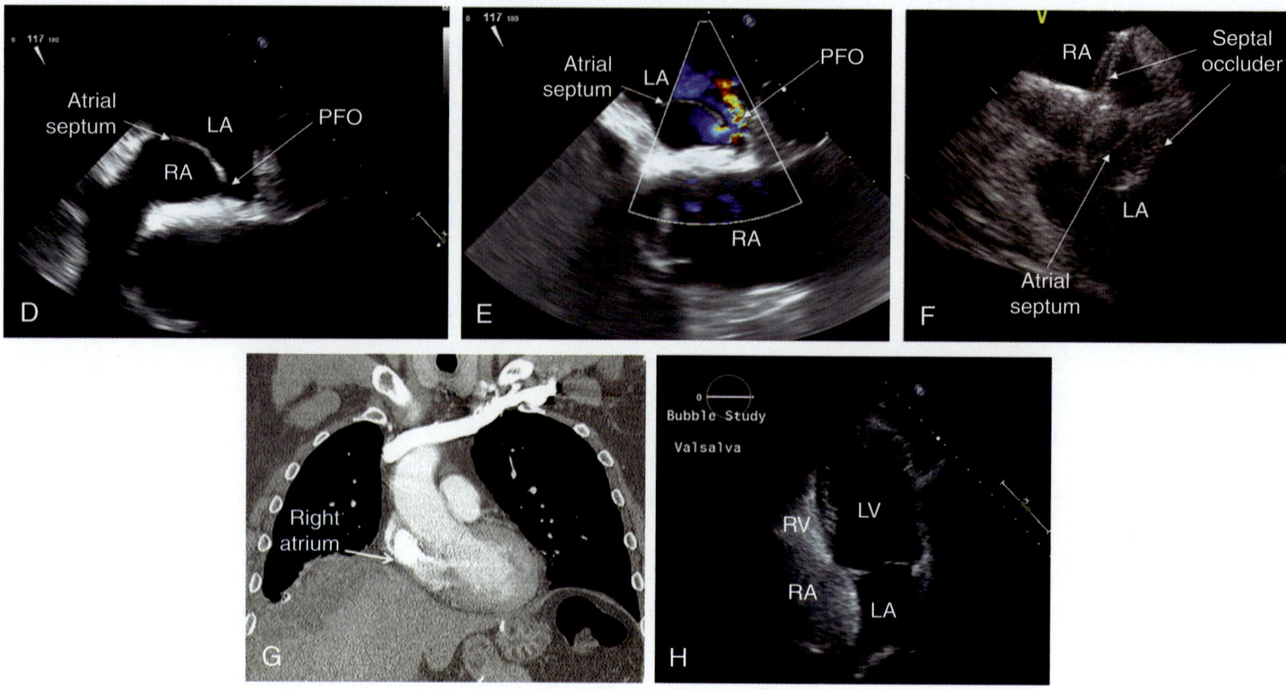

FIG. 5.2, cont'd (D and E) Interatrial septum by transesophageal echocardiography revealing PFO with right-to-left flow. (F) Intracardiac echocardiography showing deployment of Amplatzer Septal Occluder (St. Jude Medical, St. Paul, Minnesota). (G) Chest CT after diaphragmatic plication showing improvement in hemidiaphragm elevation and decreased right atrial compression. (H) Postprocedural bubble study revealing resolution of shunt, including during provocative maneuvers (Online Videos 5.2 and 5.3). *LA*, left atrium; *LV*, left ventricle; *PFO*, patent foramen ovale; *RA*, right atrium; *RV*, right ventricle.

References

1. Kaufman DA, Ravi S, Dadu R, Horowitz D, Logue MA. Severe hypoxemia and orthodeoxia following right pneumonectomy. *Am J Respir Crit Care Med.* 2011;184:e1-e2.
2. Bhattacharya K, Birla R, Northridge D, Zamvar V. Platypnea-orthodeoxia syndrome: a rare complication after right pneumonectomy. *Ann Thorac Surg.* 2009;88:2018-2019.
3. Maholic R, Lasorda D. Successful percutaneous closure of a patent foramen ovale causing hypoxia in the setting of an elevated hemidiaphragm due to Guillain-Barré syndrome. *J Invasive Cardiol.* 2006;18:434-435.
4. Sakagianni K, Evrenoglou D, Mytas D, Vavuranakis M. Platypnea-orthodeoxia syndrome related to right hemidiaphragmatic elevation and a "stretched" patent foramen ovale. *BMJ Case Rep.* 2012;2012. bcr-2012-007735.

Aortoarteritis With Chronic Total Occlusion of All Neck Vessels: Percutaneous Stenting to Salvage Intractable Syncope

Nagaraja Moorthy, DM, Rangaraj Ramalingam, DM, Subramanyam K. Setty, DM, Shivanand S. Patil, DM, Manjunath C. Nanjappa, DM

A 42-year-old woman was admitted with a history of recurrent syncope of more than 10 to 15 episodes per day for more than 3 months that worsened over 1 month. She was diagnosed with aortoarteritis type I 3 years before an angiography showed total occlusion of bilateral subclavian (Fig. 5.3A–B, Online Video 5.4A–B), bilateral vertebral, and left common carotid arteries (Fig. 5.3C, Online Video 5.4C). The right common carotid artery had diffuse 70% lesion. Her coronary arteries, renal arteries, and aorta were normal. Because she was asymptomatic and considering the discouraging results of percutaneous interventions in aortoarteritis, she was advised medical follow-up and treated with immunosuppression. Just before additional computed tomography (CT) angiography of neck vessels, she had acute left faciobrachial monoparesis. All four neck vessels were occluded (Fig. 5.3D–E) and the sole brain was supplied by tiny collaterals. CT of the brain showed right frontotemporoparietal acute infarct (Fig. 5.3F). In view of the urgency of revascularization and

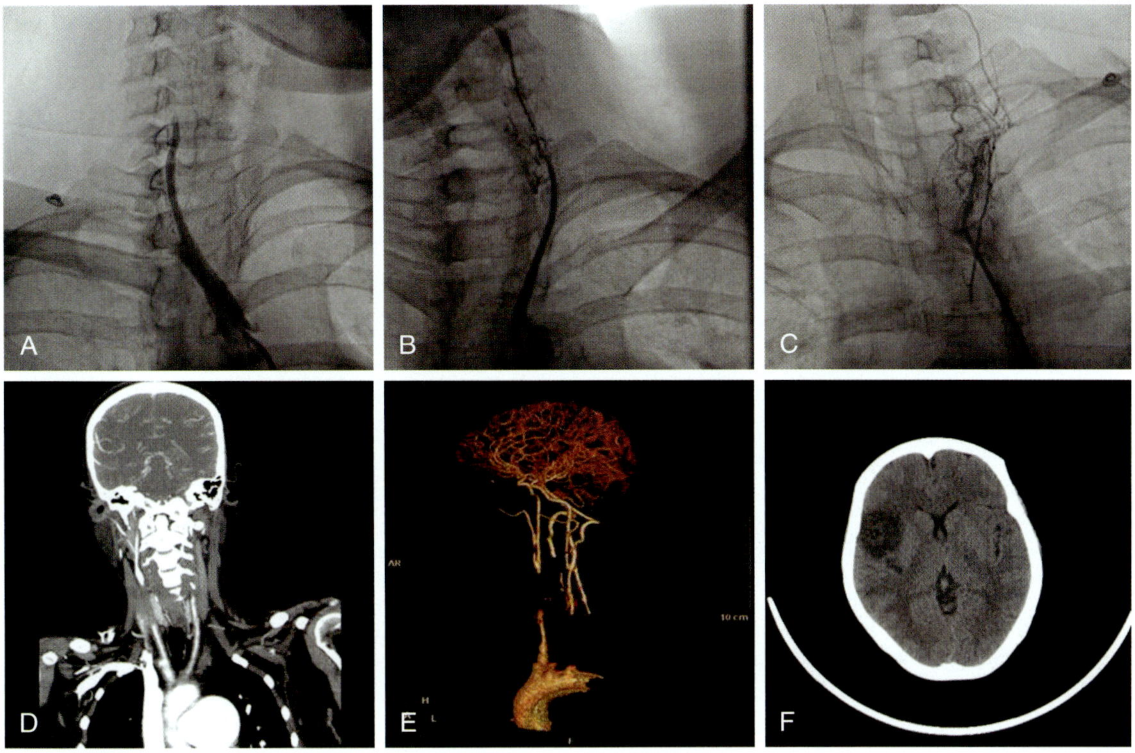

FIG. 5.3 Diagnostic Neck Vessels Angiography. (A) Right brachiocephalic injection showing total occlusion of right subclavian, right common carotid, and right vertebral arteries (Online Video 5.4A). (B) Left common carotid artery angiography showing chronic total occlusion with bridging collaterals (Online Video 5.4B). (C) Left subclavian artery angiography showing chronic total occlusion of left subclavian and left vertebral artery (Online Video 5.4C). (D) Computed tomography (CT) angiography of neck vessels showing total occlusion of all four neck vessels. (E) CT angiography volume-rendered imaging of neck vessels showing total occlusion of all four neck vessels. (F) CT of brain showing right frontotemporoparietal infarct.

risks involved in surgery, it was decided to perform urgent percutaneous angioplasty. Because the right common carotid artery was the latest to block, it was decided to open it because the success rate could be better when compared with the other three neck vessels. The right carotid artery was hooked with 6F shuttle sheath. The lesion was crossed with a 0.014-inch Pilot 150 wire (Abbott Vascular, Santa Clara, California) (Fig. 5.4A, Online Video 5.5A). However, because there was no support over this wire, it was exchanged to a 0.035-inch exchange wire (Medtronic, Inc., Minneapolis, Minnesota) to place at the distal end of the wire in the external carotid artery (Fig. 5.4B, Online Video 5.5B). In view of the patient's recent stroke and to prevent embolism, hardware manipulation was minimized and it was decided to perform direct stenting without predilation. A 6 mm × 100 mm Complete SE self-expanding stent (Medtronic, Inc.) distal edge was meticulously placed just at the bifurcation of the common carotid artery and deployed. Poststenting underexpansion of the stent was noted (Fig. 5.4C, Online Video 5.5C). Postdilation was done using a 7 mm × 20 mm NuMed (B. Braun Medical Inc., Hopkinton, New York) balloon catheter. The final result showed a well-expanded stent with significantly improved perfusion to the brain (Fig. 5.4D, Online Video 5.5D). No procedure-related complications were noted and the patient had complete relief from

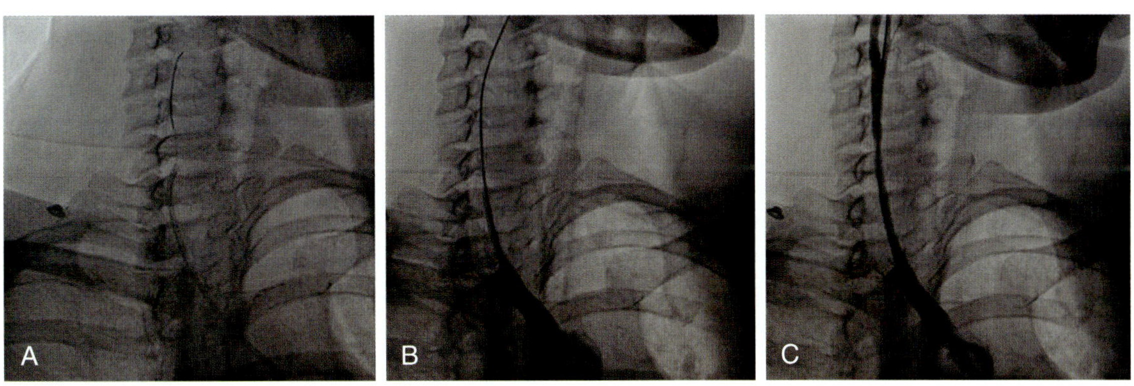

FIG. 5.4 Procedural Steps of Right Common Carotid Chronic Total Occlusion Intervention and Follow-up Carotid Doppler. (A) Pilot 150 wire crossing the total occlusion of the right common carotid artery (Online Video 5.5A). (B) The right common carotid artery lesion was crossed using a 0.35-inch exchange length wire (Online Video 5.5B). (C) Poststenting of the right common carotid artery using Complete SE stent (Medtronic, Minneapolis, Minnesota) showing an underexpanded stent (Online Video 5.5C).

Continued

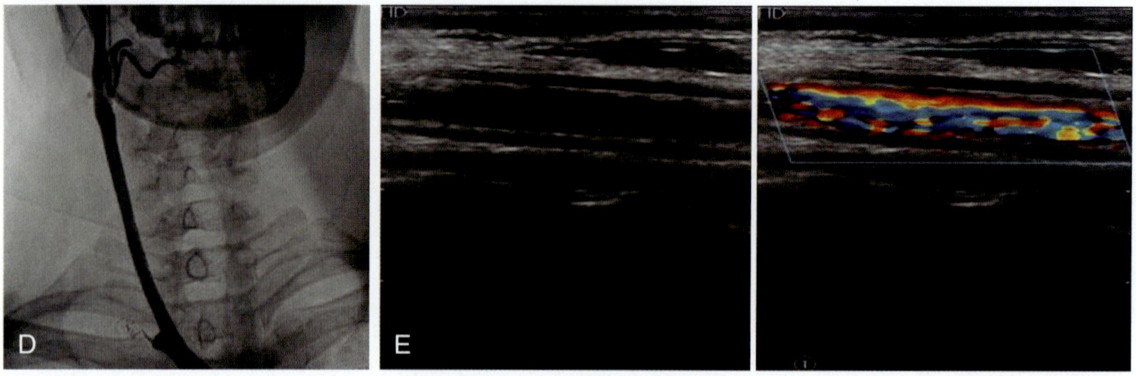

FIG. 5.4, cont'd (D) Poststenting right common carotid angiography showing fully expanded stent with improved brain perfusion (Online Video 5.5D). (E) Right common carotid Doppler at 6 months follow-up showing patent stent (Online Video 5.5E).

syncope. The carotid Doppler at 6 months follow-up showed the patent stent (Fig. 5.4E, Online Video 5.5E) and she remained asymptomatic.

Chronic total occlusions of neck vessels are not uncommon in aortoarteritis. Chronic total occlusions of all neck vessels presenting as recurrent syncope are very rare. Although percutaneous stenting of atherosclerotic total occlusion of the carotid artery is considered as contraindication, in rare conditions, such as aortoarteritis, percutaneous stenting could be considered as a safe and effective alternative to surgery.

Intraluminal Fibrous Webs in Brachial Artery Fibromuscular Dysplasia

Yoshito Kadoya, MD, Kan Zen, MD, PhD, Satoaki Matoba, MD, PhD

An 80-year-old woman diagnosed as having severe aortic stenosis underwent preoperative coronary angiography through the left radial artery for transcatheter aortic valve implantation. A 0.025-inch guidewire was advanced into the left brachial artery for sheath insertion. Upper extremity angiography was performed because it was difficult to pass the wire through the artery; the angiogram showed alternating stenoses and dilatations (i.e., a "string of beads" appearance) in the left brachial artery (Fig. 5.5A). The optical coherence tomography scan showed thickening of the middle layer (Fig. 5.5B, Online Video 5.6), causing intraluminal protrusion of the arterial segment (Fig. 5.5C). Angioscopy demonstrated intraluminal fibrous webs (arrows) as white, wall-like structures protruding into the lumen and contacting the wire (arrowheads); no thrombus was observed (Fig. 5.5D–E, Online Video 5.7). Therefore the diagnosis was brachial artery fibromuscular dysplasia (FMD). Because the patient was asymptomatic and no pressure gradient was observed across the FMD segment, no intervention or additional medical treatment was performed. Subsequently, the sheath was successfully passed through the narrowing segment, and transradial coronary angiography was completed. Further investigation showed no FMD lesions in other arterial territories.

FMD is a nonatherosclerotic, noninflammatory angiopathy that causes narrowing of medium-sized arteries, and it is characterized by fibrodysplastic changes.[1] Although catheter-based angiography is the gold standard for diagnosing FMD, it may be inadequate for visualizing intraluminal fibrous webs, whereas optical coherence tomography and angioscopic imaging can clearly show the presence of webs in the brachial artery. In the era of transradial catheter intervention, the importance of diagnosing brachial artery FMD should be recognized.

Reference

1. Olin JW, Gornik HL, Bacharach JM, et al. Fibro-muscular dysplasia: state of the science and critical unanswered questions: a scientific statement from the American Heart Association. *Circulation.* 2014;129:1048-1078.

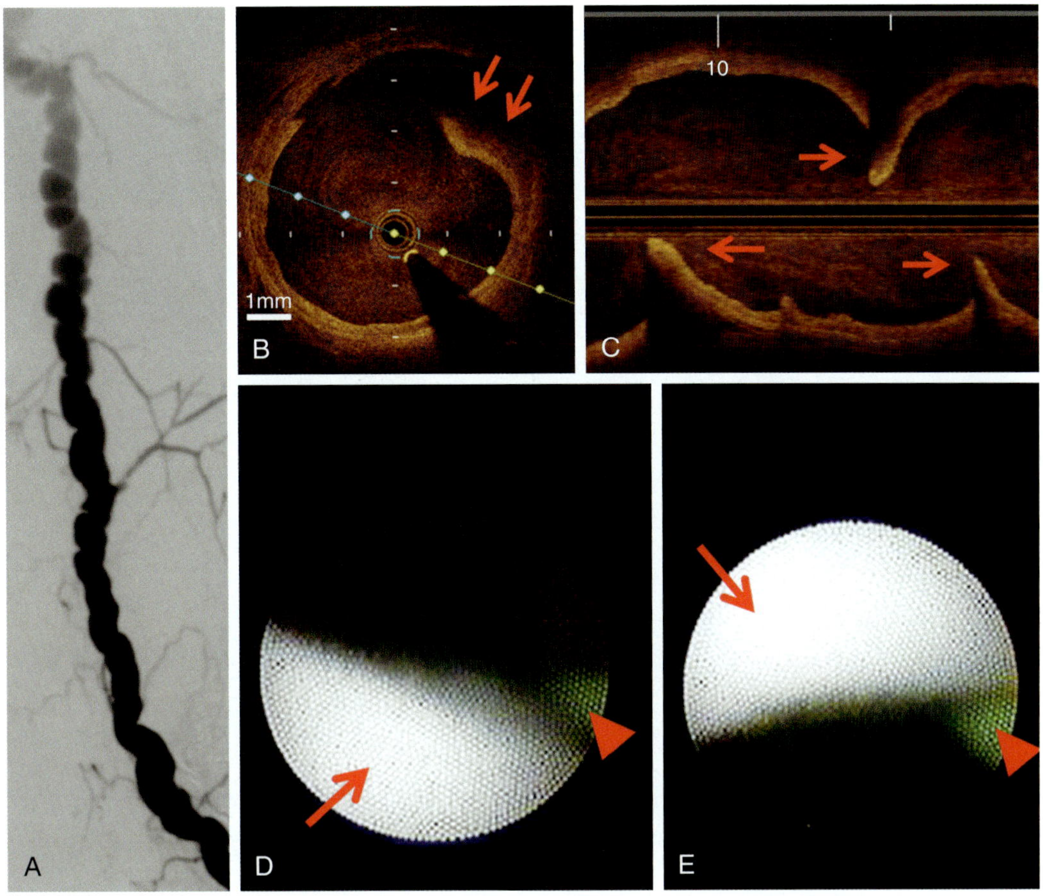

FIG. 5.5 Brachial Artery Fibromuscular Dysplasia. (A) Upper extremity angiogram showing a "string of beads" appearance in the left brachial artery. (B) Optical coherence tomography scan showing thickening of the middle layer (*arrows*) (Online Video 5.6), causing (C) intraluminal protrusion of the arterial segment (*arrows*). (D and E) Angioscopy showing intraluminal fibrous webs (*arrows*) as white, wall-like structures protruding into the lumen and contacting the wire (*arrowheads*). No thrombus is observed (See Online Video 5.7).

A Rare Radial Artery Anatomic Variant: Look for the Pulse on the Dorsum of the Wrist!

Arjun Venkatesh, BSc, Erin Wagner, RT(R), Jodi Klebe, RN, Jessica Schmidt, CVT/RCIS, Laila Payvandi, MD, Wassef Karrowni, MD

Several radial artery anatomic variations have been described.[1,2] These are especially important for the radiologists in the catheterization laboratory for troubleshooting, especially with the growing popularity of the radial artery as the preferred access site for diagnostic and interventional coronary angiographic procedures. Variation in the origin of the radial artery is a common anomaly in the upper limb. However, the distal part of its course shows a constant pattern. Here we report the unusual course of a duplicate radial artery in the lateral forearm and the dorsum of the hand.

A 56-year-old woman presented to our clinic reporting exertional chest pain. A nuclear stress test was suggestive of ischemia in the inferior wall. This was followed by cardiac catheterization, which was planned from the right radial approach. The patient had 1+ right radial pulse with normal results on Allen test. Access was obtained in the right radial artery using the Seldinger approach. A 6F Slender sheath (Terumo, Tokyo, Japan) was placed, and intraarterial nitroglycerin was infused. Advancing a Tiger catheter (Terumo) over a 0.035-inch J wire was challenging because as the wire could not be advanced past the midforearm level. Contrast injection was performed through the sheath and demonstrated a small radial artery with another larger anomalous vessel originating at the elbow level and migrating laterally (Fig. 5.6). A 2+ pulse was palpated at the dorsum of the hand. Another 6F Slender sheath was placed under ultrasound guidance in the duplicate vessel, and coronary angiography was completed with no difficulty (Fig. 5.7).

References

1. Thomas R, Newell R. Anomalous arteries in the upper limb. *Clin Anat.* 1995;7:57.
2. Chandni G, Vikram P, Murlimanju BV, Vaishali RS. A morphological study of variations in the origin and course of radial artery. *Res J Pharm Biol Chem Sci.* 2012;3:333-340.

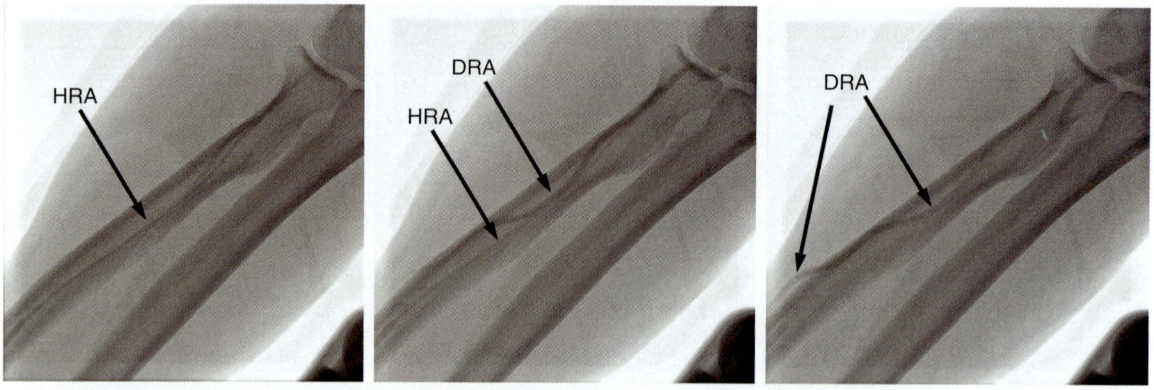

FIG. 5.6 Angiography Through Cannulated Hypoplastic Radial Artery (*HRA*) Refluxing Into Large Anomalous Duplicate Radial Artery. Contrast injection through the small, HRA at the wrist, which refluxes at the brachial artery level into a large, laterally located duplicate radial artery (*DRA*) that crosses distally to the dorsum of the wrist.

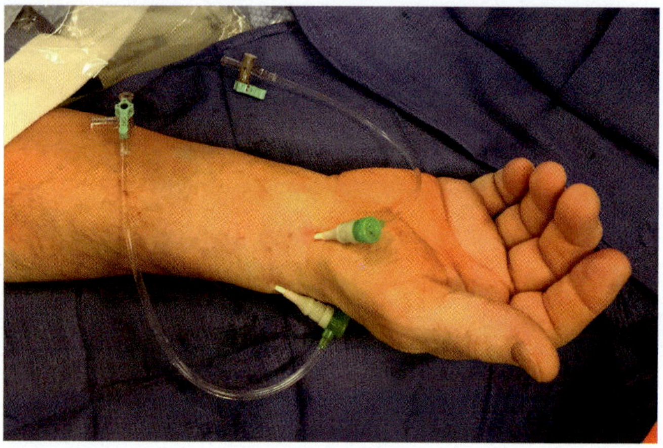

FIG. 5.7 Cannulation of a Duplicate Radial Artery at the Dorsum of the Wrist. Large duplicate radial artery cannulated at the dorsum of the wrist for successful angiography after inability to traverse the hypoplastic radial artery at the usual location.

Chronic Total Coronary Occlusion With Bronchocoronary Collateral Circulation Failed to Visualize by Conventional Angiography

Yoritaka Otsuka, MD, Hiroki Imoto, MD, Michiaki Kono, MD, Taku Koyama, MD, Keita Nakamura, MD, Sunao Kodama, MD, Hiroo Noguchi, MD, Taro Saito, MD

We describe a case of chronic total occlusion of the right coronary artery (RCA) ostium (Fig. 5.8A) in a 61-year-old man. Coronary angiography showed good collateral circulation from the left anterior descending artery via the Vieussens arterial ring to the proximal RCA and from the septal branch to the acute marginal branch, but it failed to visualize the complete course of the distal vessel segment of the RCA (Fig. 5.8B–C). Computed tomography angiography clearly demonstrated a distal vessel segment of the RCA from the in-stent occlusion previously implanted (Fig. 5.8D–F). In this patient, percutaneous coronary intervention was successfully performed, and three drug-eluting stents were implanted for the chronic total occlusion. Coronary angiography after stent implantation revealed the existence of a collateral connection to the bronchial artery (Fig. 5.9A–B). This connection, known as "bronchocoronary collateral circulation," was also confirmed by computed tomography angiography (Fig. 5.9C–D).

Coronary collateral vessels can be divided into two major classes: anastomosis via extracardiac vessels and anastomosis via intercoronary branches. Among the known extracardiac vessels as a source of collateral circulations, one is the left internal thoracic artery for the left anterior descending artery, and the other is the bronchial artery for the RCA, or the left circumflex artery. Fundamentally, the outside pericardium is supplied with blood from the left internal thoracic artery and the bronchial artery.[1,2] Therefore extracardiac anastomosis may develop when intercoronary anastomoses fail to supply blood to the peripheral coronary circulation. Computed tomography

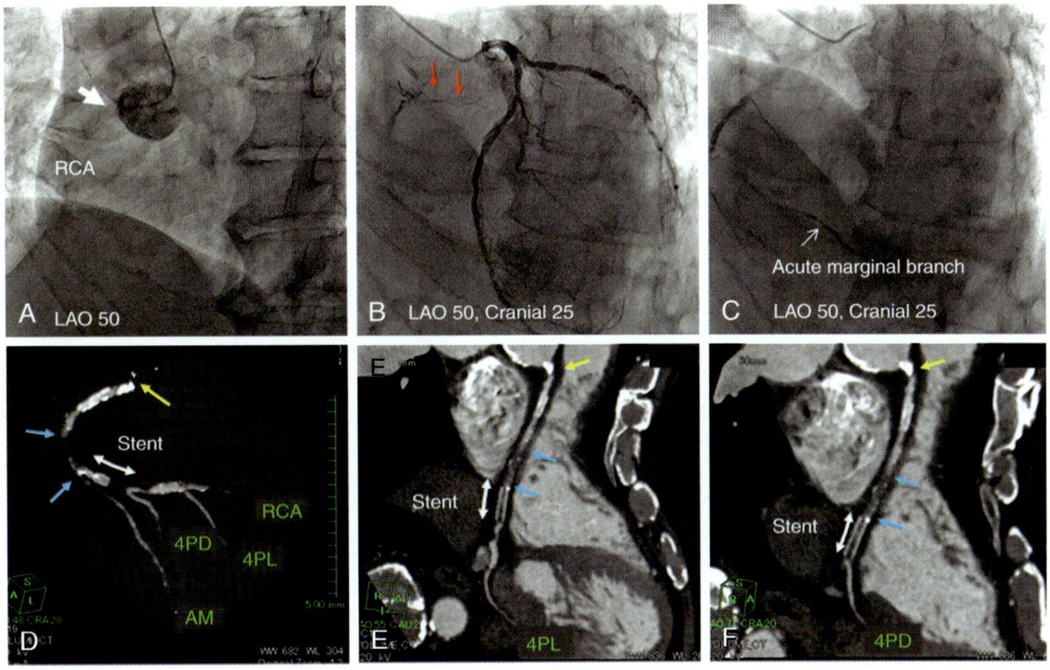

FIG. 5.8 Coronary Angiography and Computed Tomography Angiography. Coronary angiography showed chronic total occlusion (*white arrow*) of the right coronary artery (*RCA*) ostium (A) and good collateral circulation from the left anterior descending artery via the Vieussens arterial ring (*red arrows*) to the proximal RCA and from the septal branch to the acute marginal branch, but it failed to visualize the complete course of distal vessel segment of the RCA (B), (C) Delayed image of (B). (D–F) Computed tomography clearly demonstrated a vessel segment of the RCA distally from the in-stent occlusion previously implanted. The *white double-headed arrow* indicates the location of a stent previously implanted. The *yellow arrow* indicates total occlusion of the RCA ostium and the proximal RCA occlusion is represented between the *blue arrows*. *AM*, acute marginal; *LAO*, left anterior oblique; *PD*, posterodescending; *PL*, posterolateral.

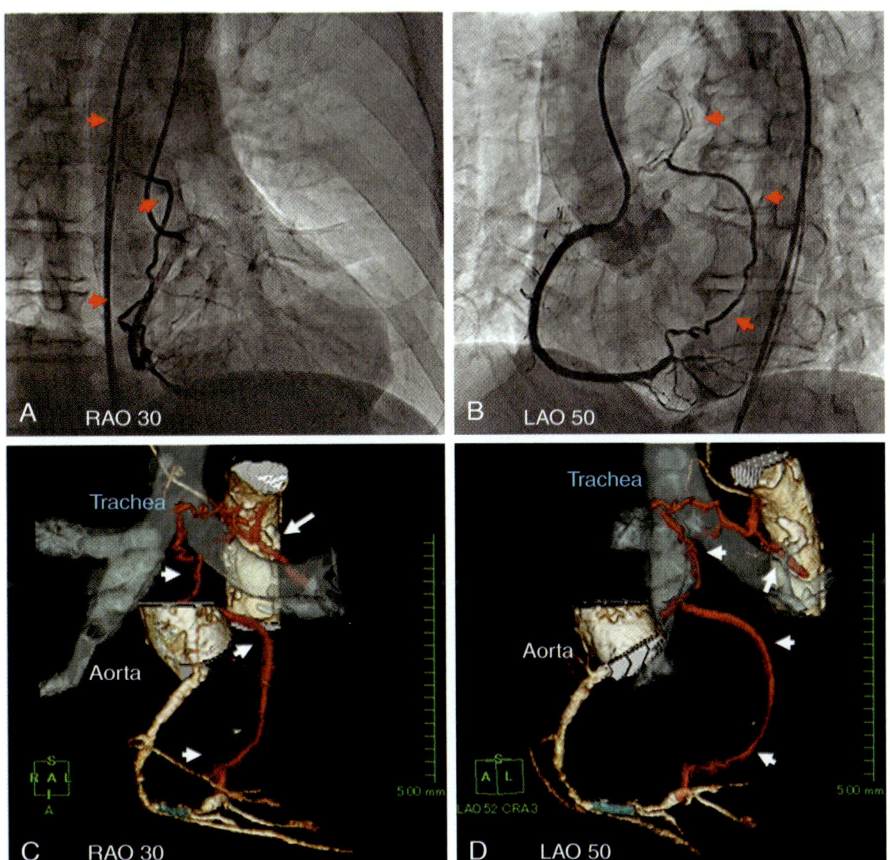

FIG. 5.9 Bronchocoronary Collateral Circulation. (A and B) Coronary angiography after stent implantation. It revealed the existence of a collateral (*red arrows*) connection to the bronchial artery. (C and D) Bronchocoronary collateral circulation (*white arrows*) on the computed tomography angiography before percutaneous coronary intervention. *LAO*, left anterior oblique; *RAO*, right anterior oblique.

angiography is useful for detecting this collateral circulation.[3,4] We should be aware of the existence of extracardiac anastomosis when a conventional coronary angiography, in the case of chronic total occlusion, fails to visualize the complete course of coronary artery.

References

1. Unger EF, Sheffield CD, Epstein SE. Creation of anastomoses between an extracardiac artery and the coronary circulation: proof that myocardial angiogenesis occurs and can provide nutritional blood flow to the myocardium. *Circulation*. 1990; 82:1449-1466.
2. White FC, Carroll SM, Magnet A, Bloor CM. Coronary collateral development in swine after coronary artery occlusion. *Circ Res*. 1992;71: 1490-1500.
3. Goetti R, Candinas R, Leschka S, Hoffmann U, Alkadhi H. Bronchocoronary collateral circulation: clinical utility of cardiac computed tomography. *Circulation*. 2010;121:180-181.
4. Pontone G, Grancini L, Andreini D, Pepi M. Detection of bronchocoronary collateral by low-dose multidetector computed tomography. *Eur J Cardiothorac Surg*. 2011; 40:272.

Corkscrew Intravascular Channels Within Chronic Common Carotid Artery Occlusions in Takayasu Arteritis That Disappear After Angioplasty

George Joseph, MD, DM, Anoop Mathew, MD, DM

In Takayasu arteritis, obliteration of the vessel lumen by mural thrombus secondary to inflammatory changes in the vessel wall is common in the aortic arch branches; the thrombus gradually undergoes organization and becomes a fibrous mass within which multiple vascular channels develop. In some cases, these channels allow partial restoration of anterograde flow through the previously occluded artery segment.[1] This phenomenon was seen angiographically in the common carotid arteries of a 43-year-old man who presented with dizziness, amaurosis fugax, and bilateral arm claudication. He met five of the six American College of Rheumatology criteria for diagnosis of Takayasu arteritis[2] and had normal levels of inflammatory markers indicating inactive disease. Both common carotid arteries exhibited diseased segments containing tangles of corkscrew channels located within the expected confines of the vessel wall (Fig. 5.10A, C, and E) with limited anterograde flow through them. The subclavian arteries had long-segment occlusions bilaterally, but these were solid occlusions without angiographic evidence of vascular channels within them. After obtaining informed consent from the patient, the diseased common carotid artery segments were traversed by fine manipulation of 0.014-inch steerable hydrophilic wires, after which balloon dilation and self-expanding stent deployment resulted in replacement of the multiple vascular channels by a single large channel with normal anterograde flow (Fig. 5.10B and D). Interventions on the two sides were performed 6 months apart without

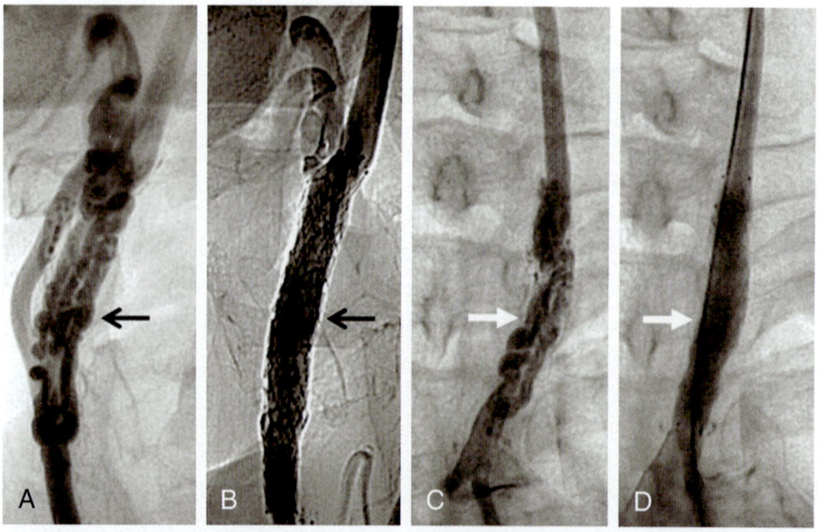

FIG. 5.10 Disappearing Corkscrew Intravascular Channels. (A and C) Baseline angiograms showing diseased arterial segments containing tangles of corkscrew channels located within the expected confines of the vessel wall in the distal right and proximal left common carotid arteries (indicated by *black arrows* and *white arrows*, respectively, throughout [A] to [F]). (B and D) Corresponding images immediately after angioplasty and stenting show replacement of the manifold channels by a single large conduit.

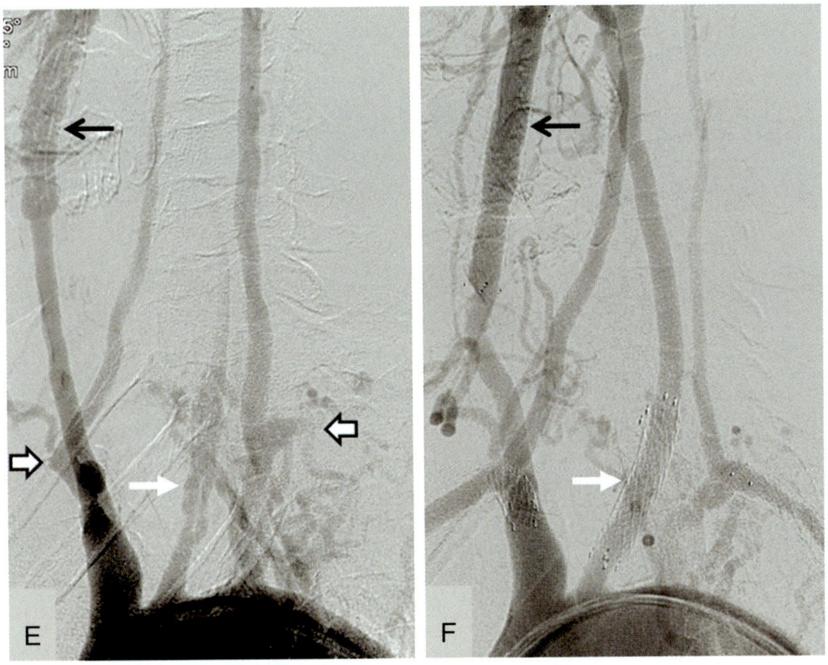

FIG. 5.10, cont'd (E) Baseline aortic arch angiogram showing the diseased common carotid artery segments and bilaterally occluded subclavian arteries (*hollow block arrows*). (F) Two-year post-intervention follow-up aortic arch angiogram showing patency of carotid and subclavian stents bilaterally.

cerebral protection and were uncomplicated; the subclavian artery occlusive lesions were concurrently recanalized and stented using standard technique. Follow-up angiography after 2 years (Fig. 5.10F) showed widely patent carotid stents and minor subclavian in-stent restenosis; the patient was asymptomatic over this period. In Takayasu arteritis, patients with inactive disease, arterial lesions with angiographic evidence of multiple vascular channels inside the expected limits of the vessel wall with limited anterograde flow, are indicative of chronic fibrous, partially recanalized occlusions that are amenable to successful percutaneous intervention.

References

1. Kinare SG, Vas GG, Gandhi M. Non-Specific Aorto-Arteritis (Takayasu's Disease): Pathology and Radiology. Mumbai, India: Quest Publications, 1998:48.
2. Arend WP, Michel BA, Bloch DA, et al. The American College of Rheumatology 1990 criteria for the classification of Takayasu arteritis. *Arthritis Rheum.* 1990;33:1129-1134.

Extreme Brachial Loop

Isaac R. Whitman, MD, Andrew J. Boyle, MBBS, PhD

A 47-year-old man with prior right ulnar collateral ligament reconstruction presented with angina and was referred for cardiac catheterization. Right radial artery angiogram was normal (Fig. 5.11A, Online Video 5.8). A J-tip guidewire met resistance just above the elbow. A subsequent brachial angiogram revealed an extremely tortuous recurrent brachial artery loop (Fig. 5.11B–C, Online Videos 5.9 and 5.10).

The transradial approach is increasingly common in coronary angiography, reducing the risk of access site complications.[1,2] Full radial artery loops occur in 1% to 2% of patients and can often be straightened with a guidewire.[3,4] However, the prevalence and challenges presented by brachial artery loops are not discussed in the literature. Furthermore, it is not known whether these tend to occur unilaterally or bilaterally, so there are no data guiding the choice between contralateral radial artery versus femoral artery as the alternative access site. Our decision was to attempt contralateral radial access. That decision proved prudent because the patient's left upper extremity demonstrated normal anatomy (Fig. 5.11D, Online Video 5.11).

References

1. Dehmer GJ, Weaver D, Roe MT, et al. A contemporary view of diagnostic cardiac catheterization and percutaneous coronary intervention in the United States: a report from the CathPCI Registry of the National Cardiovascular Data Registry, 2010 through June 2011. *J Am Coll Cardiol.* 2012;60:2017-2031.
2. Romagnoli E, Biondi-Zoccai G, Sciahbasi A, et al. Radial versus femoral randomized investigation in ST-segment elevation acute coronary syndrome: the RIFLE-STEACS study. *J Am Coll Cardiol.* 2012;60:2481-2489.
3. Valsecchi O, Vassileva A, Musumeci G, et al. Failure of transradial approach during coronary interventions: anatomic considerations. *Catheter Cardiovasc Interv.* 2006;67:870-878.
4. Lo TS, Nolan J, Fountzopoulos E, et al. Radial artery anomaly and its influence on transradial coronary procedural outcome. *Heart.* 2009;95:410-415.

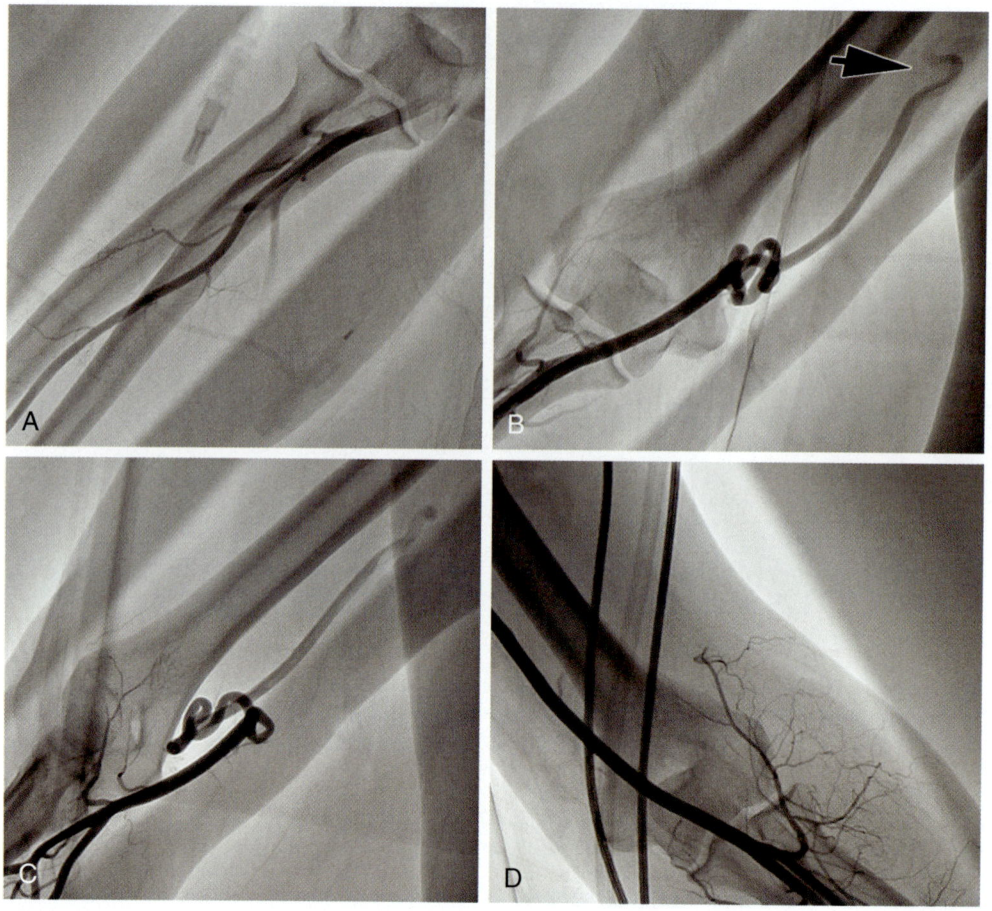

FIG. 5.11 Recurrent Brachial Loop. (A) Normal right radial angiogram. Anteroposterior (B) and lateral (C) right brachial angiograms revealing recurrent brachial artery loop. Also note there is another area of tortuosity higher in the brachial artery (*arrow*). (D) The contralateral brachial angiogram reveals no tortuosity. See Online Videos 5.8–5.11.

Internal Thoracic Artery Dissection: A Proposed Mechanistic Explanation

Xavier Freixa, MD, Richard Gallo, MD

A 61-year-old man with previous single bypass surgery of the left internal thoracic artery to the left anterior descending artery in 1996 presented to the emergency department with chest pain and anterior negative T waves. From time of surgery, the patient remained asymptomatic until the day of admission, when he experienced a sudden onset of chest pain immediately on raising and hyperextending both arms. On angiography, the native left anterior descending artery remained chronically occluded and the left internal thoracic artery showed an inferiorly displaced and flared ostium with preserved flow but a long, hazy, and severe proximal lesion. Optical coherence tomography and intravascular ultrasound showed a dissection flap and mural hematoma, respectively. To rule out the presence of subclavian dissection, a thoracic scan was done, revealing no extension of the dissection and a 10-mm area of adhesion between the internal thoracic artery and the anterior chest wall. Subsequently, the patient underwent successful angioplasty with three stents.

Spontaneous dissections of the internal thoracic artery have been described, although it remains unclear which factors can trigger this serious event (Fig. 5.12). The multiple imaging modalities used in the present case provide a new insight into the mechanism of spontaneous internal thoracic artery dissections. The upward pull on the internal thoracic artery from hyperextending the arms compounded by the downward traction of the internal thoracic artery adhering to the chest wall resulted in opposite overstretching forces that caused the internal thoracic artery to dissect. This theory is supported by the downward displacement of the internal thoracic artery ostium. Suresh and Evans[1] reported a similar case of internal thoracic artery dissection after a physical movement, but no mechanistic explanation was offered.

Reference

1. Suresh V, Evans S. Successful stenting of stenotic lesion and spontaneous dissection of left internal mammary artery graft. *Heart.* 2007;93:44.

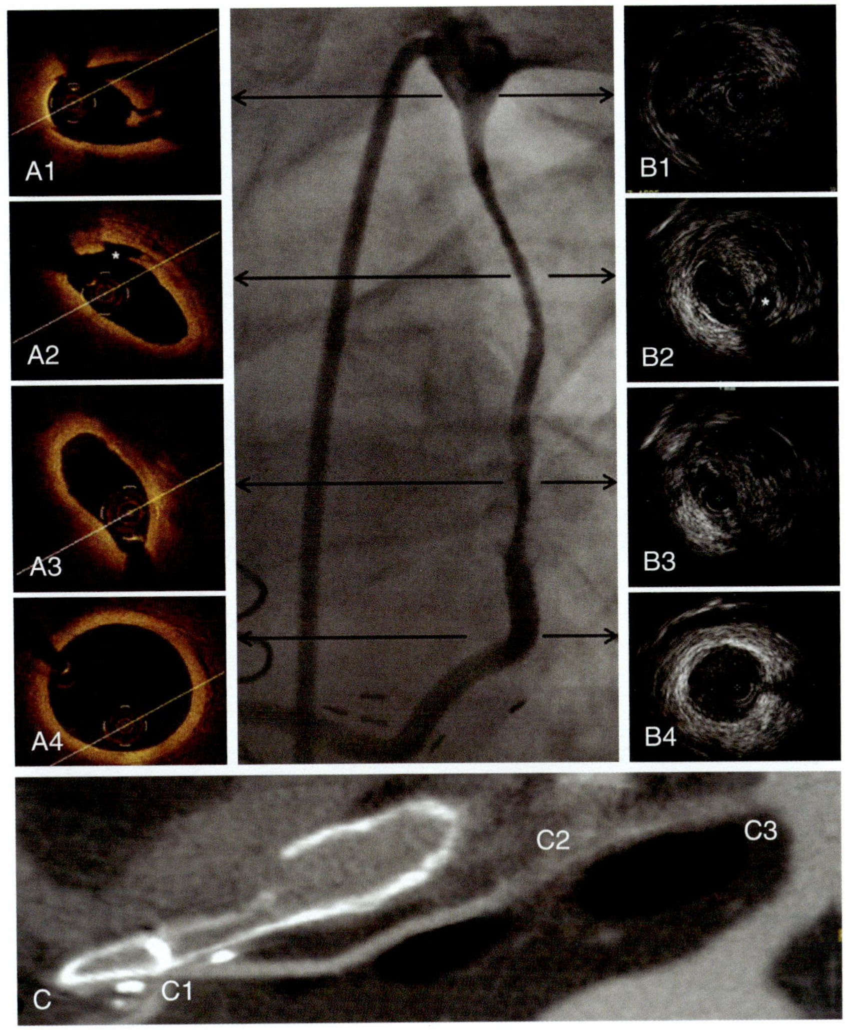

FIG. 5.12 Internal Thoracic Artery Dissection Assessed by Optical Coherence Tomography (OCT). (A) Angiography (mid). (B)I Intravascular ultrasound imaging. (C) Computed tomography. (A1) OCT provides suboptimal imaging in ostial lesions (blood interference). (B1) Ostial mural hematoma with dissection flap. (A2) Dissection flap with a clear rupture site (*asterisk*). (B2) Dissection image (*asterisk*) not as clear as OCT. (A3) Severe luminal compression suggesting intramural hematoma. OCT is unable to provide the full picture of the vessel wall and hematoma may cause shadowing/attenuation on OCT. (B3) Severe luminal compression secondary to clear intramural hematoma. (A4 and B4) Normal vessel distal to the dissection and hematoma. (C1) Adherence of the internal thoracic artery to the sternum. (C2) Internal thoracic artery dissection with intramural hematoma. (C3) No subclavian dissection.

Occlusion of Balloon-Expandable Stent in the Common Iliac Artery Due to Compression by a Spinal Spur

Hiroshi Fujita, MD, Tomomitsu Tani, MD, Tsuyoshi Ito, MD, Nobuyuki Ohte, MD

A 67-year-old man with critical limb ischemia due to left common iliac artery (CIA) occlusion underwent endovascular treatment and stent deployment (Express LD, 8.0 × 37 mm and 8.0 × 17 mm, Boston Scientific, Natick, Massachusetts) (Fig. 5.13). The symptoms of ischemia resolved after stent implantation; however, the patient felt pain in the left leg while at rest 3 years later. Angiography indicated a totally occluded left CIA at the stent site. Computed tomography angiography (CTA) revealed that the stent in the left CIA was compressed by a spinal spur (Fig. 5.14). We speculate that the following occurred. The spinal spur gradually compressed the balloon-expandable stent as the patient performed normal daily activities; eventually, it caused the stent to fracture, causing CIA reocclusion. We performed bypass surgery between the femoral arteries to obtain sufficient blood flow to the left leg, and the patient's pain was relieved.

Stent implantation for stenosis of the iliac arteries is an established procedure for limb ischemia. However, stent fracture sometimes leads to stent restenosis and reocclusion of the lesion. The fracture rate of self-expandable stents in the iliac region is 5.1%.[1] Causes of stent fracture are unknown in most cases. CTA appears to be a useful means of investigating stent fractures caused by external compression in the iliac region.

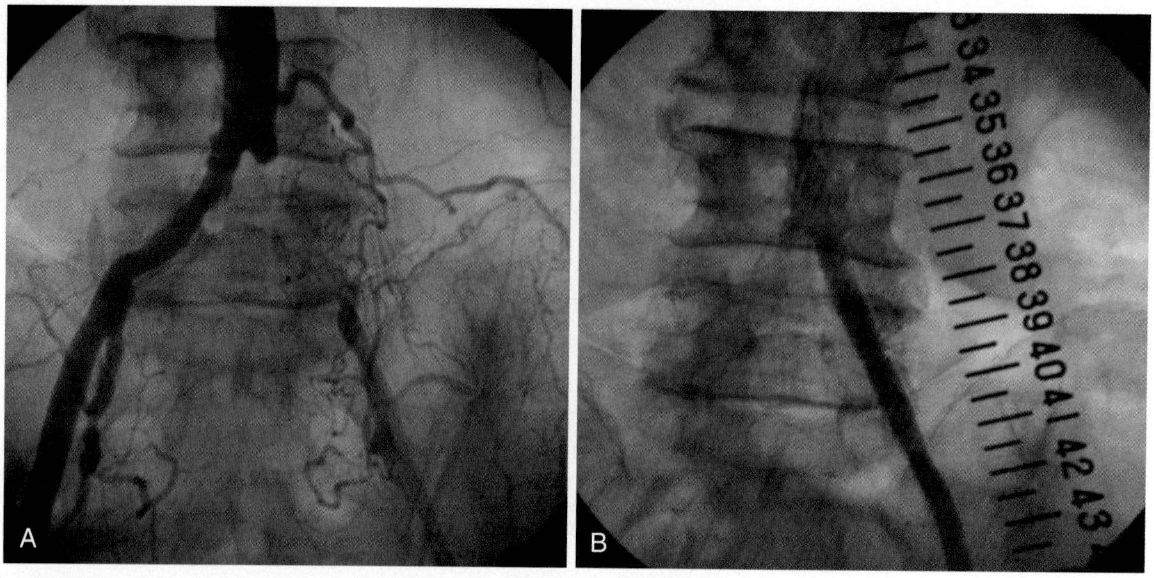

FIG. 5.13 Angiography of the Original Common Iliac Artery (CIA) Occlusion Before and After Stent Implantation. (A) Left CIA was totally occluded. (B) Blood flow at the lesion was restored by stenting.

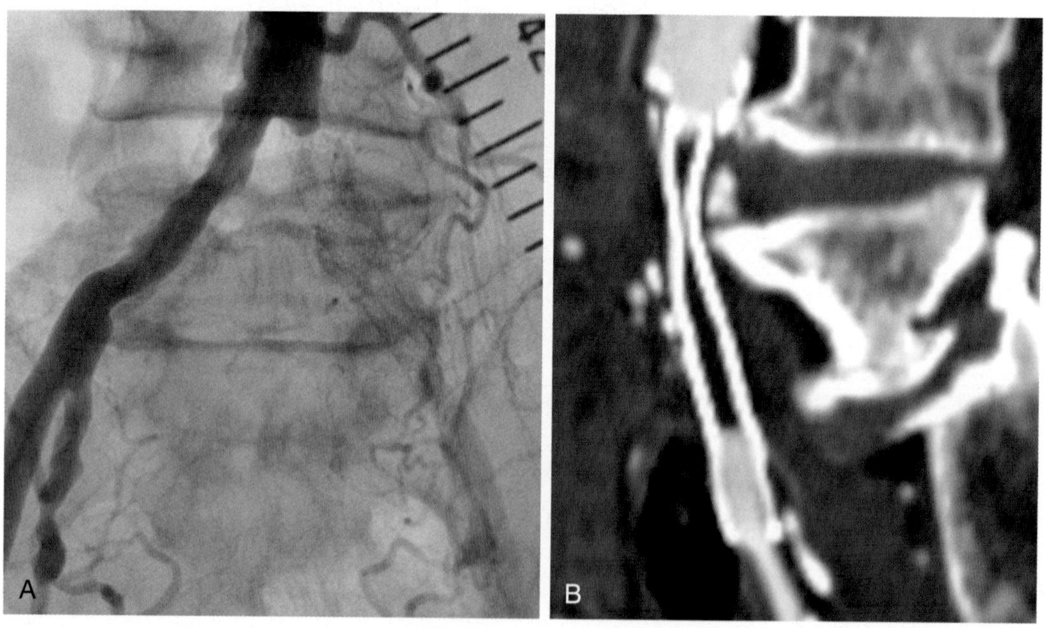

FIG. 5.14 Angiography of the Left Common Iliac Artery (CIA) Reocclusion. (A) Angiography of reocclusion at the stenting site. (B) Computed tomography angiography of spinal spur compressing the stent in left CIA.

Reference

1. Higashiura W, Kubota Y, Sakaguchi S, et al. Prevalence, factors, and clinical impact of self-expandable stent fractures following iliac stenting. *J Vasc Surg*. 2009;49:645-652.

Radial Artery Graft String Sign Due to Lumen Obliteration by Neointima: Insight From Optical Coherence Tomography

David Adlam, BM, DPhil, Keith M. Channon, MD

The radial artery is a commonly used conduit for coronary artery bypass grafting. Long-term patency rates are at least as good as and, in some series, are better than for saphenous vein grafts.[1,2] However, radial artery graft failure remains a significant problem,[3] in particular, in cases where radial conduits are used on smaller target vessels or where there is significant competitive flow from a native coronary with a relatively low-grade stenosis.[4] The string sign, where the radial graft conduit is patent but with only a thread of antegrade flow, is a well-recognized angiographic presentation of radial graft failure.[3] We describe for the first time optical coherence tomography (OCT) images of a radial conduit presenting with the string sign.

A 62-year-old man presented electively for angiographic follow-up as part of the Arterial Revascularization Trial 3 years after 4-vessel coronary artery bypass grafting, including a radial artery graft to the principle obtuse marginal branch of the circumflex coronary artery. He was clinically well and without angina at the time of the study. Angiography demonstrated the radial graft string sign with minimal contrast penetration (Fig. 5.15A–B). OCT (M3, LightLab Imaging, Westford, Massachusetts) demonstrated a thick, smooth neointima throughout the length of the radial graft almost obliterating the lumen and with no OCT features of atherosclerotic plaque formation or calcification (Fig. 5.16A, B, D, E, and G). The neointima formation in a saphenous vein graft from the same patient is shown for comparison (Fig. 5.16C and F).

OCT imaging can provide novel insights into the mechanisms underlying coronary and graft conduit pathology. Although other mechanisms may be relevant in different patients, this case suggests the radial artery string sign may result from an exaggerated neointimal reaction in the radial graft leading to a severe reduction of luminal cross-sectional area.

References

1. Hayward PA, Gordon IR, Hare DL, et al. Comparable patencies of the radial artery and right internal thoracic artery or saphenous vein beyond 5 years: results from the Radial Artery Patency and Clinical Outcomes trial. *J Thorac Cardiovasc Surg.* 2010;139:60-65, discussion 65-67.
2. Tatoulis J, Buxton BF, Fuller JA, et al. Long-term patency of 1108 radial arterial-coronary angiograms over 10 years. *Ann Thorac Surg.* 2009;88: 23-29, discussion 29-30.
3. Khot UN, Friedman DT, Pettersson G, Smedira NG, Li J, Ellis SG. Radial artery bypass grafts have an increased occurrence of angiographically severe stenosis and occlusion compared with left internal mammary arteries and saphenous vein grafts. *Circulation.* 2004;109:2086-2091.
4. Manabe S, Fukui T, Shimokawa T, et al. Increased graft occlusion or string sign in composite arterial grafting for mildly stenosed target vessels. *Ann Thorac Surg.* 2010;89:683-687.

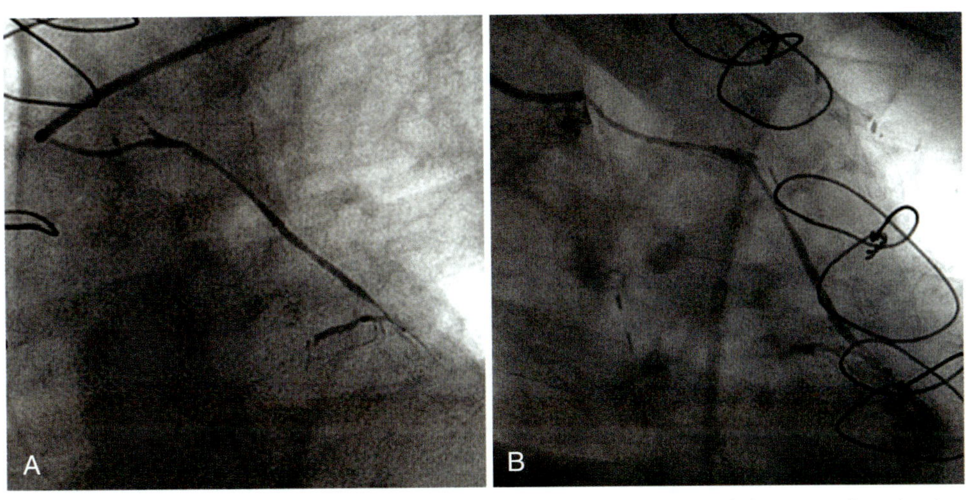

FIG. 5.15 Angiographic Appearances of the Radial Artery Graft String Sign. Aortocoronary radial artery graft to the circumflex first obtuse marginal branch with angiographic appearances of the string sign. Anteroposterior (A) and right lateral (B) projections. Although patent throughout its length, the lumen of the radial artery graft is almost completely abolished, leaving only a thread demonstrable on contrast injection.

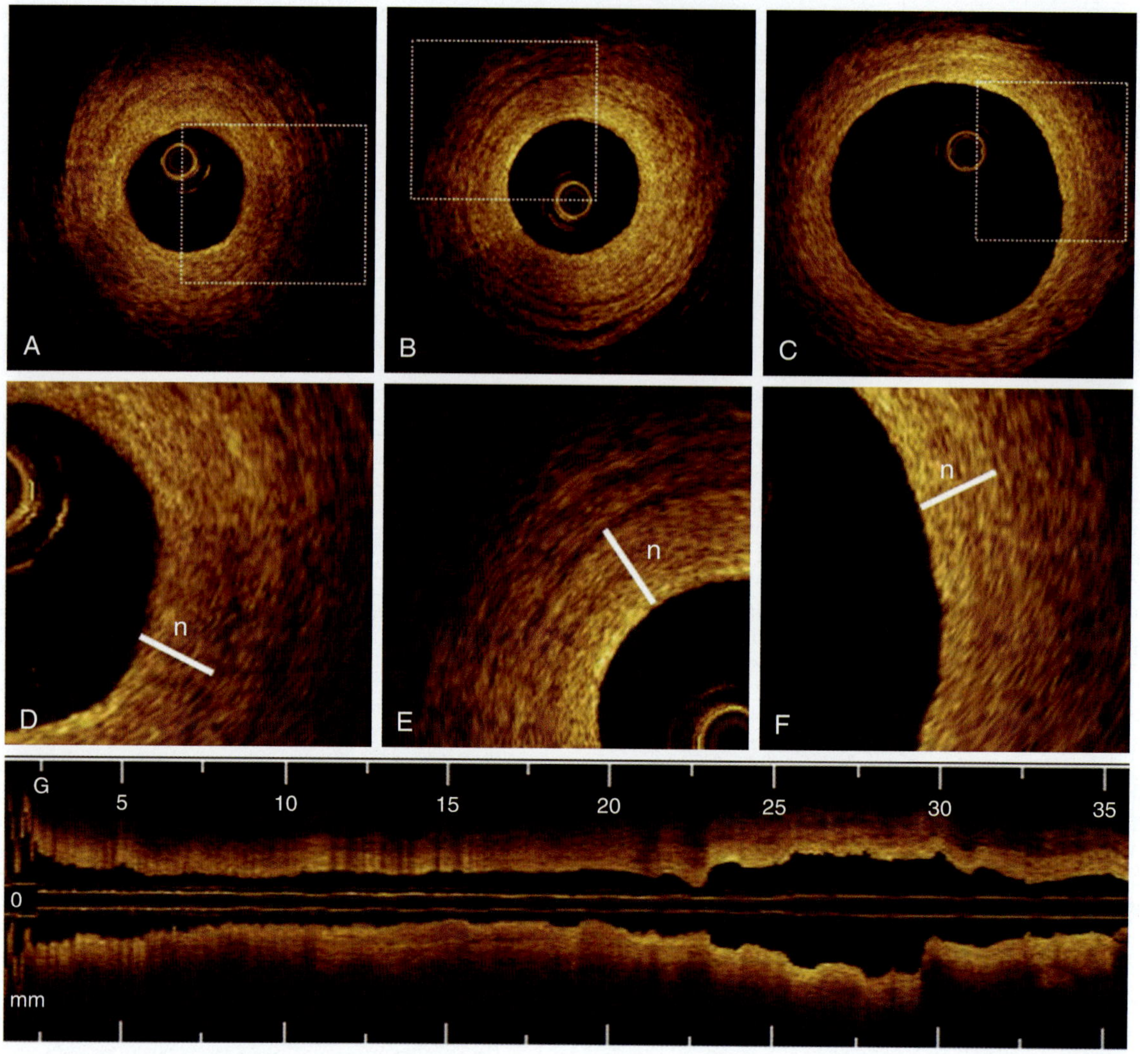

FIG. 5.16 Optical Coherence Tomography (OCT) Findings of Lumen Obliteration by Neointima. OCT cross-sectional images (A), (B), (D), and (E) and long axis (G) of the lumen and vessel wall of the radial conduit demonstrating marked concentric neointima formation (*n*) leading to severe reduction in luminal cross-sectional area. A typical OCT cross-sectional image of a saphenous vein graft from the same patient is shown for comparison in (C) and (F).

Tension Pneumopericardium Secondary to Gastropericardial Fistula Presenting as Acute Pericarditis With Cardiac Tamponade Physiology

Jacob A. Misenheimer, MD, Yan Liu, MD, Gregory Means, MD, Prashant Kaul, MD, Michael Yeung, MD

A 44-year-old man with prior Nissen fundoplication presented with chest pain, hypotension, tachycardia, and inferior ST-segment elevation on electrocardiography. Coronary angiography demonstrated normal coronaries, and left ventriculography revealed radiolucency in the pericardial space (Fig. 5.17, Online Video 5.12). Echocardiographic windows were poor. Catherization of the right side of the heart revealed diastolic equalization of pressures consistent with tamponade. The patient improved initially with intravenous fluids but developed recurrent hypotension and worsening sinus tachycardia. During pericardiocentesis, air and fluid were aspirated with immediate stabilization. Chest radiograph obtained before pericardiocentesis revealed pneumomediastinum (Fig. 5.18). Computed tomography of the chest and abdomen suggested gastropericardial fistula (Fig. 5.19), which was later repaired surgically.

Pneumopericardium typically results from chest trauma[1] but can be a complication of gastrointestinal procedures.[2] Tension

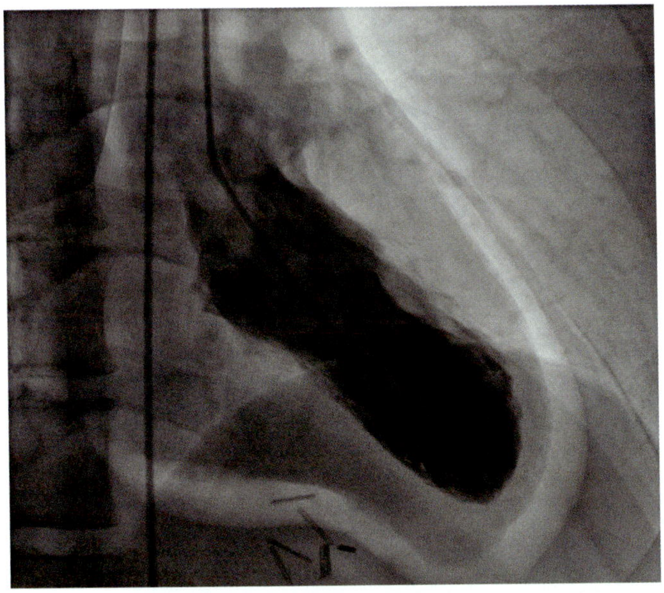

FIG. 5.17 Left Ventriculography Showing Pneumopericardium. Pneumopericardium demonstrated by radiolucency within the pericardial space. Online Video 5.12 demonstrates this finding in motion.

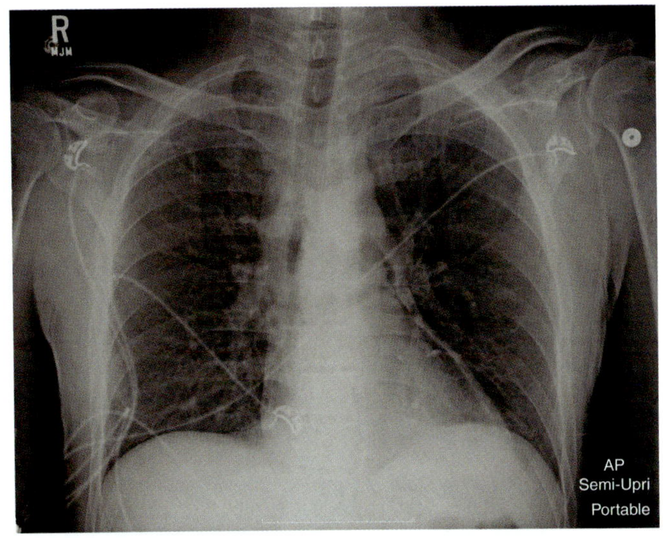

FIG. 5.18 Chest Radiography Showing Pneumopericardium. Pneumopericardium represented as a radiolucent stripe within the mediastinum.

pneumopericardium, which often mimics ST-segment elevation, myocardial infarction, and cardiac tamponade,[3] can be fatal.[1] Rapid identification and pericardiocentesis are essential. Echocardiography is seldom useful because of suboptimal windows. Computed tomography, cineangiography, and chest radiography are helpful; catheterization of the right side of the heart is sometimes necessary to confirm tamponade physiology.

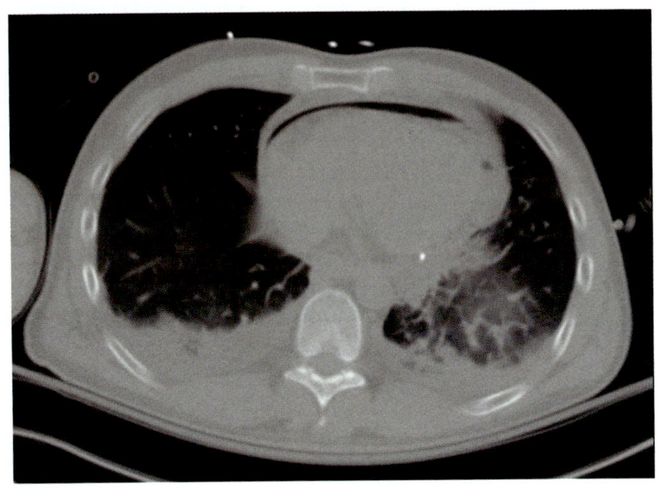

FIG. 5.19 Chest Computed Tomography With Pneumomediastinum. The pericardial space is filled with both air and dense fluid.

References

1. Nachi S, Okada H, Kato H, et al. Simple pneumopericardium due to blunt trauma progressing to tension pneumopericardium during transportation. *Am J Emerg Med.* 2016;34:933.e3-e5.
2. Kakarala K, Edriss H, Nugent K. Gastro-pericardial fistula as a delayed complication of a Nissen fundoplication. *Proc (Bayl Univ Med Cent).* 2015;28(4):478-481.
3. Ratnayake EC, Premaratne S, Lokunarangoda N, et al. Pneumopyopericardium mimicking an inferior ST elevation myocardial infarction with regional electrocardiogram changes: a case report. *BMC Res Notes.* 2015;8:173.

The Striking Interplay of Hiccup and Patent Foramen Ovale

Alessandro Colombo, MD, Paolo Danna, MD, Alessandro Cialfi, MD, Davide Sala, MD, Maurizio Viecca, MD

Previous studies have shown that reducing intrathoracic pressure during inspiration significantly increases right atrial volume (through an increase in venous return) with a slight reduction of right atrial pressure.[1] In patients with an atrial septal defect, the same phasic, inspiration-related pressure variations were noted, but right atrial volume did not change, thus indicating substantial volume shift from the right to left atrium.[2] Experimental findings in mammals also suggest that right-to-left shunting does occur in inspiration when a defect is opened in the interatrial septum.[3,4] These observations are convincing proof that right-to-left shunting might preferentially occur during inspiration also in patients with a patent foramen ovale (PFO). Indeed, the Valsalva maneuver increases the diagnostic yield of PFO diagnosis because its release phase exacerbates the hemodynamic consequences of inspiration.

A 62-year-old man with a recent transient ischemic attack and diagnosis of PFO with interatrial septal aneurysm was admitted at our center for percutaneous PFO closure.

At the beginning of the procedure, he was spontaneously hiccupping. When we injected standard saline contrast from the right femoral vein for baseline assessment of PFO, the hiccups were seen to cause three simultaneous phenomena: a sudden increase in right atrial volume, a major leftward shift of the interatrial septum, and a massive right-to-left shunt through the PFO (Fig. 5.20, Online Video 5.13).

We proceeded to PFO catheterization and were able to record the left atrial pressure during subsequent hiccups. What we saw was a series of sudden, hiccup-related sharp falls of left atrial pressure (Fig. 5.21). We did not insert an additional catheter into the right atrium, and therefore could not gauge the simultaneous pressure changes in both atria during hiccups. Anyway, massive leftward interatrial shunting concomitant to sharp pressure falls in the left atrium convincingly proves that the hiccup produces the same variations in atrial physiology as respiration does, although on higher scale and with striking consequences.

References

1. Gorgulu S, Eksik A, Eren M, et al. Assessment of the effects of various maneuvers on both atrial pressure changes. *Int J Cardiol.* 2003;92: 241-245.
2. Ferguson JJ, Miller MJ, Aroesty JM, Sahagian P, Grossman W, McKay RG. Assessment of right atrial pressure-volume relations in patients with and without an atrial septal defect. *J Am Coll Cardiol.* 1989;13:630-636.
3. Berry WB, Austen WG. Respiratory variations in the magnitude of the left to right shunt in experimental interatrial communications. *Am J Cardiol.* 1964;14:201-203.
4. Alexander JA, Rembert JC, Sealy WC, Greenfield JC. Shunt dynamics in experimental atrial septal defects. *J Appl Physiol.* 1975;39:281-286.

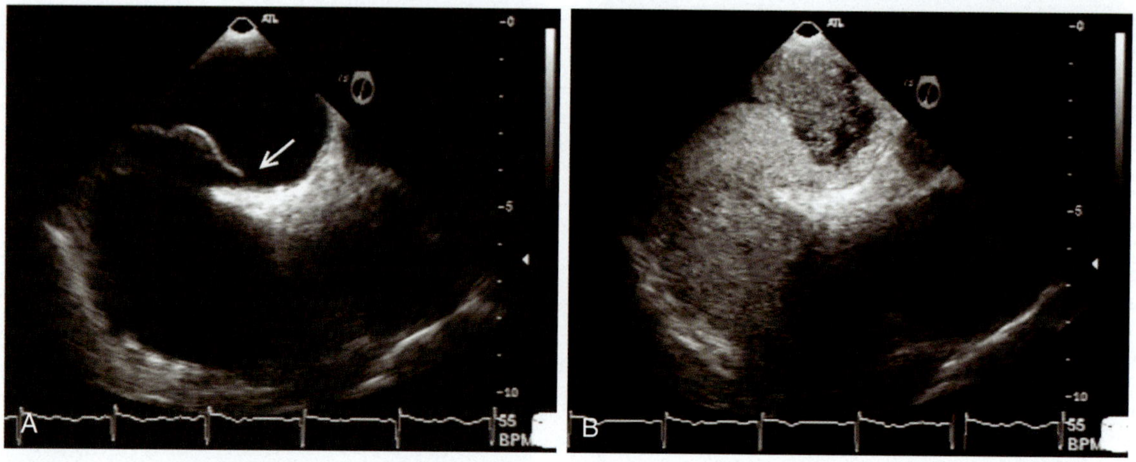

FIG. 5.20 Transesophageal Echocardiography. (A) Inferior caval view at 75° outlining the interatrial septum and the patent foramen ovale (*arrow*). (B) Same echocardiographic view. Massive microbubble shunting through the foramen ovale during hiccup. See Online Video 5.13.

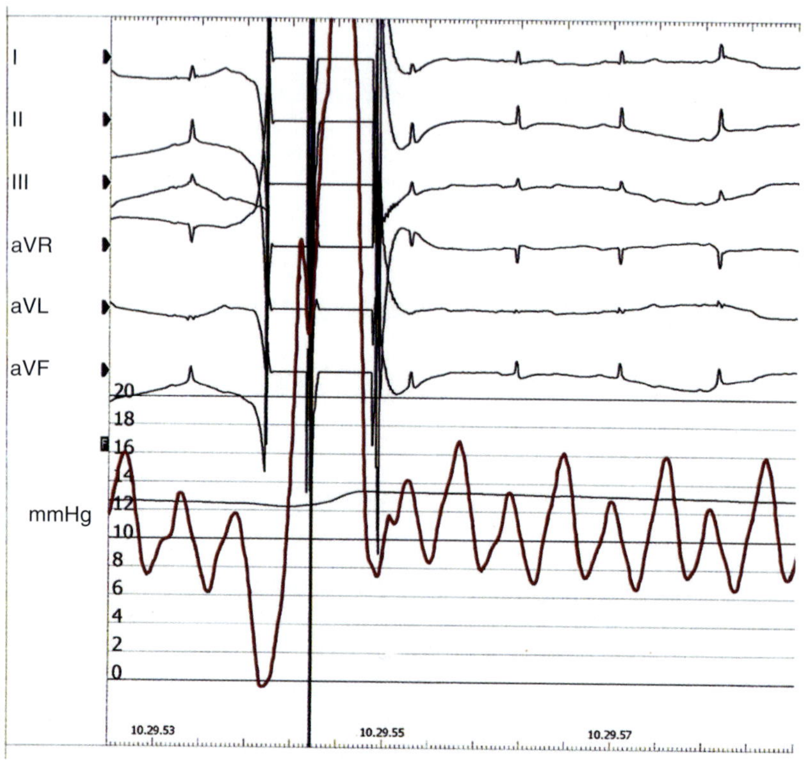

FIG. 5.21 Left Atrial Pressure Tracing. A hiccup spell (marked by artefact vertical lines through the electrocardiogram) produces a sudden and pronounced negative deflection in the pressure curve (*red line*).

Spontaneous Giant Ascending Aortic Pseudoaneurysm in a Previously Healthy Man

Dao-Kang Xiang, MD, Kui Hu, MD, Hong-Bo Luo, MD

A previously healthy 37-year-old man presented with chest pain that had lasted 2 weeks. He did not have hypertension or any other pertinent medical condition, and did not have trauma or surgical history. Chest radiograph showed a giant shadow in the right thoracic cavity (Fig. 5.22). Transthoracic echocardiography demonstrated a giant pseudoaneurysm in the ascending aorta. Contrast-enhanced computed tomography confirmed the giant ascending aortic pseudoaneurysm with diameter of 141 mm × 102 mm (Fig. 5.23A, Online Videos 5.14 and 5.15) and its breach was about 5 mm above the ostium of left coronary artery (Fig. 5. 23B) and the right lung, and the right atrium was seriously pressed (Fig. 5.23A–B).

We failed to repair the breach with a patch or do supercoronary aorta replacement due to extensive calcification of the aortic wall around the breach (Fig. 5.24A). At last, we successfully closed the breach with a 16-mm patent ductus arteriosus occluder (WBFDQ-I, Shanghai Shape Memory Alloy, China) (Fig. 5.24B). We interruptedly sutured the occluder device to the aortic wall where it was not calcified to reinforce it.

Computed tomography on the 6th day (Fig. 5.25A–B) and in 5 months postoperatively (Fig. 5.25C–D) confirmed correctly positioned occluder and the absence of endoleak as well as well reexpansion of the right lung. The patient was asymptomatic and enjoyed a good life during the follow-up.

Pseudoaneurysm rarely occurs in patients without hypertension or a history of trauma or surgical procedures. In our case, the young, previously healthy man was deemed not high risk for surgery, and open surgical repair was the first choice. However, surgical repair failed due to the extensive calcification of the aortic wall around the breach.

Our results suggest that occluder closure is safe and effective for the treatment of chronic spontaneous pseudoaneurysm.

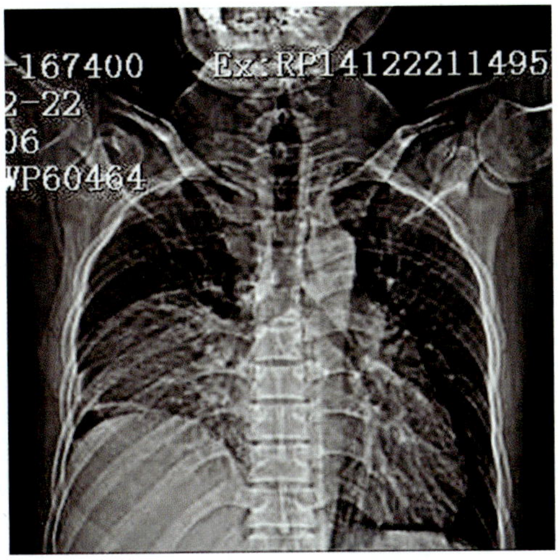

FIG. 5.22 Chest Radiograph Before Procedure.

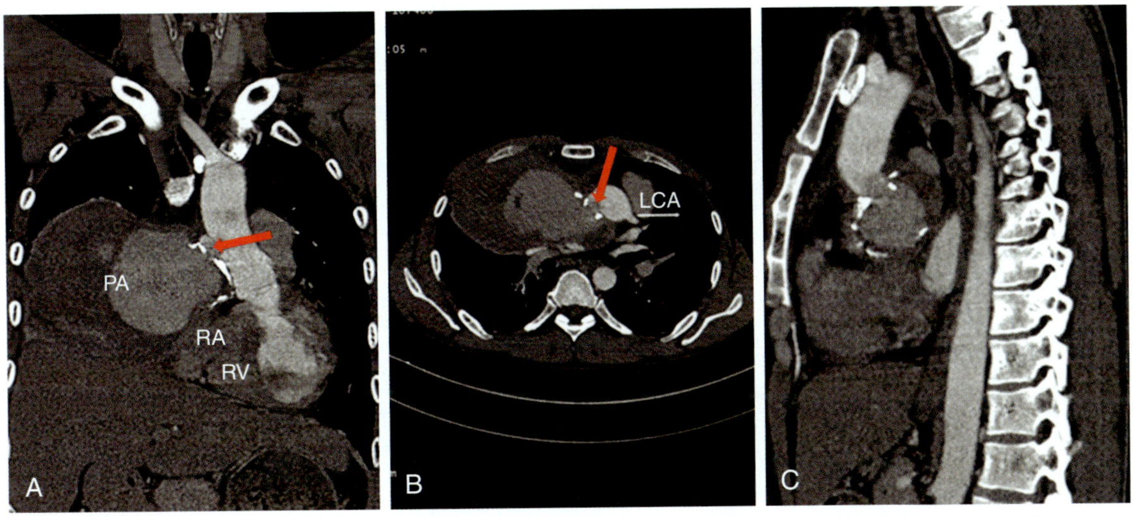

FIG. 5.23 Computed Tomography Scan Before Procedure. (A and B) Giant pseudoaneurysm compresses the right lung and right atrium (Online Videos 5.14 and 5.15). (A–C) Aortic wall around the breach was seriously calcified. *Red arrow* indicates the breach. *LCA*, left coronary artery; *PA*, pseudoaneurysm; *RA*, right atrium; *RV*, right ventricle.

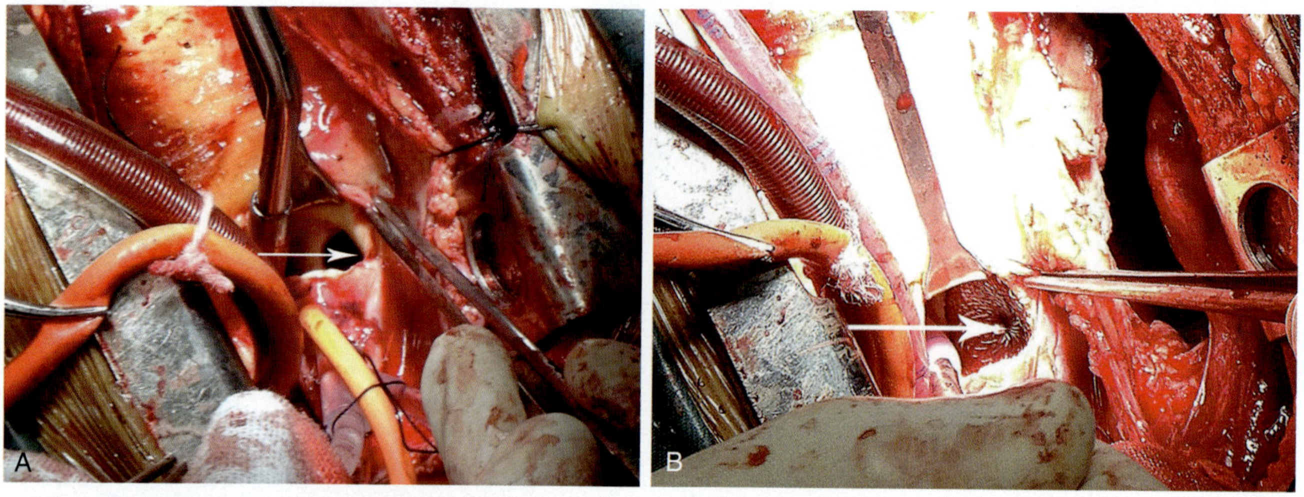

FIG. 5.24 Intraprocedural Image. (A) The breach (*white arrow*). (B) The breach was closed with a 16-mm patent ductus arteriosus occluder device (*white arrow*).

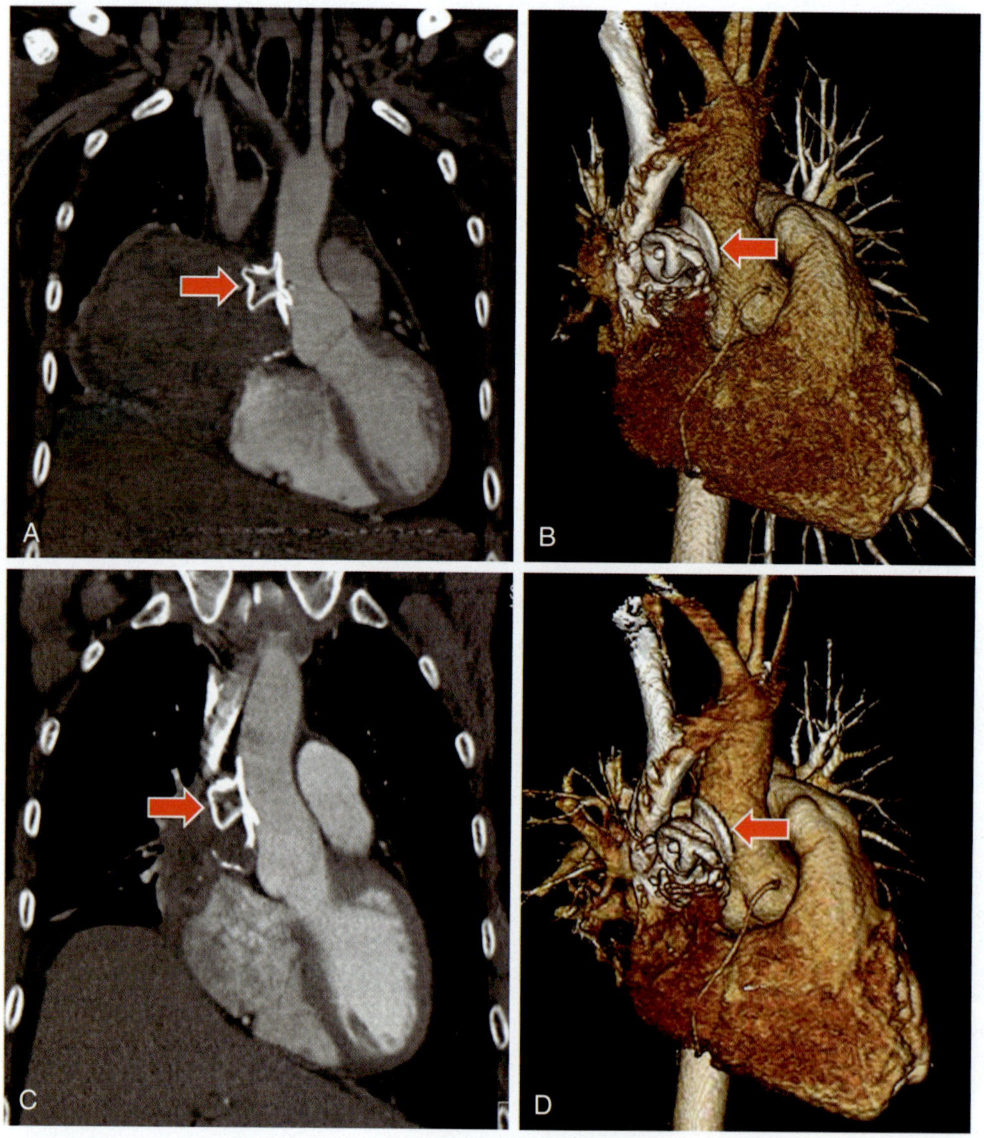

FIG. 5.25 Computed Tomography Scan and Three-Dimensional Reconstruction Postprocedure. Images from day 6 (A and B) and 5 months (C and D) postprocedure showing well-positioned occluder device without residual leak and good reexpansion of right lung and right atrium. *Red arrow* shows the patent ductus arteriosus occluder.

Chapter 6

Vascular, Congenital, and Other Interventional Complications

A Dual-Snare Percutaneous Retrieval of Venous Stent Embolization to the Right Side of the Heart

Ajay K. Sharma, MD, Sarju Ganatra, MD, James Hansen, MD, Neil Yager, DO, Thomas Piemonte, MD, Gautam Gadey, MD, Michael S. Levy, MPH, MD

A 57-year-old man with a medical history of asthma was transferred from an outside hospital for evaluation of cardiac mass where he was treated for extensive right lower extremity iliofemoral deep venous thrombosis with catheter-directed thrombolytic therapy and thrombectomy. Due to concern of compressive physiology at the site of thrombosis, two overlapping self-expanding WALLSTENT endoprostheses (Boston Scientific, Marlborough, Massachusetts) (two 10 mm ×60 mm and one 10 mm ×40 mm) were placed in the iliofemoral system. Shortly after the procedure, an incidental transthoracic echocardiogram noted a right atrial mass (Fig. 6.1). A transesophageal echocardiogram revealed a cylindrical foreign body extending from the inferior vena cava to the right atrium and across the tricuspid valve into the right ventricle. This was suspected to be a migrated venous stent (Fig. 6.2A–B). This was confirmed by a computed tomography scan of the chest, abdomen, and pelvis (Fig. 6.3). Percutaneous access was obtained in the right internal jugular vein (6F sheath) and through the right common femoral vein for a 14F Dexterity catheter (Spirus Medical, Stoughton, Massachusetts), which has the advantage of being a steerable catheter. A dual-snare approach was used: 25-mm snare from the groin and an EN Snare 18-30 (Merit Medical, South Jordan, Utah) from the right internal jugular vein. Fluoroscopy identified that two of three stents had embolized into the right atrium and right ventricle (Fig. 6.4). These were removed separately by snaring them proximally and distally and ultimately stretching and compressing the diameter of the stent so it

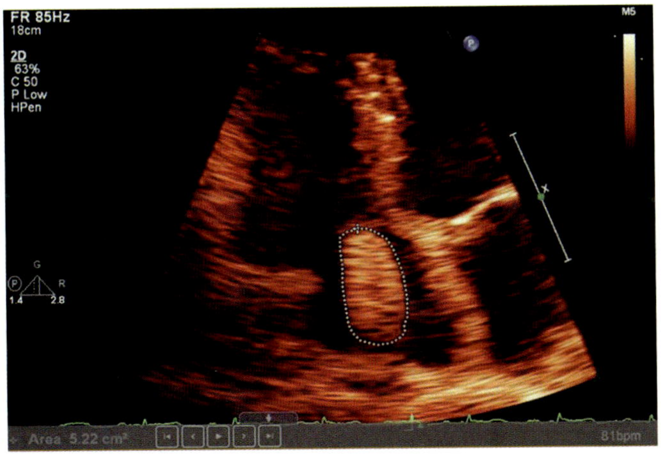

FIG. 6.1 Transthoracic Echocardiographic Image Before Intervention. Transthoracic echocardiography done at outside hospital raising suspicion for a cardiac mass.

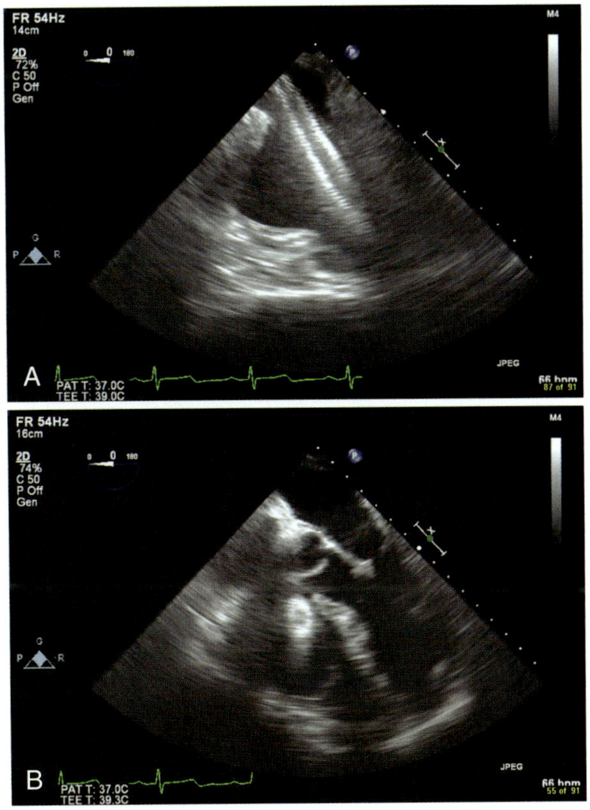

FIG. 6.2 Transesophageal Echocardiographic Images Before Intervention. (A) Transesophageal echocardiography (TEE) image showing venous stent across the tricuspid valve into the right ventricle. (B) TEE image showing venous stent in right ventricle.

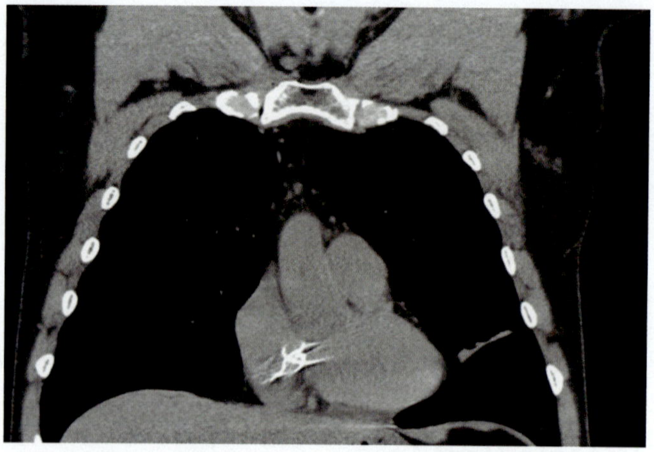

FIG. 6.3 Computed Tomography Chest Image BeforeIntervention. Computed tomography of the chest showing the two stents in right atrium and right ventricle.

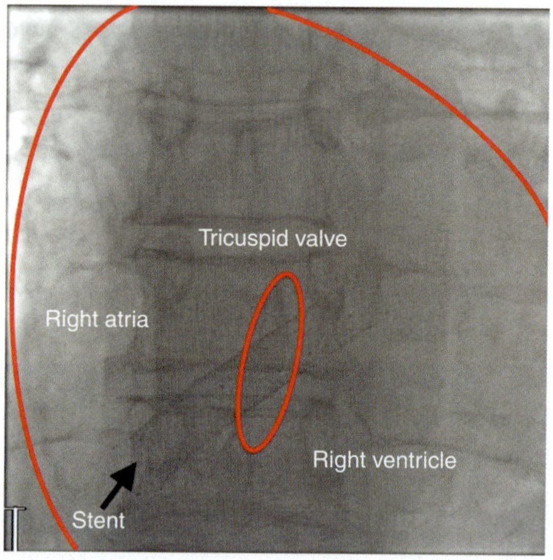

FIG. 6.4 Fluoroscopic Image Before Intervention. Fluoroscopy with pictorial representation showing the stents in the right side of the heart across the tricuspid valve.

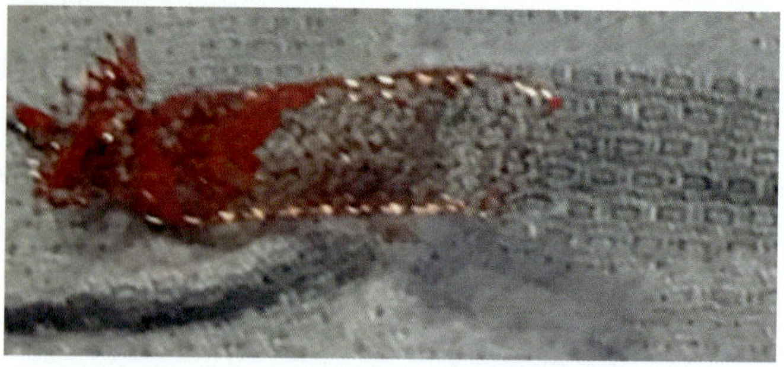

FIG. 6.5 Embolized Venous Stent After Removal. One of the venous stents after it was removed successfully (Online Video 6.1).

would fit into the 14F Dexterity catheter (Fig. 6.5, Online Video 6.1). At the end of the procedure, the femoral sheath was withdrawn and a previously placed Perclose closure (Abbott Vascular, Santa Clara, California) was used for hemostasis. The patient had an uneventful recovery and was discharged on rivaroxaban for follow-up with vascular medicine.

With the advent of self-expanding venous stents, there has been a growing enthusiasm in treating iliofemoral venous thrombosis with angioplasty and stenting when compressive physiology is suspected. This is most commonly considered in May-Thurner syndrome.[1] Several case reports[2,3] describe embolization of these stents, highlighting the need to ensure adequate oversizing in the iliofemoral vessels. Additionally, there are several cases in the literature describing various approaches to stent.

References

1. Carroll S, Moll S. Inferior vena cava filters, May-Thurner syndrome, and vein stents. *Circulation.* 2016;133:e383-e387.
2. El Feghaly M, Soula P, Rousseau H, et al. Endovascular retrieval of two migrated venous stents by means of balloon catheters. *J Vasc Surg.* 1998;28:541-546.
3. Gabelmann A, Kramer SC, Tomczak R, Gorich J. Percutaneous techniques for managing maldeployed or migrated stents. *J Endovasc Ther.* 2001; 8:291-302.

A Unique Case of May-Thurner Syndrome: Extrinsic Compression of the Common Iliac Vein After Iliac Artery Stenting

Paul L. Hermany, MD, Apurva O. Badheka, MBBS, Carlos I. Mena-Hurtado, MD, Robert R. Attaran, MBBS

A 75-year-old woman with peripheral artery disease presented with left leg discomfort and edema shortly after undergoing bilateral common iliac artery stenting. Examination revealed palpable pedal pulses, small varicose veins, and peripheral edema, most notably in the left leg. A venous duplex ultrasound ruled out lower extremity deep vein thrombosis.

The patient underwent invasive aortoiliac angiography and bilateral iliac venography (Figs. 6.6 and 6.7). Iliac artery stents were patent. Intravascular ultrasound (Volcano, San Diego, California) revealed extrinsic compression of the proximal left common iliac vein (Figs. 6.8, 6.9, and 6.10). A 14 × 60-mm WALLSTENT (Boston Scientific, Marlborough, Massachusetts) was deployed within the vein at the level of compression (Fig. 6.11). Subsequent intravascular ultrasound demonstrated improved luminal gain. At 2-week and 6-month follow-up visits, she reported complete resolution of her presenting symptoms and significant improvement in her lower extremity edema.

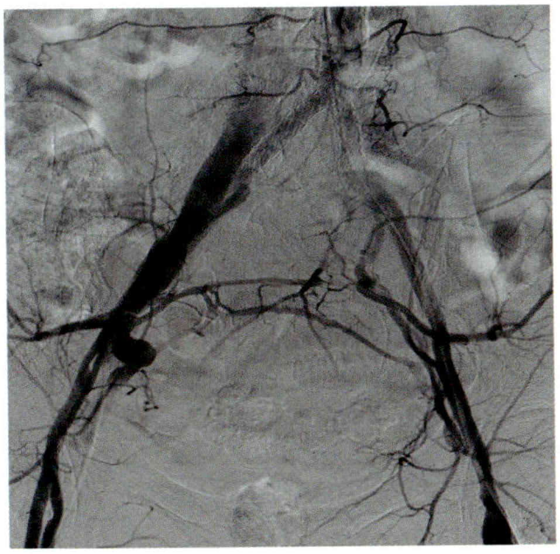

FIG. 6.6 Simultaneous Aortoiliac Arterial Angiogram and Iliac Venogram.

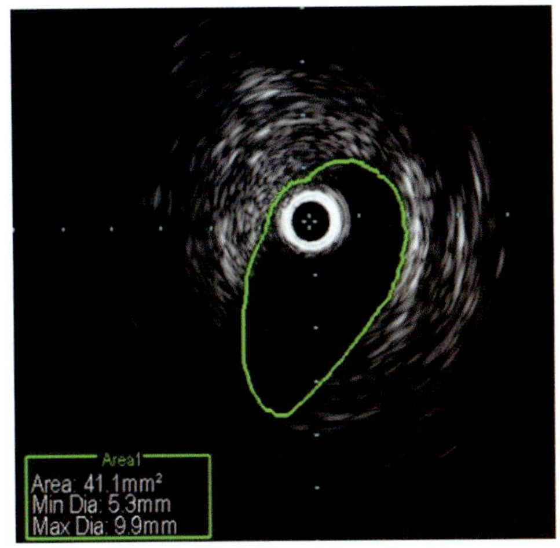

FIG. 6.9 Intravascular Ultrasound of the Proximal Left Common Iliac Vein Showing Luminal Narrowing.

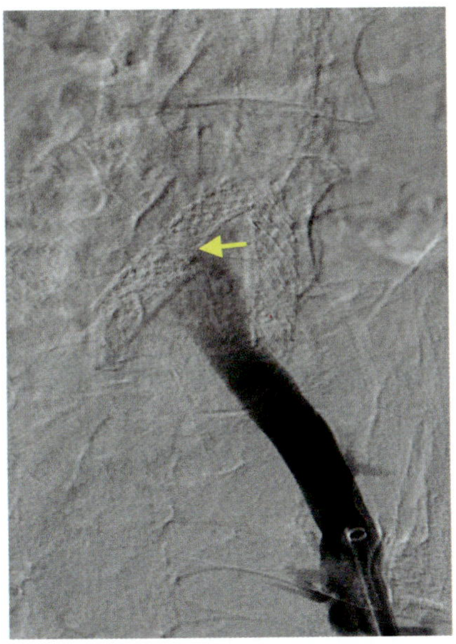

FIG. 6.7 Left Iliac Venogram Demonstrating Area of Interest at Level of Overlying Iliac Artery Stent. *Yellow arrow* indicates overlying iliac artery stent.

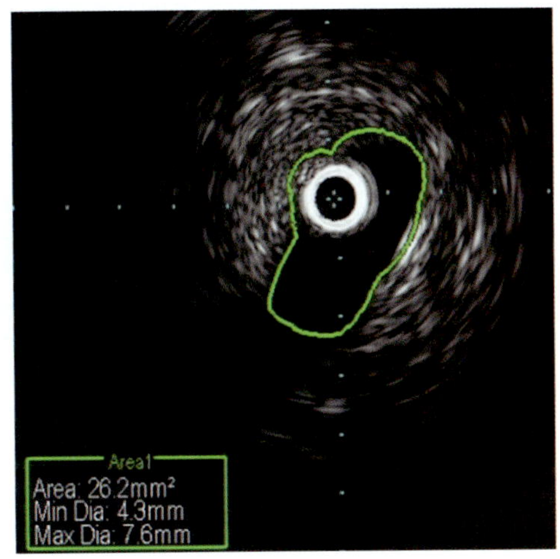

FIG. 6.10 Intravascular Ultrasound of the Proximal Left Common Iliac Vein Showing Luminal Narrowing.

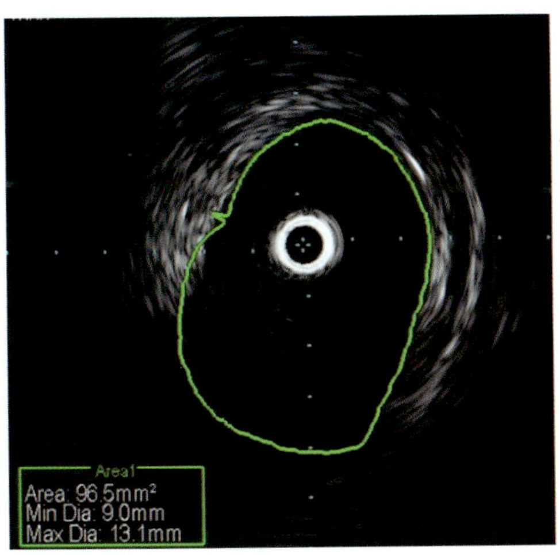

FIG. 6.8 Intravascular Ultrasound of the Mid Left Common Iliac Vein.

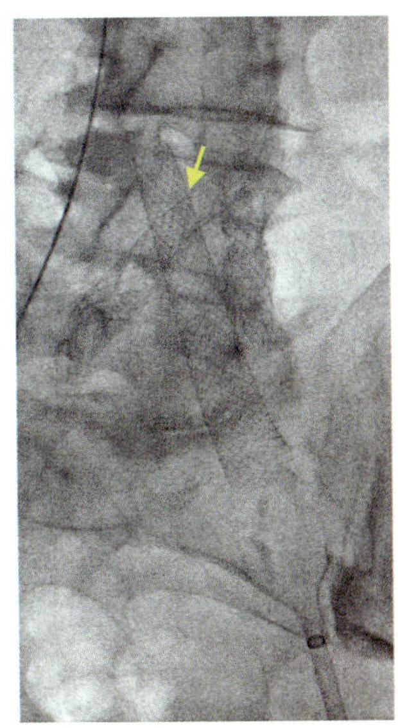

FIG. 6.11 Deployed Stent in Left Common Iliac Vein Covering Region of Compression by Right Iliac Artery Stent. *Yellow arrow* indicates right iliac artery stent now intersected beneath by left iliac vein stent.

Iliac vein compression as a consequence of arterial intervention is a rare and likely underreported entity.[1,2] These images demonstrate venous outflow obstruction due to extrinsic compression from previous arterial stenting, which responded dramatically to subsequent venous stenting.

References

1. Pandit AS, Hayes M, Guiney-Borgelt A, et al. Iatrogenic May-Thurner syndrome after EVAR. *Ann Vasc Surg.* 2014;28:739.e17-739.e20.
2. Rosen E, Groben L, George J. Rare case of bilateral common iliac vein compression by arterial stents and calcification. *Vasc Dis Management.* 2012;9:E186-E188.

Acute Pseudoaneurysm After Carotid Artery Stenting

Fabrizio Tomai, MD, Giovanni De Persio, MD, Alessandro Petrolini, MD, Luca Altamura, MD, Nicola Corcione, MD, Raoul Borioni, MD

A 73-year-old man with multidistrict artery disease was referred to our hospital for carotid artery stenting of an 85% stenosis of the right internal carotid artery (Fig. 6.12A). Protected carotid artery stenting of the right internal carotid artery was performed with a 7 × 40-mm carotid WALLSTENT (Boston Scientific, Natick, Massachusetts), postdilated with a 5 ×20-mm balloon (Fig. 6.12B). Seven days later, the patient exhibited a pulsatile neck mass and underwent computed tomography showing two large pseudoaneurysms at both proximal and distal stent edges (Fig. 6.12C), requiring urgent endovascular treatment. After diagnostic angiography (Fig. 6.12D), a 0.014-inch guidewire was positioned in the distal tract of the right internal carotid artery to facilitate distal positioning of a 0.035-inch wire. Then

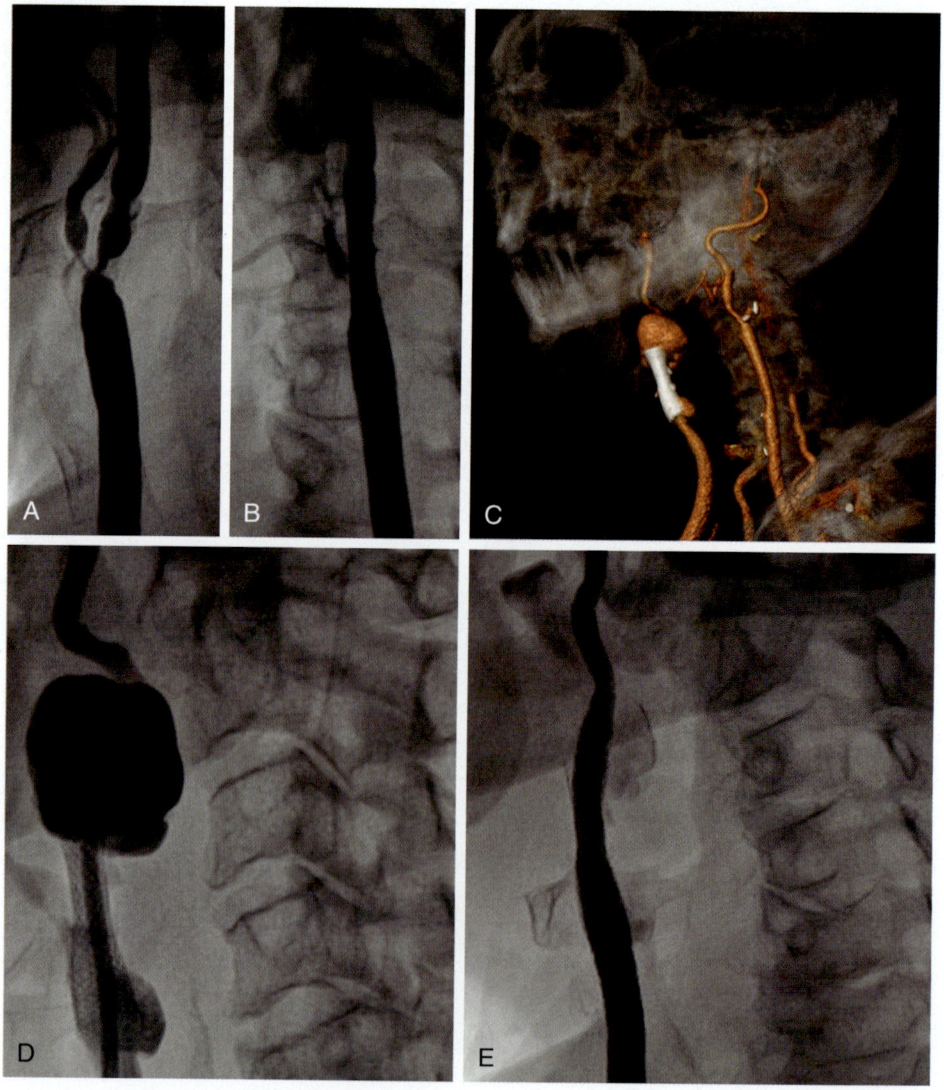

FIG. 6.12 Pseudoaneurysm After Carotid Artery Stenting. (A) Baseline angiography of severe stenosis of the right internal carotid artery. (B) Angiographic result after stenting. (C) Three-dimensional reconstruction of computed tomography showing two pseudoaneurysms at both proximal and distal stent edges. (D) Carotid angiography showing the pseudoaneurysms. (E) Angiographic result after implantation of two overlapping, covered stents with exclusion of the pseudoaneurysms.

two overlapping, covered BeGraft stents (Bentley Innomed GmbH, Hechingen, Germany) were implanted with complete exclusion of the pseudoaneurysms (Fig. 6.12E), without any complication. Extracranial carotid artery pseudoaneurysm is an infrequent lesion most commonly traumatic, spontaneous, or iatrogenic in origin.[1] Iatrogenic lesions include complications of carotid endarterectomy or central venous catheterization. The incidence of pseudoaneurysm formation secondary to carotid stenting is extremely rare. To the best of our knowledge, this is the first case of pseudoaneurysm formed at both proximal and distal carotid stent edges a few days after the procedure, successfully treated with implantation of covered stents.

Reference

1. Seward CJ, Dumont TM, Levy EI. Endovascular therapy of extracranial carotid artery pseudoaneurysm: case series and literature review. *J Neurointerv Surg.* 2015;7:682-689.

An Unusual Cause of Iatrogenic Hypertension

Shikhar Agarwal, MD, MPH, Maya Serhal, MD, Daniel Shivapour, MD, John R. Bartholomew, MD, Christopher Bajzer, MD

A 26-year-old woman was referred for management of resistant hypertension after admission for hypertensive emergency. Her medical history was notable for attention deficit hyperactivity disorder and a motor vehicle accident 6 years before presentation that was complicated by subdural hematoma and provoked deep venous thrombosis requiring placement of an inferior vena cava (IVC) filter. During her hospital admission, the patient was found to have a headache, acute kidney injury, and proteinuria in the setting of hypertensive emergency. In addition, the patient was found to be hypokalemic. Her antihypertensive agents were progressively titrated to include labetalol, amlodipine, and spironolactone. Renal artery ultrasound revealed normal velocities in the right renal artery, with dampened, monophasic, and turbulent Doppler waveforms suggestive of renal artery atherosclerotic disease. The patient was observed by the Nephrology Department as an outpatient and was found to have elevated plasma renin of 32.8 mg/L per hour (normal range, 0.8–5.8 mg/L per hour). Because of suspicion for renovascular hypertension, magnetic resonance angiography was pursued, which demonstrated severe stenosis of the mid portion of the right renal artery with associated atrophy of the kidney (Fig. 6.13). The left renal arterial system was normal. Invasive angiography was pursued and demonstrated a high-grade stenosis in the mid portion of the right renal artery (Figs. 6.14 and 6.15). Stenosis was found to be secondary to extrinsic compression by a prong of the IVC filter (Fig. 6.15). Intravascular ultrasound imaging demonstrated that the prong of the IVC filter had migrated into the media of the renal artery with resultant high-grade stenosis due to marked intimal proliferation (Fig. 6.16). The patient was subsequently referred for surgical removal of the filter and vascular reconstruction of the renal artery.

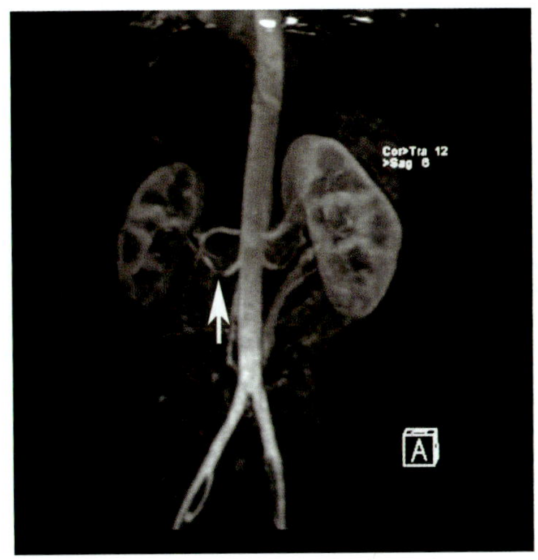

FIG. 6.13 Magnetic Resonance Angiography. Three-dimensional reconstruction from magnetic resonance angiography showing severe stenosis in the mid portion of the right renal artery (*white arrow*).

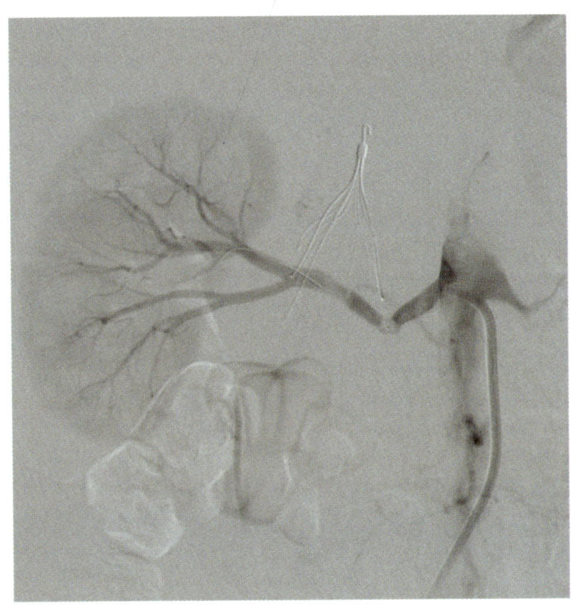

FIG. 6.14 Digital Subtraction Angiography of the Right Renal Artery. Digital subtraction angiography of the right renal artery showing severe stenosis in the right renal artery.

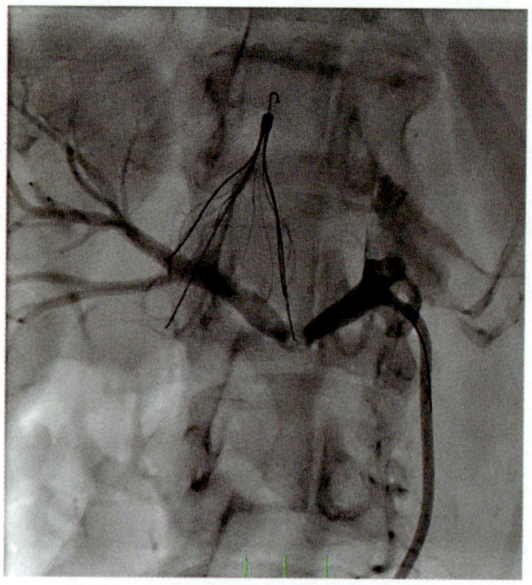

FIG. 6.15 Invasive Angiography of the Right Renal Artery. The relationship of the inferior vena cava filter prong to the right renal artery is shown, suggesting external compression of the artery.

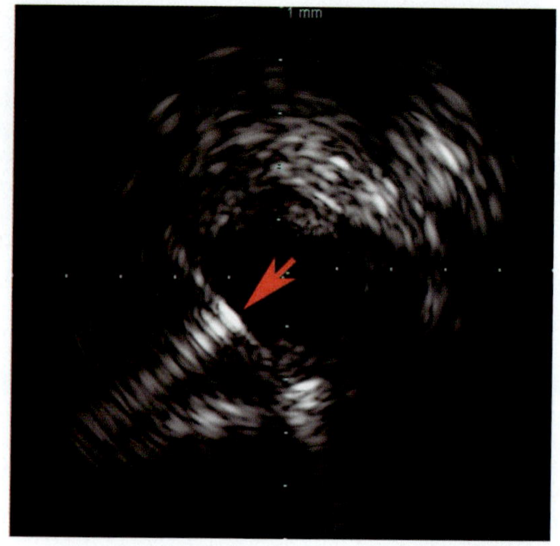

FIG. 6.16 Intravascular Ultrasound of the Right Renal Artery. Intravascular ultrasound image showing the metallic prong encroaching into the media of the renal artery (*red arrow*).

Bail-out Technique for Pulmonary Artery Rupture With a Covered Stent in Balloon Pulmonary Angioplasty for Chronic Thromboembolic Pulmonary Hypertension

Kentaro Ejiri, MD, Aiko Ogawa, MD, PhD, Hiromi Matsubara, MD, PhD

A 76-year-old male patient with inoperable chronic thromboembolic pulmonary hypertension was referred to our hospital for treatment with balloon pulmonary angioplasty (BPA). He was in World Health Organization functional class III and pulmonary artery pressure was 69/6 (34) mm Hg. We performed BPA in a staged fashion and at the fourth BPA session, we targeted the left upper lobe A1+2. Pulmonary angiography showed the ringlike stenotic lesion (*arrowhead* in Fig. 6.17A), and we evaluated the lumen size of the vessel with intravascular ultrasound. We then expanded the vessel with a balloon (5.0 × 20 mm; Bandicoot RX, Kaneka Medix, Osaka, Japan) (Fig. 6.17B). However, immediately after deflation of the balloon, severe hemosputum occurred. Pulmonary angiography showed extravasation of contrast medium (Fig. 6.17C, Online Video 6.2). We recognized that a pulmonary artery rupture had occurred and tried to stop the bleeding by balloon occlusion. However, we failed and deployed a covered stent of 3.0 × 16 mm (JOSTENT GraftMaster, Abbott Vascular, Santa Clara, California) to the rupture site. We inflated the balloon (5.0 ×20 mm) inside the stent, and pulmonary angiography showed the disappearance of extravasation of contrast medium (Fig. 6.17D, Online Video 6.3). Repeated pulmonary angiography 2 weeks later revealed no extravasation. In-stent restenosis does not occur for 2 years (Fig. 6.17E–F, Online Video 6.4).

Although pulmonary artery rupture is a rare complication during BPA, it can cause lethal bleeding. Therefore it is essential for operators of BPA to know how to handle this complication. The efficacy of coil embolization for pulmonary artery rupture was reported[1,2]; however, the embolized vessel could never be reperfused. Treatment with a covered stent could maintain the perfusion of the treated artery. Although the utility of a covered stent for pulmonary artery stenosis and aneurysm has been reported,[3,4] this is the first report to describe the management of pulmonary artery rupture by a covered stent.

References

1. Baker CM, McGowan FX Jr, Keane JF, Lock JE. Pulmonary artery trauma due to balloon dilation: recognition, avoidance, and management. *J Am Coll Cardiol.* 2000;36:1684-1690.
2. Tajima H, Murata S, Kumazaki T, Abe Y, Takano T. Pulmonary artery perforation repair during thrombectomy using microcoil embolization. *Cardiovasc Intervent Radiol.* 2006;29: 155-156.
3. Dallaudière B, Hummel V, Pierre Laissy J. The use of covered stents for treatment of pulmonary artery pseudoaneurysms. *J Vasc Interv Radiol.* 2013;24:296-298.
4. Grubstein A, Atar E, Litvin S, et al. Angioplasty using covered stents in five patients with symptomatic pulmonary artery stenosis after single-lung transplantation. *Cardiovasc Intervent Radiol.* 2014;37:686-690.

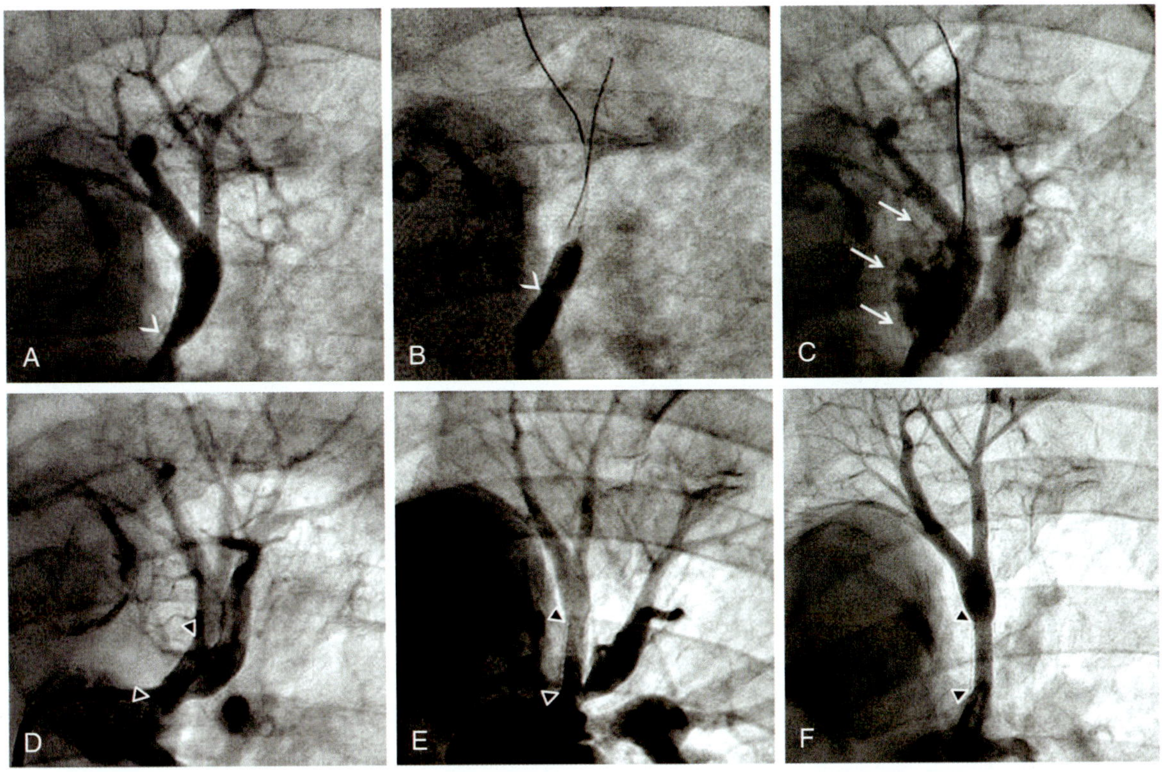

FIG. 6.17 Angiography of Pulmonary Artery Rupture During Balloon Pulmonary Angioplasty (BPA) and Treatment With a Covered Stent. (A) Pulmonary angiography before BPA shows the ringlike stenosis (*arrowhead*) of the left upper lobe A1+2. (B) Inflation of the 5.0-mm balloon to 8 atm does not expand the lesion completely (*arrowhead*). (C) Although inflation of the balloon to 14 atm expands the lesion completely, pulmonary angiography shows extravasation of contrast medium (*arrows*) (Online Video 6.2). (D) After sufficient expansion of the covered stent by the inflated balloon (between *triangles*), pulmonary angiography shows disappearance of extravasation of contrast medium (Online Video 6.3). (E) Pulmonary angiography at the 1-year follow-up after stenting shows patency of the stent with a slight neointimal formation without significant restenosis (between *triangles*). (F) Pulmonary angiography at the 2-year follow-up after stenting shows patency of the stent without significant restenosis (between *triangles*) (Online Video 6.4).

Case of Percutaneous Extracorporeal Femorofemoral Bypass for Acute Limb Ischemia From Large-Bore Access

Saurav Chatterjee, MD, Riyaz Bashir, MD, RVT, Vladimir Lakhter, DO, Brian O'Murchu, MD, Brian O'Neill, MD, Vikas Aggarwal, MD, MPH, RPVI

An 80-year-old man presented with acute inferior ST-segment elevation myocardial infarction and cardiogenic shock. Cardiac catheterization revealed 99% stenosis in the mid right coronary artery, a 95% focal severe stenosis in mid left anterior descending coronary artery, and a 60% to 70% stenosis in the proximal circumflex artery. Given advanced age and unstable hemodynamics, emergent multivessel percutaneous coronary intervention (PCI) with complete revascularization was performed. An intraaortic balloon pump was initially placed, but cardiogenic shock persisted despite this and multiple vasopressors. His femoral arteries were <5 mm bilaterally. Despite borderline access vessels, hemodynamic support with an Impella CP heart pump (Abiomed, Danvers, Massachusetts) was instituted via left common femoral access. The patient was only 4 feet 9 inches tall, weighed 50 kg, and had a body surface area of 1.4 m^2. Lack of flow distal to the common femoral arteriotomy was confirmed on duplex ultrasound examination. [1] The patient was, however, completely dependent on the Impella CP and could not be weaned off despite maximal doses of four vasopressors.[2,3]

It had already been established noninvasively and with a lower extremity angiogram (Fig. 6.18) that the patient had no antegrade distal flow beyond the site of insertion of the cannula, hence conservative management could threaten the viability of the limb. We thus decided to proceed with percutaneous temporary femorofemoral bypass establishment by placing an antegrade sheath in the left superficial femoral artery and connecting it male-to-male with the contralateral common femoral sheath. This was achieved via careful antegrade access in the left superficial femoral artery, distal to the common femoral arteriotomy, and placement of a 6F BRITE TIP

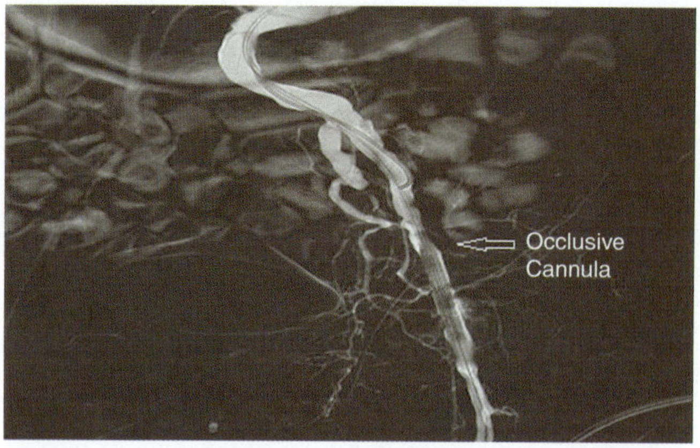

FIG. 6.18 Lower Extremity Angiogram Showing Occlusive Impella Cannula. The fluoromasked "roadmap" image shows that the 13F Impella CP cannula was occlusive for the common femoral artery of the diminutive index patient.

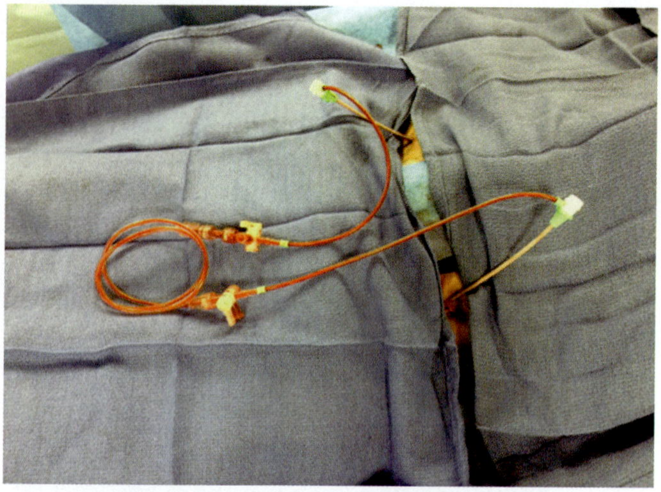

FIG. 6.19 Successful Placement of Fully Percutaneous Extracorporeal Femorofemoral Bypass for Acute Limb Ischemia From Large-Bore Access. We were able to successfully establish flow distal to the insertion site of the occlusive arterial cannula by a temporary, novel percutaneous femorofemoral bypass circuit.

Cordis sheath (Cordis Corporation, Milpitas, California). This sheath was then connected male-to-male with the contralateral 6F right common femoral artery retrograde sheath (Fig. 6.19), thereby creating a temporary, novel percutaneous femorofemoral bypass circuit.[4] Subsequently, the left popliteal pulse was confirmed on physical examination, and duplex ultrasound suggested flow reestablishment in the left lower extremity.

References

1. Abaunza M, Kabbani LS, Nypaver T, et al. Incidence and prognosis of vascular complications after percutaneous placement of left ventricular assist device. *J Vasc Surg.* 2015;62: 417-423.
2. Liu W, Mukku VK, Gilani S, Fujise K, Barbagelata A. Percutaneous hemodynamic support (Impella) in patients with advanced heart failure and/or cardiogenic shock not eligible to PROTECT II Trial. *Int J Angiol.* 2013; 22:207-212.
3. Lima B, Kale P, Gonzalez-Stawinski GV, Kuiper JJ, Carey S, Hall SA. Effectiveness and safety of the Impella 5.0 as a bridge to cardiac transplantation or durable left ventricular assist device. *Am J Cardiol.* 2016;117: 1622-1628.
4. Kizner L, Flottmann C, Horstkotte D, Gummert J. Bilateral antegrade perfusion of the superficial femoral artery to prevent limb ischaemia during combined use of Impella CP left ventricular assist device and extracorporeal life support. *Interact Cardiovasc Thorac Surg.* 2016;23:335-337.

Crushed Stent With Acute Occlusion in Superficial Femoral Artery After Enhanced External Counterpulsation

Yongsung Suh, MD, Young-Guk Ko, MD, Seung Hyun Lee, MD, PhD, Man-Deuk Kim, MD, PhD, Donghoon Choi, MD, PhD

A 60-year-old woman with hypertension was admitted because of the abrupt onset of resting pain in the left thigh, starting 2 weeks earlier. Three years earlier, she received self-expanding Nitinol stent implantation (overlapping stents, proximal 6 × 80 mm and distal 6 × 150 mm, SMART, Cordis Endovascular, Warren, New Jersey) in a totally occluded left superficial femoral artery (SFA) because of claudication (Fig. 6.20A–B). At this admission, a computed tomography angiogram showed total occlusion of the left SFA stent with a narrowed stented area in the middle portion of the stents (Fig. 6.20C). Invasive angiography revealed totally occluded SFA stents that were extensively crushed in the middle portion (Fig. 6.20D). After meticulous history taking, we found out that she took enhanced external counterpulsation in a private clinic shortly before symptom onset. For revascularization of the left SFA, we performed femoropopliteal bypass surgery with an artificial graft (Fig. 6.20E).

Compared with balloon-expanding stents, the self-expanding Nitinol stent is known to be resistant to mechanical stress, including external compression. Several mechanisms such as joint flexion, external muscular compression, or metal fatigue related with pulsatile blood flow were suggested as causes of stent fracture or compression. In this report, we demonstrated a case of Nitinol stent compression as an iatrogenic cause of restenosis, resulting from medical external compression. Even after Nitinol stent implantation, a caution to avoid excessive external compression seems to be necessary to prevent restenosis related to stent deformity.

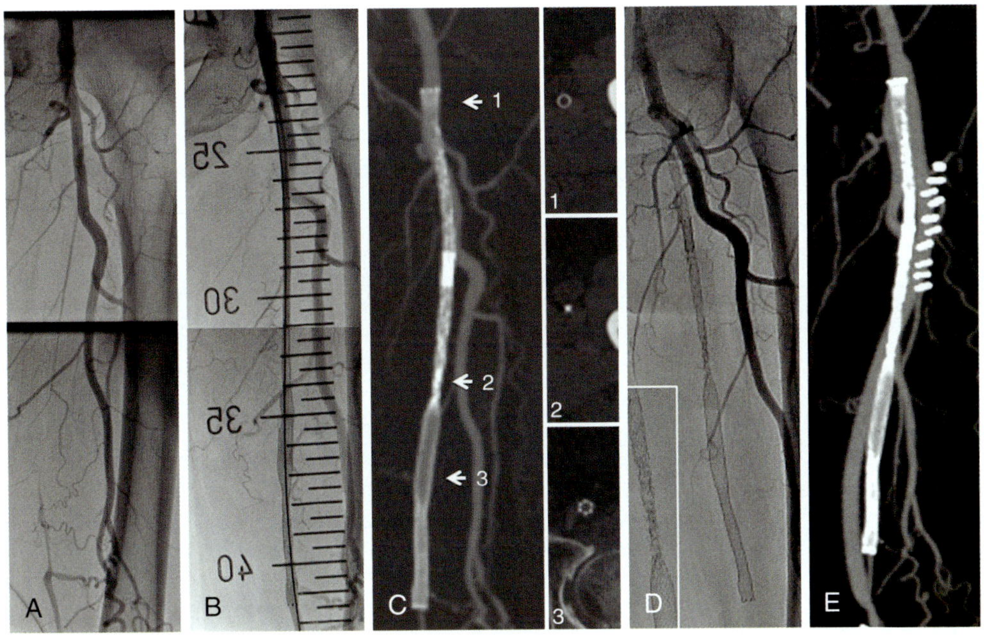

FIG. 6.20 A 60-Year-Old Woman With Resting Pain in the Left Thigh After Enhanced External Counterpulsation. (A) Left superficial femoral artery (SFA) was totally occluded. (B) Two SMART stents, 6 × 150 mm and 6 ×80 mm, were implanted from the proximal to middle segments of the left SFA 3 years earlier. (C) Computed tomography (CT) angiogram showed left SFA stent occlusion with a narrowed stented area of the middle portion of two stents. (D) Left SFA stents were occluded and extensively crushed in the middle portion. (E) CT angiogram after femoropopliteal bypass.

Cutaneous Radiation Injury After Complex Coronary Intervention

David P. Slovut, MD, PhD

A 57-year-old man who presented with exertional chest discomfort underwent stenting of a high-grade, calcified lesion in the distal right coronary artery (RCA). An ostial dissection, which resulted from deep intubation of the guiding catheter during delivery of the stent, was also treated. The procedure time was 171 min with 59.1 min of fluoroscopy recorded. Thirty-four of the 47 cine runs were performed in left anterior oblique 39, caudal 0 projection. One week later, the patient presented with recurrent chest pain. Repeated angiography revealed a filling defect within the distal RCA stent. The stent was redilated. The second procedure required 108 min with 34.6 min of fluoroscopy recorded. Of the 38 cine runs, 27 were obtained in left anterior oblique 32, caudal 0. The estimated skin dose from both interventions was 3.75 Gy.

The patient presented to his primary care physician 5 weeks later complaining of a rash over his right scapula. Topical steroids were prescribed. Later that week, he again developed exertional chest pain. Physical examination revealed a 5 ×10-cm area of erythema and dry desquamation over the patient's right scapula (Fig. 6.21A–B). A grade I cutaneous radiation injury was diagnosed. The affected area was marked with radiopaque rulers (Stent Guide, LeMaitre, Burlington, Massachusetts). Diagnostic angiography was performed, taking care to avoid exposing the demarcated area to additional radiation. Severe in-stent restenosis was observed in both the proximal and distal RCA stents. The patient was referred for surgical bypass of the RCA and left anterior descending coronary artery. The radiation injury was treated with topical Silvadene and resolved over the next month.

In contemporary practice, operators routinely perform complex interventions in the coronary and peripheral circulation that may expose patients to large radiation doses. Patients who receive a skin dose of >2 Gy may develop cutaneous radiation injury (CRI). The incidence of CRI is thought to be less than 0.01% but is likely underreported because radiation burns may be unrecognized or misdiagnosed.[1] In grade I CRI, a prodromal phase consisting of pruritis, tingling, or transient erythema may be observed 1 to 2 days after exposure. After a latent phase of 2 to 5 weeks, cutaneous erythema, slight edema, and increased pigmentation may be seen. Dry desquamation is observed 6 to 7 weeks after exposure. Mainstay therapy for grade I CRI includes controlling pain and preventing infection. Complete recovery is expected 3 to 6 months after exposure. Larger radiation doses produce greater injury. In grade IV CRI, which is associated with skin dose >550 Gy, patients develop blisters and ischemia 1 to 4 days after exposure. Within 2 weeks, skin necrosis may occur. The affected area may require skin grafting.

Patient and operator exposure to radiation may be decreased by minimizing source-to-image distance, angling the tube toward right anterior oblique projection or using less steep left anterior oblique angles, collimating the fluoroscopy beam, and avoiding high-intensity fluoroscopy mode.[2] During lengthy procedures, the tube angle should be altered periodically. In cases where patients have received high-dose radiation and are slated to undergo additional intervention, the skin entrance site should be excluded from the fluoroscopy field to decrease the cumulative skin dose.[3]

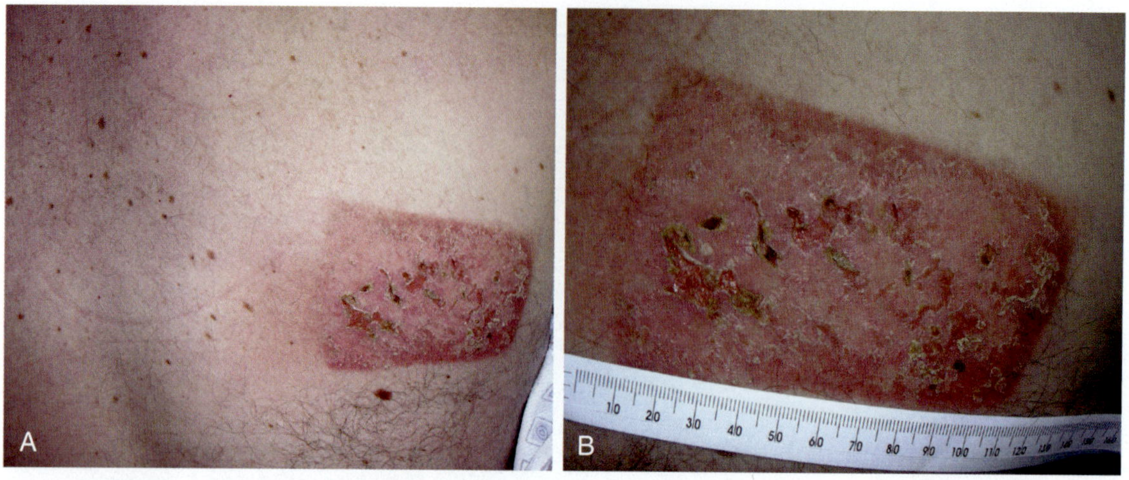

FIG. 6.21 Photograph and Close-up of Cutaneous Radiation Injury. (A) Grade I cutaneous radiation injury over scapula. Photograph showing a 5 × 10-cm rectangular area of erythema over the right scapula of a patient 7 weeks after 2 complex percutaneous coronary interventions of the right coronary artery. The index procedure was performed principally in left anterior oblique 39, caudal 0 projection, the second procedure was performed primarily in left anterior oblique 32, caudal 0. The estimated skin dose from both interventions was 3.75 Gy (1 Gy = 100 rads, a unit of absorbed dose that reflects the amount of energy deposited in a mass of tissue). (B) Close-up photograph of grade I cutaneous radiation injury. The burned skin is sharply demarcated and features dry desquamation. A lighter area of erythema is present medially (left edge of photograph) that reflects the damage produced during the second procedure when the camera angle was shallower. Several blisters have resolved. There was no evidence of infection.

References

1. Vlietstra RE, Wagner LK, Koenig T, Mettler F. Radiation burns as a severe complication of fluoroscopically guided cardiological interventions. *J Interv Cardiol.* 2004;17:131-142.
2. Kuon E, Dahm JB, Empen K, Robinson DM, Reuter G, Wucherer M. Identification of less-irradiating tube angulations in invasive cardiology. *J Am Coll Cardiol.* 2004;44:1420-1428.
3. Suzuki S, Furui S, Isshiki T, et al. Methods to reduce patients' maximum skin dose during percutaneous coronary intervention for chronic total occlusion. *Catheter Cardiovasc Interv.* 2008;71:792-798.

Delayed Displacement of Aortic Coarctation Stent

Taner Seker, MD, Armagan Acele, MD, Mustafa Topuz, MD, Yucel Colkesen, MD

We describe a case of postoperative displacement of an aortic coarctation (CoA) stent, which was determined 6 months after deployment. A 21-year-old woman with history of surgery for CoA in early childhood presented with fatigue and shortness of breath. Cardiac catheterization and aortography showed a recurrence of CoA. An 18 × 42-mm sinus-XL (Optimed XL, Ettlingen, Germany) self-expandable stent was implanted at the narrowing segment with a good outcome (Fig. 6.22A–B). The patient was asymptomatic at the 1-month follow-up. Six months later she became symptomatic, and continuous Doppler echocardiography showed a peak systolic gradient of 70 mm Hg in the aorta. Additional aortography showed migration of the stent distally from its normal position (Fig. 6.22C). We deployed a new self-expandable stent at the CoA site and performed balloon angioplasty for complete sealing to the wall (Fig. 6.22D). A stent with an antimigration design may be preferred to prevent displacement. If self-expandable stents are used for CoA, postdilation must be performed with adequate balloon angioplasty. To our knowledge, this is the first report of late slippage of a self-expandable stent after successful deployment in a patient with CoA recurrence.

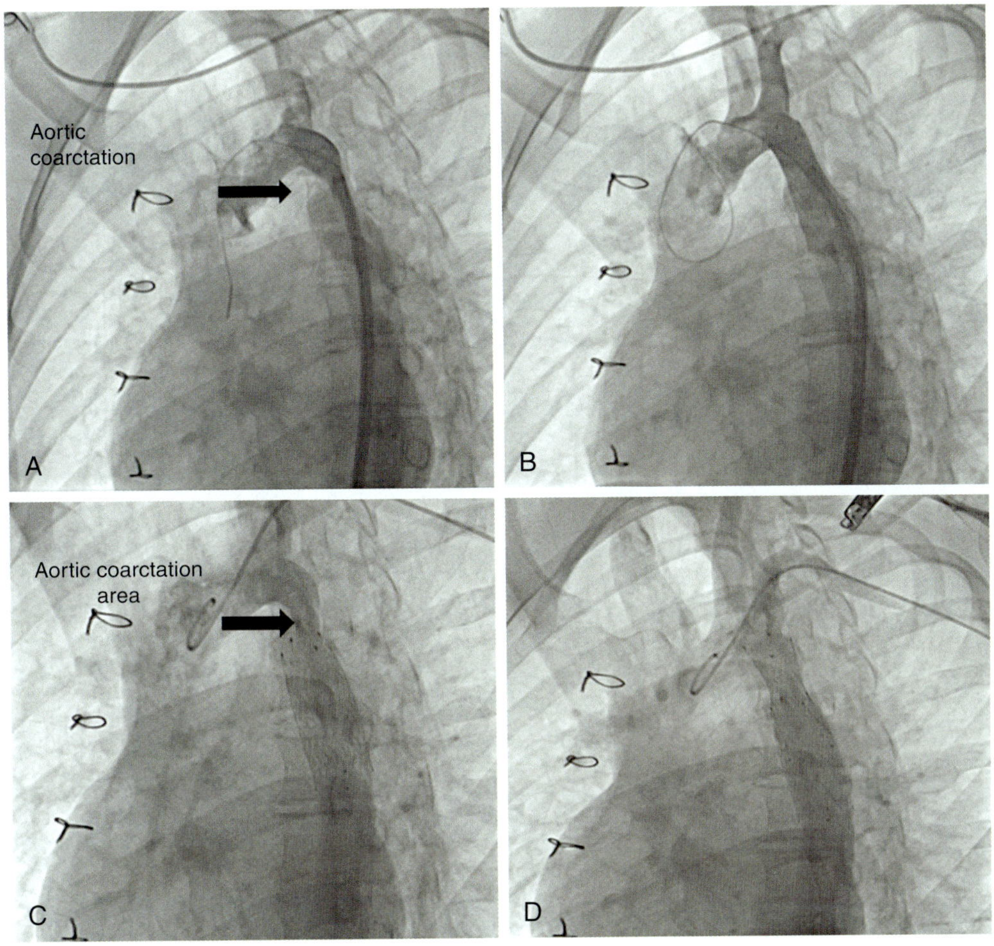

FIG. 6.22 Intervention to Aortic Coarctation. (A) Aortic recoarctation (*arrow*). (B) An 18 × 42-mm self-expandable stent deployed successfully. (C) Stent migrated distally, and coarctation area (*arrow*) is not covered. (D) Final result of procedure.

Delayed Left Main Coronary Artery Obstruction After Radiofrequency-Induced Coronary Dissection and Spasm: Insights From Optical Frequency-Domain Imaging and Intravascular Ultrasound Imaging

Umihiko Kaneko, MD, Yoshifumi Kashima, MD, Daitaro Kanno, MD, Takayuki Kitai, MD, Hiroshi Taniguchi, MD, Kikuya Uno, MD, Tsutomu Fujita, MD

A 70-year-old woman underwent second radiofrequency ablation at the left coronary cusp for recurrent and drug-refractory premature ventricular contractions arising from the left coronary cusp. Preprocedural coronary angiography showed no stenosis in either coronary artery. Radiofrequency energy application (30 W/50°C/30 s) with an open-irrigated catheter resulted in premature ventricular contraction suppression (Fig. 6.23A). No catheter insertion into the left main coronary artery (LMCA) was observed during ablation. However, the patient suddenly developed severe hypotension and escaped junctional rhythm. Angiography revealed an acute critical true bifurcation lesion in the LMCA (Fig. 6.23B). Optical frequency-domain imaging (LUNAWAVE, Terumo, Tokyo, Japan) demonstrated significant medial thickening, suggestive of severe coronary spasm (Fig. 6.23A–C, Online Video 6.5). Furthermore, intravascular ultrasound (IVUS) revealed acute dissection into the media in the proximal left anterior descending artery, in addition to medial

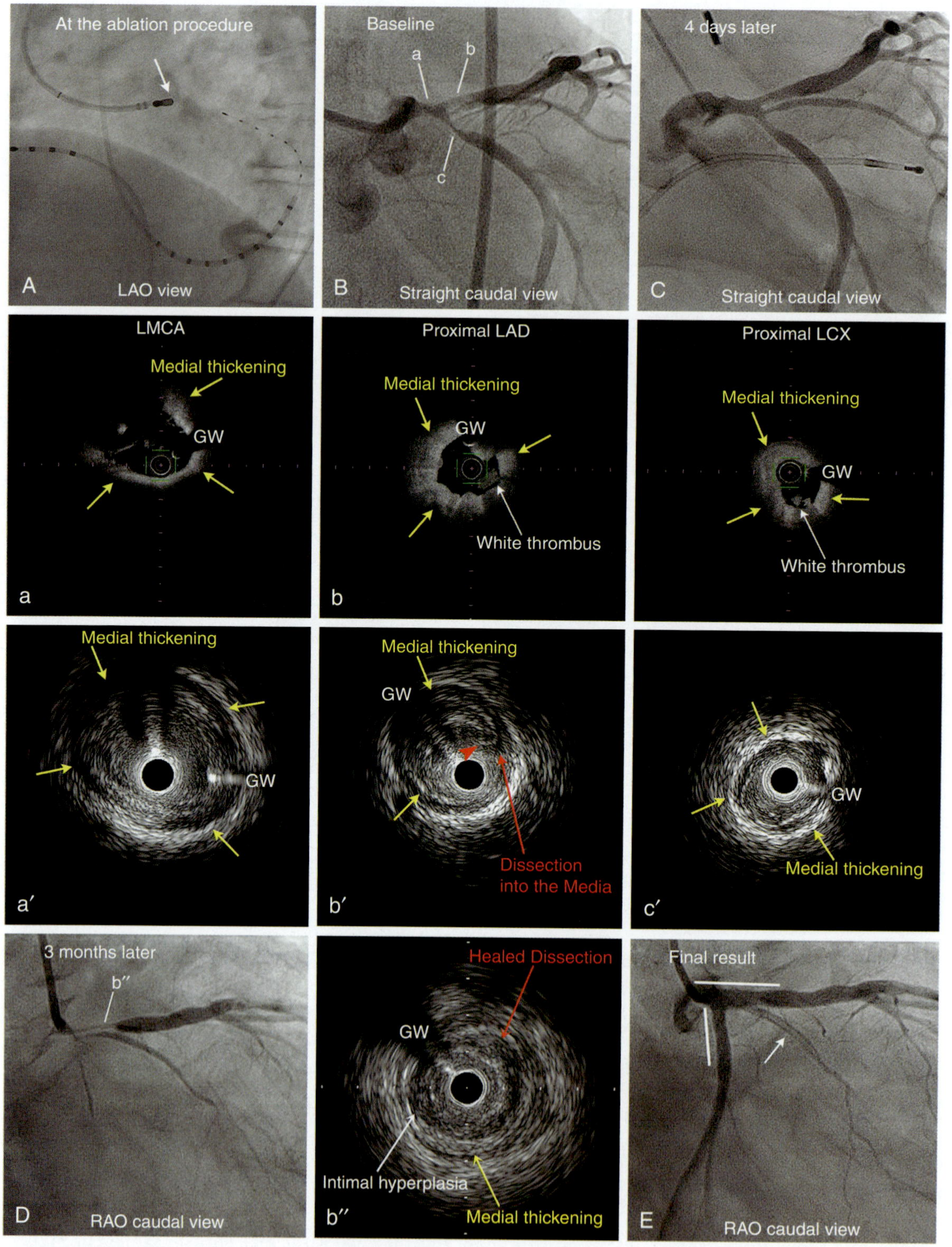

FIG. 6.23 Angiography, Intravascular Ultrasound (IVUS), and Optical Frequency-Domain Imaging (OFDI) Assessment of the Coronary Artery Dissection and Spasm After Radiofrequency Ablation. (A) Radiofrequency ablation was performed at the left coronary cusp for recurrent premature ventricular contraction. The *white arrow* shows the tip of the ablation catheter. (B) Coronary angiography revealed subocclusive stenosis of the distal left main coronary artery (LMCA) bifurcation, involving the left anterior descending artery (*LAD*) and the left circumflex artery (LCX) ostium. (a–c) OFDI (Online Video 6.5) and (a′–c′) IVUS images (Online Video 6.6) demonstrated severe medial thickening (*yellow arrows*), causing luminal compromise and white thrombus (*white arrow*). (b′) IVUS image of LAD revealed propagation of the coronary dissection into the media (*red arrow*). The *red arrowhead* denotes the mobile flap. (C) Angiography taken 4 days postoperatively showed improvement in the LMCA lesion. (D) Emergent angiography obtained 3 months later showed total occlusion in the LMCA. (b″) High-definition 60-MHz IVUS demonstrated persistent medial thickening (*yellow arrow*) covered with homogeneous intimal hyperplasia (*white arrow*) and mixed thrombus at the occluded proximal LAD lesion. The *red arrow* denotes previously dissected part, namely chronic healed dissection (Online Video 6.7). (E) Excellent angiographic results were obtained after the bifurcation reconstruction with modified T-stenting. The *white line* shows the location of the implanted stents. The *white arrow* shows coronary dissection induced by kissing balloon dilation in the first obtuse margin. The (a)–(c) OFDI and (a′)–(c′) IVUS images at baseline and (b″) IVUS image 3 months later correspond to each other. *GW*, guidewire; *LAO*, left anterior oblique; *RAO*, right anterior oblique.

thickening (Fig. 6.23a′–1c′, Online Video 6.6). After repeated intracoronary injections of nitroglycerin and intraaortic balloon pump insertion, the patient gained hemodynamic stability. She was managed medically with nifedipine, isosorbide mononitrate, pravastatin, and aspirin. Angiography at 4 days postoperatively showed improvement in the LMCA lesion with thrombolysis in myocardial infarction (TIMI) flow grade 3 (Fig. 6.23C). Although localized acute coronary dissection had been detected on baseline IVUS, substantial improvement of the coronary spasm was confirmed under medical therapy with TIMI flow grade 3 on a subsequent angiogram. Therefore she had been treated medically. However, 3 months later, she developed non–ST-segment elevation myocardial infarction and cardiogenic shock due to total occlusion in the LMCA (Fig. 6.23D). High-definition 60 MHz IVUS (Alta View, Terumo) demonstrated a persistent medial thickening covered with homogeneous intimal hyperplasia and healed dissection (Fig. 6.23b″, Online Video 6.7). Bifurcation reconstruction with two drug-eluting stents was successfully performed (Fig. 6.23E).

This is the first report demonstrating acute coronary dissection into the media, in addition to severe spasm, as the primary mechanism of radiofrequency-induced coronary artery injury, successfully demonstrated by IVUS and optical frequency-domain imaging.[1] Acute coronary dissection and spasm led to residual medial thickening with gradual reorganization and intimal hyperplasia, and finally, to delayed LMCA obstruction. This case also highlights the importance of bail-out stenting in the setting of radiofrequency-induced coronary artery injury.

Reference

1. Viles-Gonzalez JF, de Castro Miranda R, Scanavacca M, Sosa E, d'Avila A. Acute and chronic effects of epicardial radiofrequency applications delivered on epicardial coronary arteries. *Circ Arrhythm Electrophysiol.* 2011; 4:526-531.

Downstream Panniculitis Secondary to Drug-Eluting Balloon Angioplasty

Tareq Ibrahim, MD, Ralf Dirschinger, MD, Rüdiger Hein, MD, Juliane Jaitner, MD

A 72-year-old woman with peripheral arterial disease presented with a 5-day history of rest pain of the left lower leg. Nine years earlier, she had undergone left-sided femoropopliteal bypass surgery, with multiple endovascular procedures thereafter. Examination revealed absent popliteal and pedal pulses in the symptomatic leg and an ankle-brachial pressure index of 0.44. Magnetic resonance angiography revealed thrombotic occlusion of the bypass graft and multiple subsequent stenoses (Fig. 6.24). The patient underwent endovascular mechanical thrombectomy of the bypass graft plus angioplasty of the distal bypass anastomosis and popliteal artery using two paclitaxel-eluting balloons (IN.PACT Admiral, Medtronic, Minneapolis, Minnesota) (Fig. 6.25).

Two weeks later, the patient developed a painful rash completely restricted to her left lower limb. She consulted numerous physicians, but no diagnosis could be made. Three months later, she visited our outpatient clinic for a regular follow-up, still presenting with the

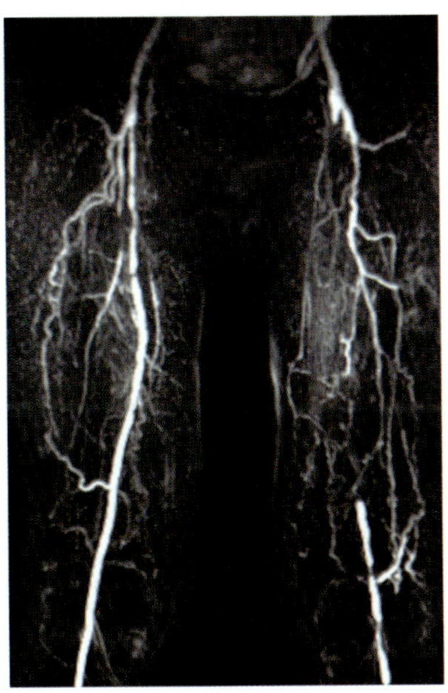

FIG. 6.24 Magnetic Resonance Imaging. Magnetic resonance angiography of the upper leg region revealed left-sided graft occlusion and subsequent stenoses of the femoropopliteal vasculature.

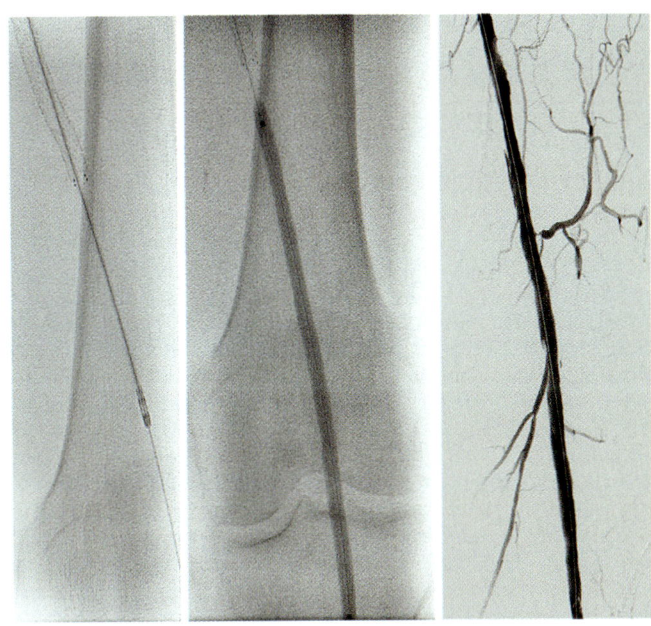

FIG. 6.25 Endovascular Therapy. Thrombectomy of the bypass graft (*left*) and drug-eluting balloon angioplasty of the subsequent femoropopliteal vasculature (*middle*), with restoration of flow (*right*).

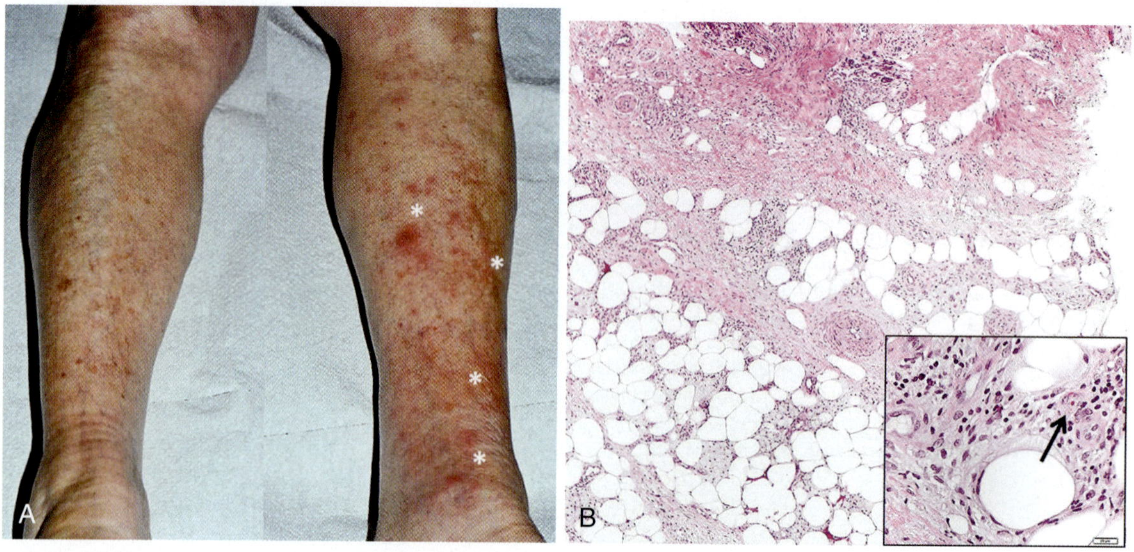

FIG. 6.26 Effect on the Skin. (A) Rash consisting of multiple livid skin nodules (*asterisks*) solely on the left lower leg. (B) Biopsy revealed diffuse subcutaneous inflammation with perivascular evidence of eosinophilic granulocyte (*arrow*), consistent with panniculitis.

localized rash, whereupon skin biopsy yielded a diagnosis of panniculitis (Fig. 6.26A–B). With oral steroid treatment, the rash gradually resolved after 3 months.

In view of the histologic findings, the regional distribution of the rash, and the temporal relationship to the procedure, this reaction is compatible with panniculitis secondary to particle embolization of the drug-eluting balloon coating, including paclitaxel and urea components. This adverse event should be considered because of the widespread application of drug-eluting balloons in patients with peripheral arterial disease.[1]

Reference

1. Cortese B, Granada JF, Scheller B, et al. Drug-coated balloon treatment for lower extremity vascular disease intervention: an international positioning document. *Eur Heart J.* 2016;37:1096-1103.

Left Ventricular Perforation During Ventriculogram Using an Optitorque Tiger Catheter

Jarrod D. Frizzell, MD, MS, Munif Alkouz, MD, Mark W. Sheldon, MD

A 76-year-old woman underwent catheterization and coronary angiography of the left side of the heart for a non–ST-segment elevation myocardial infarction. A transradial approach with an Optitorque Tiger (Terumo, Somerset, New Jersey) catheter was used. Angiography was significant for only moderate nonobstructive disease in the right coronary artery. The Tiger catheter crossed the aortic valve and was used to obtain left-sided heart pressures. After the pressure waveform and a small test injection appeared to show adequate positioning, a planned injection of 30 mL of contrast delivered over 10 s was begun. The patient developed chest discomfort and contrast appeared to dissect through the anterolateral wall and entered the pericardium (Figs. 6.27 and 6.28, Online Video 6.8). The injection was promptly stopped and the catheter withdrawn. Approximately 4 mL of contrast were delivered. Postinjection myocardial staining and the presence of dye in the pericardium were noted (Figs. 6.29 and 6.30, Online Video 6.9). She was hemodynamically stable and was monitored uneventfully in the catheterization laboratory for 30 min after a transthoracic echocardiogram showed a small effusion and no signs of tamponade. Shortly after transfer to the cardiac floor, she decompensated and underwent emergent pericardiocentesis. Nearly 250 mL of frank blood were drained. The patient subsequently had an uneventful recovery.

Transradial catheters, such as the Optitorque Jacky and Tiger shapes, have the promise of being "multipurpose" catheters for obtaining left- and right-sided coronary angiography as well as left ventriculography.[1] Ours is not the first report of complications during ventriculography using such catheters.[2] We hypothesize that whereas the end hole was directly juxtaposed against the endocardium, the side hole allowed for adequate transmission of pressure waveforms and the appearance of safe position during the test

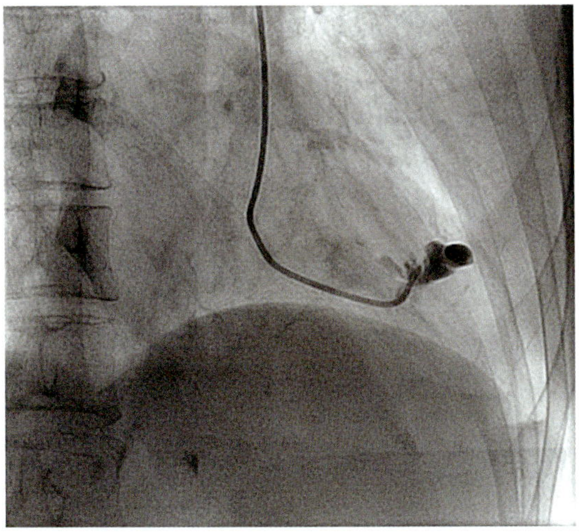

FIG. 6.27 Intramyocardial Extravasation. Early still-frame image showing the dye dissecting through the anterolateral myocardium. See Online Video 6.8.

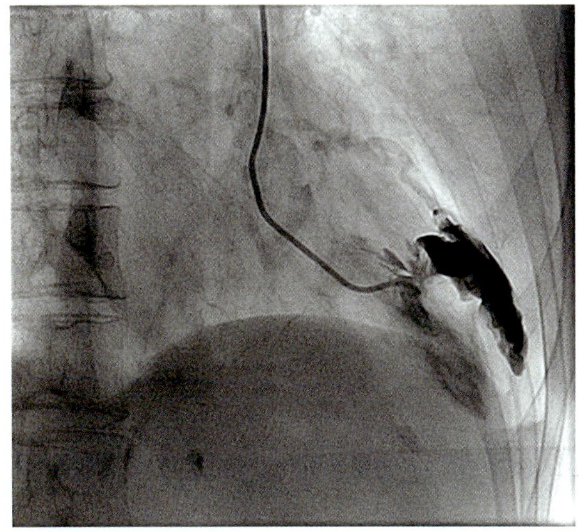

FIG. 6.28 Dye Entering Pericardium. The tract of dye through the myocardium can be seen, and the dye appears to enter the pericardium. See Online Video 6.8.

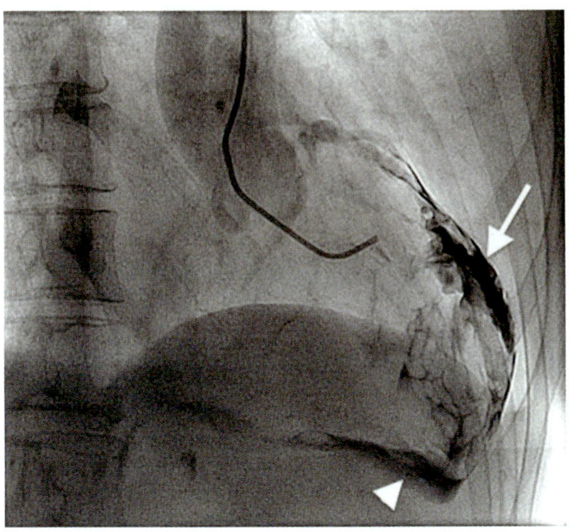

FIG. 6.29 Dye Extent on Cessation. Still-frame image as the catheter begins to be retracted, showing dark myocardial staining (*arrow*) and dye in the pericardium (*arrowhead*). See Online Video 6.9.

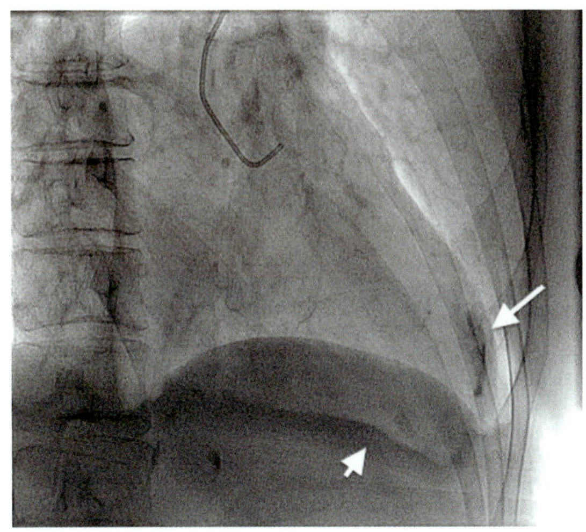

FIG. 6.30 Residual Myocardial Staining Post-Injection. Still-frame image after aborted left ventriculography, showing continued staining of the myocardium (*arrow*) and pericardial dye (*arrowhead*). See Online Video 6.9.

injection. Although perforation is a rare but well-recognized complication of left-sided heart catheterization,[3] the growing use of transradial catheterization leads to an insufficient literature documenting complications with transradial-specific catheters.

References

1. Caputo RP, Tremmel JA, Rao S, et al. Transradial arterial access for coronary and peripheral procedures: executive summary by the Transradial Committee of the SCAI. *Catheter Cardiovasc Interv.* 2011;78:823-839.
2. Basit A, Nazir R, Hahn H. Myocardial and pericardial staining by transradial Optitorque Jacky shape catheter during left ventriculogram. *J Invasive Cardiol.* 2012;24:128.
3. Friedrich SP, Berman AD, Baim DS, Diver DJ. Myocardial perforation in the cardiac catheterization laboratory: incidence, presentation, diagnosis, and management. *Cathet Cardiovasc Diagn.* 1994;32:99-107.

Massive Left Pulmonary Artery Pseudoaneurysm in a Young Child

Sivasubramanian Ramakrishnan, MD, DM, Shyam S. Kothari, MD, DM, Sanjiv Sharma, MD

Pulmonary artery (PA) pseudoaneurysm is a rare but life-threatening disorder. We describe an unusually large PA pseudoaneurysm in a young child that posed diagnostic and therapeutic challenges.

An 18-month-old male child, weighing 7 kg, had presented with recurrent hemoptysis. Chest x-ray showed complete opacification of the left hemithorax (Fig. 6.31). A computerized tomography angiogram (Figs. 6.32 and 6.33) revealed a massive pseudoaneurysm arising from the left lower PA. The sheer size of the pseudoaneurysm made conventional surgical approach difficult. A hybrid strategy of percutaneous closure of the pseudoaneurysm followed by surgical removal was considered.

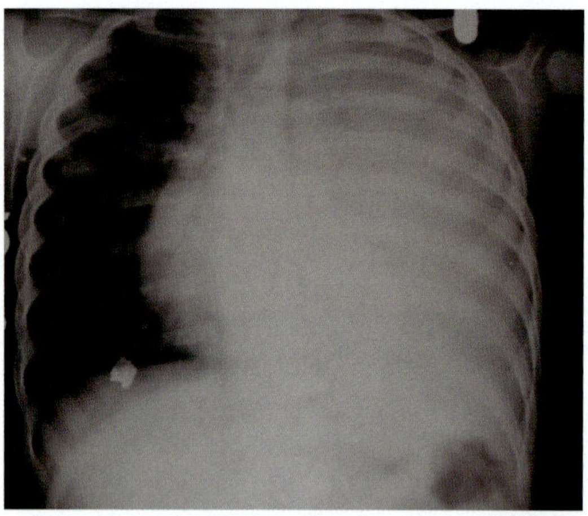

FIG. 6.31 Chest X-ray, Pulmonary Artery View. Opaque left hemithorax. There is tracheal shift to the right. The border of the left side of the heart is faintly visualized, suggesting that the lesion is not in contact with the heart.

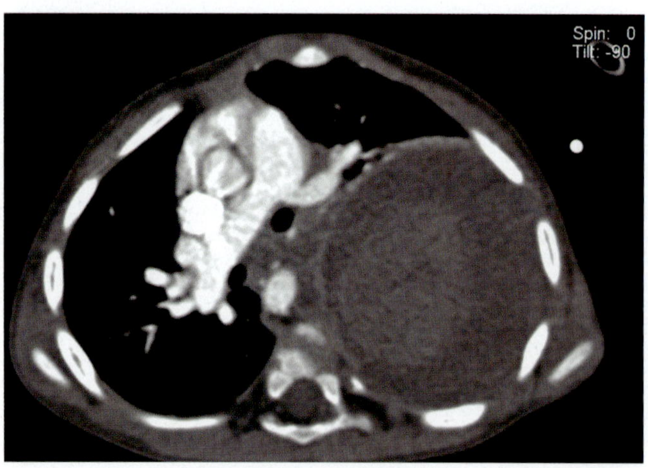

FIG. 6.32 Computed Tomography Angiogram in the Axial Plane. Large vascular lesion with peripheral thrombus, involving the left lower lobe, causing mediastinal shift (including descending aorta) to the right and resulting in collapse of the left lung.

A selective left PA angiogram clearly delineated the anatomy (Fig. 6.34). A 6F right coronary guiding catheter (Judkins right 3.5, Cordis Corp., Miami, Florida) was introduced across the neck of the pseudoaneurysm with the help of a 4F multipurpose catheter (catheter-in-catheter). An Amplatzer vascular plug (9-PLUG-012,

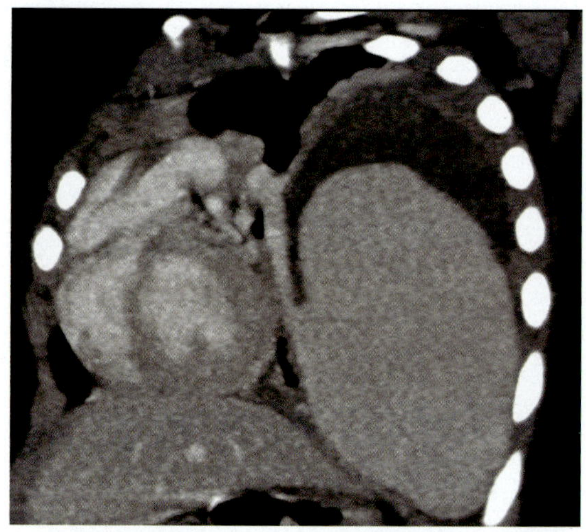

FIG. 6.33 Delayed Phase of Computed Tomography Angiogram in the Coronal Oblique Plane. CT angiogram coronal oblique plane (delayed phase) showing a giant pseudoaneurysm originating from the descending lower lobe branch of left pulmonary artery. The pseudoaneurysm is partially filled with thrombus.

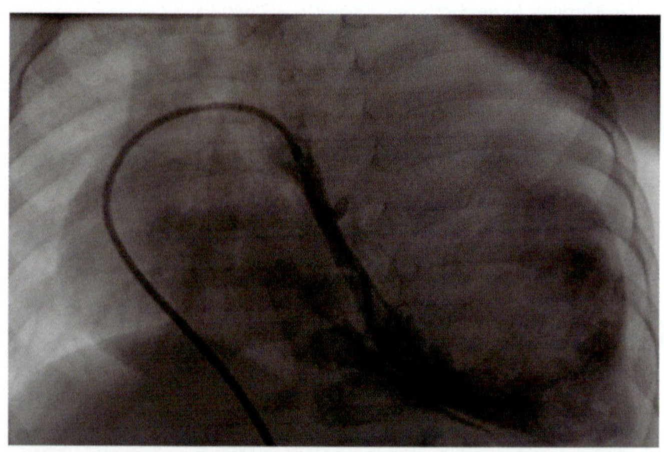

FIG. 6.34 Selective Pulmonary Artery Angiogram Showing the Giant Left Pulmonary Artery Pseudoaneurysm and Its Narrow Neck. Selective angiography of the left descending pulmonary artery confirms the computed tomography angiography findings. It shows the narrow neck of the giant pseudoaneurysm and additionally reveals the lesion to arise distal to the takeoff of most of the lower lobe branches.

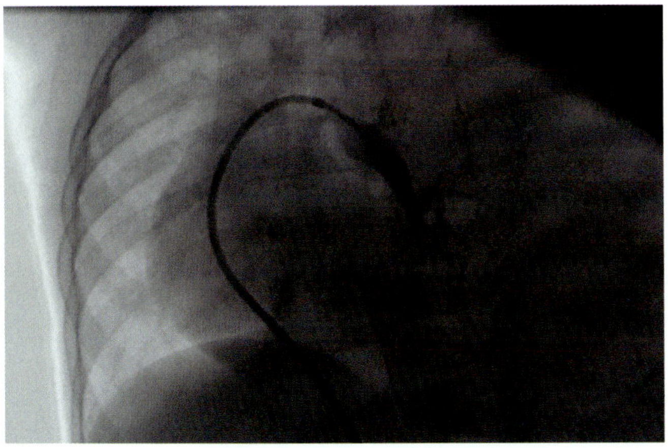

FIG. 6.35 Selective Pulmonary Artery Angiogram After Successful Device Deployment. Complete abolition of flow into the pseudoaneurysm.

AGA Medical Corporation, Minneapolis, Minnesota) was successfully deployed (Fig. 6.35). The flow across the pseudoaneurysm was completely abolished, and the left lung was expanded. The aneurysm significantly decreased in size at short-term follow-up.

Pulmonary artery pseudoaneurysms commonly result from infection, trauma, or interventional procedures on the pulmonary artery.[1] The cause of pseudoaneurysm in our case remains unclear. This might be the largest pseudoaneurysm reported in the published data in a young child. Percutaneous coil occlusion of the feeding artery of the pseudoaneurysm is standard treatment.[2] Percutaneous injection of thrombin glue, stent graft, and covered stent have also been used in the management of PA pseudoaneurysm.[3] In our case, the larger size of the pseudoaneurysm and smaller size of the patient were the major challenges. We initially even considered a combined approach. However, complete closure was achieved with an Amplatzer vascular plug alone.

In conclusion, a massive pseudoaneurysm of left pulmonary artery in a young child was successfully treated nonsurgically with a vascular plug.

References

1. Nguyen ET, Silva CI, Seely JM, Chong S, Lee KS, Müller NL. Pulmonary artery aneurysms and pseudoaneurysms in adults: findings at CT and radiography. *AJR Am J Roentgenol.* 2007;188:W126-W134.
2. Shin TB, Yoon SK, Lee KN, et al. The role of pulmonary CT angiography and selective pulmonary angiography in endovascular management of pulmonary artery pseudoaneurysms associated with infectious lung diseases. *J Vasc Interv Radiol.* 2007;18:882-887.
3. Lee K, Shin T, Choi J, Kim Y. Percutaneous injection therapy for a peripheral pulmonary artery pseudoaneurysm after failed transcatheter coil embolization. *Cardiovasc Intervent Radiol.* 2008;31:1038-1041.

Severe Renal Artery Stenosis After Renal Sympathetic Denervation

Alejandro Diego-Nieto, MD, PhD, Ignacio Cruz-Gonzalez, MD, PhD, Javier Martin-Moreiras, MD, Juan C. Rama-Merchan, MD, PhD, Javier Rodriguez-Collado, MD, Pedro L. Sanchez-Fernandez, MD, PhD

We present the case of a 73-year-old woman scheduled for renal angiography for severe recurrent refractory arterial hypertension 2 months after sympathetic renal denervation with the EnligHTN multielectrode catheter system (St. Jude Medical, Saint Paul, Minnesota).

The angiogram confirmed right renal artery subocclusive stenosis at the site of previous radiofrequency application (Fig. 6.36). After catheter-balloon dilation to advance the imaging catheter, optical coherence tomography showed severe diffuse neointimal hyperplasia (Fig. 6.37).

Since 2012, several cases of renal stenosis after renal denervation have been reported, demonstrating a wide spectrum of clinical presentation, but presenting recurrent hypertension as the most relevant finding.[1]

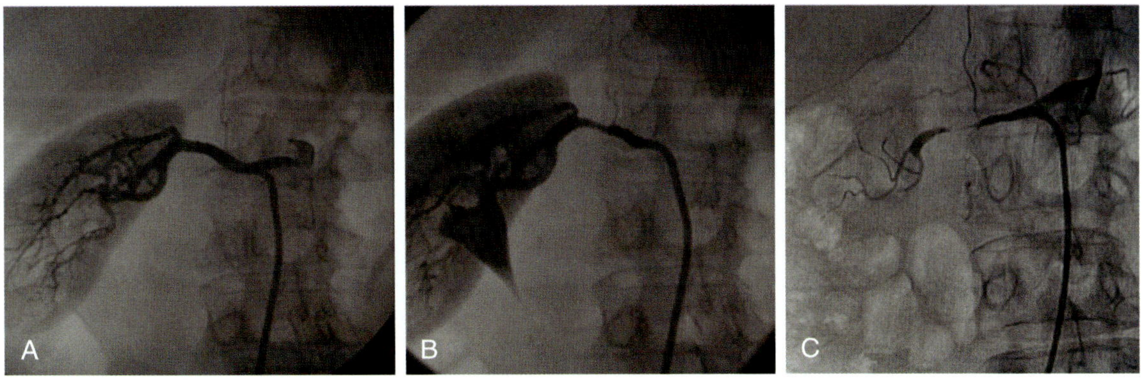

FIG. 6.36 Renal Angiogram. Right renal artery angiogram showing (A) the absence of angiographic preexisting stenosis, (B) vessel irregularities immediately after radiofrequency delivery, and (C) severe restenosis 2 months after the procedure.

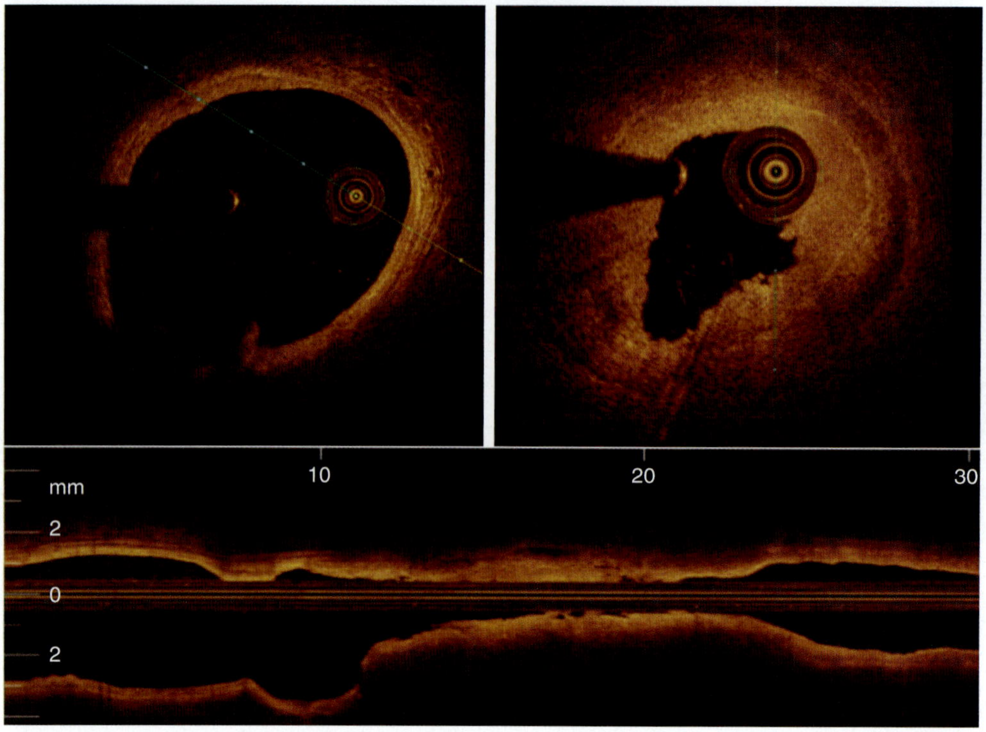

FIG. 6.37 Optical Coherence Tomography of the Right Renal Artery. Optical coherence tomography findings after dilation showing severe concentric neointimal hyperplasia.

In the previous trials HTN-1 (Symplicity Renal Denervation in Patient With Refractory Hypertension)[2] and EnligHTN-I (Safety and Efficacy of Study of Renal Artery Ablation in Resistant Hypertension Patients),[3] renal artery stenosis had been attributed mainly to preexisting artery stenosis worsening and not to a de novo procedure-related adverse event. The increasing reports of the last call into question the safety of this procedure and point to this complication as a possible cause of therapy ineffectiveness.

References

1. Cordeanu ME, Gaertner S, Bronner F, et al. Neointimal thickening resulting in artery stenosis following renal sympathetic denervation. *Int J Cardiol.* 2014;177:e117-e119.
2. Krum H, Schlaich MP, Sobotka PA, et al. Percutaneous renal denervation in patients with treatment-resistant hypertension: final 3-year report of the Symplicity HTN-1 study. *Lancet.* 2014;383:622-629.
3. Papademetriou V, Tsioufis CP, Sinhal A, et al. Catheter-based renal denervation for resistant hypertension: 12-month results of the EnligHTN I first-in-human study using a multielectrode ablation system. *Hypertension.* 2014;64:565-572.

Successful Coronary Angioplasty via the Radial Approach After Sealing a Radial Perforation

Gianluca Rigatelli, MD, Fabio Dell'Avvocata, MD, Federico Ronco, MD, Alexander Doganov, MD

A 78-year-old woman with Canadian Cardiovascular Society class III angina, despite maximal medical therapy, was admitted to our center for elective coronary angiography. The clinical history was remarkable for smoking, hypertension, hypercholesterolemia, and severe peripheral atherosclerosis with moderate bilateral carotid stenosis. The coronary angiography revealed a critical stenosis in the middle portion of the right coronary artery. Stable selective cannulation of the right coronary artery could not be achieved via the femoral approach because of severe tortuosity of the diseased iliac arteries and abdominal aorta. Coronary angioplasty was scheduled for the next day via the left radial artery approach (the Allen test was abnormal on the right radial artery).

Because of difficult advancement of the standard guidewire through the needle, a short 2.7F pressure catheter (Vygon, Ecouen, France) was inserted over a short guidewire as previously described,[1] and an intraarterial cocktail of verapamil plus nitrate was administered. A gentle contrast injection through the arterial sheath revealed a diffuse spasm of the proximal portion of the vessel

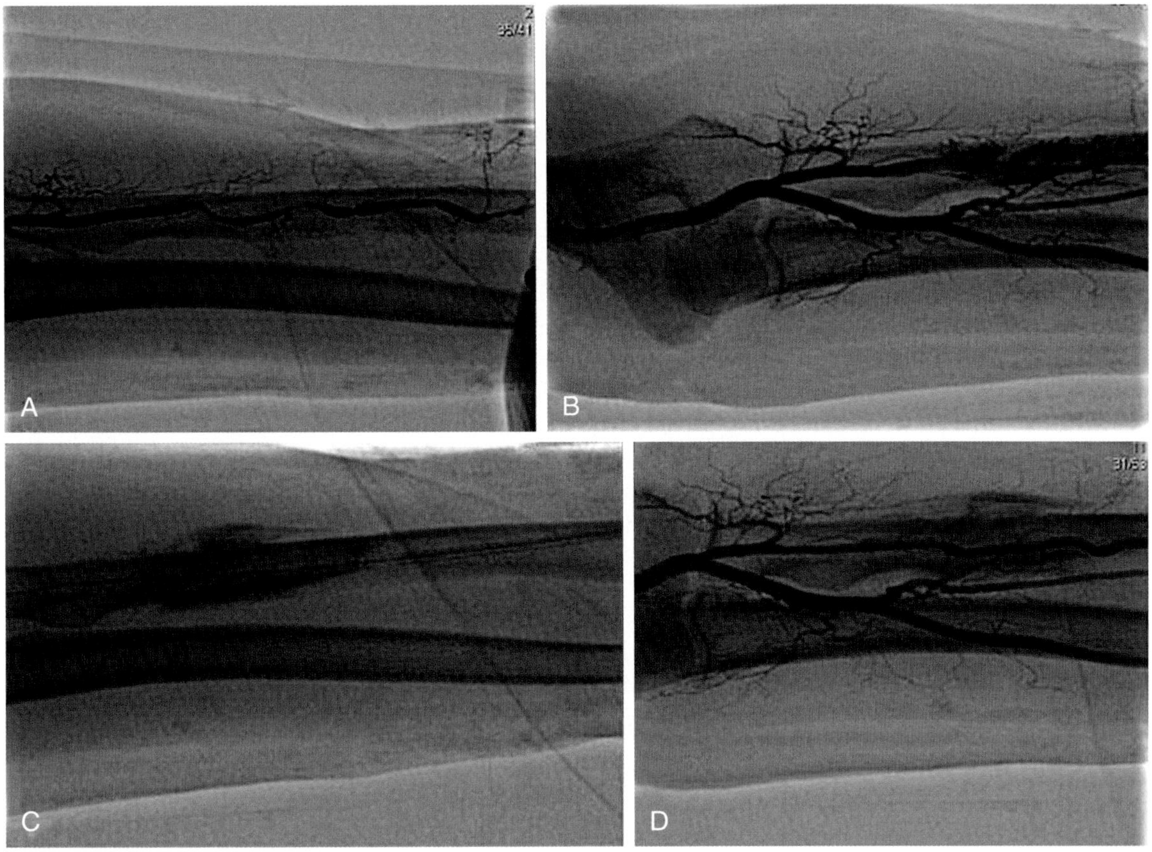

FIG. 6.38 Radial Artery Rupture and Salvage During Coronary Intervention Through the Radial Artery. (A) Radial artery angiography through a 2.7F pressure arterial sheath after generous intraarterial nitroglycerin and verapamil administration, revealing diffuse spasm of the entry site and stenosis of the middle portion of the radial artery. (B) Radial artery angiography through a 6F sheath, revealing rupture of the radial artery. (C) Prolonged balloon inflation. (D) Sealing and stenosis resolution after prolonged balloon inflation.

associated with multiple long stenosis of the middle radial artery (Fig. 6.38A). The arterial sheath was exchanged for a standard radial artery sheath, but the first attempt to advance an Emerald 0.35-inch wire (Cordis, Miami, Florida) failed, and on the subsequent contrast injection, a dissection and rupture of the radial artery in its middle portion (Fig. 6.38B) was observed. Despite a well-functioning palmar arch as demonstrated by the Allen test before the procedure, the patient experienced pain in the left arm and hand. A Pilot 50 guidewire (Guidant, Santa Clara, California) was passed through the ruptured radial artery to the subclavian artery, and a peripheral Submariner balloon 2 × 60 mm (Invatec, Roncadelle, Brescia, Italy) was inflated for 5 min at the bleeding site at 8 atm (Fig. 6.38C). Sealing and hemostasis of the artery and dilation of stenotic segments was documented with pain resolution (Fig. 6.38D). Then, a standard JR 6F guiding catheter (Cordis) with gentle manipulation was advanced over the guidewire, and the procedure was accomplished without other complications with direct stenting of the right coronary artery via the same access. Three days later the patient was discharged totally asymptomatic with no ischemia of the left arm and normal velocity wave on radial artery Doppler ultrasound.

Atherosclerotic disease of the radial artery associated with diffuse spasm is unusual but still possible in elderly patients[2]; the availability of peripheral balloons and knowledge of simple peripheral intervention techniques might help to resolve the otherwise painful consequences of radial artery rupture.

References

1. Rigatelli G, Magro B, Maronati L, et al. An improved technique for gaining radial artery access in endovascular interventions. *Cardiovasc Revasc Med.* 2006;7:46-47.
2. Lo TS, Nolan J, Fountzopoulos E, et al. Radial artery anomaly and its influence on transradial coronary procedural outcome. *Heart.* 2009;95: 410-415.

Successful Percutaneous Device Closure of Right Ventricular Perforation During Pericardiocentesis

Anita Saxena, MD, DM, Suman Karmakar, MD, Rajiv Narang, MD, DM

A 47-year-old woman with known metastatic ovarian carcinoma presented to the emergency department with cardiac tamponade. During pericardiocentesis using subxiphoid approach and a 6F sheath, the guidewire was noted to go into the right ventricle (RV) and pulmonary artery, indicating perforation of the RV, which was confirmed by contrast injection (Fig. 6.39A). The patient remained hemodynamically stable, and there was no increase in pericardial effusion. It was decided to close the perforation with an occluder device. There are only occasional previous reports of device closure of RV perforation.[1–4] A 6 × 4 (waist 6 mm, length 4 mm) Amplatzer duct occluder II device (St. Jude Medical, St. Paul, Minnesota) was chosen because this device has expanded skirts on both sides, reducing the chance of embolization. Moreover, only a device that could be delivered through a 6F sheath alongside a 0.028-inch wire could be used. The wire was kept in place before loading the device to ensure that access to perforation remains available. The positioning of the device across the RV wall was challenging in the absence of any fluoroscopic landmarks. It was guided by transthoracic echocardiography and RV angiography in two orthogonal views performed though femoral venous access (Fig. 6.39B). The distal disk of the device was deployed in the RV, keeping it very close to the perforation (Fig. 6.39C). The sheath was gently withdrawn and the proximal disk was deployed under echo guidance (Fig. 6.39D). The 0.028-inch wire remained across the perforation site. This wire was gradually pulled out and placed into the pericardial cavity. Its position in the pericardium was confirmed on fluoroscopy (Fig. 6.39E). A 5F pigtail catheter was passed over it and 500 mL of hemorrhagic pericardial fluid was drained. The patient's heart rate and blood pressure improved with the drainage of pericardial fluid. A follow-up echocardiography done 4 days after the procedure showed minimal pericardial effusion. There was no drainage after 3 days and the pigtail was removed after 5 days. Echocardiography and fluoroscopy performed 2 weeks later showed the device to be in the proper place (Fig. 6.39F).

We conclude that device closure is feasible for inadvertent perforation of the RV during pericardiocentesis and should be considered as an alternative to surgery in such patients.

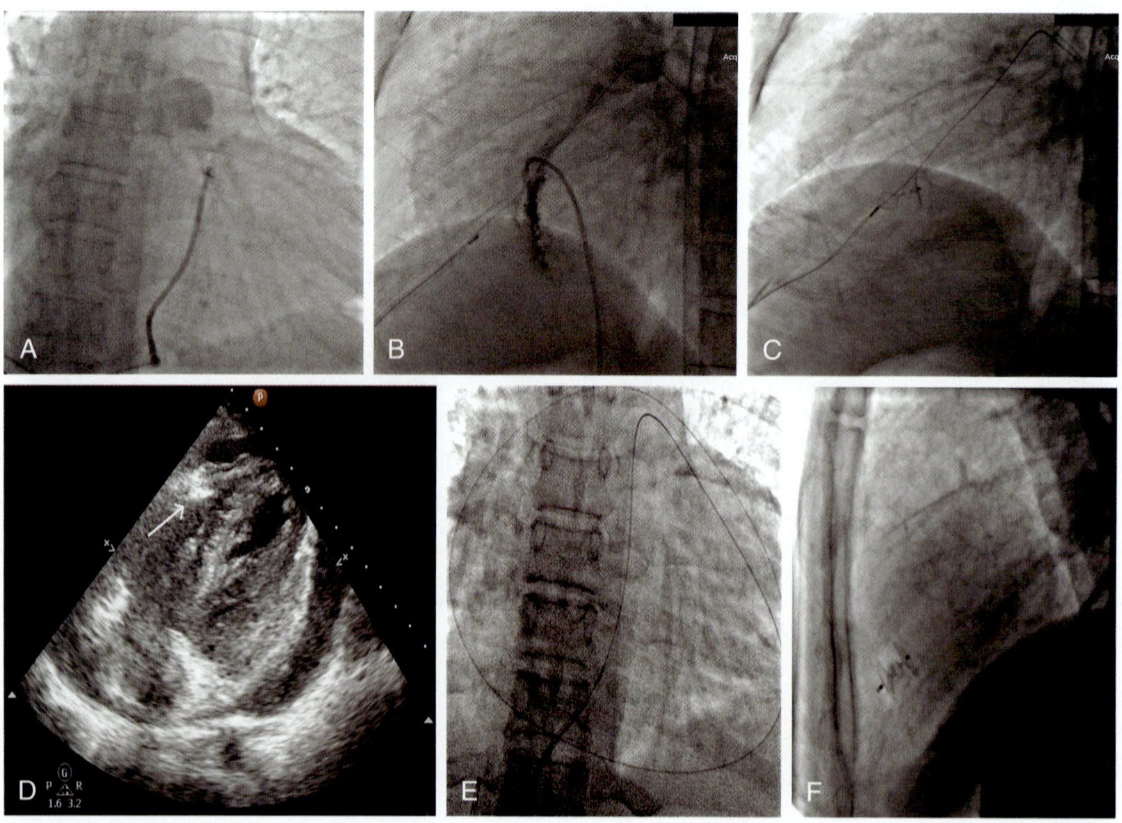

FIG. 6.39 Fluoroscopic, Angiographic, and Echocardiographic Images at Different Stages of the Procedure. (A) Contrast injected through the right ventricular sheath opacifies pulmonary arteries. (B) The device being localized using contrast injected into right ventricle using a catheter passed into it from femoral vein. (C) The distal disk deployed in the right ventricle. (D) Device (arrow) localization confirmed by transthoracic echocardiography. (E) The guidewire positioned in the pericardial cavity after device deployment. (F) The fully deployed device in lateral view.

ACKNOWLEDGMENTS

The authors are grateful to Dr. Rajnish Juneja for his contribution in managing this case.

REFERENCES

1. Stolt V, Cook S, Räber L, et al. Amplatzer septal occluder to treat iatrogenic cardiac perforations. *Catheter Cardiovasc Interv.* 2012;79:263-270.
2. Petrov I, Dimitrov C. Closing of a right ventricle perforation with a vascular closure device. *Catheter Cardiovasc Interv.* 2009;74:247-250.
3. Eshtehardi P, Garachemani A, Meier B. Percutaneous closure of a postinfarction ventricular septal defect and an iatrogenic left ventricular free-wall perforation using two Amplatzer muscular VSD occluders. *Catheter Cardiovasc Interv.* 2009;74:243-246.
4. Pawelec-Wojtalik M, Antosik P, Wasiatycz G, Wojtalik M. Use of muscular VSD Amplatzer occluder for closing right ventricular free wall perforation after hybrid procedure. *Eur J Cardiothorac Surg.* 2004;26:1044-1046.

UNRAVELING A KNOT IN THE HEART: TACKLING AN UNANTICIPATED COMPLICATION

Deepa Sasikumar, MD, Narayanan Namboodiri, MD, K.M. Krishnamoorthy, MD

A 1-year-old girl underwent catheterization before device closure of a large patent ductus arteriosus with pulmonary artery hypertension. The entry of the Goodale-Lubin catheter into the right ventricle was difficult and required excessive manipulations involving repetitive withdrawal and advancement of the catheter into the right atrium. After one such attempt, it was noted that the Goodale-Lubin catheter (Fig. 6.40A, *white arrow*) had formed a knot in the right atrium (Fig. 6.40A, *black arrow*). Gently pushing the catheter to loosen the knot was not successful, nor was it possible to pass a guidewire through the catheter (Fig. 6.40B, *white arrow*), because the knot was very tight. After repeated attempts, we were able to pass a Terumo wire (Terumo Interventional Systems, Somerset, New Jersey) through the knot, and we then threaded a 5F Judkins right catheter (Fig. 6.40B, *black arrow*, Online Videos 6.10 and 6.11) over the wire and into the knot. We passed a superstiff exchange wire through the Judkins catheter and gently withdrew the Judkins catheter. We then passed a size 10 (length 2 cm) Tyshak balloon (B. Braun Interventional Systems, Chicago, Illinois) (Fig. 6.40C, *arrow*, Online Video 6.12) over the superstiff wire and inflated it gently within the knot. As the balloon expanded, the knot loosened, and we were able

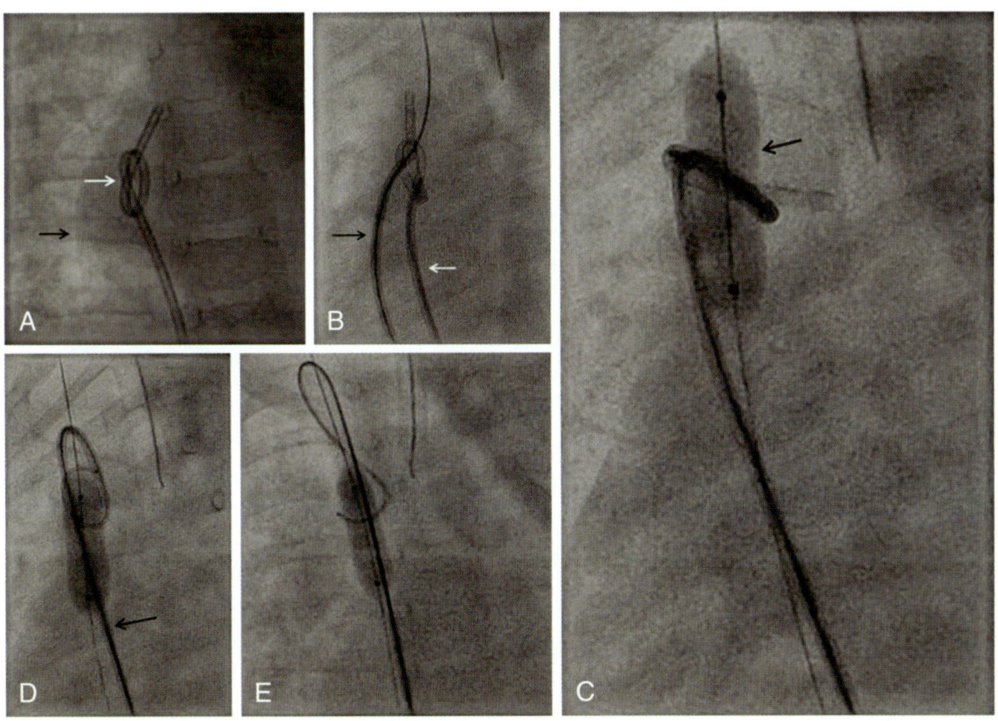

FIG. 6.40 Fluoroscopic Images Showing the Knot in the Atrium and the Unraveling of the Knot. (A) Anteroposterior view showing the Goodale-Lubin catheter, which has formed a knot (*white arrow*) in the right atrium (*black arrow*). (B) A guidewire (*white arrow*) is seen at the beginning of the knot in the Goodale-Lubin catheter; a Terumo wire (Terumo Interventional Systems, Somerset, New Jersey) is seen passing through the knot (*black arrow*), over which a Judkins right catheter is passed (Online Videos 6.10 and 6.11). (C) A Tyshak balloon (B. Braun Interventional Systems, Chicago, Illinois) (*black arrow*) is inflated inside the knot (Online Video 6.12). (D) A guidewire (*arrow*) is passed through the lumen of the Goodale-Lubin catheter, and the knot is untied. (E) The knot is untied and the catheter is withdrawn (Online Videos 6.13 and 6.14).

to pass a guidewire (Fig. 6.40D, *arrow*) through the Goodale-Lubin catheter, thus unfolding the knot (Fig. 6.40E, Online Videos 6.13 and 6.14).

Knotting of a pulmonary artery flotation catheter is well described and has been ascribed to excessive looping and repetitive manipulations; it has been managed in various ways, including balloon inflation inside the knot, as in our case. Knotting of catheters other than flotation catheters is rare but can occur when the catheters are stressed beyond their operative design. The operator using the catheter should be well versed in techniques in managing complications related to catheters such as breakage and embolization, knotting, or entrapment. In all cases of catheterization, manipulation of catheters should be gentle and controlled to avoid complications.

Thrombus in the Aorta: Late Complication After Percutaneous Closure of Ruptured Sinus of Valsalva Aneurysm

Robert Sabiniewicz, MD, PhD, Jarosław Meyer-Szary, MD, Piotr Siondalski, MD, PhD, Magdalena Kołaczkowska, MD, PhD, Rafał Gałąska, MD, PhD

A 35-year-old woman with no medical history presented after experiencing 6 months of progressive fatigue (New York Heart Association functional class II). Diagnostic two-dimensional echocardiography (2DE) revealed a 7-mm hemodynamically significant noncoronary ruptured sinus of Valsalva aneurysm into the right atrium. Workup revealed a normal coagulation profile and no comorbidities. Percutaneous closure of the aneurysm was performed uneventfully via femoral access using the self-expandable ADO 9-PDA-004 (AGA Medical Corporation, Golden Valley, Minnesota) (4/6/10 mm). The aortic retention disk was deployed with full contact with minimal residual shunt postprocedure (Fig. 6.41A–B, Online Video 6.15). The patient took aspirin for 6 months. Follow-up 2DE at 0, 1, 3, 6, and 12 months documented proper implant placement without residual shunt or thrombosis.

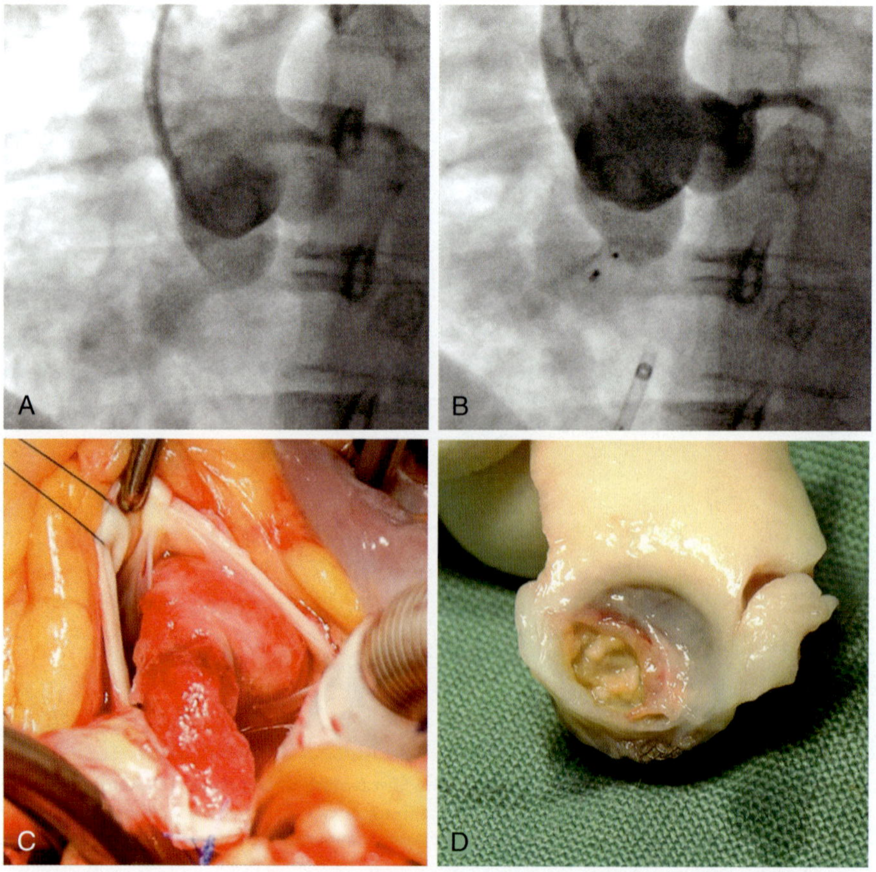

FIG. 6.41 Fluoroscopic and Surgical Findings. Fluoroscopy of the shunt through ruptured sinus of Valsalva aneurysm (A) and the effect of device implantation (B). Thrombus in situ (C). Aortic side of the sinus with the site of origin of the thrombus (D). See Online Video 6.15.

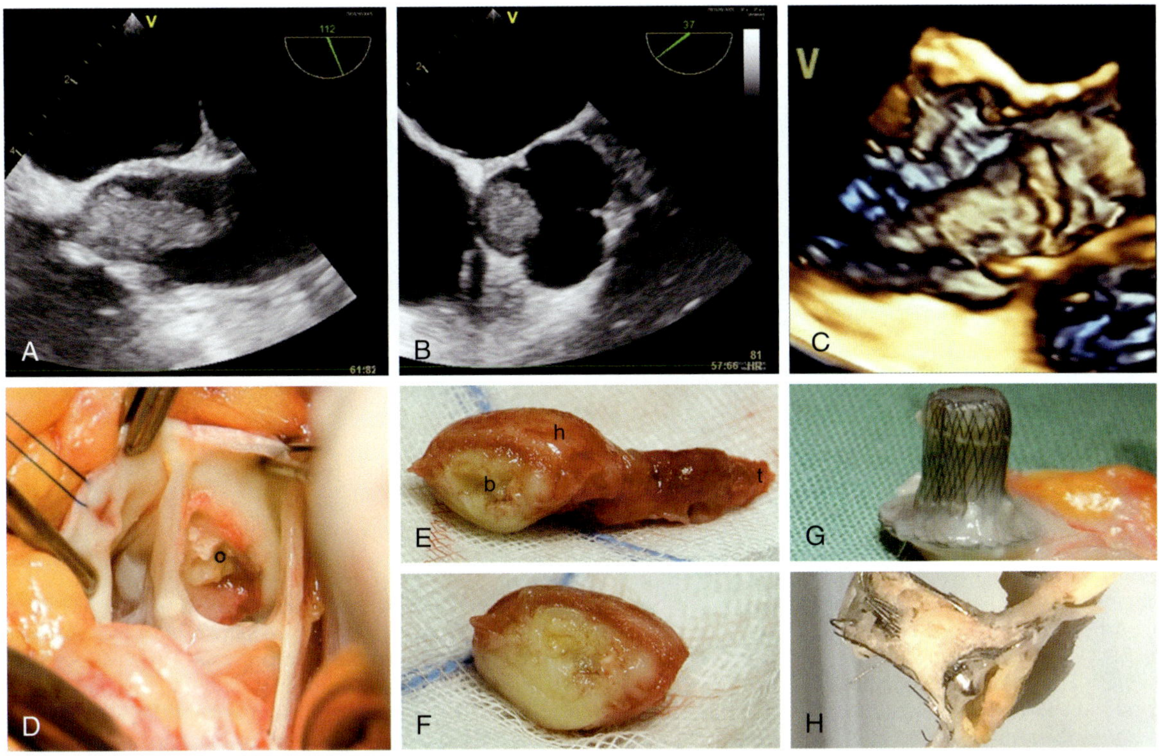

FIG. 6.42 Echocardiographic and Surgical Findings. Transthoracic echocardiography revealed a massive thrombus at the noncoronary sinus of the Valsalva at the short (A) and longitudinal (B) axis and three-dimensional (C) (Online Video 6.16). (D) The origin (*o*) of the thrombus in the noncoronary sinus at the time of surgery. (E) The base (*b*), head (*h*), and a tail (*t*) of the thrombus. (F) Cross section at the head level revealing a fibrous nucleus. (G) Properly endothelialized device from the right atrial side. (H) Cross section of the device.

Nearly 2 years later, the patient underwent popliteal endarterectomy for acute thromboembolism. Evaluation with 2DE revealed a massive (13 × 16 × 37 mm) thrombus originating at the noncoronary sinus of Valsalva (Fig. 6.42A–D, Online Video 6.16). No aortic regurgitation, aortic stenosis, or residual shunt at the site of the device was detected. The thrombus and the device were surgically extracted, and the noncoronary sinus of Valsalva was reconstructed uneventfully, with no shunt or aortic valve dysfunction on follow-up 2DE. Pathologic evaluation of the extracted specimen (Fig. 6.41C–D, Fig. 6.42D–H) revealed proper endothelialization of the device on the right atrial side and a thrombus with a well-organized fibrous nucleus originating at the aortic disk of the implant, consistent with a chronic process lasting approximately 3 to 6 months. A hypercoagulable state is suspected.

Chapter 7
Vascular, Congenital, and Other Interventional Techniques

A Magic Port-A-Cath

Ming-Chih Lin, MD, PhD, Te-Kau Chang, MD, Yun-Ching Fu, MD, PhD, Sheng-Ling Jan, MD

A 7-year-old boy with Burkitt lymphoma was referred by pediatric oncologists for severe chest pain when flushing a Port-a-cath catheter. Chest x-ray showed a dislodged Port-a-cath catheter and cardiomegaly (Fig. 7.1A) compared with the last film taken 6 months earlier (Fig. 7.1B). Echocardiography revealed pericardial effusion and a dislodged catheter in the pericardium.

To avoid surgical removal, access was established using a 7F sheath via the subxiphoid approach into the pericardium (Fig. 7.2A). A 5F end-hole catheter was then introduced through the sheath, and a 25-mm AndraSnare catheter (Andramed, Reutlingen, Germany) was used to capture the dislodged Port-a-cath catheter (Fig. 7.2B), which was then retrieved through the sheath (Fig. 7.2C)

After the procedure, the 7F sheath was changed to a 6F pigtail drainage catheter (Fig. 7.2D), and a total of 170 mL of bloody fluid was drained. The procedure took about 14 min, and fluoroscopy time was 1.6 min. The drainage tube was removed 3 days later after confirming there was no more hemopericardium by echocardiography (Online Video 7.1).

Port-a-cath catheter dislodgment is not an unusual complication. The reported incidence rate ranges from 1.4% to 4.1%.[1-3] Transcatheter retrieval was introduced in 1967,[4] and after the invention of the Amplatz Goose Neck snare catheter (ev3 Endovascular, Plymouth, Minnesota), the procedure has since become very effective, with almost a 100% success rate.[3] However, transcutaneous retrieval of a Port-a-cath catheter from the pericardium has not been previously reported. The possible mechanism is the vigorous flushing of the thrombosed catheter, causing it to disconnect and penetrate the thin wall of the right atrium like an arrow. The negative pressure of the thorax then caused the entire catheter to migrate into the pericardium. This case emphasizes that flushing of a Port-a-cath catheter should be gently done, and percutaneous retrieval may be a safe and effective method.

References

1. Babu R, Spicer RD. Implanted vascular access devices (ports) in children: complications and their prevention. *Pediatr Surg Internat.* 2002;18:50-53.
2. Dillon PA, Foglia RP. Complications associated with an implantable vascular access device. *J Pediatr Surg.* 2006;41:1582-1587.
3. Ho CL, Chou CM, Chang TK, Jan SL, Lin MC, Fu YC. Dislodgment of port-a-cath catheters in children. *Pediatr Neonatol.* 2008;49:179-182.
4. Massumi RA, Ross AM. Atraumatic, nonsurgical technique for the removal of broken catheters from cardiac cavities. *N Engl J Med.* 1967; 277:195-196.

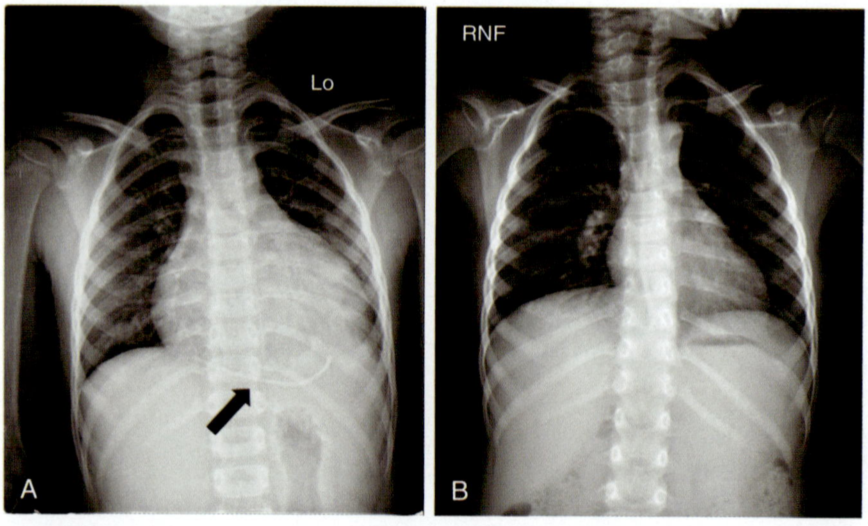

FIG. 7.1 The Patient's Chest X-Ray Findings. (A) Chest x-ray on presentation revealed a dislodged Port-a-cath catheter and cardiomegaly *(black arrow)*. (B) Previous chest x-ray taken 6 months before showed the Port-a-cath catheter positioned at the superior vena cava (Online Video 7.1).

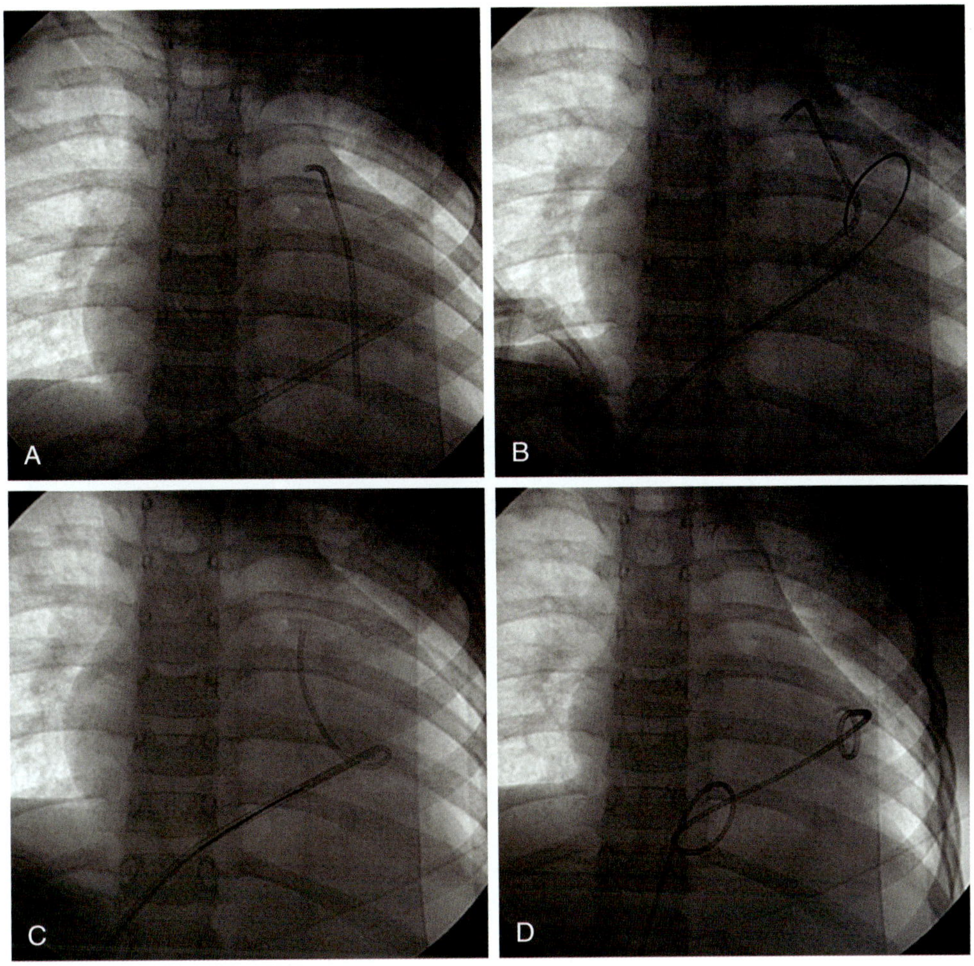

FIG. 7.2 Interventional Procedure. (A) A 7F short sheath was introduced into the pericardium via the subxiphoid approach. (B) A 25-mm snare catheter was used to capture the catheter. (C) The dislodged catheter was pulled out of the pericardium through the sheath along with the snare catheter. (D) The 7F sheath was changed to a pigtail drainage tube.

A New Tool to Manage Side-Branch Occlusion After Covered-Stent Implantation for Vascular Complications: The Neocarina Reconstruction Technique

Chiara Bernelli, MD, Francesco Maisano, MD, Alaide Chieffo, MD, Matteo Montorfano, MD, Jaclyn Chan, MBBS, Davide Maccagni, RT, Antonio Colombo, MD

Endovascular stent-graft implantation can be used to manage access site vascular complications during transcatheter aortic valve implantation.[1] Nonetheless, the deployment of these devices may be technically challenging.

An 85-year-old man underwent a transfemoral transcatheter aortic valve implantation using a 29-mm CoreValve ReValving system (Medtronic Inc., Minneapolis, Minnesota). After failure of therapeutic access preclosure by Prostar XL (Abbott Vascular Devices, Redwood City, California), a Viabahn endoprosthesis (W.L. Gore & Associates, Flagstaff, Arizona) was deployed. However, because the previous contralateral wire was inadvertently positioned in the profunda, the Viabahn occluded the superficial femoral artery (Fig. 7.3A). Therefore, to reaccess the superficial femoral artery, a Brockenbrough needle and Mullins sheath (Medtronic, Minneapolis, Minnesota) were used to perforate the covered stent (Fig. 7.3B–C). After puncture, a 0.014-inch wire was advanced in the superficial femoral artery and dilation of the covered stent with a 5.5- × 20-mm balloon was performed (Fig. 7.3D). Branch patency was restored with thrombolysis in myocardial infarction flow grade 3 and a "neofemoral carina" was created (Fig. 7.3E).

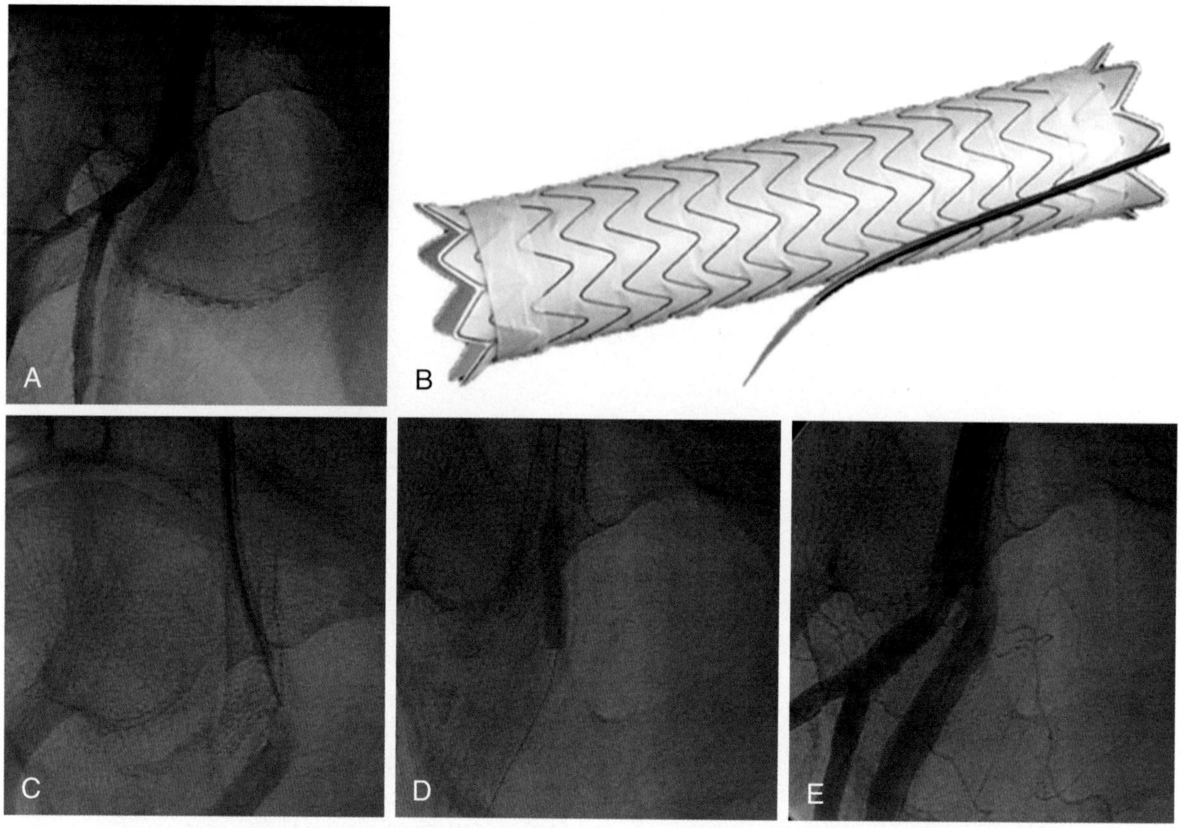

FIG. 7.3 The Neocarina Reconstruction Technique. (A) Femoral contrast angiography via the crossover sheath demonstrating superficial femoral artery (SFA) occlusion after Viabahn implantation. Schematic (B) and angiographic (C) representation of the Brockenbrough needle and Mullins sheath used to pass through Viabahn endoprosthesis. (D) Dilation with 5.5- × 20-mm balloon through the endoprosthesis. (E) Restoration of SFA patency with thrombolysis in myocardial infarction flow grade 3.

This "neocarina reconstruction" technique may be applied to manage vascular complications in various interventional procedures. However, the clinical impact of this new technique on the long-term patency of the stent graft and the need for close surveillance remain unclear.

Reference

1. Stortecky S, Wenaweser P, Diehm N, et al. Percutaneous management of vascular complications in patients undergoing transcatheter aortic valve implantation. *J Am Coll Cardiol Intv.* 2012;5:515-524.

Ascending Aorta to Main Pulmonary Artery Fistula After Orthotopic Heart Transplantation: Successful Percutaneous Closure Employing an Amplatzer Duct Occluder

Todd L. Kiefer, MD, John P. Vavalle, MD, Adam Devore, MD, Chetan B. Patel, MD, Joseph Rogers, MD, Carmelo Milano, MD, Thomas R. Gehrig, MD, J. Kevin Harrison, MD

A 60-year-old man with end-stage heart failure underwent orthotopic heart transplantation. Before transplantation, he had elevated pulmonary artery (PA) pressures (60/17 mm Hg; mean PA, 35 mm Hg) and pulmonary vascular resistance (PVR) (6.6 Wood units). After transplantation, he initially did well, with normalization of PA pressures (27/13 mm Hg; mean PA, 20 mm Hg). Several months later, however, he developed overt right-sided heart failure. Invasive hemodynamic evaluation demonstrated severe pulmonary hypertension (92/51 mm Hg; mean PA, 66 mm Hg) with a PVR of 10 Wood units. There was no evidence of allograft rejection or pulmonary embolism. Transthoracic echocardiogram demonstrated right ventricular (RV) systolic dysfunction and enlargement. Color flow Doppler imaging demonstrated continuous flow from the ascending aorta into the main PA. The anatomy was confirmed by computed tomographic angiographic imaging (Fig. 7.4).

Oximetry measured a modest left-to-right shunt at the PA level and no right-to-left shunt (Qp/Qs shunt fraction = 1.2:1). Percutaneous closure of the aorta-to-PA fistula was recommended.

A 6F Judkins Left 3.5 (Cordis Inc., Miami, Florida) guide catheter inserted via the right femoral artery engaged the fistula origin in the ascending aorta. Biplane angiography demonstrated the fistulous connection (Fig. 7.5 and Online Video 7.2, and Fig. 7.6 and Online Video 7.3).

A 0.035-inch Glidewire (Terumo Medical Corporation, Somerset, New Jersey) was advanced via the guide catheter through the fistulous connection into the PA and externalized out the right femoral vein using a 25-mm loop snare (ev3 Endovascular, Plymouth, Minnesota).

Based on computed tomographic and angiographic measurements (a sizing balloon would not cross the fistula), a 12/10 mm Amplatzer Duct Occluder was selected and deployed via a TorqVue delivery sheath (St. Jude Medical, St. Paul, Minnesota) (Fig. 7.7). Aortography confirmed stable and ideal positioning of the device within the fistula, with dramatic reduction of flow into the PA (Fig. 7.8, Online Video 7.4). The patient did well postprocedure without complications. At follow-up evaluation 4 months after the procedure, the patient reported improvement in his dyspnea, increased energy, and diminished peripheral edema. In addition, transthoracic echocardiogram demonstrated decreased RV size and Doppler-derived RV systolic pressure with no residual shunt.

Review of the literature failed to reveal a report of the posttransplantation complication described in our patient: formation of a fistula between the aorta and PA after heart transplantation. The approach described for percutaneous closure represents a novel and less morbid solution compared with further open cardiac surgery.

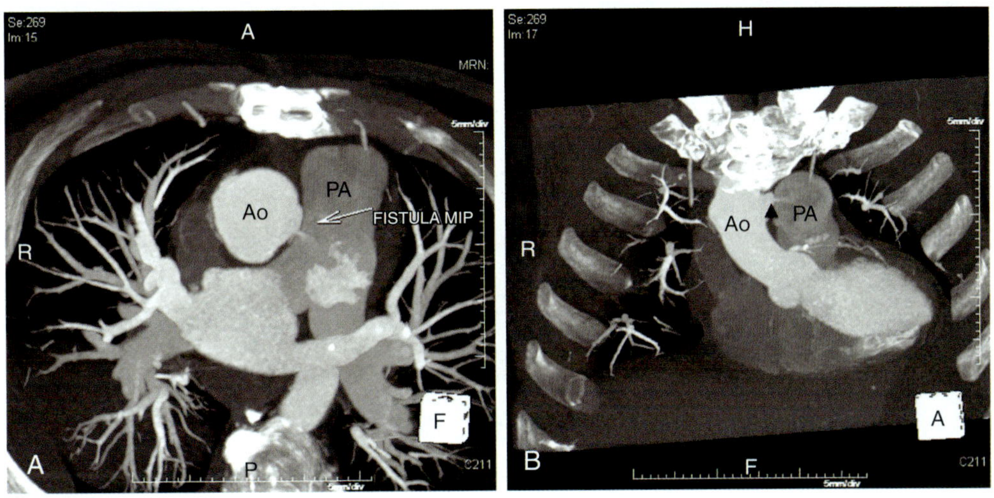

FIG. 7.4 Computed Tomographic Angiography (CTA) Imaging of the Aorta-to-Pulmonary Artery Fistula. (A) Axial oblique CTA image demonstrating contrast flow from the ascending aorta (*Ao*) into the distal main pulmonary artery (*PA*). (B) Coronal CTA image demonstrating contrast flow from the ascending Ao into the PA at a site of out-pouching along the inner curvature of the Ao (*arrowhead*). *A*, anterior; *F*, feet; *H*, head; *L*, left; *MIP*, maximum-intensity projection; *P*, posterior; *R*, right.

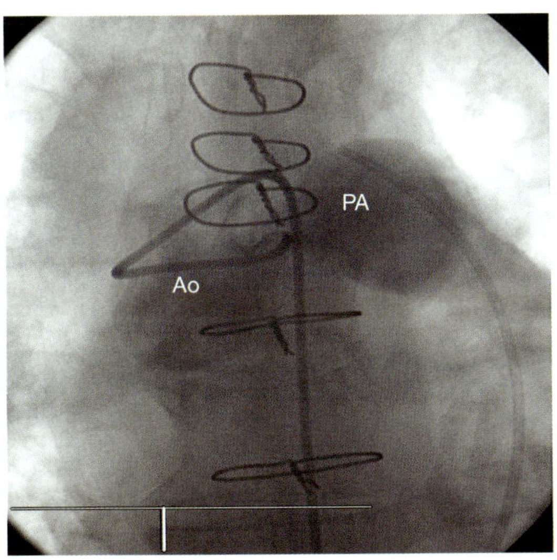

FIG. 7.5 Still Cineangiographic Image in the Straight Anterior-Posterior Projection. Note the flow from the ascending aorta (*Ao*) to the pulmonary artery (*PA*) (Online Video 7.2).

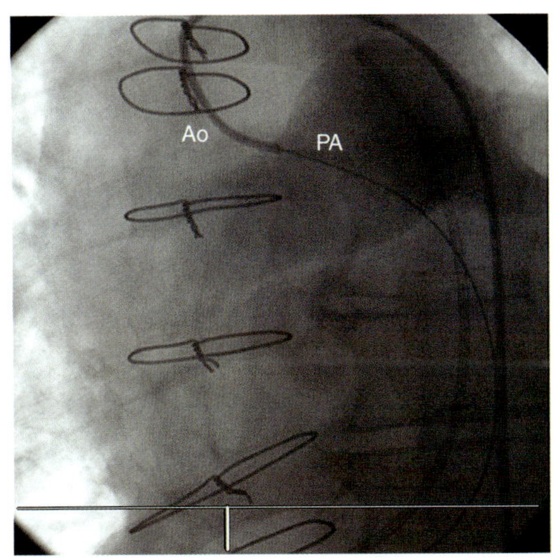

FIG. 7.6 Still Cineangiographic Image in the 16° Left Anterior Oblique Projection. Note the Judkins Left 3.5 guide catheter entering the fistula from the ascending aorta (*Ao*) and contrast opacifying the pulmonary artery (*PA*) (Online Video 7.3).

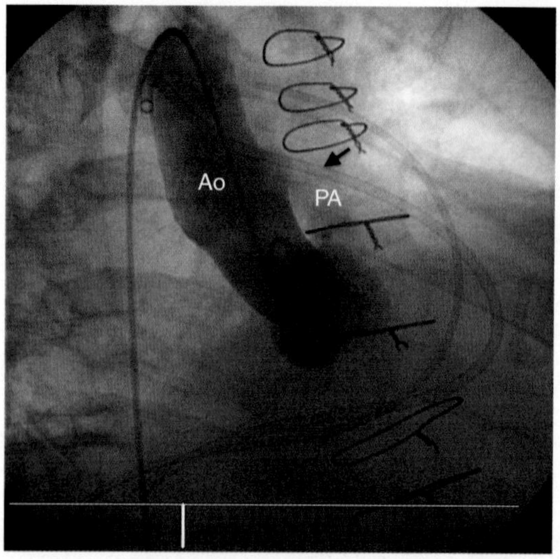

FIG. 7.7 Still Cineangiographic Image of the Ascending Aorta Viewed from 32° Right Anterior Oblique. Note the course of the 9F, 45° TorqVue delivery sheath (*arrow*) from the pulmonary artery (*PA*) into the aorta (*Ao*).

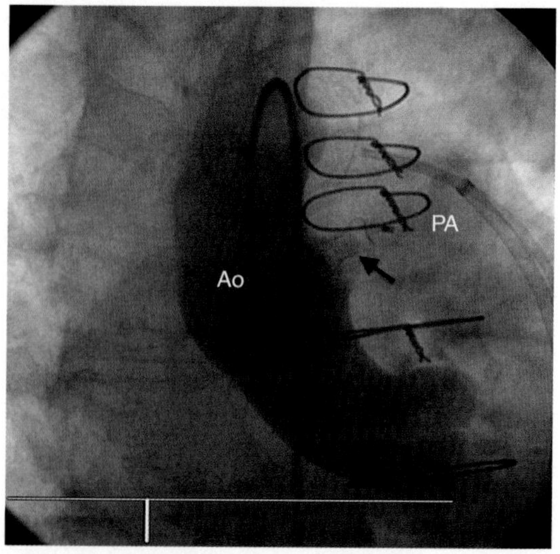

FIG. 7.8 Still Cineangiographic Image of the Ascending Aorta (18° Right Anterior Oblique). Note the stable position of the deployed 12/10 mm Amplatzer Duct Occluder device (*arrow*) and the absence of contrast flow from the aorta (*Ao*) into the pulmonary artery (*PA*) (Online Video 7.4).

Embolotherapy in Giant Pulmonary Arteriovenous Malformations: Blocking the Exit—Reducing the Risk of Periinterventional Stroke?

Christoph M. Happel, MD, PhD, Kamal Nashwan, MD, Harald Bertram, MD

Several publications report strokes early after embolotherapy for pulmonary arteriovenous malformations (pAVM).[1-3] Various mechanisms are discussed for this event, including embolization of newly formed thrombotic material originating from the aneurysmal sac after occlusion of the arterial feeder.[2]

To reduce the risk of periinterventional stroke in a 22-year-old woman with a giant pAVM (66 × 47 × 70 mm^3) (Fig. 7.9A–B, Online Video 7.5), after occlusion of the main feeding artery (16-mm vascular plug II), we additionally blocked the draining vein via a transseptally advanced 18-mm vascular plug II (both devices: AGA Medical Corporation, Plymouth, Minnesota) (Fig. 7.9C, Online Video 7.6). The patient recovered uneventfully; pulse oximetry rose from approximately 85% before intervention to 98%. Four months after embolotherapy, a computed tomography scan confirmed the excellent result (Fig. 7.9D). A minor residual pAVM was not targeted, because the patient refused a second procedure. Two years after embolotherapy, the patient is in good clinical condition with no neurologic sequelae.

References

1. Felix S, Jeannin S, Goizet C, et al. Stroke following pulmonary arteriovenous fistula embolization in a patient with HHT. *Neurology.* 2008;71:2012-2014.
2. Mager JJ, Overtoom TTC, Blauw H, Lammers JWJ, Westermann CJJ. Embolotherapy of pulmonary arteriovenous malformations: long-term results in 112 patients. *J Vasc Interv Radiol.* 2004;15: 451-456.
3. Dutton JAE, Jackson JE, Hughes JMB, et al. Pulmonary arteriovenous malformations: results of treatment with coil embolization in 53 patients. *AJR Am J Roentgenol.* 1995;165:1119-1125.

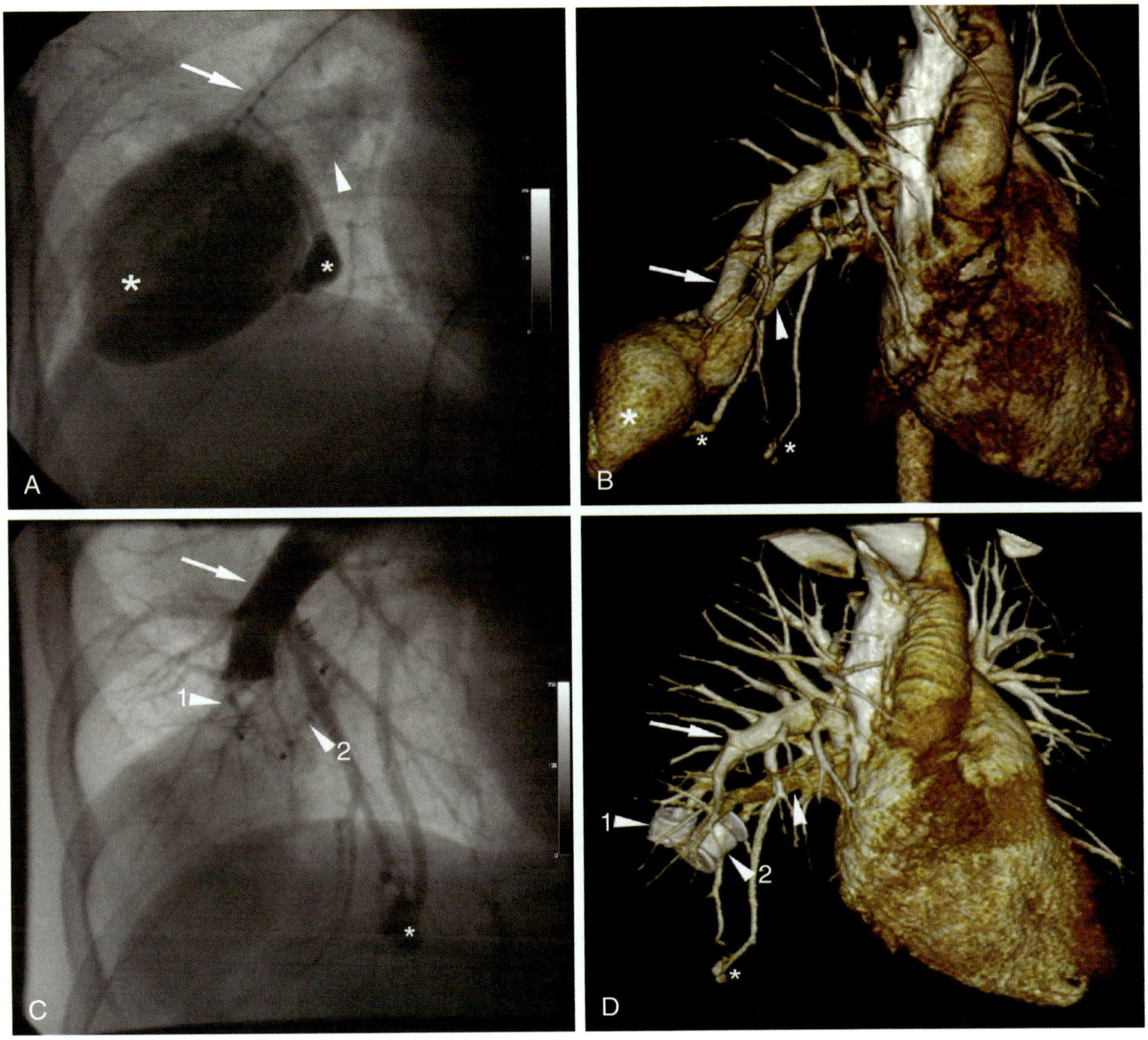

FIG. 7.9 Pulmonary Arteriovenous Malformation (pAVM) Before and After Intervention. (A) Angiography demonstrating the giant pAVM and an additional pAVM (Online Video 7.5). (B) Three-dimensional computed tomography (3D-CT) reconstruction before intervention. (C) Angiography after placement of both vascular plugs (Online Video 7.6). (D) 3D-CT reconstruction 4 months after occlusion showing complete occlusion of the giant pAVM, a residual smaller pAVM, and normal-sized pulmonary vessels. *Arrow*, feeding artery; *arrowhead*, draining vein; *large asterisk*, giant pAVM; *small asterisks*, additional pAVMs; *arrowhead 1*, arterial vascular plug; *arrowhead 2*, venous vascular plug.

Endovascular Repair of Ruptured Pseudoaneurysm of Left Internal Mammary Graft After Redo Aortic Valve Replacement and Coronary Artery Bypass Grafting

Sanjeev U. Nair, MBBS, MD, Nainesh C. Patel, MD, David A. Cox, MD

Pseudoaneurysm of internal mammary arteries may be asymptomatic or present within weeks after a sternotomy procedure with features such as chest swelling, atypical chest pain, and angina or rarely with rupture and exsanguination.[1–3]

A 62-year-old man who had undergone coronary artery bypass grafting and aortic mechanical valve replacement presented a decade later with angina and dyspnea. He was found to have a partially thrombosed aortic prosthetic valve. The patient underwent a reoperation with aortic bioprosthetic valve replacement. Two weeks later the patient was readmitted with acute chest pain and ST-T changes on the electrocardiogram. Urgent coronary angiography showed the previously placed coronary artery grafts to be patent. However, there was a large (1 × 1 cm) pseudoaneurysm of the left internal mammary artery (LIMA) graft with leakage of contrast into the mediastinum at the site of the pseudoaneurysm, suggesting an associated rupture (Fig. 7.10, Online Video 7.7). Utilizing the femoral arterial approach, a 7F LIMA guide was used to wire the LIMA, and a 3.0- × 26-mm covered Jostent stent graft (Jomed International AB, Helsingborg, Sweden) was placed and inflated to 19 atm. This completely sealed the ruptured pseudoaneurysm, and postdilation was done with a 3.0 Quantum balloon to 20 atm (Fig. 7.11, Online Video 7.8). An excellent result was obtained, with thrombolysis in myocardial infarction flow grade 3 distally. There was good flow down to the left anterior descending coronary artery (LAD) with some evidence of wire spasm, which improved with intracoronary nitroglycerine. The LAD diagonal, as well as the collaterals to the right coronary artery, were patent. Multiple angiographic views were taken that showed no evidence of further extravasation of contrast (Fig. 7.12, Online Video 7.9). The patient was eventually discharged home on dual-antiplatelet therapy (aspirin and clopidogrel).

Thus, a ruptured pseudoaneurysm of an internal mammary graft can be successfully and safely repaired percutaneously using a covered stent; this avoids the risks and complications associated with sternotomy.

References

1. Martin A, Ross BA, Braimbridge MV. Peristernal wiring in closure of median sternotomy. False aneurysm of the internal mammary artery. *J Thorac Cardiovasc Surg.* 1973;66:145-146.
2. Frank MW, Alexander JC Jr., Pineless GR, Votapka TV, Curran RD. False aneurysm of the right internal mammary artery. Late rupture after sternotomy. *Tex Heart Inst J.* 1998;25:86-87.
3. Kamath S, Unsworth-White J, Wells IP. Pseudoaneurysm of the internal mammary artery as an unusual cause of post-sternotomy hemorrhage: the role of multislice computed tomography in the diagnosis and treatment planning. *Cardiovasc Intervent Radiol.* 2005;28:246-248.

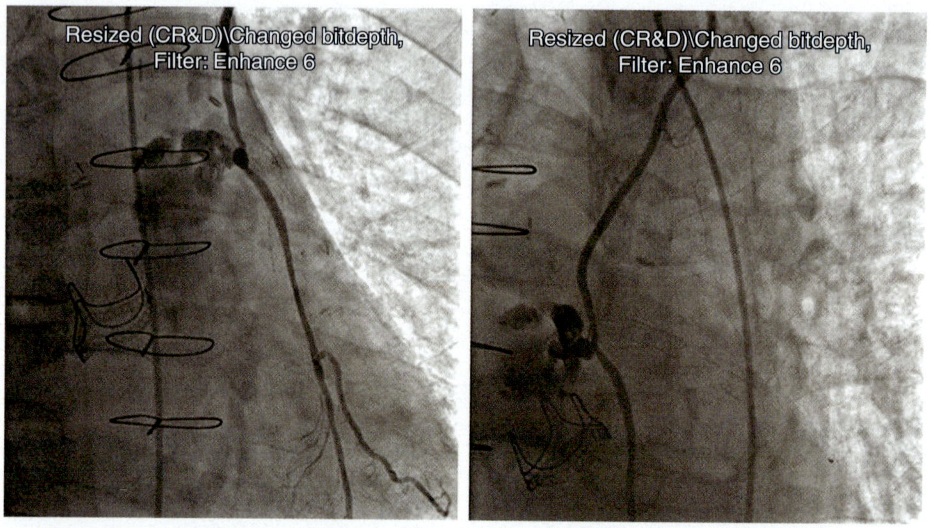

FIG. 7.10 Right Anterior Oblique and Left Anterior Oblique Views, Respectively, by Coronary Angiography. These views demonstrate a large (1 × 1 cm) pseudoaneurysm in the midsection of the left internal mammary artery graft with associated rupture as suggested by contrast leakage into the mediastinum (Online Video 7.7). The *left panel* shows the right anterior oblique view, and the *right panel* shows the left anterior oblique view.

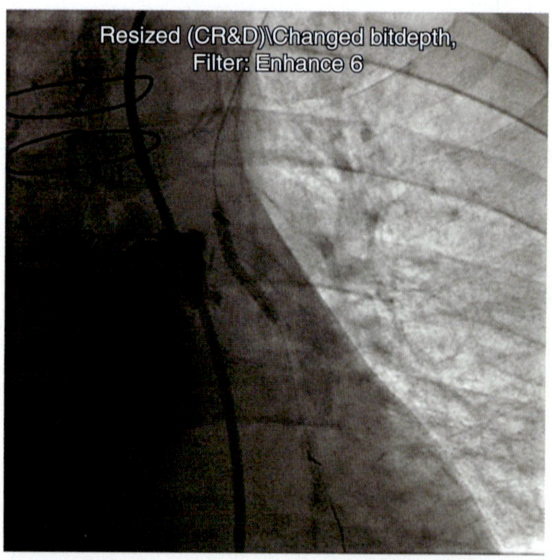

FIG. 7.11 Covered Stent (Jostent) Placement at the Site of the Ruptured Pseudoaneurysm in the Left Internal Mammary Artery (LIMA) Graft. By the femoral arterial route, a 7F LIMA guide was used to wire the LIMA. A 3.0- × 26-mm covered Jostent stent (Jomed International AB, Helsingborg, Sweden) was placed at the site of the rupture and inflated to 19 atm pressure (Online Video 7.8).

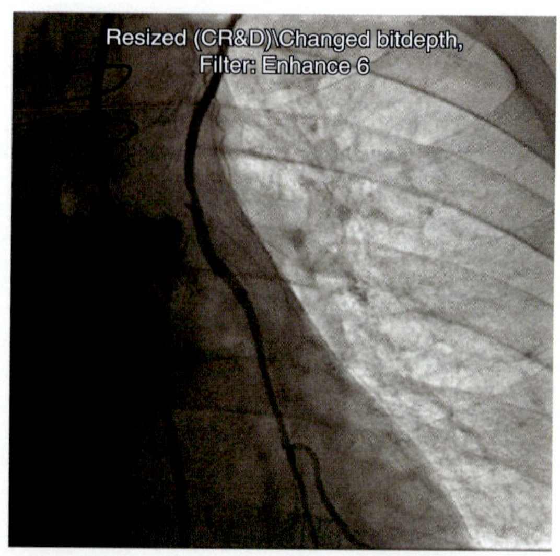

FIG. 7.12 Poststent Left Internal Mammary Artery (LIMA) Graft With Good Distal Thrombolysis In Myocardial Infarction (TIMI) Flow. TIMI flow grade 3 was obtained distally after placement of covered stent (Jostent) at the site of the ruptured LIMA graft pseudoaneurysm (Online Video 7.9). The associated rupture is completely sealed off as evidenced by lack of contrast extravasation.

Endovascular Stenting of Suture Line Supravalvular Pulmonic Stenosis After Orthotopic Heart Transplantation Using Rapid Pacing Stabilization

Justin Z. Lee, MD, Kwan S. Lee, MD, Aiden Abidov, MD, Ricardo A. Samson, MD, Kapildeo Lotun, MD

A 61-year-old woman, 6 months after orthotopic heart transplantation (OHT), presented with gradual-onset class III dyspnea and fatigue for 4 months. Her transplantation procedure was significant for right ventricular sternal adhesions after left ventricular assist device placement and significant size mismatch between the donor and recipient aortas, requiring fashioning of the donor aorta to correct the mismatch. A computed tomography angiogram (Fig. 7.13) showed an eccentric anastomotic line supravalvular stenosis 1.5 cm distal to the pulmonic valve, 1.4 × 2.0 cm at the narrowest portion with poststenotic dilation of 4.0 cm. Right ventricular systolic pressure (RVSP) was 60 mm Hg + central venous pressure with supravalvular flow acceleration.

The proximity of the stenosis to the pulmonary valve led to an unsuccessful initial angioplasty attempt because there was persistent distal migration of the balloon during inflation and an inability to maintain a stable balloon position. The procedure was reattempted with angioplasty and stenting using a Palmaz 39 10-mm balloon-expandable stent (Cordis, Miami, Florida) mounted on a balloon-in-balloon 20- × 40-mm balloon (NuMED, Hopkinton, New York) using a rapid pacing stabilization technique with transesophageal echocardiographic guidance (Figs. 7.14, 7.15). Postdilation was then performed with a Tyshak II 25- × 40-mm balloon (B. Braun, Bethlehem, Pennsylvania) (Fig. 7.16). The procedure was successful with reduction of the peak gradient from 22 mm Hg to 3 mm Hg and

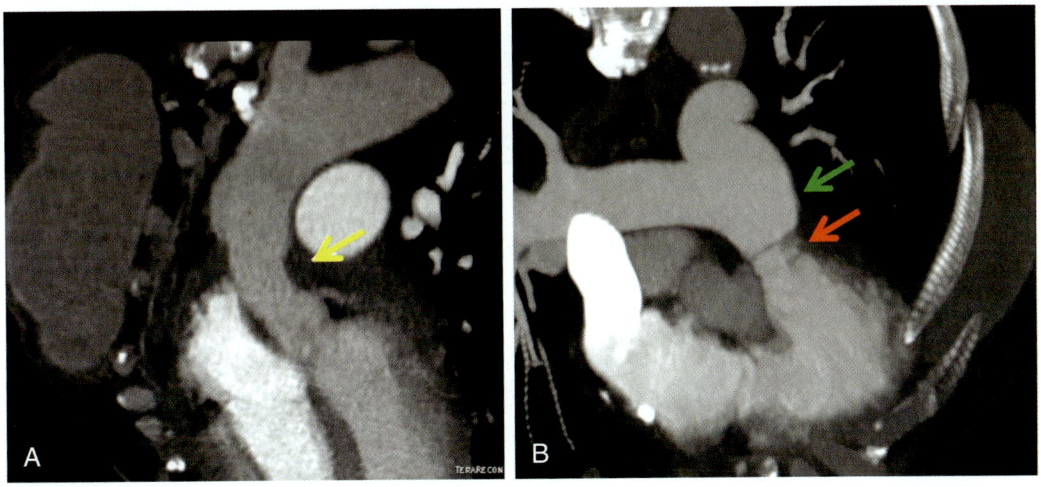

FIG. 7.13 Computed Tomography Angiogram Showing Pulmonary and Aortic Anastomosis Stenotic Lesions After Orthotopic Heart Transplantation. Computed tomography angiogram showing great vessel anastomotic lesions after orthotopic heart transplantation. (A) Focal proximal aortic stenosis (*yellow arrow*) that was hemodynamically insignificant. (B) Proximal main pulmonary artery stenosis (*red arrow*) with poststenotic dilation (*green arrow*). The stenosis was hemodynamically significant, with a gradient across the lesion of 22 mm Hg, and a right ventricular systolic pressure of 60 mm Hg + central venous pressure.

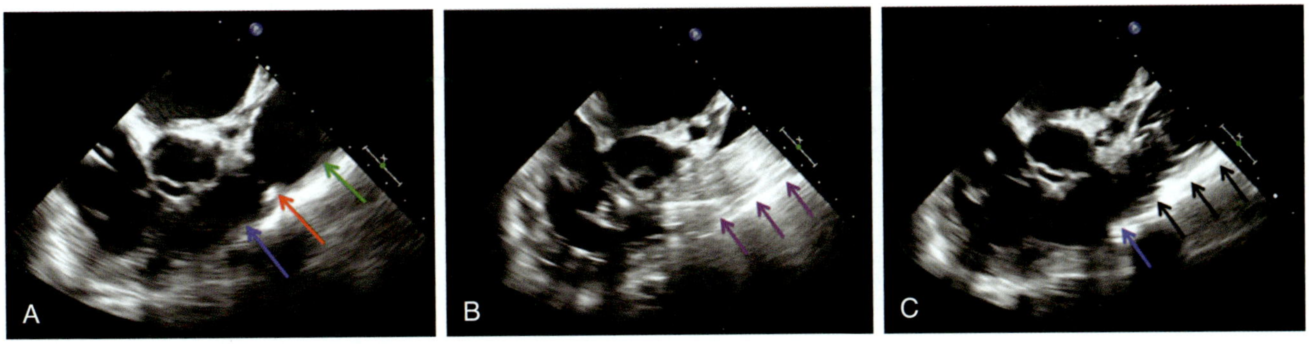

FIG. 7.14 Intraprocedural Transesophageal Echocardiographic Images of Pulmonary Stenosis Intervention. (A) Preprocedural modified mid upper esophageal transesophageal echocardiographic view of the great vessels showing supravalvular pulmonic stenosis in the area of surgical anastomosis after orthotopic heart transplantation (*red arrow*), 15 mm distal to the pulmonary valve (*blue arrow*). Poststenotic dilation of main pulmonary artery (*green arrow*) is also seen in this view. (B) Tyshak II balloon deployment (*purple arrows*). (C) Final stent position (*black arrows*) above pulmonary valve (*blue arrow*).

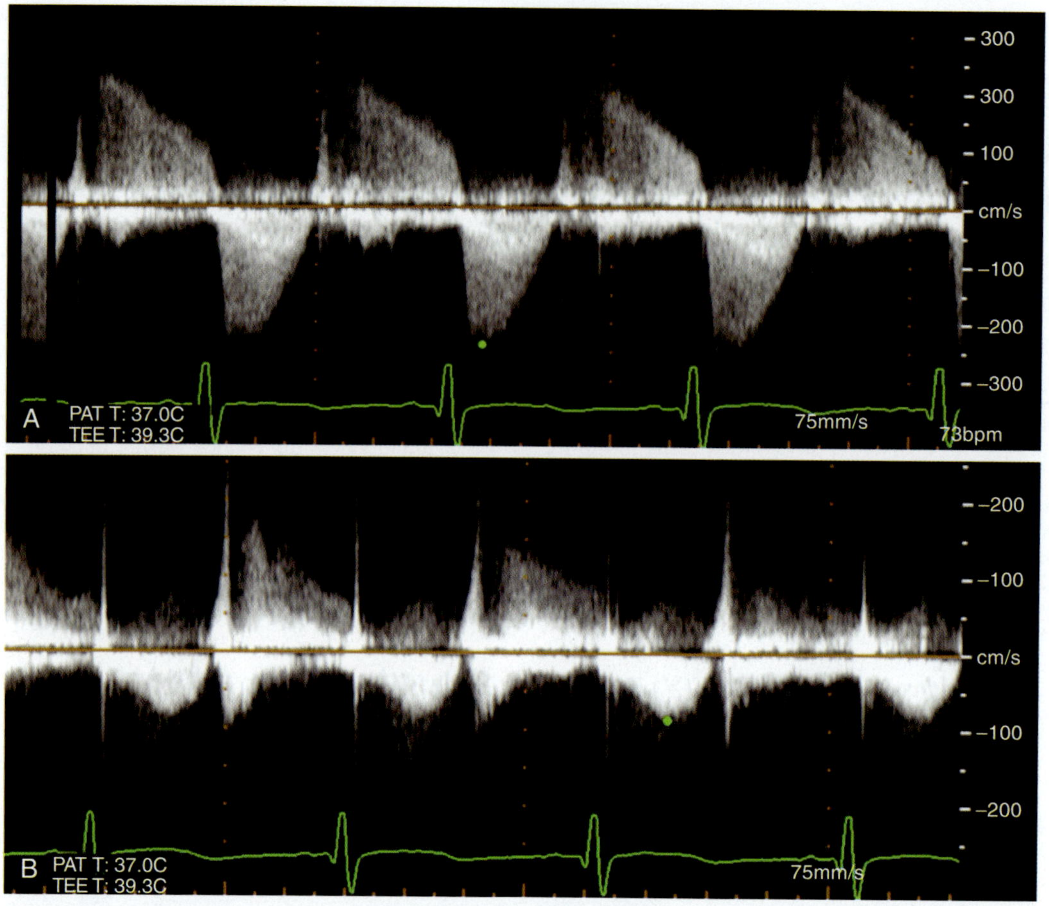

FIG. 7.15 Translesional Stenosis Gradients by Doppler Assessment Before and After Procedure. Images show continuous-wave (CW) Doppler findings across the main pulmonary artery lesion before the intervention (A) and immediately after the balloon valvuloplasty and stent implantation (B). CW recordings document a decrease in pressure gradient across the lesion from 22 to 3 mm Hg. There was evidence of mild pulmonary regurgitation before the procedure with no worsening after the procedure.

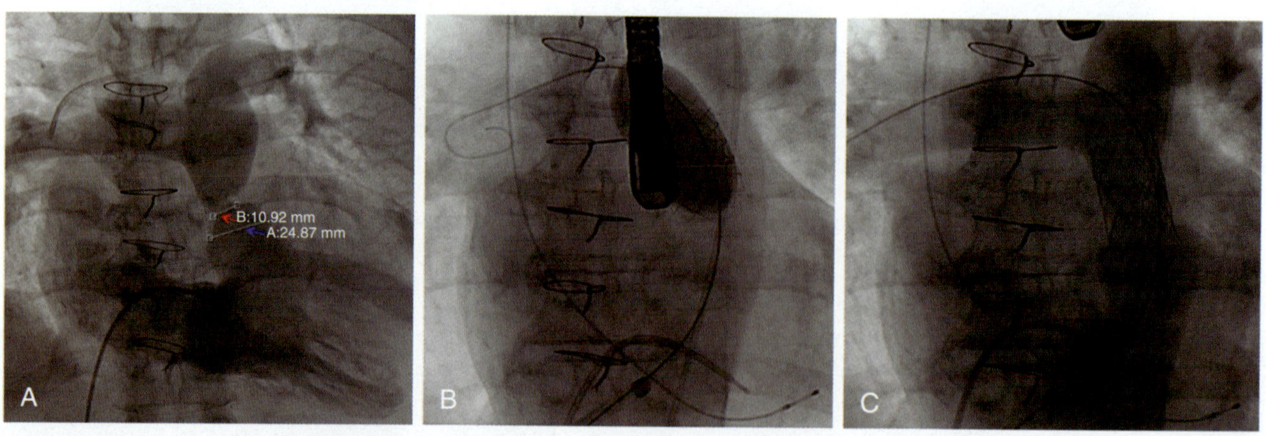

FIG. 7.16 Right-Sided Heart Angiography Before and After Stent Deployment. (A) Initial right ventriculogram showing normal pulmonary valve annulus (*blue arrow, A*: 24.9 mm) and supravalvular pulmonic stenosis (*red arrow, B*: 10.9 mm). (B) Postdilation of a Palmaz 39- × 10-mm stent with a Tyshak II 25- × 40-mm balloon during rapid ventricular pacing. (C) Poststent right ventriculogram.

resulting peak RVSP reduction from 70 mm Hg to 51 mm Hg with minimal pulmonary artery diameter increase from 1.4 cm to 2.2 cm. The patient's fatigue and dyspnea resolved.

This is the first described case of suture line supravalvular pulmonic stenosis post-OHT and highlights the possibility of successful endovascular therapy using rapid pacing as a stabilization technique for device deployment. Intraprocedural transesophageal echocardiographic imaging was instrumental in positioning the stent secondary to the proximity of the pulmonary valve.

Extravasation From an Accessory Renal Artery: A Critical Complication Associated With Percutaneous Coronary Intervention

Nobuaki Kobayashi, MD, Noritake Hata, MD, Tomoyuki Kuwako, MD, Wataru Shimizu, MD

A 72-year-old woman was admitted with acute anterior ST-segment elevation myocardial infarction and underwent emergency primary percutaneous coronary intervention (PCI) at the mid portion of the left anterior descending coronary artery. After the procedure, she suffered from shock and severe abdominal pain. Enhanced computed tomography showed marked perirenal hematoma (Fig. 7.17). An aortogram revealed that the left kidney was supplied by double renal arteries and that an accessory renal artery originated from the L3-L4 intervertebral disk level and traveled in parallel with the aorta (Fig. 7.18A, Online Video 7.10). Furthermore, a selective injection demonstrated that the extravasation occurred from the left accessory renal artery (Fig. 7.18B–C, Online Video 7.11). Transcatheter embolization with Gelfoam (Pfizer, Tokyo, Japan) was performed, and final angiograms showed complete embolization of the left accessory renal artery in the absence of extravasation (Fig. 7.19A–C, Online Videos 7.12 and 7.13).

In the present case, it was suspected that the extravasation was caused during the primary PCI when a 0.035-inch guidewire was used to advance a guiding catheter. Guidewire penetration into the left accessory renal artery went undetected because the accessory renal artery originated from a lower level and traveled in parallel with the aorta. Renal artery variations are common; in a previous report, the frequency of a left accessory renal artery was found to be 13%.[1] However, the frequency of left accessory renal arteries originating from regions lower than lumbar spine L3 has been reported to be only 6% of all left accessory renal arteries.[1]

Reference

1. Özkan U, Ogvuzkurt L, Tercan F, Kizilkiliç O, Koç Z, Koca N. Renal artery origins and variations: angiographic evaluation of 855 consecutive patients. *Diagn Interv Radiol.* 2006;12:183-186.

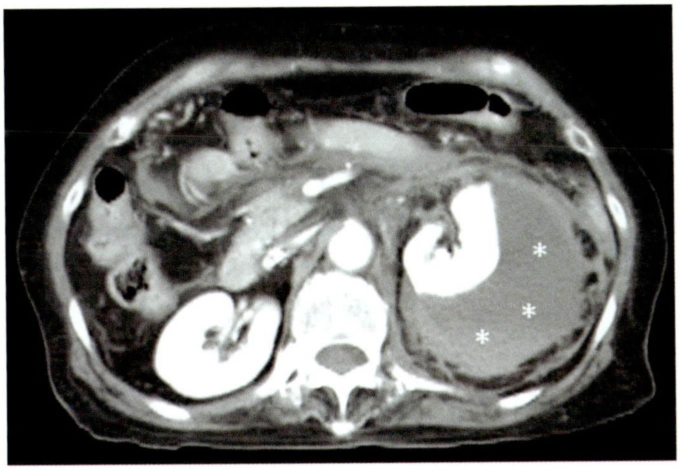

FIG. 7.17 Enhanced Abdominal Computed Tomography. Computed tomography showed marked left perirenal hematoma (*asterisks*).

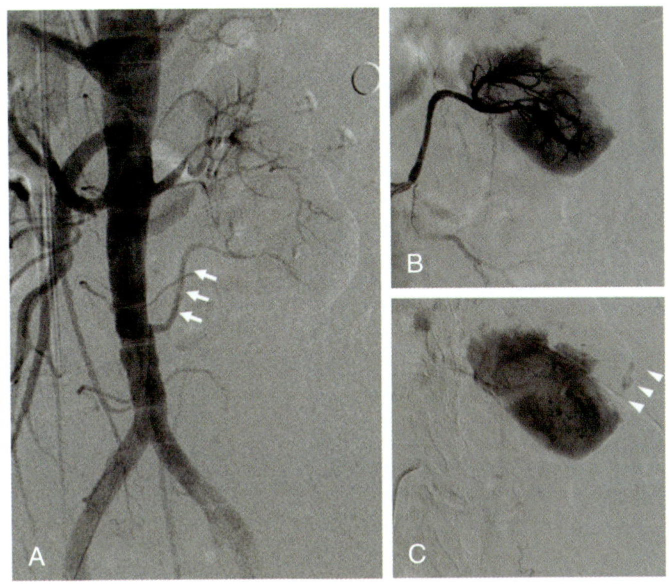

FIG. 7.18 Initial Angiograms of Abdominal Arteries. (A) An abdominal aortogram. The left kidney is supplied with double renal arteries. *White arrows* show the left accessory renal artery originating from the L3-L4 intervertebral disk level and traveling in parallel with the aorta (Online Video 7.10). Early- (B) and late- (C) phase selective left accessory renal arteriograms (Online Video 7.11). *White arrowheads* show extravasation from the left accessory renal artery.

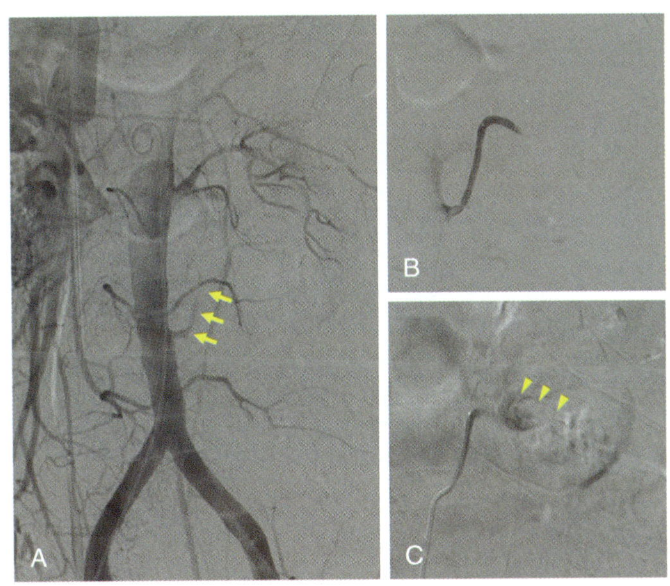

FIG. 7.19 Posttranscatheter Embolization Angiograms for Abdominal Arteries. An abdominal aortogram (A) (Online Video 7.12) and early- (B) and late- (C) phase selective left accessory renal arteriograms (Online Video 7.13). *Yellow arrows* show the complete embolization of the accessory renal artery. Extravasation is not observed (*yellow arrowheads*).

Iatrogenic Aortocoronary Arteriovenous Fistula: Percutaneous Management of a Surgical Complication

Zaher Fanari, MD, Jhapat Thapa, MD, Armin Barekatain, MD, MSC, Kevin Copeland, DO, James T. Hopkins, MD

Iatrogenic aortocoronary arteriovenous fistula (ACAVF) resulting from placement of an arterial graft to a cardiac vein is a rare complication of coronary artery bypass grafting (CABG).[1,2] Most patients present postoperatively with angina as a result of residual ischemia that is due to either an unbypassed artery or a coronary steal syndrome (CSS). A 74-year-old woman presented with recurrence of angina with a history of multivessel coronary artery disease after CABG in 2006 with a left internal mammary artery (LIMA) Y graft to the left anterior descending and first diagonal coronary arteries, and sequential saphenous vein graft (SVG) to the circumflex obtuse marginal and the posterior descending arteries, and recurrent angina secondary to an occluded SVG resulting in a second CABG with a free radial graft anastomosed to the LIMA and then placed sequentially to the obtuse marginal and posterior descending arteries. Coronary angiography showed that the radial graft was in reality anastomosed to the left circumflex vein (Fig. 7.20A–B). This iatrogenic fistula resulted in a dilated tortuous LIMA and radial grafts with possible CSS that explained the ischemia. Given that the patient was not a candidate for a third surgery and that medical therapy was not controlling the patient's angina, a decision for percutaneous closure was made. An initial attempt with coil embolization of the coronary vein was unsuccessful because the interlock coils did not deploy appropriately. A deployment of a 3-mm Amplatzer vascular plug II (St. Jude Medical, Saint Paul, Minnesota) was successful, with no residual flow into the coronary sinus from the radial graft (Fig. 7.20C–F). In summary, ACAVF is a rare but serious complication of CABG that may result in ischemia secondary to CSS or high-output heart failure when a significant degree of left-to-right shunting develops over time. Percutaneous closure by embolization with either detachable balloons or coils[3] or deployment of a vascular plug offers an effective and safe management for symptomatic patients.

References

1. Seabra-Gomes R, Ross DN, Gonzalez-Lavin L. Iatrogenic left ventricular–right atrial fistula following mitral valve replacement. *Thorax.* 1973;28:235-241.
2. Renard VP, Vandenbogaerde J. Fistula between the left internal thoracic artery and the coronary sinus. *N Engl J Med.* 2000;343:149-150.
3. White RW, Sivananthan MU, Kay PH. Aorto-coronary bypass graft fistula after surgical treatment of circumflex coronary artery fistula: a unique variation of a rare condition successfully treated with percutaneous embolization. *Interact Cardiovasc Thorac Surg.* 2010;10:256-257.

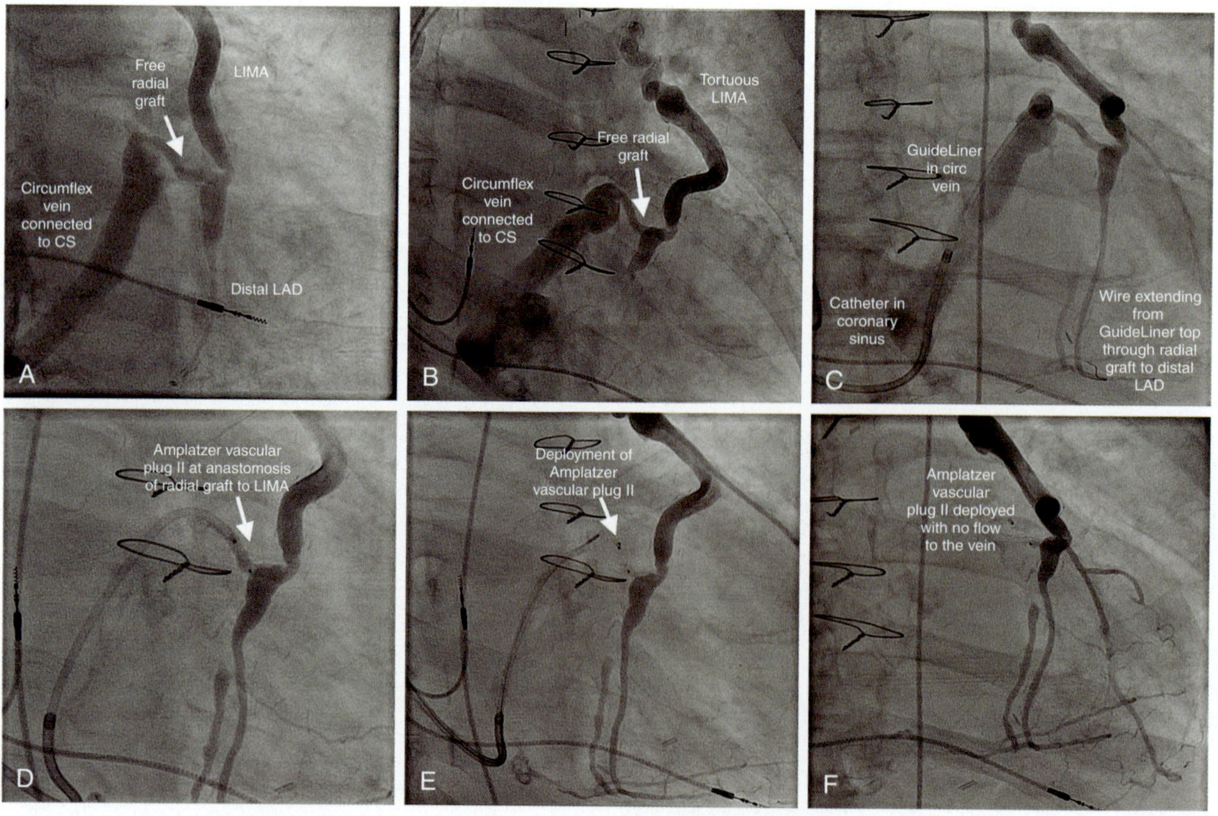

FIG. 7.20 Selective Left Internal Mammary Artery (LIMA) Graft Angiography Showing Iatrogenic Aortocoronary Arteriovenous Fistula. (A) Free radial graft connecting the LIMA graft to the circumflex vein. *CS*, coronary sinus, *LAD*, left anterior descending coronary artery. (B) Large tortuous LIMA filling a large circumflex vein draining to the CS. (C) Percutaneous procedure with a catheter placed through the CS with the GuideLiner XL catheter (Vascular Solutions Inc., Minneapolis, Minnesota) extending beyond the catheter tip to the level of the radial graft–vein anastomosis. *Circ*, circumflex. (D) The Amplatzer vascular plug II at the level of LIMA–radial graft anastomosis. (E) Deployment of the Amplatzer vascular plug II. (F) Amplatzer vascular plug II in place with no residual flow from the LIMA to the circumflex vein.

Percutaneous Plugging of an Ascending Aortic Pseudoaneurysm

Ravinay Bhindi, MBBS, PhD, James Newton, MB ChB, Neil Wilson, MBBS, Oliver J. Ormerod, DM

A 76-year-old woman presented to hospital with a 1-month history of progressively worsening central chest pain. Her medical history was remarkable for a previous aortic valve replacement with an ascending aortic interposition graft 10 years earlier.

A computed tomography (CT) scan showed a large ascending aortic pseudoaneurysm with aortic communication through a defect at the superior aspect of the structure, below the level of the innominate vessels. Given the position of the pseudoaneurysm, the risk of repeat sternotomy was thought too high. Furthermore, the abdominal aorta was severely diseased and tortuous, making potential delivery of a covered stent difficult. It was therefore decided to attempt to close the mouth of the defect percutaneously.

Vascular access was achieved via the right brachial artery, and aortography showed moderate dehiscence at the posterior aspect of the superior margin of the interposition graft (Fig. 7.21A, Online Video 7.14). Adjuvant intracardiac echocardiography (ICE) was performed with the imaging catheter in the superior vena cava and showed a leak from the true aortic lumen into the false cavity (Fig. 7.21B). A 6F Judkins Right catheter was used with a 0.035-inch exchange-length wire to enter the defect, and contrast injection through the catheter further defined the anatomy of the cavity (Fig. 7.21C). Balloon sizing was performed with a 10-mm Cristal balloon (Fig. 7.21C), and a 7F Amplatzer TorqVue sheath was then used to deliver a 10-mm Amplatzer atrial septal defect device. This resulted in immediate reduction in flow into the defect by repeat aortography and ICE (Fig. 7.21D–E; Online Videos 7.15 and 7.16). A second CT scan 2 days later confirmed obliteration of the defect and thrombosis of the cavity (Fig. 7.21G).

Focal percutaneous sealing of ascending thoracic aneurysms has been successfully used previously by others[1]; however, to our knowledge this is the first case to use the brachial access approach in the setting of previous aortic graft surgery with adjuvant ICE imaging. In cases where surgical correction is deemed too high-risk and stent coverage not feasible, such an approach can be considered.

Reference

1. Kanani RS, Neilan TG, Palacios IF, Garasic JM. Novel use of the Amplatzer septal occluder device in the percutaneous closure of ascending aortic pseudoaneurysms: a case series. *Catheter Cardiovasc Interv.* 2007;69:146-153.

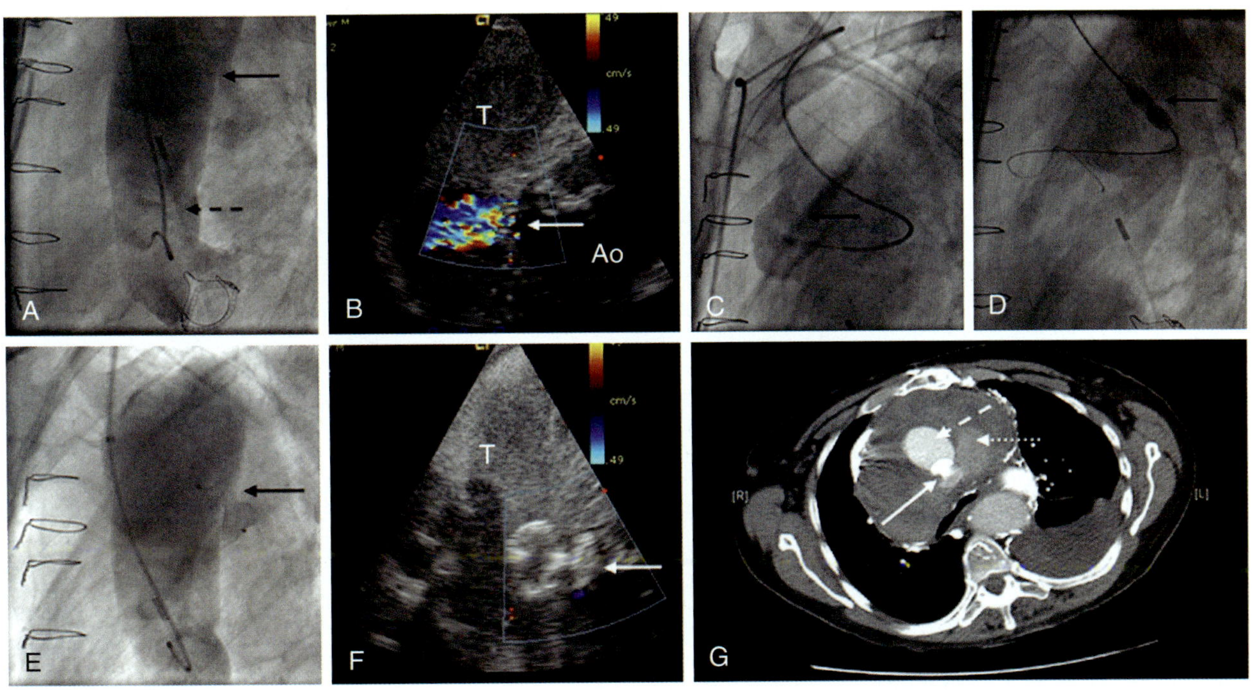

FIG. 7.21 Images Illustrating Percutaneous Closure of the Aortic Pseudoaneurysm. (A) Ascending thoracic aortography performed via the right brachial artery shows a leak (*solid arrow*) into a pseudoaneurysm cavity. An intracardiac echocardiography (ICE) probe (*dashed arrow*) is shown in the superior vena cava. (B) The ICE appearances of the pseudoaneurysm cavity, which are partly thrombosed (*T*). Blood is seen flowing through the defect in the aortic wall (*arrow*), from the true aortic lumen (*Ao*) into the false cavity. (C) Contrast opacification of the pseudoaneurysm cavity (*arrow*) via a Judkins Right catheter placed inside the defect shows its large size. (D) Balloon sizing (*arrow*) of the defect, showing the position of the orifice of the cavity. (E) An Amplatzer atrial septal defect (ASD) device (*arrow*) is shown deployed across the defect with a second aortogram showing no significant filling of the pseudoaneurysm. (F) An ICE showing position of the device across the defect with abolition of flow on color flow Doppler. Organizing thrombus (*T*) is also seen within the pseudocavity. (G) Computed tomography scan demonstrating thrombosis of the pseudocavity (*dotted arrow*) with the ASD occlusion device (*solid arrow*) seen in position (the true lumen of the ascending thoracic aorta is shown by the *dashed arrow*).

Inferior Vena Cava Filter Thrombosis and Suprarenal Caval Stenosis: A Double Whammy

Mohamad Alkhouli, MD, Irfan Shafi, MD, Riyaz Bashir, MBBS

Inferior vena cava (IVC) thrombosis associated with filters is not uncommon in clinical practice. However, suprarenal extension of the thrombosis to the hepatic segment of the IVC is very rare, particularly in the absence of renal or hepatic tumors.[1] Benign intrinsic IVC stenosis is a rare anomaly that has been associated with IVC thrombosis.[2] We describe a case of extensive IVC thrombosis secondary to perihepatic IVC stenosis (documented by intravascular ultrasound [IVUS]) and a permanent IVC filter, which was successfully treated by endovascular techniques.

A 38-year-old male smoker presented with back pain and left leg swelling for 1 week. He had no medical or surgical history except for a motor vehicle accident 18 years previously, which led to left hip surgery and a prophylactic IVC filter placement. He was not taking any medications and had no family history of venous thromboembolism or hypercoagulable state. On physical examination, he had a markedly swollen and tender left leg and thigh with moderate skin erythema. He had normal pulses and no evidence of skin breakdown or ulceration. Duplex ultrasound showed acute deep vein thrombosis (DVT) of the left common femoral vein, and no evidence of DVT in the right leg. A computed tomography venogram showed massive IVC filter–associated thrombosis with totally occluded infrarenal IVC and suprarenal extension of the thrombus all the way up to hepatic segment. It also suggested a possible stenosis of the perihepatic IVC (Fig. 7.22).

In view of the severe and disabling symptoms in this young man, we decide to proceed with catheter-directed thrombolysis (CDT). A 50-cm EKOS catheter (EKOS, Bothell, Washington) was positioned from the hepatic segment of the IVC to the left femoral vein, and tissue plasminogen activator was infused over 16 h. While undergoing CDT, he noted complete resolution of his back pain. Post-CDT venography showed complete lysis of the thrombus above the IVC filter and a severe stenosis of the IVC just below the hepatic veins (Fig. 7.23, Online Video 7.17). The latter was confirmed by IVUS, as well as pressure gradient measurement (Fig. 7.23, Online Video 7.18). Minimal clot lysis was noted below the filter and was treated with mechanical thrombectomy followed by balloon angioplasty and stenting. In view of the IVUS findings and a pressure gradient of 18 mm Hg across the lesion in the hepatic IVC, we went on to treat it with a self-expanding (24 × 70 mm) wall stent with excellent angiographic and hemodynamic results (Fig. 7.23). On 1-week follow-up, he had complete resolution of his lower extremity swelling and pain. At 6 months, he continued to be asymptomatic with patent stents and no evidence of recurrent DVT (Fig. 7.24). In most cases, IVC filter–related thrombosis is seen below or a few centimeters above the filter.[1] Extension of clot all the way up to the

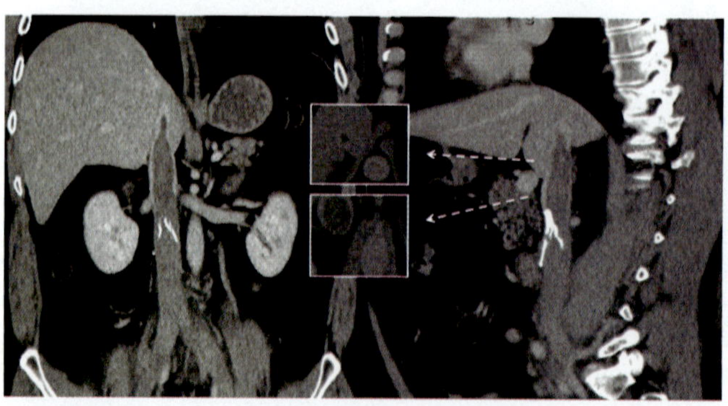

FIG. 7.22 Computed Tomography Scan (Coronal and Lateral Views) Showing Massive Inferior Vena Cava Thrombosis Extending to the Hepatic Segment. *Upper inset* is a cross-sectional view showing severe stenosis/near obliteration of the inferior vena cava. *Lower inset* is a cross-sectional view of the suprarenal inferior vena cava showing severe thrombosis.

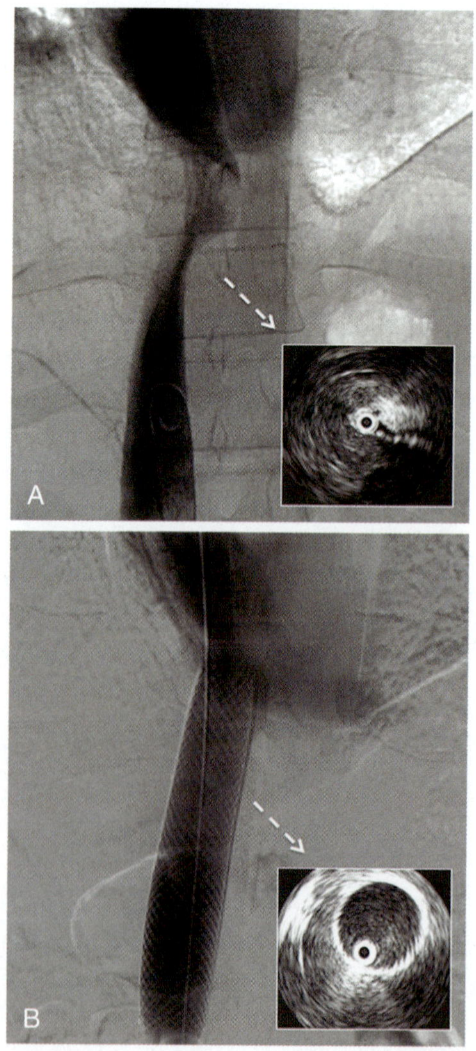

FIG. 7.23 Inferior Vena Cava Stenosis Below the Hepatic Veins. (A) Cavogram (Online Video 7.17) and intravascular ultrasound (Online Video 7.18) after catheter-directed thrombolysis showing inferior vena cava stenosis below the hepatic veins. (B) Poststent imaging showed excellent angiographic and ultrasonographic results. *Insets* are intravascular ultrasound cross-sectional views of the inferior vena cava before (A) and after (B) stenting.

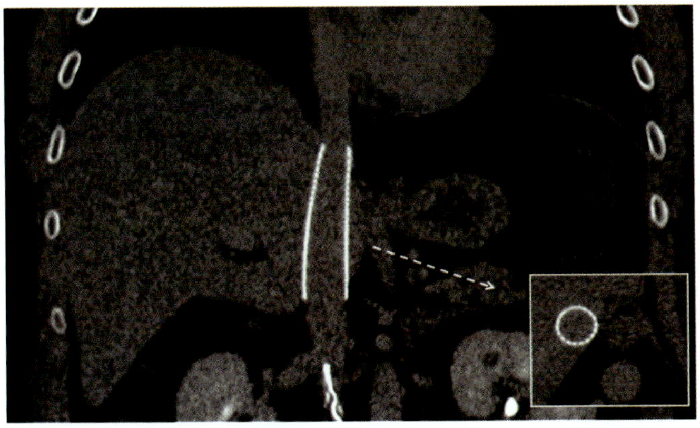

FIG. 7.24 Patent Stent at 3 Months. Computed tomography scan at 3 months showing a well-opposed patent stent in the suprarenal inferior vena cava. *Inset* is a cross-sectional view.

hepatic segment is usually seen in patients with hepatic or nephric tumors, which either invade or compress the IVC.[1,2] Benign intrinsic IVC stenosis is very rare (<0.1%) but is known to be associated with massive caval thrombosis.[2] The most common location for this stenosis is around the perihepatic region of the IVC. The exact pathogenesis of such lesions is not well understood. Some authors suggest that it is a congenital anomaly related to abnormal fusion of the vitelline and the subcardinal veins in utero,[3] whereas others propose that it is an acquired condition caused by healed thrombosis producing intravascular membrane or web formations.[4]

This case suggests that patients with IVC stenosis who are undergoing IVC filter placement may be at particularly high risk for extensive IVC thrombosis, including very high suprarenal extension. Hence there is a need for the very judicious use of IVC filters in these patients and timely retrieval if they are absolutely indicated. In addition, this case highlights the feasibility of catheter-based treatment of this rare but debilitating complication.

References

1. McAree BJ, O'Donnell ME, Fitzmaurice GJ, Reid JA, Spence RA, Lee B. Inferior vena cava thrombosis: a review of current practice. *Vasc Med.* 2013;18:32-43.
2. Koc Z, Oguzkurt. Interruption or congenital stenosis of the inferior vena cava: prevalence, imaging, and clinical findings. *Eur J Radiol.* 2007;62:257-266.
3. Watkins E Jr., Fortin CL. Surgical correction of a congenital coarctation of the inferior vena cava. *Ann Surg.* 1964;159:536-541.
4. Okuda K. Membranous obstruction of the inferior vena cava (obliterative hepatocavopathy, Okuda). *J Gastroenterol Hepatol.* 2001;16: 1179-1183.

Neurovascular Rescue for Thrombus-Related Embolic Stroke During Transcatheter Aortic Valve Implantation

Pablo Salinas, MD, Raul Moreno, MD, PhD, Remedios Frutos, MD, Jose Luis Lopez-Sendon, MD, PhD

An 88-year-old woman with critical aortic stenosis was scheduled for transfemoral transcatheter aortic valve implantation (TAVI). She received preprocedural aspirin plus clopidogrel, and 100 IU/kg unfractionated heparin during the procedure. The procedure was uneventful, and the balloon-expandable valve was successfully deployed. After deflating the balloon, an echo-dense mobile mass was seen in the left ventricular outflow tract (Fig. 7.25, Online Video 7.19), probably attached to the intraventricular portion of the guidewire. This mass was not present after valvuloplasty, so torn leaflets from the native valve were unlikely. Activated clotting time was 270 s. When the balloon catheter and guidewire were withdrawn, the mass disappeared.

The patient remained stable with nice prosthesis gradients. All pulses were palpable, but after prompt reversal of anesthesia, a complete left hemiparesis was found. A brain computed tomography scan confirmed a large right middle cerebral artery (RMCA) stroke. Immediate mechanical neurovascular rescue was attempted. In the initial angiography, there was a complete occlusion of the M1 branch of the RMCA with thrombus in the A1 branch (Fig. 7.26). Mechanical thrombectomy was performed with a Solitaire AB device (ev3, Endovascular Inc., Plymouth, Minnesota), extracting a 13-mm thrombus (Fig. 7.27). The control angiogram shows complete RMCA reperfusion (Fig. 7.28). The neurologic deficit improved to modified Rankin scale 1 at discharge and remained unchanged after 6 months of follow-up.

Strokes during TAVI are attributed to calcific debris embolization, native valve guidewire crossing, and aortic balloon valvuloplasty.[1] Catheter-related thrombus is a known cause of stroke during percutaneous coronary intervention, with an incidence of approximately 0.4%.[2] However, catheter-related thrombus during a TAVI procedure has not been previously reported and merits a few forethoughts. First, the optimal level of anticoagulation remains uncertain. Second, it is important to promptly reverse anesthesia/sedation to assess any potential neurologic deficit. Finally, interventional treatment for embolic strokes should be considered in selected cases.

References

1. Stortecky S, Windecker S, Pilgrim T, et al. Cerebrovascular accidents complicating transcatheter aortic valve implantation: frequency, timing and impact on outcomes. *EuroIntervention.* 2012;8:62-70.
2. Hamon M, Baron JC, Viader F, Hamon M. Periprocedural stroke and cardiac catheterization. *Circulation.* 2008;118:678-683.

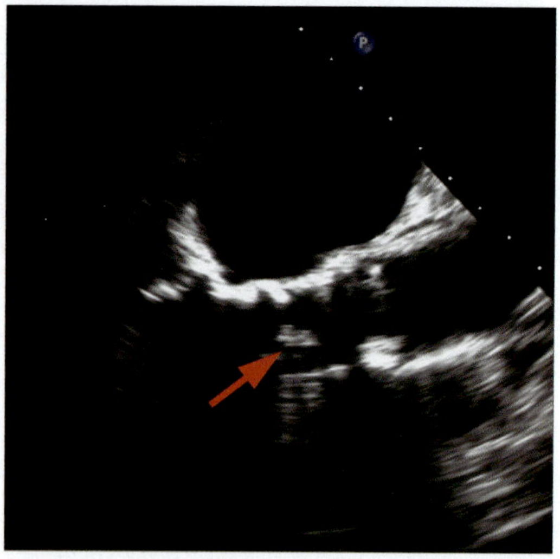

FIG. 7.25 Transesophageal Echocardiogram After Prosthesis Deployment. Echo-dense mobile mass (*arrow*) in the left ventricular outflow tract after transcatheter valve deployment. This is best seen in Online Video 7.19.

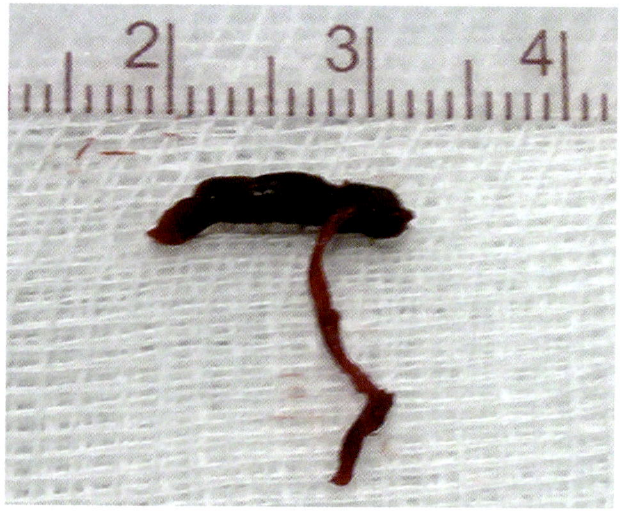

FIG. 7.27 Retrieved Thrombus. Thrombus retrieved from the right middle cerebral artery.

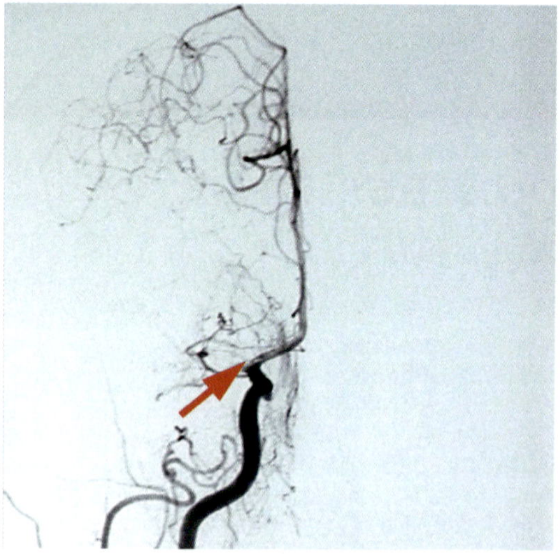

FIG. 7.26 Initial Selective Cerebral Angiogram. Selective cerebral angiogram showing complete occlusion of the M1 branch (*arrow*) of the right middle cerebral artery and some thrombus in the A1 branch.

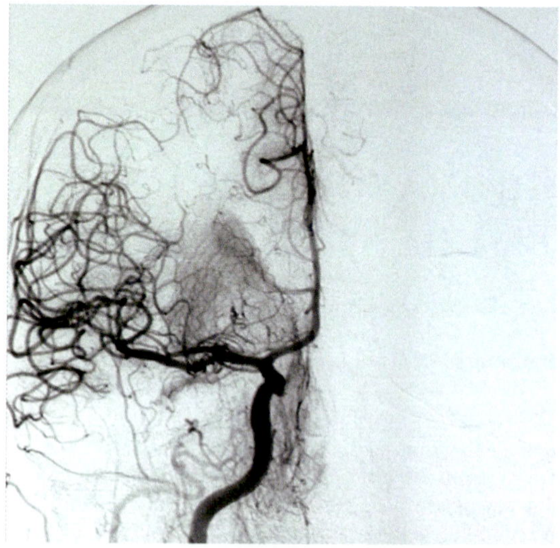

FIG. 7.28 Control Cerebral Angiogram After Neurovascular Intervention. Control selective cerebral angiogram showing reperfusion of occluded arteries.

Percutaneous Closure of a Large Ascending Aorta Pseudoaneurysm Due to Mediastinitis Using an Amplatzer Occluder Device

Manolis Vavuranakis, MD, PhD, Konstantinos Kalogeras, MD, Carmen Moldovan, MD, Sophia Vaina, MD, PhD, Dimitrios Vrachatis, MD, Maria Kariori, MD, Evelina Mpei, MD, Dimitrios Tousoulis, MD, PhD, Christodoulos Stefanadis, MD, PhD

A 63-year-old man presented with chest pain. He had undergone coronary artery bypass graft surgery 15 years earlier and mitral valve repair due to severe regurgitation 6 months earlier with a simultaneous right internal mammary artery (RIMA) to left anterior descending artery graft. The early postoperative period was complicated by mediastinitis, which required surgical drainage. Due to persistent infection, a vacuum device was used to drain inflammatory fluid.

During the present admission, the patient was afebrile with mild right arm edema, right jugular vein distention, and audible systolic murmur. A computed tomography (CT) scan exposed a large aortic pseudoaneurysm with communication 1 cm below the innominate artery, probably as a result of inflammation, cannulation, and vacuum tubing (Fig. 7.29A–B, Online Video 7.20).

Because of the two sternotomies, the RIMA graft across the sternum, and the position of the pseudoaneurysm, surgical treatment was not considered by the heart team. Thus, percutaneous closure of the pseudoaneurysm mouth with an Amplatzer septal occluder was selected.

However, there were concerns regarding the stability of the surrounding orifice aortic rims and the support they could provide. Defect sizing was based on multisliced CT angiography, which showed the orifice to be 10 mm.

Via femoral access, a 0.035-inch guidewire was inserted into the pseudoaneurysm, and over that, a 5F multipurpose catheter was advanced into its cavity (Fig. 7.30A, Online Video 7.21). The procedure was guided by angiography and transthoracic echocardiography (TTE). Finally, a 12-mm Amplatzer atrial septal defect device was successfully delivered (Fig. 7.30B, Online Video 7.22). This resulted in immediate flow elimination confirmed by Doppler (Fig. 7.30C, Online Video 7.23). A second CT scan 10 days later confirmed a pseudoaneurysm size reduction by thrombus development in the cavity (Fig. 7.31A–B).

In our case, the pseudoaneurysm cavity had relatively postinflammatory fragile rims and large dimensions, which resulted in adjacent great vessel compression. Device implantation was even more challenging without TEE guidance because of the high orifice location. In conclusion, large postinflammatory pseudoaneurysms can be successfully closed with off-label use of available equipment.[1,2] However, the development of specific devices for on-label use is required.

References

1. Hussain J, Strumpf R, Wheatley G, Diethrich E. Percutaneous closure of aortic pseudoaneurysm by Amplatzer occluder device-case series of six patients. *Catheter Cardiovasc Interv.* 2009;73:521-529.
2. Bhindi R, Newton J, Wilson N, Ormerod OJ. Percutaneous plugging of an ascending aortic pseudoaneurysm. *J Am Coll Cardiol Intv.* 2008;1:327-328.

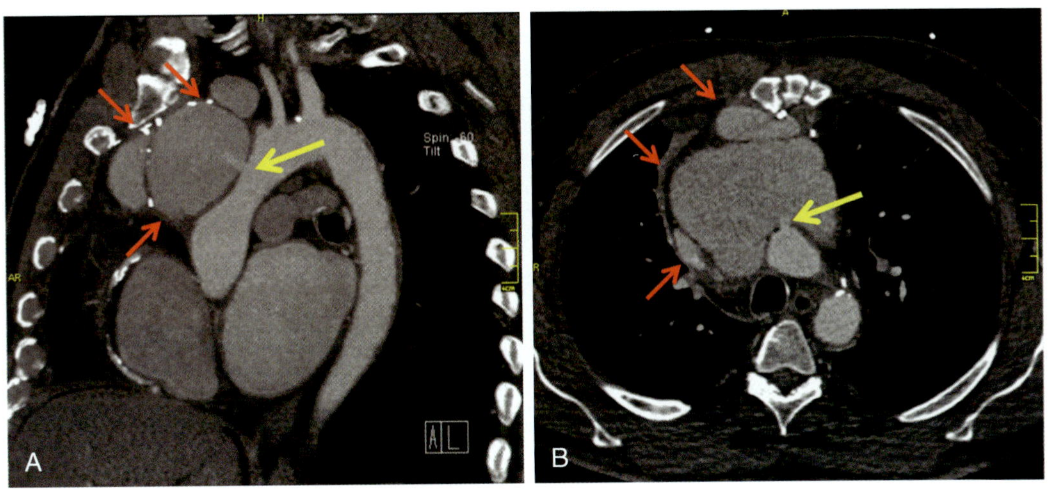

FIG. 7.29 Computed Tomography Images Before Implantation. (A and B) Computed tomography scan demonstrating the pseudoaneurysm cavity (*red arrows*) and its orifice (*yellow arrow*) close to the innominate artery before intervention (Online Video 7.20).

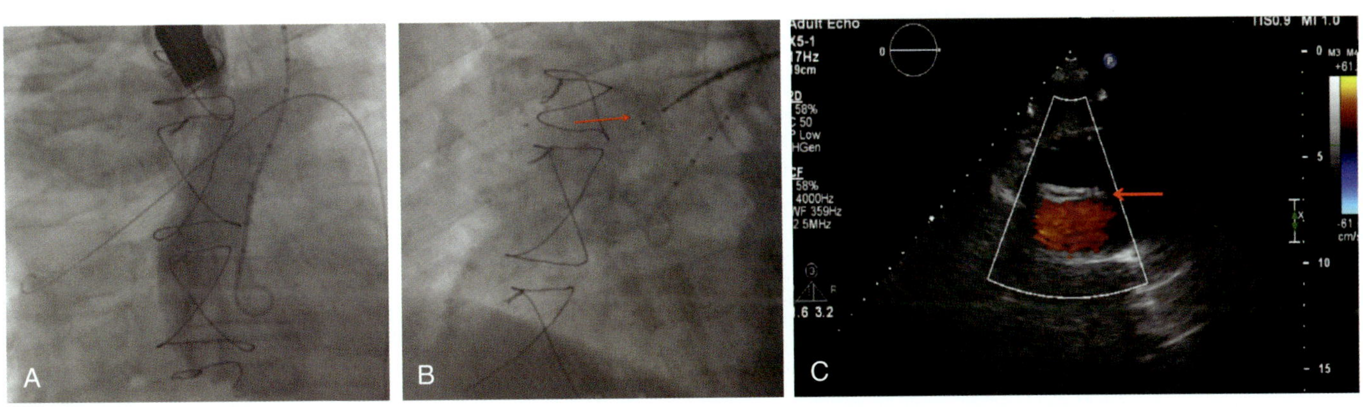

FIG. 7.30 Amplatzer Occluder Device Implantation. (A) Aortography of the ascending aorta with a guidewire passed through the pseudoaneurysm mouth into its cavity during implantation (Online Video 7.21). (B) Angiographic image of the Amplatzer occluder device (*red arrow*) successfully implanted at the orifice of the aortic pseudoaneurysm (Online Video 7.22). (C) Transthoracic Doppler ultrasound image demonstrating the implanted device (*red arrow*) in the ascending aorta (Online Video 7.23).

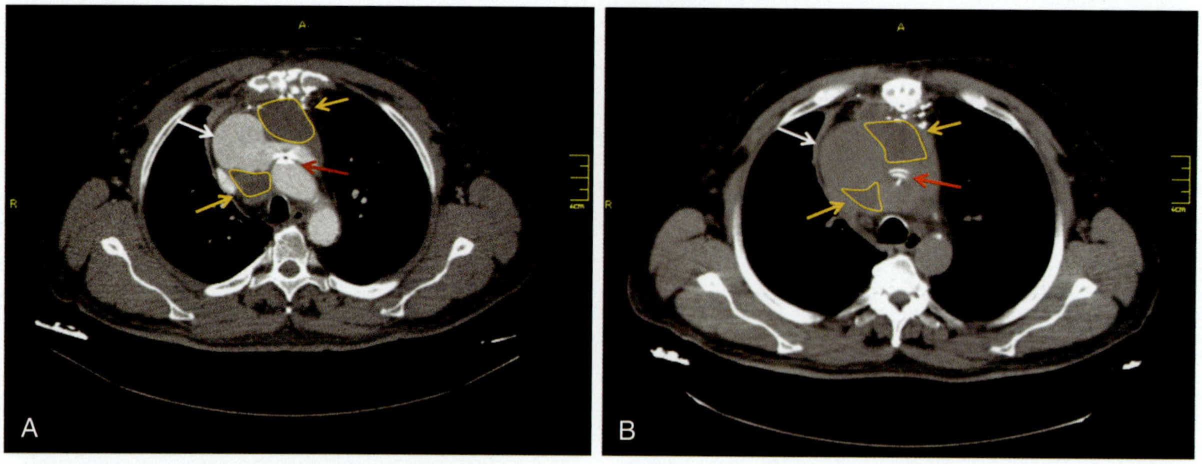

FIG. 7.31 Computed Tomography Images After Implantation. (A and B) Computed tomography scan demonstrating Amplatzer occluder device (*red arrow*), thrombus formation in the cavity (*yellow outline* and *arrow*), and the remaining pseudoaneurysm cavity (*white arrow*) shortly after intervention.

Percutaneous Closure of a Pulmonary Arteriovenous Malformation in a Young Patient With Cryptogenic Stroke

Giuseppe Patti, MD, Luca D'Antonio, MD, Pietro Sedati, MD, Simona Mega, MD, Germano Di Sciascio, MD

A 44-year-old woman had a transient ischemic attack in 2010 and a subsequent ischemic stroke (while on a regimen of aspirin therapy) in May 2012 with evidence of an ischemic cerebral lesion at magnetic resonance imaging. Thrombophilic screening tests showed factor V Leiden homozygosis. Transesophageal echocardiography revealed an atrial septum aneurysm without shunt during Valsalva maneuver after injection of agitated saline solution in the right antecubital vein; however, there was a late (after five cardiac cycles) appearance of agitated saline microbubbles in the left atrium through a pulmonary vein (Fig. 7.32A–B). An arteriovenous malformation was thus suspected, and this was confirmed by computed tomography imaging, showing a simple communication in the right lower pulmonary lobe between an inferior lobar artery of the right pulmonary artery and a vein draining in the lower right pulmonary vein (Fig. 7.32C). Percutaneous closure of the malformation was considered indicated and successfully performed with implantation of a 7-mm Amplatzer vascular plug 4 (St. Jude Medical, St. Paul, Minnesota) (Fig. 7.33). Prevalence of pulmonary arteriovenous malformations is approximately 2 to 3 per 100,000 persons, but this is higher in patients with cryptogenic stroke.[1] These malformations are usually congenital, and 47% to 80% of the cases are associated with Osler-Weber-Rendu disease.[1] The presence of a pulmonary arteriovenous malformation has to be kept in mind as a possible cause of paradoxic embolism, especially in young adults with cryptogenic stroke,[2] particularly in

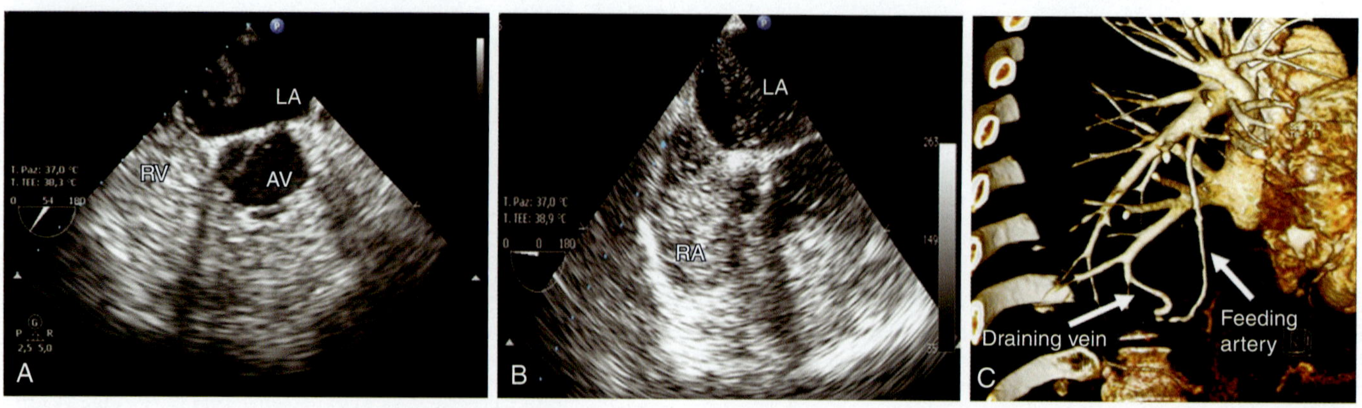

FIG. 7.32 Preprocedural Diagnostic Evaluations. (A and B) Multiplane transesophageal echocardiography. This examination showed late appearance of agitated saline microbubbles in the left atrium (*LA*) through a pulmonary vein in the short-axis view (A) and in the four-chamber view (B). The lack of shunt across the atrial septum during Valsalva maneuver excluded the presence of patent foramen ovale. (C) Computed tomography imaging showed a simple pulmonary arteriovenous malformation involving a feeding artery originating from the inferior lobar artery of the right pulmonary artery and a vein draining in the lower right pulmonary vein. *AV*, aortic valve; *RA*, right atrium.

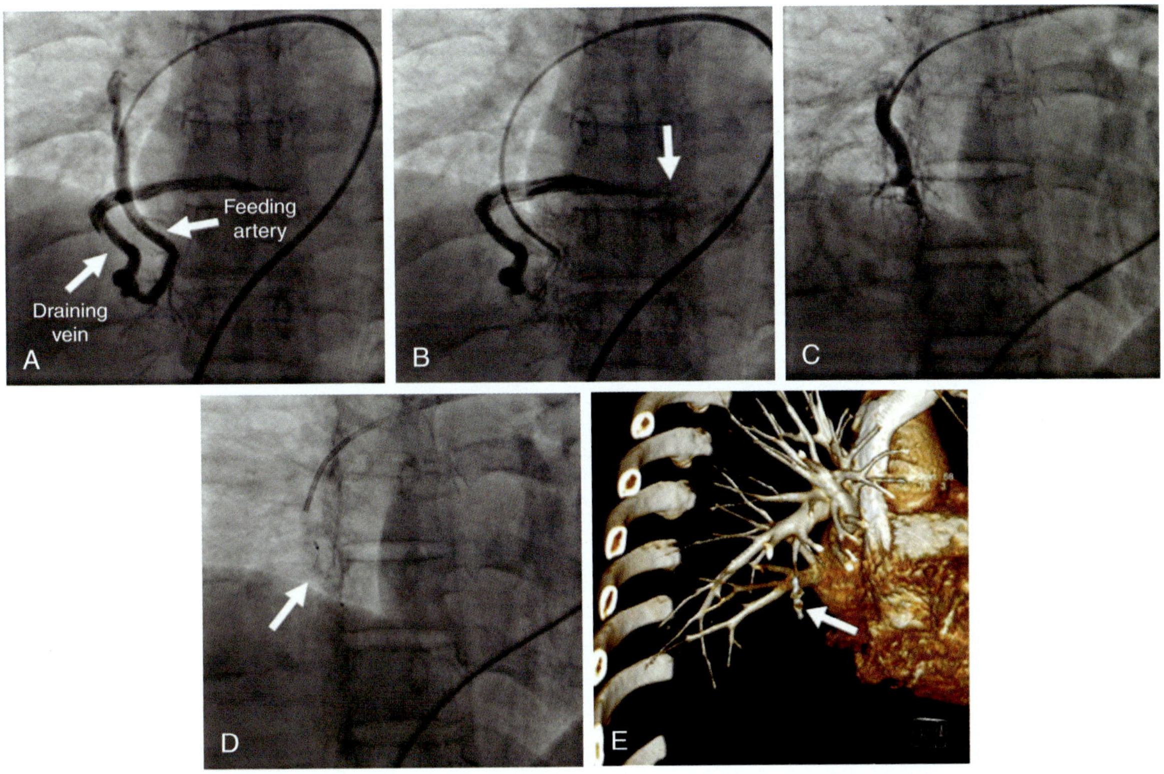

FIG. 7.33 Periprocedural and Postintervention Images. (A) Preprocedural selective angiography with the feeding artery and the draining vein of the pulmonary arteriovenous malformation. (B) Drainage of the vein in the left atrium (*arrow*). (C) Postprocedural angiography showing complete closure of the anomaly. (D) Implanted vascular plug (*arrow*). (E) Computed tomography imaging confirming complete closure of the anomaly by the vascular plug (*arrow*).

the presence of a thrombophilic genetic pattern. In our patient, transesophageal echocardiography—initially performed to possibly diagnose a patent foramen ovale—strongly suggested the presence of a pulmonary arteriovenous malformation, which was confirmed at computed tomography imaging. According to guidelines[3] that recommend treatment of these malformations when considered responsible for a cerebral ischemic event, we performed percutaneous closure of the anomaly for secondary prevention.

References

1. Khurshid I, Downie GH. Pulmonary arteriovenous malformation. *Postgrad Med J.* 2002;78:191-197.
2. Trerotola SO, Pyeritz RE. PAVM embolization: an update. *AJR.* 2010;195:837-845.
3. Faughnan ME, Palda VA, Garcia-Tsao G, et al. International guidelines for the diagnosis and management of hereditary haemorrhagic telangiectasia. *J Med Genet.* 2011;48:73-87.

Percutaneous Palliation of Right Ventricular Outflow Tract Obstruction Caused by Metastatic Malignancy

George Joseph, DM, Sujith Thomas Chacko, DM, Elizabeth Joseph, DNB, Vishnu Chandra Kumar, MD

A 52-year-old man was evaluated for dry cough, progressive breathlessness, and exertional syncope. He had distended neck veins, bilateral leg edema, and a grade 3/6 ejection systolic murmur in the left parasternal region. Transthoracic echocardiography (Fig. 7.34A) and cardiac magnetic resonance imaging (Fig. 7.34B) revealed an obstructive intracavitary mass in the right ventricular outflow tract (RVOT) and pulmonary artery producing a peak systolic pressure gradient of 75 mm Hg. The mass did not infiltrate adjacent structures, but multiple subcentimeter nodules were present in both lungs consistent with metastases. Positron emission tomography (Fig. 7.34C–E) showed the mass and metastatic nodules to be metabolically active, but an active primary focus could not be detected. Fluoroscopy-guided transjugular endomyocardial biopsy of the lesion was performed. Histopathologic findings obtained from the biopsy specimens, including spindle cell morphology and positive staining for pancytokeratin and vimentin (Fig. 7.34F–H), and the immunohistochemical profile, suggested a metastatic sarcomatoid carcinoma.

Because the patient's clinical condition was deteriorating rapidly, a palliative stenting procedure (Fig. 7.34I–J) was performed. A 22- ×

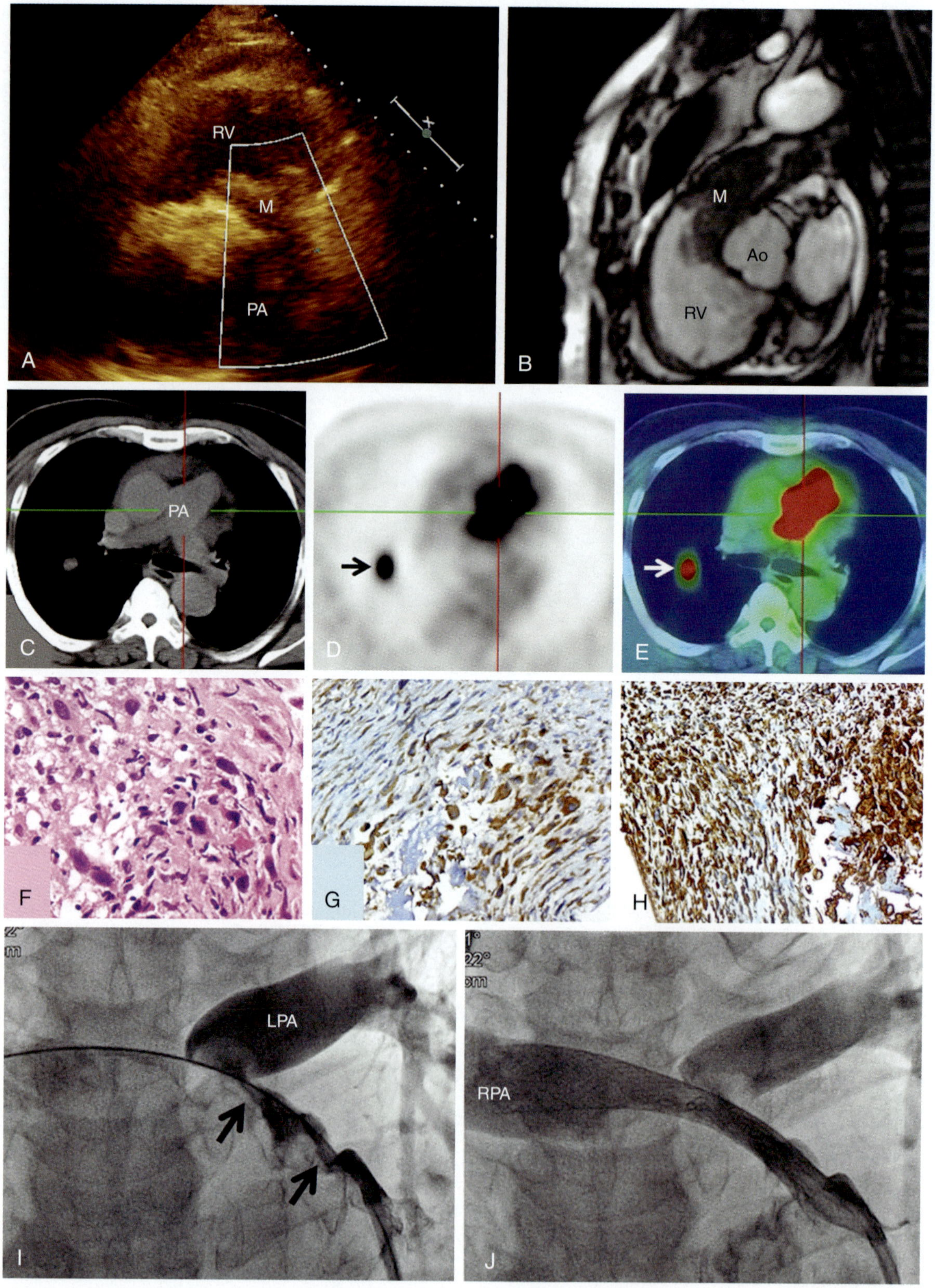

FIG. 7.34 Malignant Right Ventricular Outflow Tract Obstruction. (A) Transthoracic echocardiogram in parasternal short-axis view shows dilatation of the right ventricle (*RV*) and an obstructive mass (*M*) in the RV outflow tract (RVOT) and pulmonary artery (*PA*). (B) Cardiac magnetic resonance imaging in sagittal section shows the RVOT mass to be large, hypodense, and almost occlusive. *Ao,* aortic root. Computed tomography (C), positron emission tomography (D), and fusion of both modalities (E) shows increased fluorodeoxyglucose uptake (*black* and *red areas* in D and E, respectively) in the RVOT mass and lung nodules (*black* and *white arrows*, respectively). Histopathologic sections of endomyocardial biopsy specimens obtained from the RVOT mass stained with hematoxylin and eosin (F), pancytokeratin (G), and vimentin (H) suggest a metastatic sarcomatoid carcinoma. (I) Conventional RV angiogram shows severe luminal narrowing (*arrows*) of the RVOT and main PA caused by the intracavitary tumor and preferential flow into the left PA (*LPA*). (J) Poststenting RV angiogram shows luminal widening of the RVOT and improved flow into the right PA (*RPA*).

45-mm self-expanding stent (WALLSTENT, Boston Scientific, Natick, Massachusetts) was deployed across the RVOT extending into the right pulmonary artery. This improved flow through the RVOT significantly and produced dramatic resolution of the patient's symptoms. He was discharged from the hospital after receiving three cycles of palliative chemotherapy. However, the symptoms recurred after 3 months, at which time he died. The primary focus remained undetected because an autopsy was not performed.

Most cardiac tumors are metastatic and the right side of the heart is more often involved than the left because it receives the systemic venous and lymphatic drainage.[1] Metastatic RVOT obstruction is rare, and may occur in the absence of widespread malignancy; new-onset right-sided heart failure and left parasternal systolic murmur should arouse clinical suspicion.[1] The prognosis is generally poor. Palliative RVOT stenting[2] is useful for symptomatic relief.

References

1. Labib SB, Schick EC Jr, Isner JM. Obstruction of right ventricular outflow tract caused by intracavitary metastatic disease: analysis of 14 cases. *J Am Coll Cardiol.* 1992;19:1664-1668.
2. Balkin PW, Imoto EM. Treatment of malignant obstruction of the right ventricular outflow tract and pulmonary artery with metallic stents. *AJR Am J Roentgenol.* 1997;169:439-440.

Percutaneous Recanalization of Occluded Brachiocephalic Vein–Superior Vena Cava Connection After Resection of Mediastinal Mass

Michael D. Seckeler, MD, MSc, Chet Villa, MD, Russel Hirsch, MD

A 15-year-old male patient underwent removal of chronic mediastinal histoplasmosis with residual superior vena cava (SVC) stenosis and brachiocephalic vein (BCV) obstruction. He developed significant dizziness after surgery that was attributed to an inability to increase preload during activity. He underwent catheterization for attempted percutaneous BCV recanalization.

Under general anesthesia, vascular access was obtained in the right femoral and left subclavian veins. Simultaneous contrast injections in the SVC and BCV revealed SVC narrowing and a 12-mm gap between the veins with decompressing venous flow (Fig. 7.35, Online Video 7.24). The SVC was stented from the femoral approach.

From the subclavian vein, a 56-cm transseptal needle in a 7F introducer sheath was advanced, while staining with contrast, across the fibrous tissue from the BCV to SVC. The tract was dilated with a 7-mm Conquest balloon (Bard Peripheral Vascular, Tempe, Arizona), stented with a 7- × 22-mm Atrium iCAST covered stent (Atrium Medical Corporation, Hudson, New Hampshire), and post-dilated with a 9-mm Conquest balloon. Final angiography demonstrated flow from the BCV into the SVC with diminished collateral flow (Fig. 7.36, Online Video 7.25). There were no procedural complications. He was discharged on clopidogrel 75 mg daily and warfarin with a target international normalized ratio of 2 to 2.5.

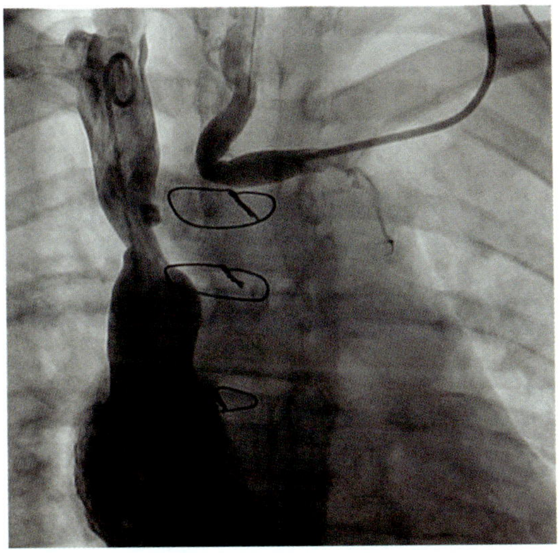

FIG. 7.35 Baseline Angiography. Simultaneous contrast injections in the superior vena cava (SVC) and brachiocephalic vein (BCV) reveal SVC narrowing and a 12-mm gap with a venous collaterals from the BCV (Online Video 7.24).

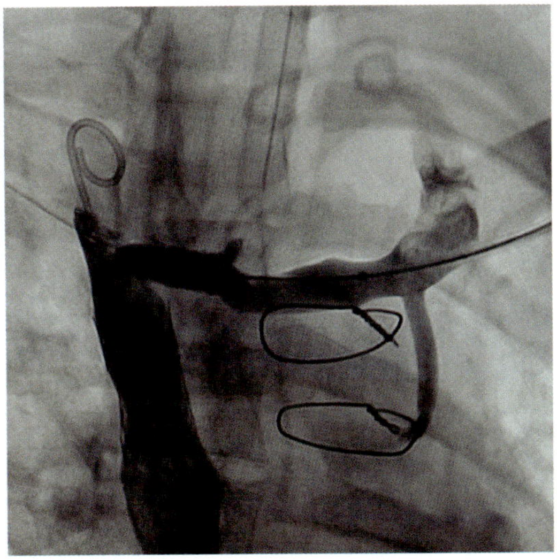

FIG. 7.36 Postintervention Angiography. Contrast injection in the brachiocephalic vein (BCV) after recanalization and covered-stent placement in the superior vena cava–BCV connection with much decreased flow through the venous collaterals (Online Video 7.25).

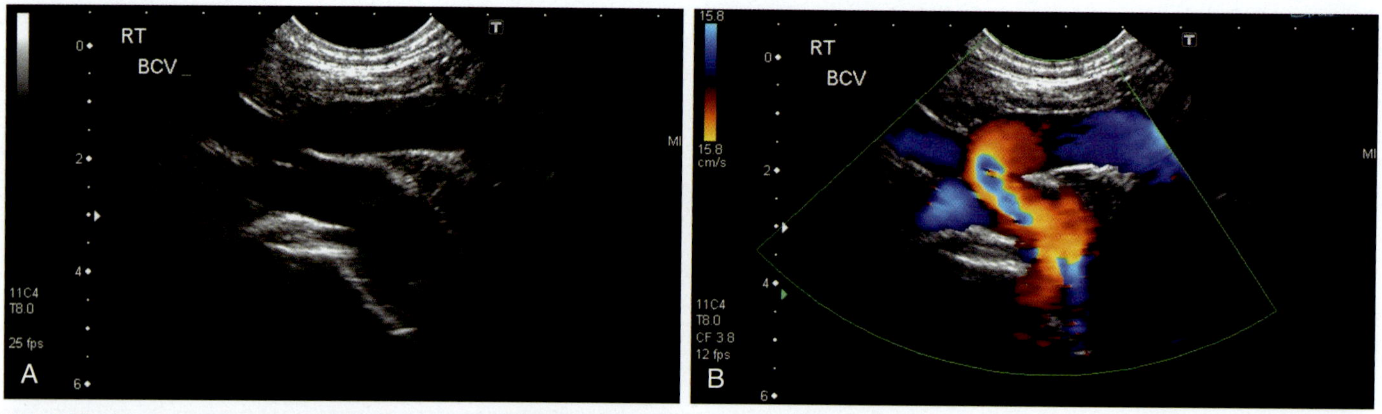

FIG. 7.37 Follow-up Venous Ultrasound and Color Doppler. Two-dimensional (A) and color Doppler (B) ultrasound showing patency of the stented superior vena cava–brachiocephalic vein (*BCV*) connection without significant flow acceleration. *RT*, right.

There was a marked improvement in symptoms. Follow-up venous ultrasound and Doppler demonstrated continued patency of the connection with no gradient (Fig. 7.37).

Occluded systemic central veins pose a therapeutic challenge. Surgery and balloon angioplasty have modest acute success with frequent restenosis,[1,2] whereas percutaneous vascular stenting provides higher rates of long-term patency.[3] Successful percutaneous recanalization of occluded central systemic veins, with the aim of normalizing ventricular preload, is possible with careful mapping and understanding of the surrounding tissue substrate. Careful follow-up and anticoagulation are vital to ensure continued patency of recanalized vessels.

References

1. Shimizu N, Date H, Moriyama S, Ando A, Teramoto S. Reconstruction of the superior vena cava in patients with mediastinal malignancies. *Eur J Cardiothorac Surg.* 1991;5:575-578.
2. Wisselink W, Money SR, Becker MO, et al. Comparison of operative reconstruction and percutaneous balloon dilatation for central venous obstruction. *Am J Surg.* 1993;166:200-204.
3. Ing FF, Fagan TE, Grifka RG, et al. Reconstruction of stenotic or occluded iliofemoral veins and inferior vena cava using intravascular stents: re-establishing access for future cardiac catheterization and cardiac surgery. *J Am Coll Cardiol.* 2001;37:251-257.

Percutaneous Transluminal Pulmonary Angioplasty for Central-Type Chronic Thromboembolic Pulmonary Hypertension

Haruhisa Ishiguro, MD, Masaharu Kataoka, MD, Takumi Inami, MD, Ryoji Yanagisawa, MD, Nobuhiko Shimura, MD, Hiroki Taguchi, MD, Hideyasu Kohshoh, MD, Hideaki Yoshino, MD, Toru Satoh, MD

A 76-year-old man had severe pulmonary artery stenosis in the main tract of the right pulmonary artery (Fig. 7.38, Online Video 7.26), suggesting central-type chronic thromboembolic pulmonary hypertension (CTEPH). Percutaneous transluminal pulmonary angioplasty (PTPA) was strategized because he was excluded from surgical pulmonary endarterectomy due to his severe chronic obstructive pulmonary dysfunction and poor physical condition.

The procedure was divided into two staged sessions performed on different days to prevent large-scale pulmonary edema due to acute revascularization. During the first session, the right pulmonary artery was incompletely dilated using a 2.5- to 6-mm monorail balloon catheter (Fig. 7.39A–B). The first PTPA session was stopped in an insufficient state of pulmonary flow (Fig. 7.39C). One week later, the mean pulmonary arterial pressure (PAP) had decreased to 29 mm Hg just before the second session (baseline, 41 mm Hg). The main lesion was dilated further using a 10-mm balloon catheter, and pulmonary blood flow was significantly improved, with rapid increases in flow (Fig. 7.40A–B, Online Video 7.27). No major complications, including reperfusion pulmonary edema, occurred. There was no pulmonary restenosis seen on 6-month follow-up (mean PAP, 23 mm Hg).

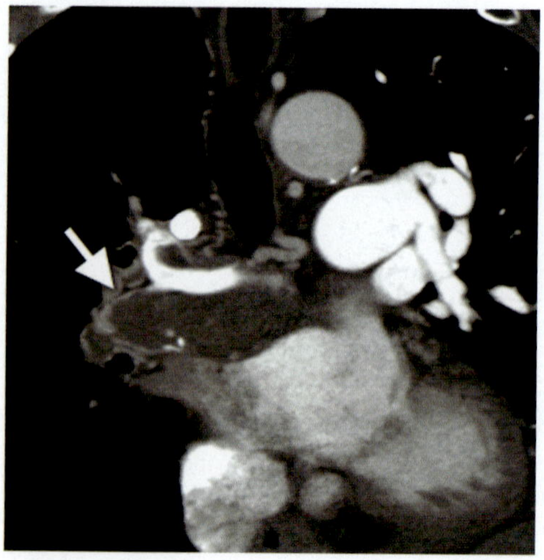

FIG. 7.38 Chest Computed Tomography Before Percutaneous Transluminal Pulmonary Angioplasty. *Arrow* indicates a large thrombosis in the main tract (Online Video 7.26).

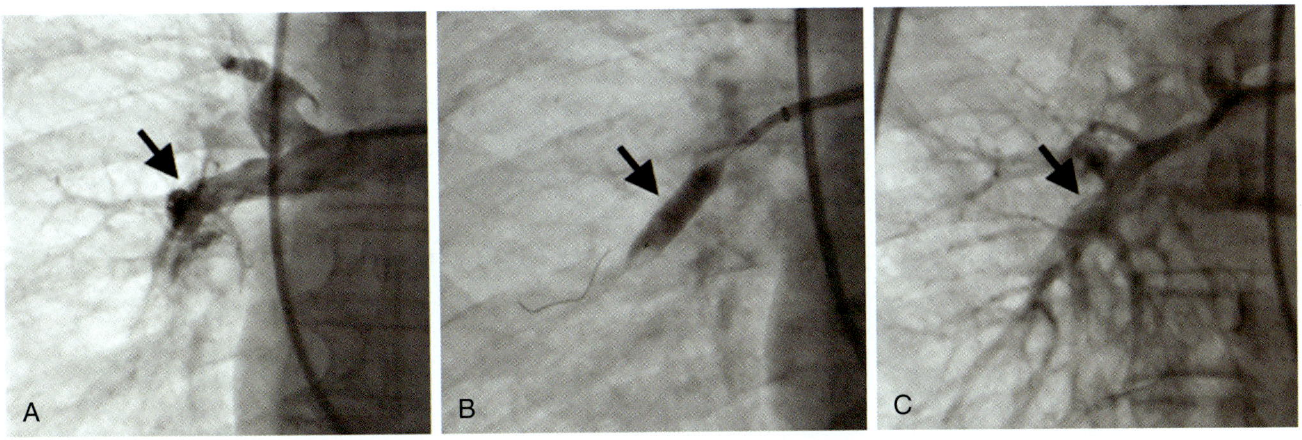

FIG. 7.39 Angiographies at the First Session. Angiographies before percutaneous transluminal pulmonary angioplasty (PTPA) (A), during dilation of the target lesion by the small-size balloon catheter (B), and after the first session of PTPA (C).

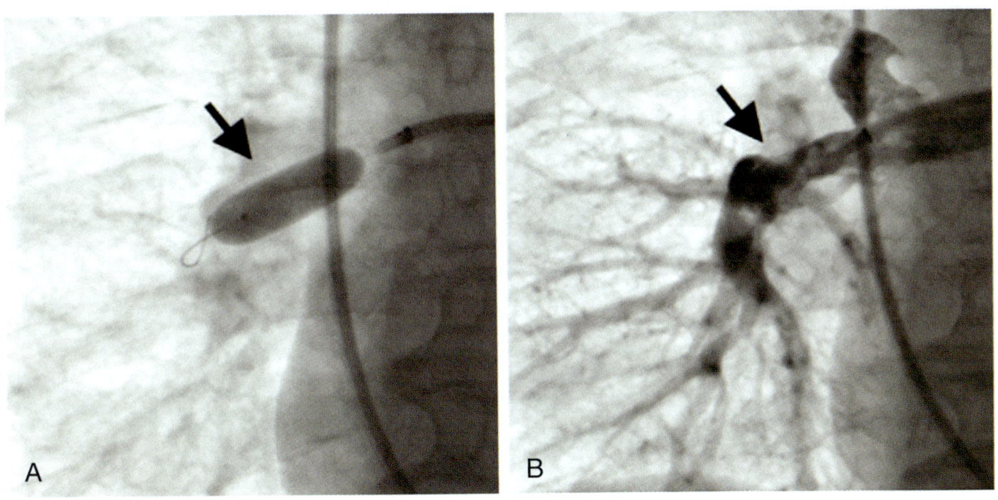

FIG. 7.40 Angiographies at the Second Session. Angiographies during dilation by a larger balloon catheter (A) and after the second session of percutaneous transluminal pulmonary angioplasty (B) (Online Video 7.27).

Patients with central-type CTEPH have been excluded from PTPA because it would have resulted in large-scale pulmonary edema, with grave consequences in terms of morbidity and mortality.[1,2] However, we have demonstrated that staged revascularization by PTPA is effective in the treatment of central-type CTEPH and therefore may be a therapeutic option for these patients.

References

1. Kataoka M, Inami T, Hayashida K, et al. Percutaneous transluminal pulmonary angioplasty for the treatment of chronic thromboembolic pulmonary hypertension. *Circ Cardiovasc Interv.* 2012;5:756-762.
2. Feinstein JA, Goldhaber SZ, Lock JE, Ferndandes SM, Landzberg MJ. Balloon pulmonary angioplasty for treatment of chronic thromboembolic pulmonary hypertension. *Circulation.* 2001;103:10-13.

Percutaneous Treatment of Chronic Distal Aortic Occlusion: A Viable Option

Mohamad Alkhouli, MD, Irfan Shafi, MD, Pravin Patil, MD, Riyaz Bashir, MBBS

A 55-year-old woman presented with severe lifestyle-limiting bilateral calf and thigh claudication (Rutherford stage III). She had history of aortobifemoral bypass 13 years previously, which had occluded since then. Her ankle brachial index (ABI) was 0.67 on the right and 0.69 on the left. Computed tomography (CT) and digital subtraction angiograms showed an occluded infrarenal aorta (Figs. 7.41A and 7.42A, Online Video 7.28). She was deemed to be a poor candidate for surgical revascularization secondary to her comorbidities (uncontrolled diabetes and severe coronary artery disease) and the need for redo surgery.

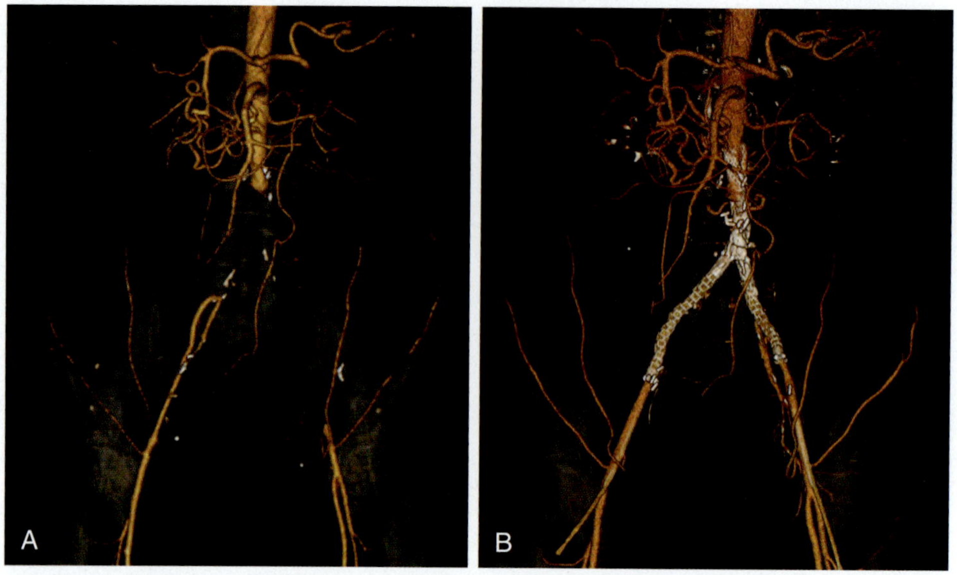

FIG. 7.41 Computed Tomography Angiogram Three-Dimensional Volume Rendering Reconstruction Image. (A) Occluded infrarenal aorta, with distal reconstitution (Online Video 7.28). (B) Reconstruction of the distal aorta with kissing stents (Online Video 7.29).

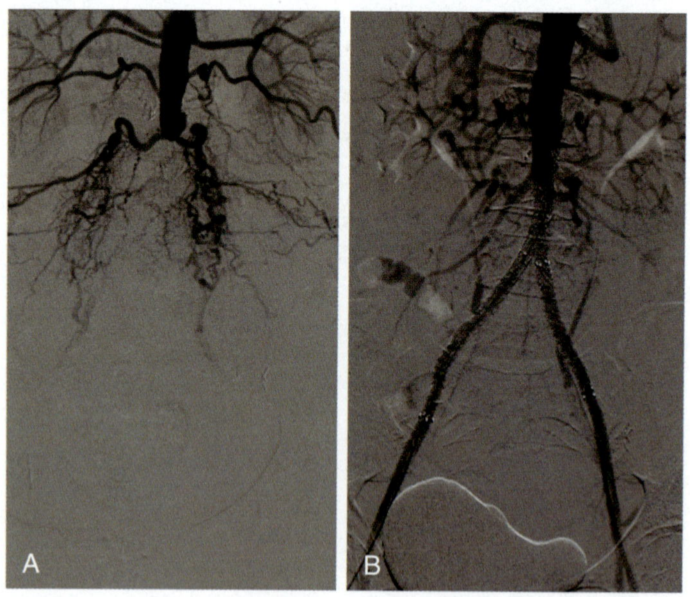

FIG. 7.42 Aortoiliac Angiogram. (A) Occluded distal aorta. (B) Reconstruction of the aortoiliac bifurcation with kissing stents.

She was treated successfully with percutaneous bilateral kissing aortoiliac stenting using bilateral femoral and left radial approaches. The left aortoiliac occlusion was successfully traversed in a retrograde fashion from the left femoral access using a Pioneer reentry catheter (Volcano, San Diego, California). The right aortoiliac occlusion was traversed in an antegrade fashion from the left radial approach using an 0.018-inch Victory wire (Boston Scientific, Natick, Massachusetts) that was externalized via the right femoral sheath. The aortoiliac bifurcation was reconstructed with kissing balloon angioplasty and stenting with balloon-expandable Assurant Cobalt stents (Medtronic, Langhorne, Pennsylvania) and self-expanding LifeStar stents (Bard Peripheral Vascular, Tempe, Arizona) with excellent angiographic and hemodynamic results (Figs. 7.41B and 7.42B, Online Video 7.29). The following day, the patient was walking without any claudication and continued to be free of symptoms at 3-month follow-up. Follow-up ABI measurements were completely normal (1.17 on the left and 1.19 on the right).

Surgical revascularization is considered to be the preferred treatment of infrarenal aortic occlusion (TASC-D lesion).[1] However, with current advances in percutaneous technologies such as intravascular ultrasound–guided reentry devices, endovascular treatment seems to be a very reasonable first-line approach particularly in high-risk surgical patients.[2,3]

References

1. Norgren L, Hiatt WR, Dormandy JA, et al. Inter-Society Consensus for the Management of Peripheral Arterial Disease (TASC II). *Eur J Vasc Endovasc Surg.* 2007;33:Suppl 1:S1-S75.
2. Moise MA, Alvarez-Tostado JA, Clair DG, et al. Endovascular management of chronic infrarenal aortic occlusion. *J Endovasc Ther.* 2009;16:84-92.
3. Kim TH, Ko YG, Kim U, et al. Outcomes of endovascular treatment of chronic total occlusion of the infrarenal aorta. *J Vasc Surg.* 2011;53:1542-1549.

Shortcut Under Pressure: Stenting the Tortuous Neonatal Duct Involves Induced Spasm

Mieke Roggen, MD, Filip Rega, MD, PhD, Marc Gewillig, MD, PhD

A neonate (3410 g) presented with a duct-dependent complex pulmonary atresia (double discordance, ventricular septal defect, right aortic arch).

The duct originated with an obtuse angle from the inner curvature of the aorta facing the right carotid artery (Fig. 7.43A, Online Video 7.30); it was long and tortuous with a cumulative angulation of 360 degrees (Fig. 7.43B). By cutdown, a 4F sheath was positioned in the right carotid artery. A soft Progreat coaxial wire (Terumo Medical, Tokyo, Japan) was advanced through the tortuous duct into the left pulmonary artery. The total duct length was 26 mm; however, the "direct distance" between the aorta and the pulmonary artery was only 13 mm. A 4/18-mm stent was prepared because we anticipated straightening the curve that would shorten and kink the duct with critical spasm. The 0.018-inch inner probing wire was exchanged for a more rigid coronary wire: Iron Man 0.014 inch (Abbott Vascular, Santa Clara, California). The duct kinked and spasmed as expected (Fig. 7.43C–D, Online Videos 7.31 and 7.32); oxygen levels dropped from 81% to well below 60%. The stent was forced through the duct. Great care was taken to cover the duct completely with little protrusion in both aorta and pulmonary artery. After stent deployment, the saturation quickly rose to 93% (Fig. 7.43E, Online Video 7.33).

Three months later, the duct was restented with a 4.5/16-mm stent followed by a Glenn shunt after 8 months on well-developed pulmonary arteries. This case illustrates the critical steps: choose the right access to allow forcing the stent through a spastic duct, have an adequately sized stent prepared, and properly position the stent at deployment.

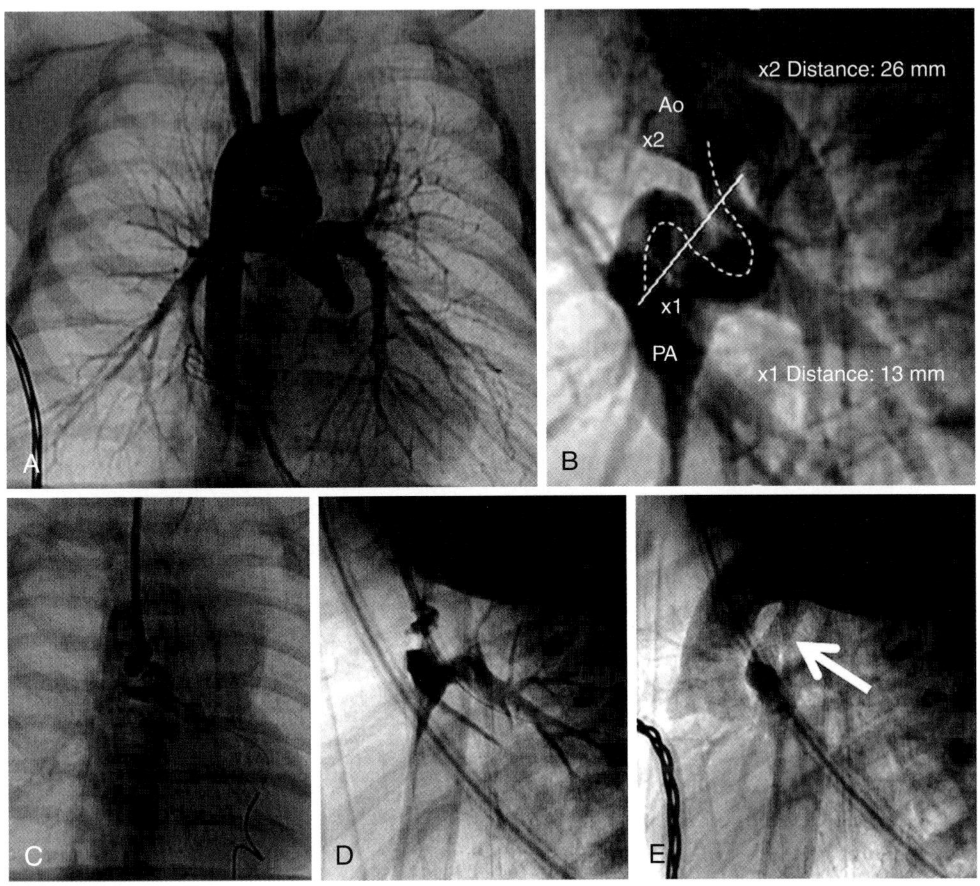

FIG. 7.43 Sequence of Stenting the Tortuous Neonatal Duct. (A) Aortogram through the 4F sheath from the right carotid artery. The duct originates just across the right carotid artery in a right arch. (B) Lateral view of aortogram. The duct originates from the cross of the aorta in a vertical way, followed by a very tortuous course with a cumulated angulation of 360 degrees. The total length of the duct (*dotted line*) is 26 mm, the direct distance between aorta and pulmonary artery (*solid line*) measures only 13 mm. (C and D) After insertion of a stiff 0.014-inch coronary wire through the duct until the distal left pulmonary artery, the duct straightens and shortens, but with significant spasm and subtotal obstruction. (E) Aortogram after deployment of a 4/18-mm stent: the stented duct (*arrow*) now has a straight course; the stent covers the full length of the duct from the aortic lumen to the pulmonary artery. *Ao*, aorta; *PA*, pulmonary artery. See Online Videos 7.30–7.33.

Stenting for Juxtarenal Abdominal Aortic Occlusion

Tetsuya Nadahama, MD, Osami Kawarada, MD, PhD, Kaho Shibata, MD, Koichiro Harada, MD, PhD, Teruo Noguchi, MD, PhD, Kenji Minatoya, MD, PhD, Hisao Ogawa, MD, PhD, Satoshi Yasuda, MD, PhD

Tremendous advancements in endovascular intervention have opened the door for treating distal abdominal aortic occlusion percutaneously.[1,2] "Juxtarenal" abdominal aortic occlusion is one of the final frontiers in endovascular intervention.

An 83-year-old man with a history of hypertension, dyslipidemia, and percutaneous coronary intervention was referred to our vascular team for treatment of severe progressive bilateral intermittent claudication (Rutherford category 3). Although blood testing revealed no abnormalities, his ankle-brachial index was 0.2/0.2. Enhanced computed tomography demonstrated complete occlusion of the juxtarenal abdominal aorta. The occlusion was connected to a right iliac artery occlusion and left iliac artery stenosis (Fig. 7.44A–B). Because a recent study demonstrated that the in-hospital 30-day mortality rate was relatively high (17%) for axillofemoral bypass,[3] this patient was considered a poor candidate for surgical revascularization because of his age and concomitant coronary artery disease status. Multidisciplinary discussion led to the decision to attempt endovascular therapy. Diagnostic digital subtraction angiography findings via the right brachial artery were consistent with the computed tomography findings (Fig. 7.45A, Online Video 7.34). Immediately after successful retrograde crossing of the guidewire from the left groin, direct abdominal aortic stenting with self-expanding stents (12 × 40 mm and 12 × 60 mm) was performed from just below the ostium of the renal artery to the terminal aorta without pre- and postdilation to prevent shifting of the plaque or thrombus into the renal artery or significant distal embolization. After successful crossing of the right iliac artery occlusion using a rendezvous technique, kissing stenting with self-expanding stents followed by postdilation was performed. The final angiography demonstrated excellent revascularization (Fig. 7.45B, Online Video 7.35). The patient's ankle-brachial index increased to 0.8/0.8, and he was uneventfully discharged with a dramatic relief of claudication.

Contemporary endovascular intervention might be a viable option even for juxtarenal abdominal aortic occlusion in high-risk surgical patients.

References

1. Alkhouli M, Shafi I, Patil P, Bashir R. Percutaneous treatment of chronic distal aortic occlusion: a viable option. *J Am Coll Cardiol Intv.* 2014;7:e185-e186.
2. Mujtaba M, Chhabra L, Abdulbaki AM, Sadiq I. Balloon angioplasty with secondary stenting for chronically occluded abdominal aorta in a high-risk patient. *BMJ Case Rep.* 2014;2014.
3. Liedenbaum MH, Verdam FJ, Spelt D, de Groot HG, van der Waal J, van der Laan L. The outcome of the axillofemoral bypass: a retrospective analysis of 45 patients. *World J Surg.* 2009;33:2490-2496.

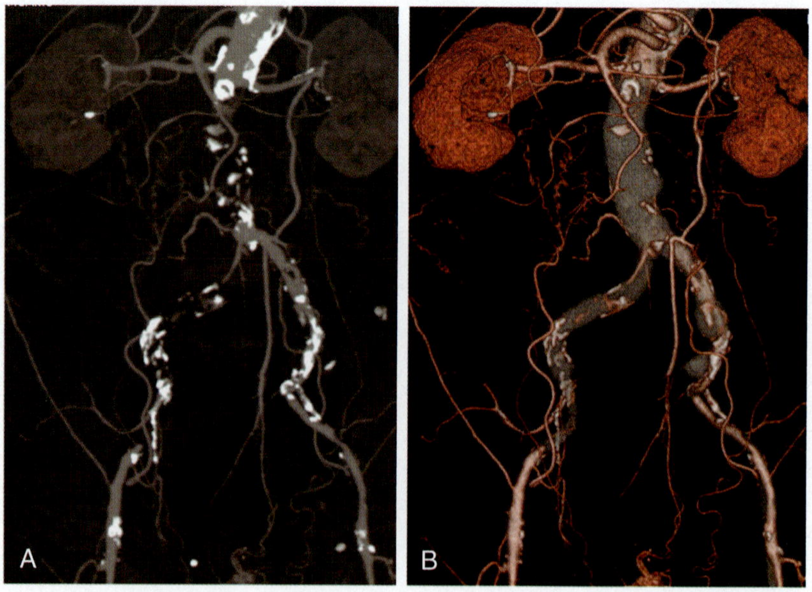

FIG. 7.44 Contrast-Enhanced Computed Tomography. (A) A juxtarenal abdominal aortic occlusion with vessel calcification that connects to a right iliac artery occlusion and left iliac artery stenosis. (B) A complex of plaque and mural thrombus in the vessel, shown in *gray*.

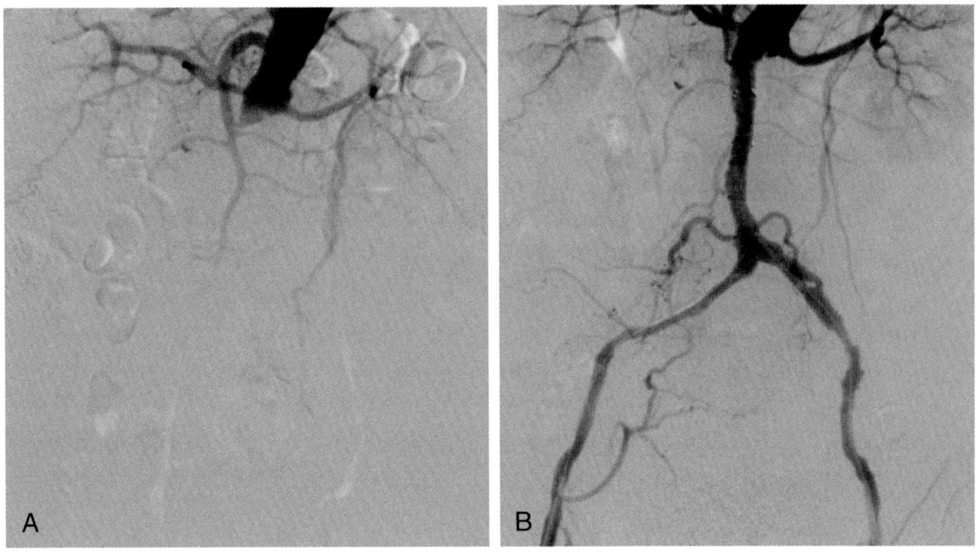

FIG. 7.45 Before and After Juxtarenal Abdominal Aortic Stenting. (A) Aortography of the abdominal aorta that yielded findings consistent with enhanced computed tomography findings (Online Video 7.34). (B) Final angiography after serial abdominal stenting and kissing iliac stenting showing an excellent result without any significant distal embolization and compromising renal artery (Online Video 7.35).

Successful Balloon Mitral Valvotomy in a Case of Inferior Vena Cava Obstruction: Where There Is a Will, There Is a Way

Madan Tarun, MD, DNB, Garg Rajiv, MD, DM, Thakkar Bhavesh, MD, DM

A 30-year-old woman with known rheumatic heart disease presented with New York Heart Association functional class III dyspnea. The patient had undergone balloon mitral valvotomy 14 years previously. Transthoracic echocardiography demonstrated severe mitral stenosis with mean gradient of 18 mm Hg across the mitral valve and a pulmonary artery pressure of 70 mm Hg.

The patient was to undergo balloon mitral valvotomy, but the lower limb venous access was not giving way. A venous angiogram showed a partially obstructed right external iliac vein and complete occlusion of the right common iliac vein and inferior vena cava in the infrahepatic segment (Fig. 7.46). The option of performing the balloon mitral valvotomy via the internal jugular vein or femoral route was evaluated. The inferior vena cava route was thought to be more appropriate.

After accessing the right internal jugular vein and right common femoral vein, a road map was created of the occluded inferior vena cava segment. The occluded segment of the inferior vena cava was crossed with 0.035-inch J-tipped Terumo wire (Terumo Interventional Systems, Somerset, New Jersey) via right femoral venous access. Balloon angioplasty of the right external iliac vein, right common iliac vein, and inferior vena cava was done sequentially using a 4- × 150-mm Admiral Xtreme balloon (Invatec, Roncadelle, Italy), an 8- × 40-mm OPTA Pro balloon (Cordis Corporation, San Jose, California), and a 24-mm SYM balloon (Lifetech Scientific, Shenzhen, China) (Fig. 7.47). After the balloon angioplasty, there was brisk flow in the right common iliac vein and inferior vena cava. Successful venous access for balloon mitral valvotomy was established from the right lower limb, and balloon mitral valvotomy was done successfully in a conventional manner using a 26-mm SYM balloon (Lifetech Scientific), and the transmitral gradient decreased from 18 mm Hg to 4 mm Hg (Fig. 7.48).

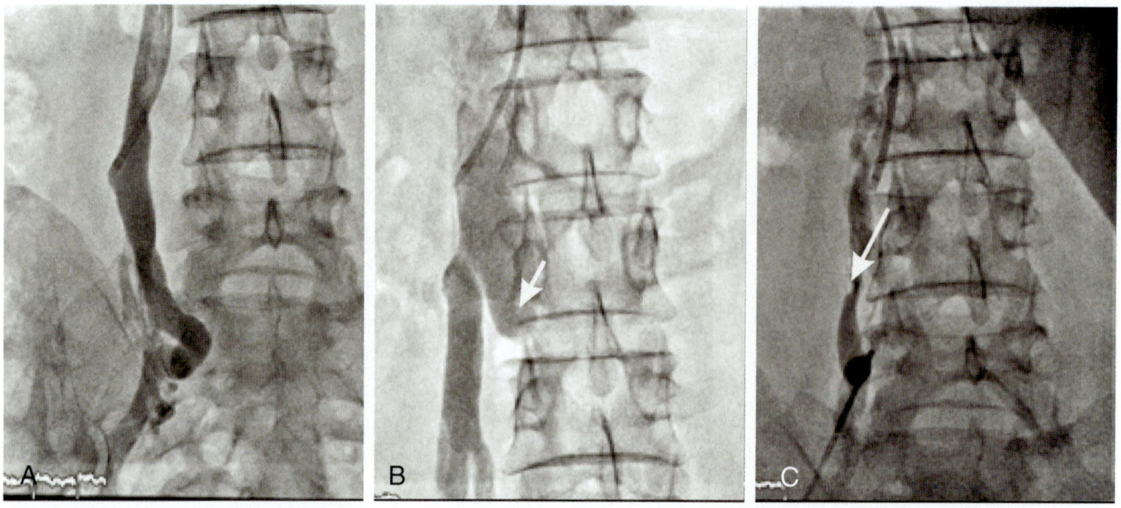

FIG. 7.46 Preprocedure Venous Angiogram. (A) Right iliac venous angiogram demonstrating partially obstructed right common iliac vein and collaterals reforming distally into inferior vena cava. (B) Total occlusion of the inferior vena cava (*arrow*). (C) Two catheters (one each via the jugular and femoral access) are seen, showing complete occlusion of the inferior vena cava and venous collateral (*arrow*).

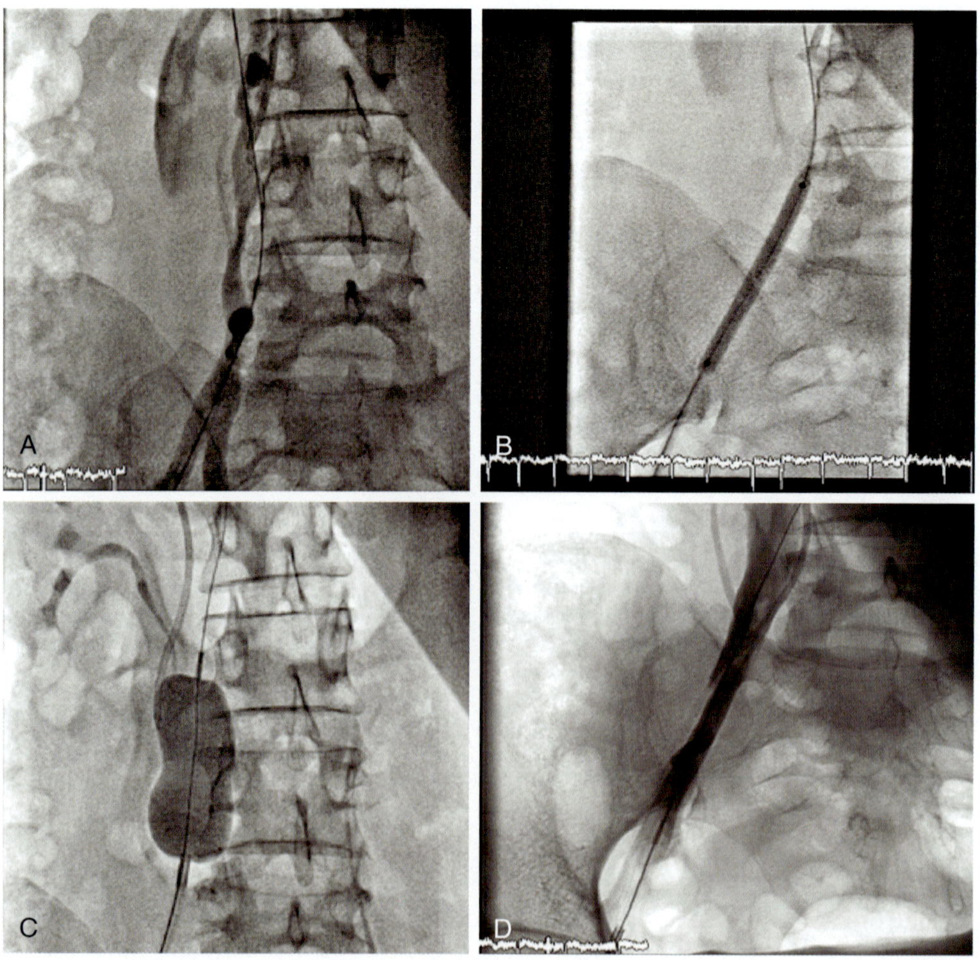

FIG. 7.47 Balloon Angioplasty of the Common Iliac Vein and Inferior Vena Cava. (A) Terumo wire crossed from the right femoral vein into the inferior vena cava via the occluded segment. (B) Balloon angioplasty of the right common iliac vein done using an OPTA Pro balloon (Cordis Corporation, San Jose, California). (C) Balloon angioplasty of the vena cava and proximal right common iliac vein using the SYM balloon (Lifetech Scientific, Shenzhen, China). (D) Brisk flow in the inferior vena cava after balloon angioplasty.

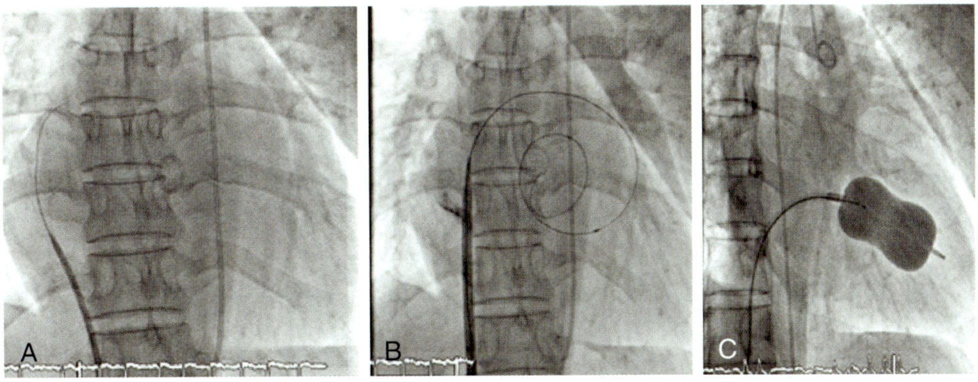

FIG. 7.48 Balloon Mitral Valvotomy via the Interior Vena Cava. (A) A Mullins dilator passed from the inferior vena cava into the left atrium through a transseptal puncture. (B) A 0.025-inch coiled tip wire placed in the left atrium through the Mullins dilator. (C) Mitral valve being dilated with the SYM balloon (Lifetech Scientific, Shenzhen, China).

A New Method for Hemostasis of a Pseudoaneurysm Using Autologous Blood

Daisuke Ueno, MD, Kenji Yanishi, MD, PhD, Kan Zen, MD, PhD, Satoaki Matoba, MD, PhD

A 70-year-old female dialysis patient underwent percutaneous coronary intervention using the right common femoral approach because of effort angina. She reported pain and a hematoma in the right femoral region a few hours after compression by hand. Abdominal computed tomographic angiography showed a pseudoaneurysm and retroperitoneal bleeding near the right common femoral artery. We attempted hemostasis for the pseudoaneurysm without an anticoagulant agent, but we could not stop the bleeding with hand compression and balloon inflation (Fig. 7.49A). Hence, we attempted a novel method of hemostasis for the pseudoaneurysm. First, the sheath was inserted and approximately 20 mL of the patient's own blood was drawn. This autologous blood was separated into serum and clotted blood, and the clotted blood was subsequently transferred into a syringe (Fig. 7.49B). After we confirmed the pseudoaneurysm by angiography, the syringe with an 18-gauge needle was advanced while applying negative pressure toward the pseudoaneurysm. The draining site of the contrast medium was within the pseudoaneurysm, so we injected the clotted autologous blood directly into the pseudoaneurysm while inflating the balloon (Fig. 7.49C). Hemostasis was

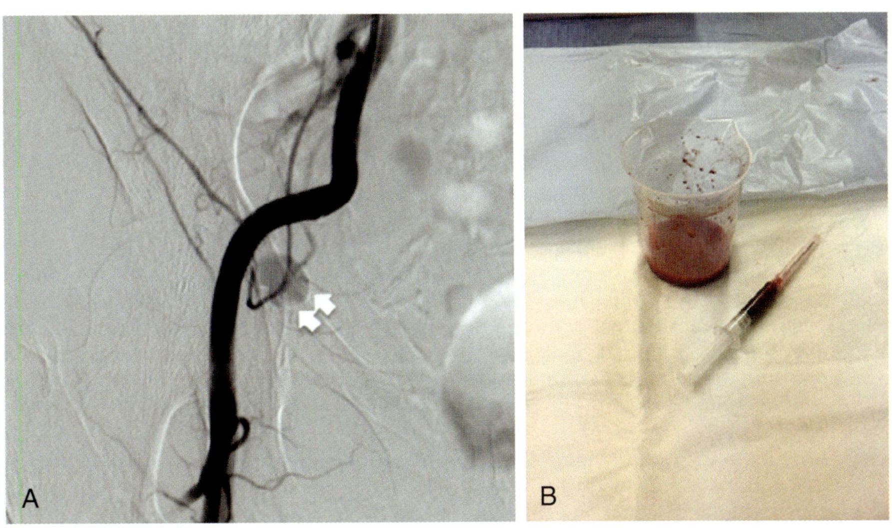

FIG. 7.49 Hemostasis Using Clotted Autologous Blood for a Pseudoaneurysm. (A) Lower extremity angiography shows a pseudoaneurysm and bleeding near the right common femoral artery (*arrows*). (B) The patient's own blood, which was drawn upon insertion of the sheath and the syringe into which the clotted autologous was transferred.

Continued

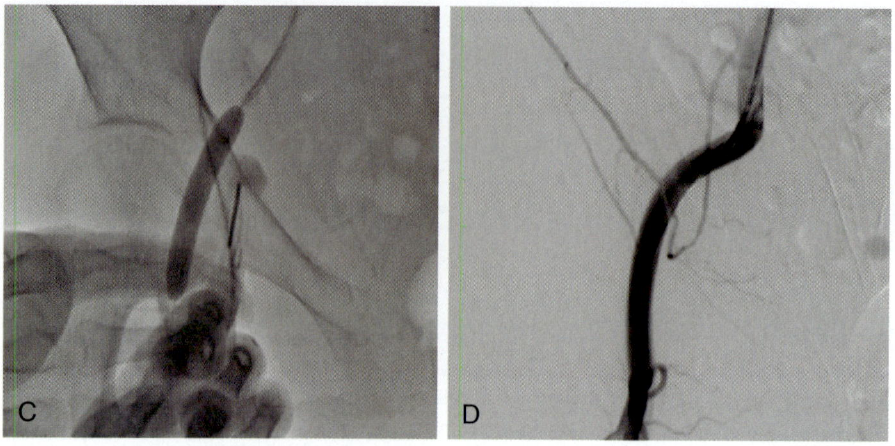

FIG. 7.49, cont'd (C) The clotted blood was directly injected into the pseudoaneurysm using the syringe with an 18-gauge needle. (D) Lower extremity angiography shows hemostasis after injection of the clotted autologous blood.

successful immediately after injection of the clotted blood (Fig. 7.49D). We speculated that the blood flow into the pseudoaneurysm became stagnated by the injection of the blood clot, and the fibrin contained in the clot promoted hemostasis.

Hemostasis by direct injection of thrombin reportedly has a high success rate, but complications, such as thrombosis and allergies,[1,2] can occur. Hemostasis by autologous blood is simpler and safer than that by thrombin with respect to the occurrence of thrombosis due to intraarterial infusion and allergy. Hemostasis using clotted autologous blood may become an effective treatment for some pseudoaneurysms for which it is difficult to stop bleeding.

References

1. Perna L, Olin JW, Goines D, Childs MB, Ouriel K. Ultrasound-guided thrombin injection for the treatment of postcatheterization pseudoaneurysms. *Circulation.* 2000;102:2391-2395.
2. Shah KJ, Halaharvi DR, Franz RW, Jenkins J II. Treatment of iatrogenic pseudoaneurysms using ultrasound-guided thrombin injection over a 5-year period. *Int J Angiol.* 2011;20:235-242.

"Protruding Myocardium" as a Target for Percutaneous Transluminal Septal Myocardial Ablation in a Case of Hypertrophic Obstructive Cardiomyopathy

Yuichiro Maekawa, MD, PhD, Keitaro Akita, MD, Hikaru Tsuruta, MD, Fumiaki Yashima, MD, Mai Kimura, MD, Yoshitake Yamada, MD, PhD, Takashi Kawakami, MD, Hideaki Kanazawa, MD, PhD, Kentaro Hayashida, MD, PhD, Shinsuke Yuasa, MD, PhD, Mitsushige Murata, MD, PhD, Masahiro Jinzaki, MD, PhD, Keiichi Fukuda, MD, PhD

A 57-year-old woman with known hypertrophic obstructive cardiomyopathy presented with dyspnea and fatigue, consistent with New York Heart Association functional class III heart failure. The patient had previously undergone percutaneous transluminal myocardial ablation (PTSMA) twice at another hospital. Echocardiography revealed a "protruding myocardium," systolic anterior motion of the mitral valve, and mild mitral regurgitation (Fig. 7.50A–B, Online Videos 7.36 and 7.37). The protruding myocardium adjoined the basal and mid portion of the ventricular myocardium that had been previously ablated. At rest, the left ventricular outflow tract (LVOT) gradient was 109 mm Hg. Comparison of the coronary angiography that we performed with that performed previously at another hospital confirmed that one of the two proximal septal branches could not be used in PTSMA because the guidewire could not be passed. The patient declined open surgery; therefore, PTSMA was performed. Selective alcohol ablation was performed in the first branch of the identified target vessel guided by real-time two-dimensional echocardiography to the enhanced saturation of each vascular bed (Fig. 7.50C). The postprocedural LVOT gradient was 7 mm Hg. Three months later, her symptoms improved to New York Heart Association functional class I, and echocardiography revealed the disappearance of the protruding myocardium (Fig. 7.50D, Online Video 7.38). Target vessel selection is the most important step in PTSMA.[1] Misidentification of the correct target vessel is a potential cause of PTSMA failure. In addition, the guidewire can occasionally fail to pass due to technical difficulties despite correct identification of the target septal branches. Our case highlights the importance of target vessel selection and complete myocardial ablation.

Reference

1. Maekawa Y, Jinzaki M, Anzai A, et al. Successful second attempt multidetector computed tomography-guided percutaneous transluminal septal myocardial ablation for an octogenarian with hypertrophic obstructive cardiomyopathy. *Int J Cardiol.* 2014;176:e131-e132.

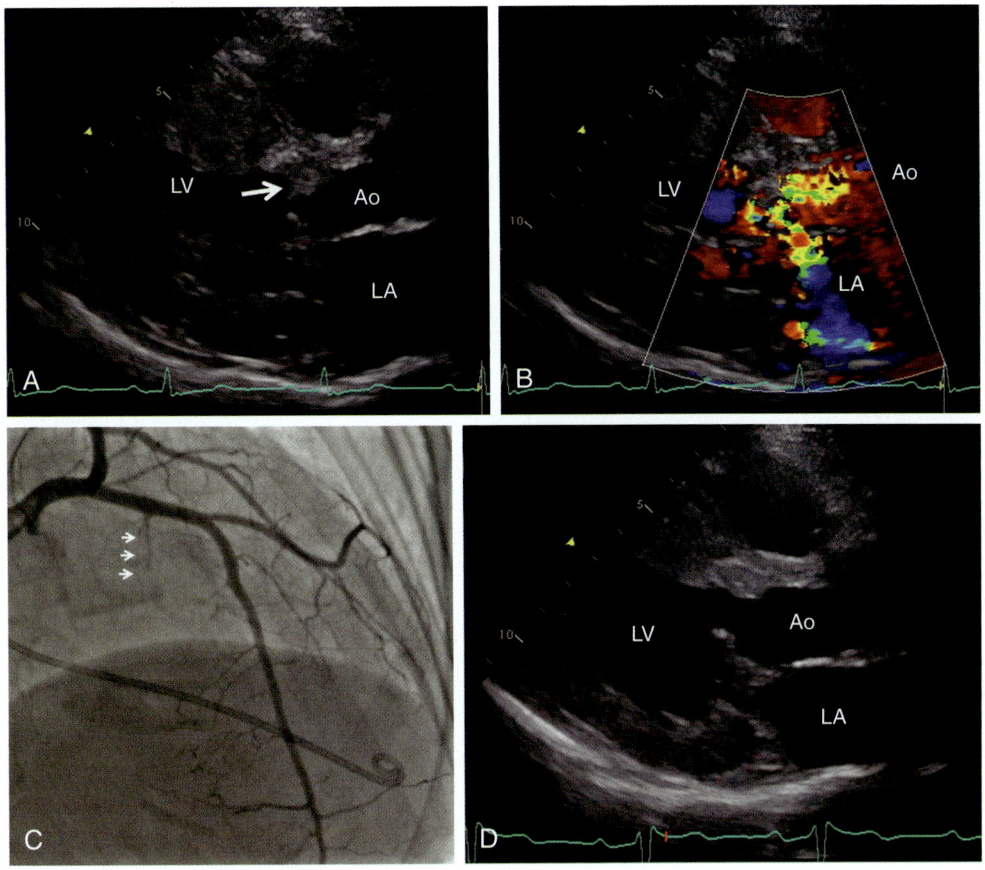

FIG. 7.50 Transthoracic Echocardiographic Images and Coronary Angiogram. (A) Two-dimensional (Online Video 7.36) and (B) color Doppler (Online Video 7.37) images of the parasternal long axis view demonstrating systolic anterior motion of the mitral valve, mild mitral regurgitation, and a "protruding myocardium" (*white arrow*). (C) Coronary angiogram of the right anterior oblique cranial projection showing the first septal branch of the identified target vessels (*white arrows*). (D) Two-dimensional image of the parasternal long-axis view taken 3 months after percutaneous transluminal myocardial ablation demonstrating the disappearance of the ablated protruding myocardium (Online Video 7.38). *Ao*, aorta; *LA*, left atrium; *LV*, left ventricle.

Angio-Seal–Assisted Closure of Iatrogenic Refractory Femoral Arterial Pseudoaneurysm: A Novel Technique

Adnan Hadziomerovic, MD, Prasad Jetty, MD, Ashish Gupta, MBBS, MD

A 63-year-old woman presented 20 days after a coronary artery angiogram with a pulsatile mass in the right groin. Doppler ultrasound confirmed the presence of a 4.5-cm-diameter pseudoaneurysm arising from the superficial femoral artery (SFA) (Fig. 7.51).

The patient was on full anticoagulation for a recent episode of unprovoked massive pulmonary embolism. It was decided to attempt percutaneous thrombin injection with balloon protection.

The contralateral common femoral artery was accessed, an angiogram was performed (Fig. 7.52), and a 5- × 40-mm balloon was placed across the neck of the pseudoaneurysm. Using ultrasound guidance, the pseudoaneurysm was accessed with a 22-gauge needle. The balloon was inflated across the neck, and a total of 3000 U of thrombin (TISSEEL fibrin sealant kit, Baxter Healthcare, Deerfield, Illinois) was injected without success, likely due to full anticoagulation.

Because the neck of the pseudoaneurysm was quite narrow and the diameter of the SFA was adequate, it was decided to attempt

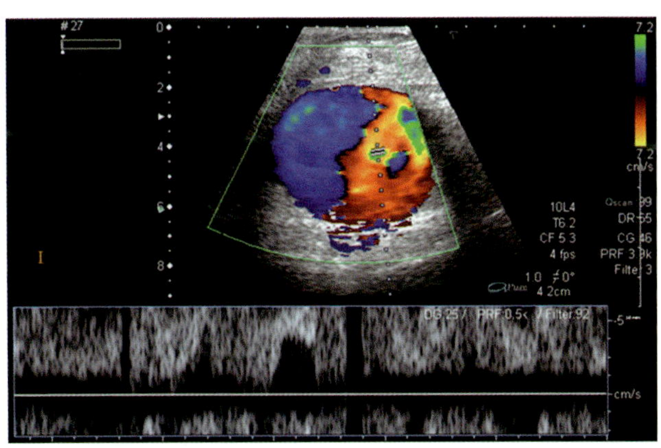

FIG. 7.51 Doppler Ultrasound. Large pseudoaneurysm with "to-and-fro" flow on color Doppler.

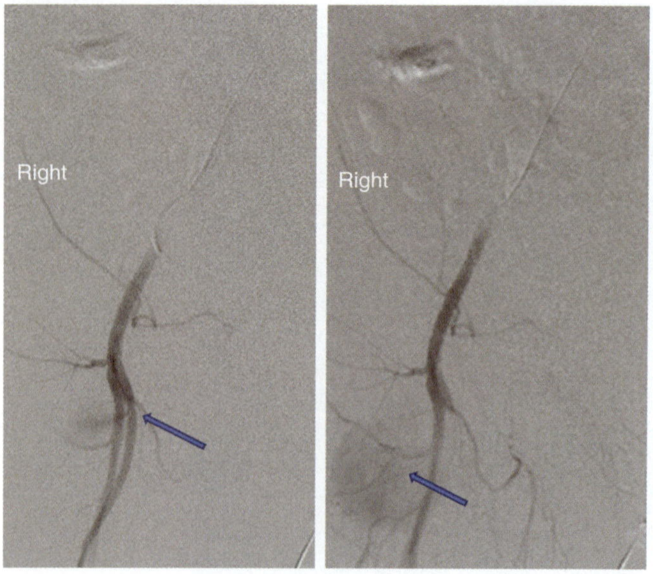

FIG. 7.52 Predeployment Angiogram. Narrow neck pseudoaneurysm (*arrows*) arising from superficial femoral artery.

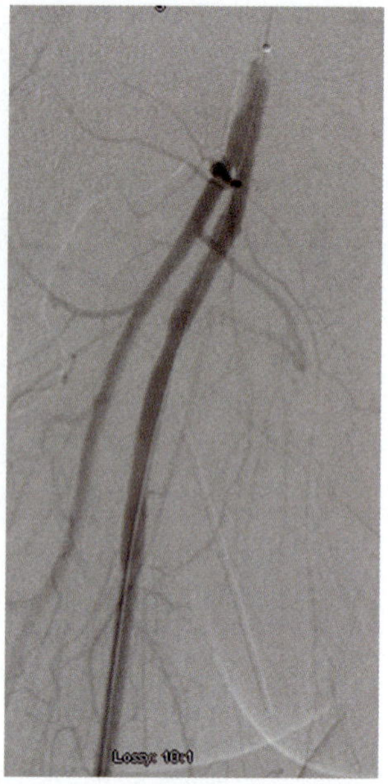

FIG. 7.53 Postdeployment Angiogram. Nonfilling of the pseudoaneurysm and patent superficial femoral artery.

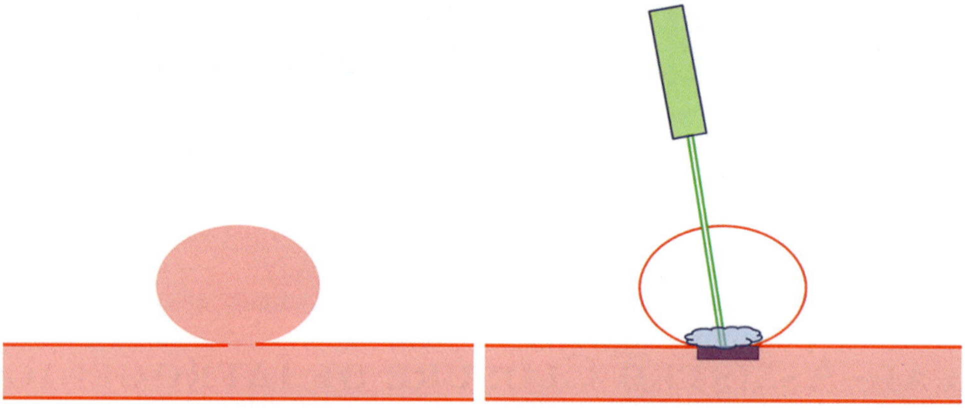

FIG. 7.54 Diagram of the Angio-Seal Deployment. The concept of deployment of the Angio-Seal across the neck of the pseudoaneurysm.

deployment of a 6F Angio-Seal closure device (St. Jude Medical, Minnetonka, Minnesota) across the neck.

The pseudoaneurysm was accessed with 22-gauge needle; a microwire was negotiated through the neck into the proximal SFA and was then exchanged for a 0.035-inch J wire. A sheath from the Angio-Seal device was advanced over the wire into the SFA, and the closure device was deployed with the footplate in the SFA and the collagen plug in the pseudoaneurysm. Once the tamping tube was removed, no further filling was identified on angiography (Fig. 7.53), and no flow was present on color Doppler examination (Fig. 7.54).

The left common femoral artery puncture site was also closed with a 6F Angio-Seal device. The patient was discharged home 6 h after the procedure and was asymptomatic on follow-up.

Endovascular Repair for Pulmonary Artery and Aortic Dissection Associated With Patent Ductus Arteriosus

Yinsu Zhu, MD, Lijun Tang, MD, PhD, Haibin Shi, MD, PhD

A 26-year-old female patient was admitted to our center with chest pain and dyspnea. She had a 2-year history of hypertension (highest systolic pressure was 180 mm Hg) and retrosternal chest pain for more than 1 year without any previous interventional procedure. Thoracic computed tomography angiography (CTA) revealed a Stanford type B aortic dissection and main pulmonary artery dissection accompanied with patent ductus arteriosus (PDA) (Fig. 7.55). The aortic angiogram confirmed the diagnosis (Fig. 7.56A). Consequently, endovascular aortic stent-graft implantation was performed successfully (Fig. 7.56B). The patient's postoperative course was uneventful without any noteworthy symptoms. A follow-up CTA scan at 16 months showed no migration of the covered stent with partial false lumen thrombosis, closure of PDA, and still the existence of pulmonary artery dissection (Fig. 7.56C).

Aortic dissection with concomitant pulmonary artery dissection is a rare entity associated with high mortality. It is a lethal complication of PDA, and the dissection usually occurs as a result of chronic pulmonary hypertension or Eisenmenger syndrome.[1] We speculated that the infiltration could have dissected the layers of the pulmonary artery and aortic wall through the PDA.

The optimal management of this disease has not been defined because of limited cases in the published data. On the basis of anecdotal reports, surgical repair and heart-lung transplantation have been performed occasionally[2,3]; otherwise, the outcome is fatal. In our patient, the fully closed PDA was revealed by follow-up CTA after the aortic stent-graft implantation. To our knowledge, this is the first case of a patient with pulmonary artery and aortic dissection using an endovascular procedure and remaining well during follow-up. Therefore, in comparison with surgery, endovascular treatment could be an attractive option for pulmonary artery and aortic dissection associated with PDA.

References

1. Westaby S, Evans BJ, Ormerod O. Pulmonary artery dissection in patients with Eisenmenger's syndrome. *N Engl J Med.* 2007;356:2110-2112.
2. Tonder N, Kober L, Hassager C. Pulmonary artery dissection in a patient with Eisenmenger syndrome treated with heart and lung transplantation. *Eur J Echocardiogr.* 2004;5:228-230.
3. Yaman M, Arslan U, Ates AH, et al. Pulmonary arterial dissection in a post-partum patient with patent ductus arteriosus: case report and review of the literature. *World J Cardiol.* 2015;7:101-103.

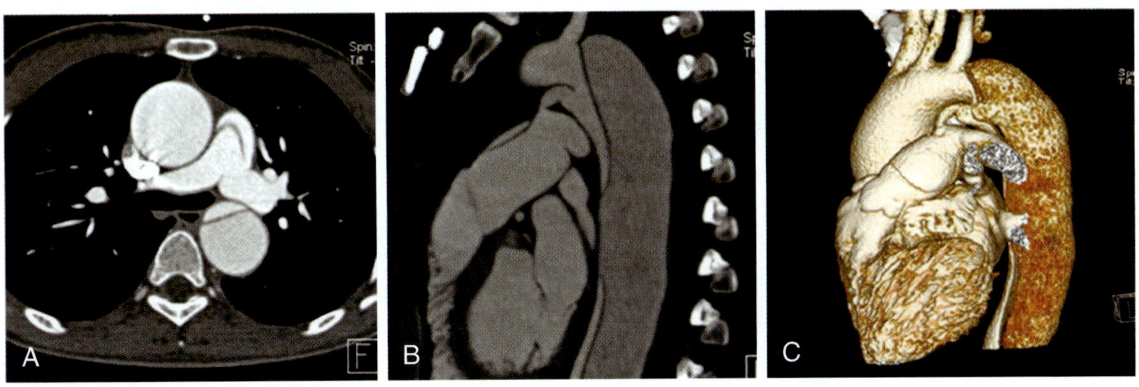

FIG. 7.55 Thoracic Computed Tomography Angiography. Thoracic computed tomography angiography showing Stanford type B aortic dissection and main pulmonary artery dissection accompanied with patent ductus arteriosus. (A) Axial, (B) sagittal, and (C) volume-rendering images.

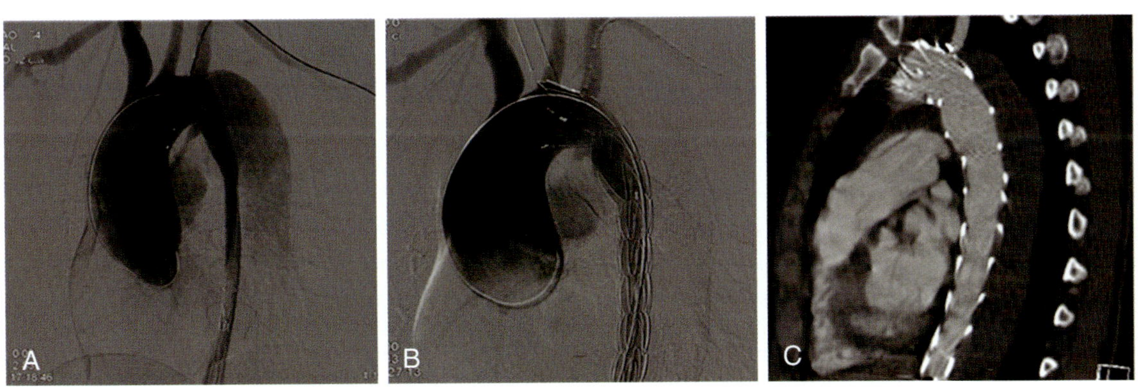

FIG. 7.56 Aortic Angiogram and Follow-up Thoracic Computed Tomography Angiography. Aortic angiogram showing Stanford type B aortic dissection accompanied with patent ductus arteriosus (A) and aortic stent-graft implantation (B). (C) At 16-month follow-up, computed tomography angiography shows stent deployed into the aorta with partial false lumen thrombosis, closure of patent ductus arteriosus, and continued pulmonary artery dissection.

Mesenteric Ischemia Secondary to Paroxysmal Atrial Fibrillation: Percutaneous Recanalization of Superior Mesenteric Artery via Simultaneous Stenting and Inflated Jailed Balloon for Ileal Branch Protection

Yucel Colkesen, MD, Mustafa Topuz, MD, Durmus Yildiray Sahin, MD

We describe a case of thrombotic occlusion of the superior mesenteric artery (SMA) associated with paroxysmal atrial fibrillation (AF). A 74-year-old patient presented with abdominal pain secondary to acute mesenteric ischemia resulting in ischemic gut injury. Electrocardiographic recordings revealed paroxysmal AF, which terminated spontaneously to normal sinus rhythm. Computed tomography demonstrated a luminal filling defect within the SMA (Fig. 7.57A). An exploratory laparotomy was not necessary because of the absence of peritonism. Selective angiography via the transfemoral approach revealed thrombotic occlusion of the SMA at the ileal and ileocolic bifurcation (Fig. 7.57B). The SMA was engaged with a 7F Judkins Right coronary catheter, and a 0.014-inch floppy coronary guidewire (Choice; Boston Scientific, Natick, Massachusetts) was used to cross the lesion. We performed ad hoc thrombectomy by using a thrombus aspiration catheter (Export AP aspiration catheter; Medtronic Vascular, Minneapolis, Minnesota) (Fig. 7.57C). Despite numerous attempts, the flow-limiting lesion remained distally. We decided to perform direct stenting via deployment of a balloon-expandable coronary stent. An additional 0.014-inch floppy coronary guidewire was placed at the ileal branch. A 5- × 30-mm balloon-expandable stent (Liberté Monorail Stent; Boston Scientific) was placed across the occlusion (Fig. 7.57D). For side-branch protection, a 2- × 20-mm monorail balloon (Invader percutaneous transluminal coronary angioplasty balloon; Alvimedica, Assen, the

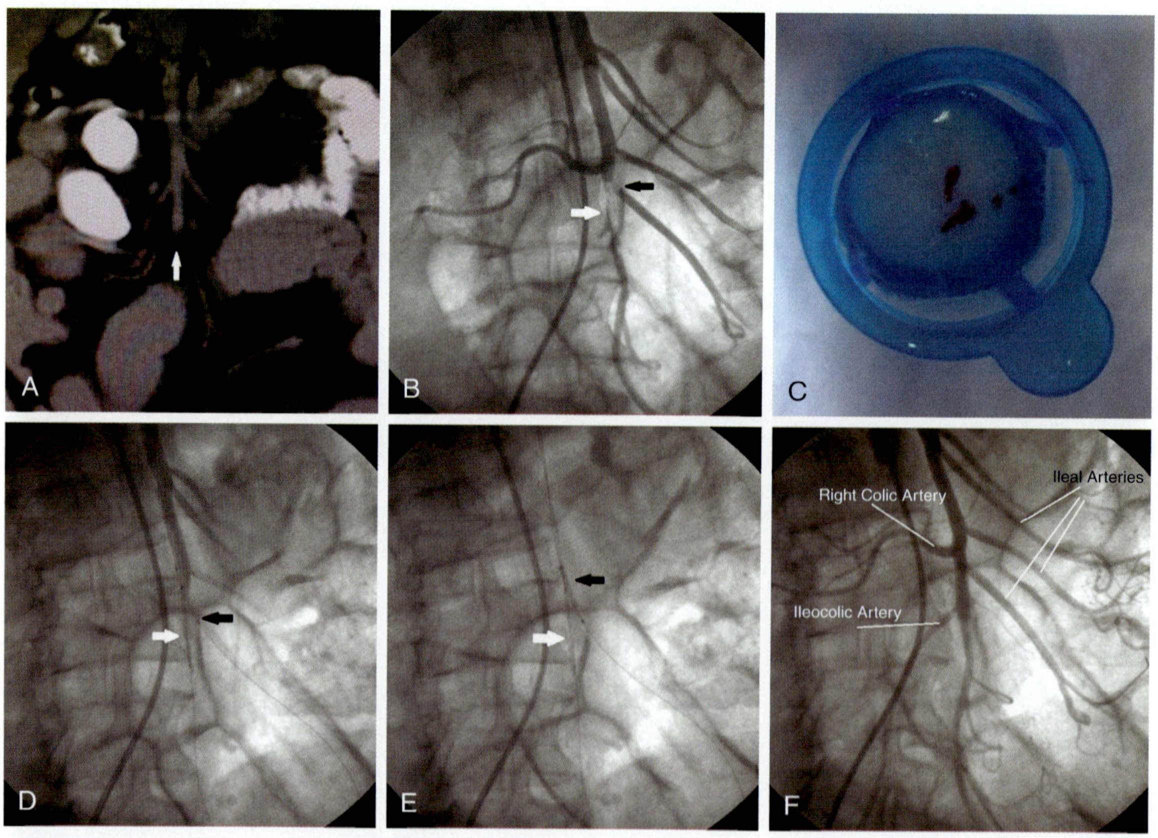

FIG. 7.57 Computer Tomography Scan and Angiographic Views. (A) Coronal reconstruction of contrast-enhanced computed tomography of the abdomen demonstrates luminal filling defect within the superior mesenteric artery (SMA) (*arrow*). (B) Angiographic image in an anteroposterior view showing thrombus occluding the SMA (*white arrow*) and compromising the ileal branch (*black arrow*). (C) Thrombi extracted after catheter aspiration. (D) Balloon-expandable stent in the SMA (*white arrow*) and monorail balloon in the ileal branch (*black arrow*). (E) Stent (*white arrow*) and semiinflated balloon at the ileal branch (*black arrow*). (F) Final angiogram showing the SMA and its branches with satisfactory outcome.

Netherlands) was placed at the bifurcation toward the ileal branch and inflated up to 4 atm to eliminate the side-branch loss and thrombus emboli to the ileal branch during provisional stenting (Fig. 7.57E). Completion angiography showed a widely open SMA with normal filling of its branches (Fig. 7.57F). The patient was successfully discharged and remained asymptomatic at 3-month follow-up.

Paroxysmal AF has not generated as much concern as permanent AF, although no significant differences in thromboembolic event rates between AF types exist.[1] In patients without gut necrosis, a patient-based endovascular intervention appears practicable, and early treatment is advised.[2]

References

1. Disertori M, Franzosi MG, Barlera S, et al., for the GISSI-AF Investigators. Thromboembolic event rate in paroxysmal and persistent atrial fibrillation: data from the GISSI-AF trial. *BMC Cardiovasc Disord.* 2013;13:28-36.
2. Colkesen Y, Seker T, Kuloglu O, Çayli M. TAP-stenting technique for bifurcation stenosis of celiac artery. *Case Rep Vasc Med.* 2015;2015:468561.

Minichimney Technique for Subclavian Artery Iatrogenic Bleeding

Davide Tavano, MD, Marco Pocar, MD, PhD, Flavio Airoldi, MD

An 87-year-old woman with symptomatic severe aortic stenosis was admitted to our institution for transcatheter aortic valve implantation. After an unsuccessful attempt of right internal jugular vein cannulation, the anesthesiologist observed a neck hematoma. The 7F catheter was retrieved and the valve procedure aborted. Duplex scan was immediately performed and showed active arterial bleeding. Contrast-enhanced computed tomography documented a pseudoaneurysm originating from the subclavian artery at the level of the vertebral artery ostium (Fig. 7.58). Catheterization was indicated for endovascular repair[1] and angiography confirmed the active bleeding from a laminar damage of the anterior subclavian arterial wall adjacent to the vertebral and internal thoracic artery ostia (Fig. 7.59, Online Video 7.39). A minichimney technique[2] was chosen to preserve vertebral arterial flow and to prevent reverse flow from the vertebral artery with the potential for a type II residual endoleak. Two stents were deployed simultaneously: a 3.5- × 20-mm nonwoven, electrospun polyurethane-covered coronary stent (Papyrus, Biotronik, Berlin, Germany) was implanted in the ostial vertebral artery through a 90-cm, 6F femoral sheath, whereas a 10- × 59-mm balloon-expandable, polytetrafluoroethylene-covered stent (E-ventus, Jotec, Hechingen, Germany) was implanted in the subclavian artery through a 12-cm, 7F radial sheath. The proximal edges of both stents were aligned and slightly overlapped in the proximal subclavian artery (Fig. 7.60). Control angiograms showed no residual bleeding and a patent vertebral artery (Fig. 7.61, Online Video 7.40).

The chimney technique, most commonly adopted for endovascular aortic aneurysm repair, may also offer a straightforward solution to interrupt active hemorrhage, preserving the patency of noble arterial branches.

References

1. Cayne NS, Berland TL, Rockman CB, et al. Experience and technique for the endovascular management of iatrogenic subclavian artery injury. *Ann Vasc Surg.* 2010;24:44-47.
2. Moulakakis KG, Mylonas SN, Avgerinos E, et al. The chimney graft technique for preserving visceral vessels during endovascular treatment of aortic pathologies. *J Vasc Surg.* 2012;55:1497-1503.

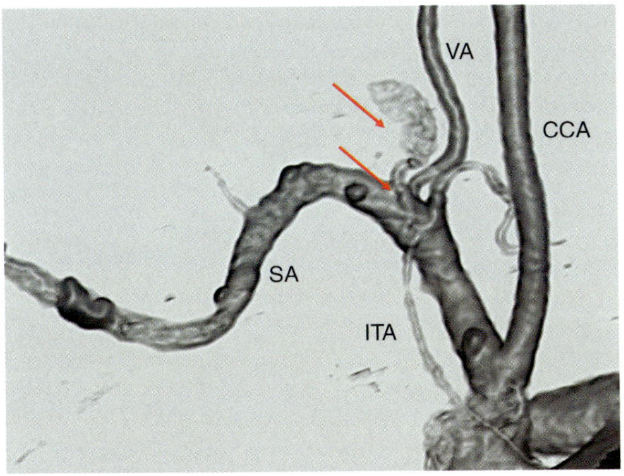

FIG. 7.58 Three-Dimensional Contrast-Enhanced Computed Tomography Scan Reconstruction. Bleeding originating from the anterior wall of the right subclavian artery (*red arrows*). *CCA*, common carotid artery; *ITA*, internal thoracic artery; *SA*, subclavian artery; *VA*, vertebral artery.

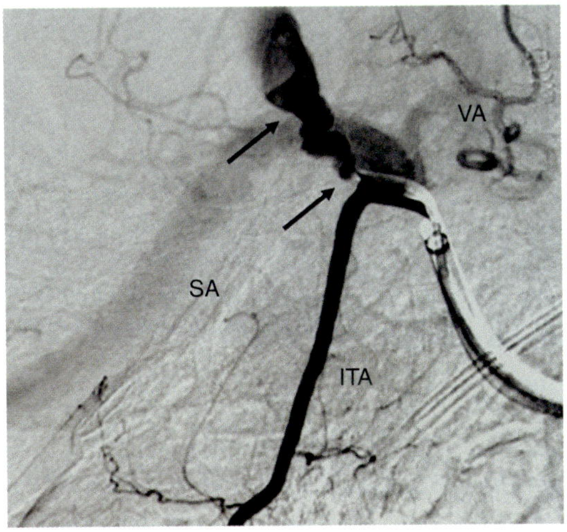

FIG. 7.59 Right Subclavian Artery Angiography. Selective injection with a diagnostic catheter next to the ITA ostium showing the pseudoaneurysm (*arrows*) (Online Video 7.39). *ITA*, internal thoracic artery; *SA*, subclavian artery; *VA*, vertebral artery.

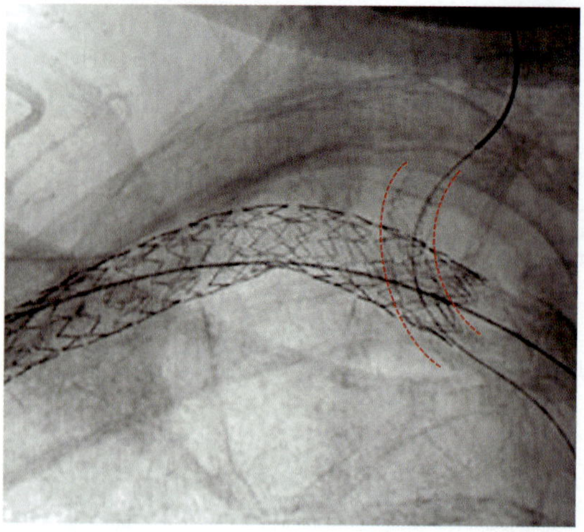

FIG. 7.60 Minichimney Technique for Subclavian (SA) and Vertebral Artery (VA) Stent Implantation. A 10- × 59-mm balloon-expandable stent graft and a 3.5- × 20-mm coronary stent graft (*red dashed lines*) were respectively implanted in the proximal and mid segments of the SA and in the proximal VA. Stent dilations were performed simultaneously.

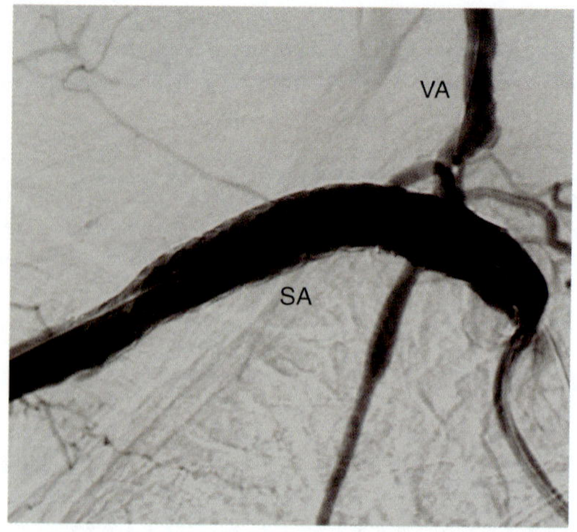

FIG. 7.61 Control Angiography. Final angiogram showing covered stents sealing the vascular injury, maintaining both vessels perfused (Online Video 7.40). *SA*, subclavian artery; *VA*, vertebral artery.

Percutaneous Coronary Intervention for Treatment of Paraganglioma With Coronary Vascularization

Rocío González-Ferreiro, MD, Emilio Rodriguez-Ruiz, MD, Diego López-Otero, MD, PhD, Amparo Martínez Monzonís, MD, PhD, María Álvarez Barredo, MD, Ramiro Trillo-Nouche, MD, José Ramón González Juanatey, MD, PhD

A 58-year-old man was referred to the cardiology outpatient clinic because of palpitations. Physical examination highlighted the presence of mitral early systolic click. Transthoracic echocardiography showed a retrocardiac mass that was compressing the left atrium and surrounding the pulmonary artery and the aorta. Cardiac computed tomography demonstrated a mass extended from the upper mediastinum to the cardiac region, with invasion of the pericardium, the wall of both atria, both pulmonary arteries, and the ascending aorta (Fig. 7.62). Histologic diagnosis of paraganglioma was made by endovascular ultrasound–guided biopsy.

On coronary angiography, vascularization of the mass by coronary fistulas was shown, principally dependent on the anterior descending coronary artery, intermediate branch, and right coronary artery and less importantly on the left circumflex coronary artery (Fig. 7.63).

In further interventions, we proceeded to implant multiple embolization coils on the coronary fistulae (Figs. 7.64 and 7.65).

High vascularization and adherence to surrounding structures are characteristic of paragangliomas, making fatal hemorrhagic complications a serious risk during surgery. Preoperative embolization has a proven role in minimizing bleeding and facilitating resection. Partial surgical excision was performed and currently is being followed up in the oncology department, where the patient is undergoing chemotherapy.

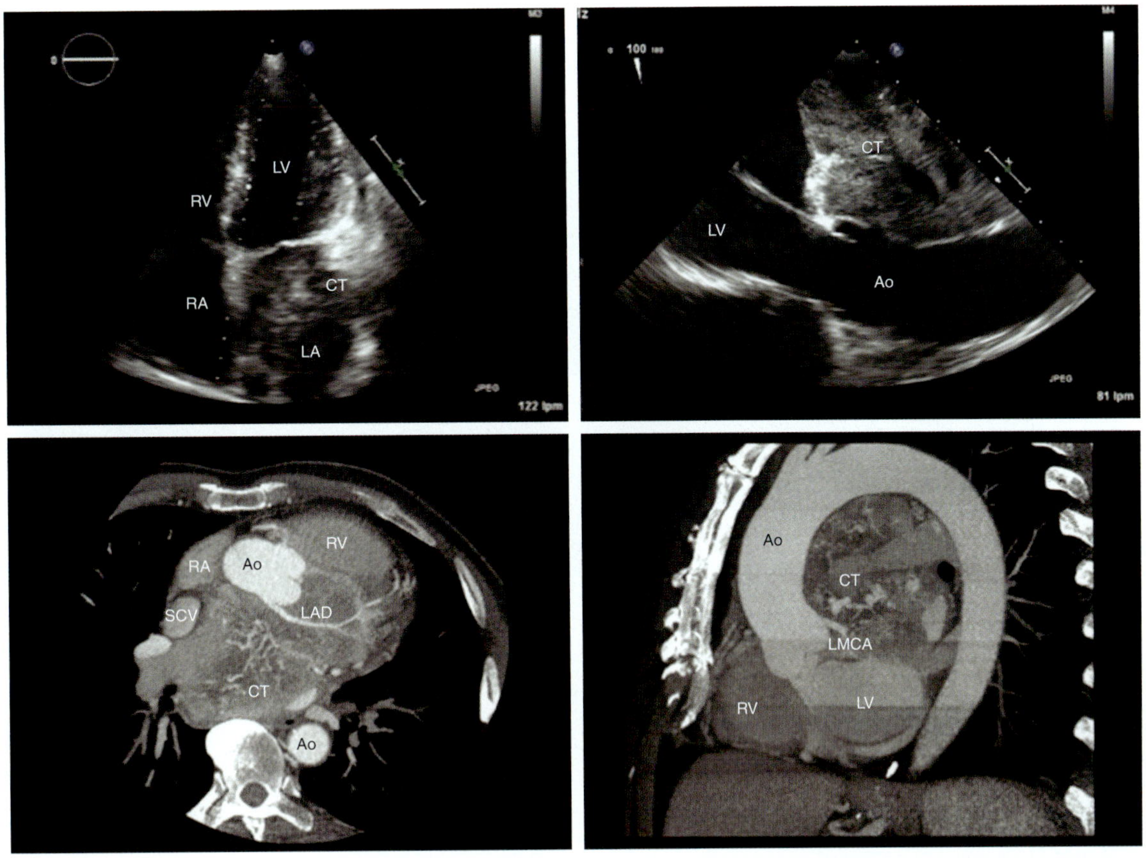

FIG. 7.62 Images of Transthoracic (*top left*) and Transesophageal Echocardiography (*top right*) and Cardiac Computed Tomography (*bottom*). The images show a mass of 13.5 × 14.3 cm, with extensive microvasculature, extending from the upper mediastinum to the cardiac region, with invasion of the pericardium, the wall of both atria, both pulmonary arteries, and the ascending aorta. *Ao*, aorta; *CT*, cardiac tumor; *LA*, left atrium; *LAD*, left anterior descending coronary artery; *LMCA*, left main coronary artery; *LV*, left ventricle; *RA*, right atrium; *RV*, right ventricle; *SCV*, superior vena cava.

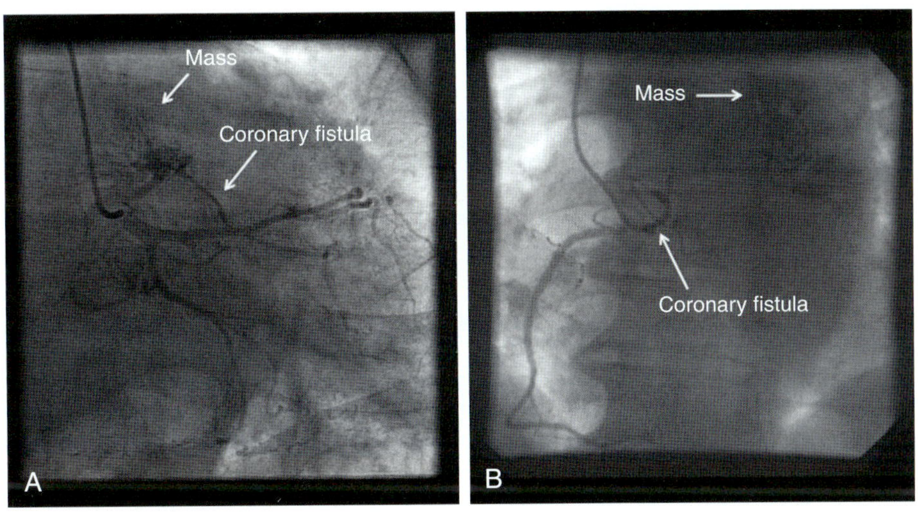

FIG. 7.63 Coronary Angiography. Initial coronary angiography showing irrigation of tumor mass by anterior descending coronary artery, intermediate branch, circumflex coronary artery (A), and right coronary artery (B).

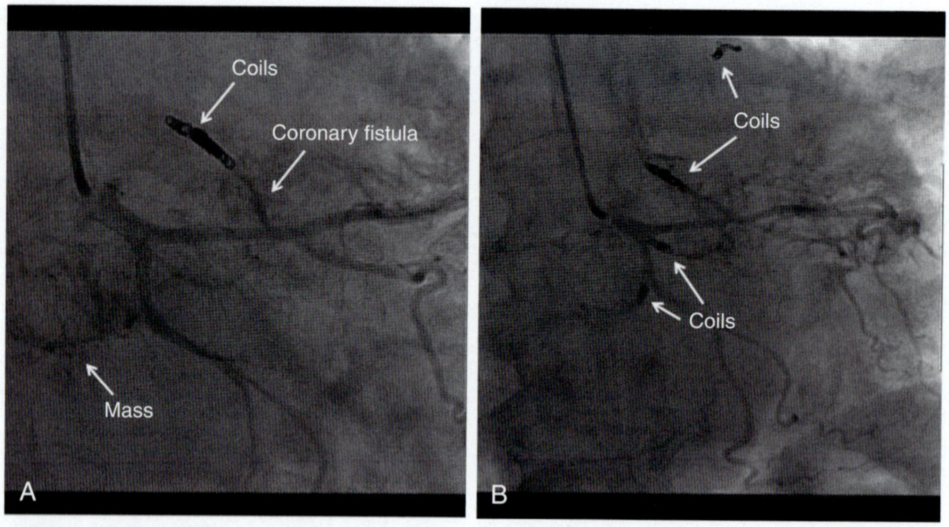

FIG. 7.64 Intracoronary Coil Implantation. Embolization of fistulas by coils with origin in proximal anterior descending coronary artery (A) and intermediate branch, and proximal circumflex (B).

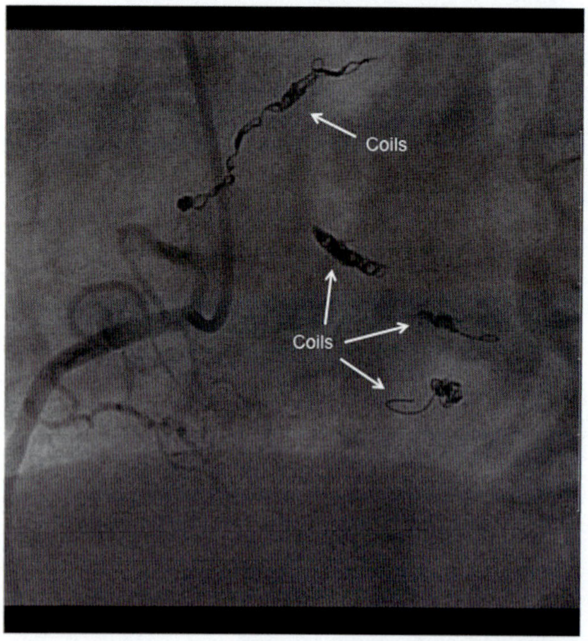

FIG. 7.65 Coronary Angiography. Complete embolization of fistula with origin in the right coronary artery.

Retrograde Approach in Balloon Pulmonary Angioplasty: A Useful Novel Strategy for Chronic Total Occlusion Lesions in Pulmonary Arteries

Takashi Kawakami, MD, Masaharu Kataoka, MD, Takahide Arai, MD, Ryo Yanagisawa, MD, Yuichiro Maekawa, MD, Keiichi Fukuda, MD

A 61-year-old man with chronic thromboembolic pulmonary hypertension underwent balloon pulmonary angioplasty (BPA).[1–3] Antegrade approach for a chronic total occlusion (CTO) lesion in an inside subsegmental branch of the left A9 pulmonary artery (A9b branch) was attempted (Fig. 7.66A), but the hydrophilic and hard guidewire (tip load, 10 gf; Chevalier PL-X, Cordis, Tokyo, Japan) could not pass through this CTO lesion. Hence another tight lesion in an outside subsegmental branch of the left A9 pulmonary artery (A9a branch) was treated (Fig. 7.66B).

Four months later, angiography revealed well-developed collaterals (Fig. 7.66C, Online Video 7.41). Because a retrograde approach in percutaneous coronary intervention can be successful in some cases

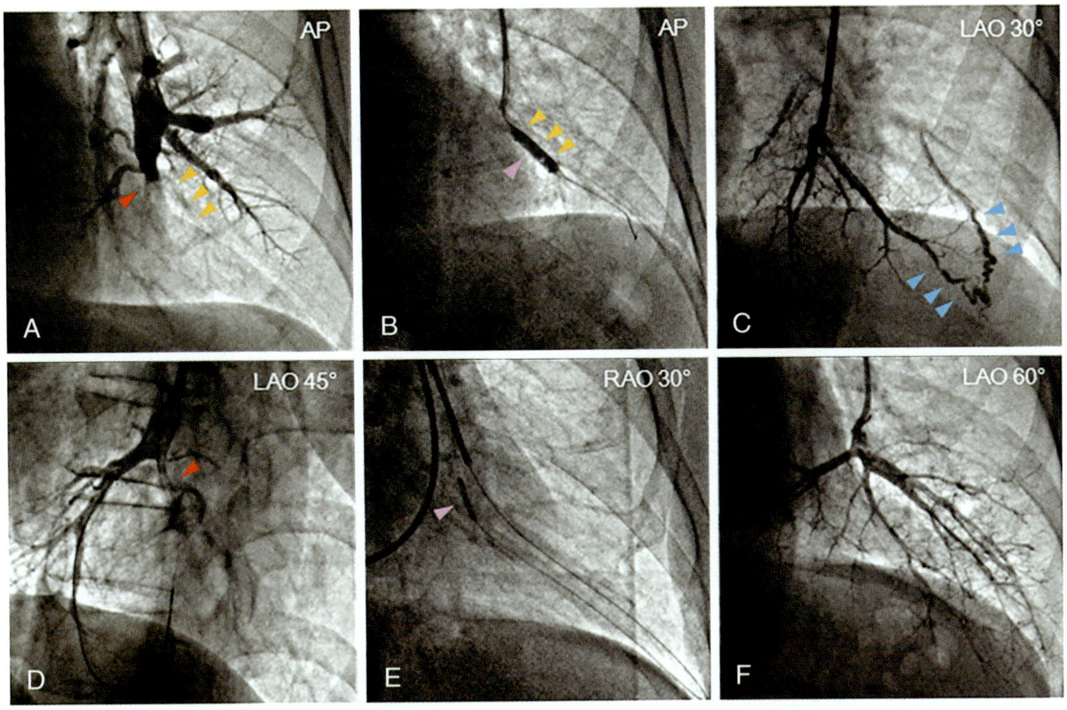

FIG. 7.66 Angiography Images Before and During Balloon Pulmonary Angioplasty (BPA). Angiography was performed on a 61-year-old man with chronic thromboembolic pulmonary hypertension. Images from the first balloon pulmonary angioplasty (BPA) session show a chronic total occlusion (CTO) lesion in an inside subsegmental branch of the left A9 pulmonary artery (A9b branch) (A) and balloon dilation for another stenotic lesion in an outside subsegmental branch of the left A9 pulmonary artery (A9a branch) (B). Images from the next BPA session, 4 months later, show flows of the A9a branch and well-developed collaterals shot by the guiding catheter (Online Video 7.41) (C), successful passing of the guidewire into the target CTO lesion in the A9b branch by the retrograde approach (Online Video 7.42) (D), over-the-wire balloon dilation in the CTO lesion (E), and good antegrade flow of the A9b branch (F). *Red arrowheads* indicate the positions of the CTO lesion in the A9b branch, *orange arrowheads* indicate the positions of the A9a branch, *blue arrowheads* indicate collaterals from peripherals of the A9a branch to the distal area of CTO lesion in A9b branch, and *pink arrowheads* indicate balloon catheters. *AP*, anteroposterior view; *LAO*, left anterior oblique view; *RAO*, right anterior oblique view.

of coronary CTO lesions,[4] we attempted the retrograde approach in BPA through these collaterals. A hydrophilic guidewire (tip load, 0.7 gf; SION, Asahi Intecc, Aichi, Japan) supported by a microcatheter (Corsair PV, Asahi Intecc) was advanced into the distal area of the A9a branch and passed through collaterals to the distal area of the target CTO lesion.

The hydrophilic and intermediate guidewire (tip load, 3 gf; Gladius, Asahi Intecc) passed into the target lesion (Fig. 7.66D, Online Video 7.42). An over-the-wire balloon catheter (Amphirion Plus 2.0- × 14-mm, Medtronic, Tokyo, Japan) was then inserted by the retrograde approach and dilated in the target lesion (Fig. 7.66E). The guidewire was again passed through the lesion by the antegrade approach for additional balloon dilation, and finally angiography revealed good antegrade flow through the target lesion (Fig. 7.66F). Mean pulmonary arterial pressure was 35 mm Hg at baseline and improved to 28 mm Hg after BPA in this CTO lesion.

This suggests that the retrograde approach in BPA could be used in similar cases where the antegrade approach is difficult and good collaterals can be visualized by angiography.

References

1. Kataoka M, Inami T, Hayashida K, et al. Percutaneous transluminal pulmonary angioplasty for the treatment of chronic thromboembolic pulmonary hypertension. *Circ Cardiovasc Interv.* 2012;5:756-762.
2. Inami T, Kataoka M, Shimura N, et al. Pulmonary edema predictive scoring index (PEPSI), a new index to predict risk of reperfusion pulmonary edema and improvement of hemodynamics in percutaneous transluminal pulmonary angioplasty. *J Am Coll Cardiol Intv.* 2013;6:725-736.
3. Kawakami T, Kataoka M, Nakahara T, et al. Usefulness of 3D SPECT/CT fusion image in CTEPH. *Int J Cardiol.* 2015;194:39-40.
4. Galassi AR, Sianos G, Werner GS, et al. Retrograde recanalization of chronic total occlusions in Europe: procedural, in-hospital, and long-term outcomes from the multicenter ERCTO registry. *J Am Coll Cardiol.* 2015;65:2388-2400.

Ultrasound-Assisted Catheter-Directed Thrombolysis in Pulmonary Embolism in Transit

Andrew Boshara, MD, Sushruth Edla, MD, Saroj Neupane, MD, Howard Rosman, MD, Antonious Attallah, MD

Pulmonary emboli (PE) in transit are associated with high mortality (27%).[1] Current treatment modalities have not been studied in randomized trials and carry exorbitant risks.[2] We encountered a 78-year-old man with a history of gallbladder cancer who presented after a ventricular fibrillation arrest. On arrival he was normotensive, tachycardic, and tachypneic. Computed tomography angiogram of the chest demonstrated bilateral upper and lower lobe pulmonary emboli (Fig. 7.67A) and a right ventricle to left ventricle diameter ratio ≥0.90 (Fig. 7.67B). Unfractionated heparin was initiated with an intravenous bolus dose of 80 IU/kg followed by infusion with a targeted activated partial thromboplastin time of 1.5 to 2 times the laboratory control. Transthoracic echocardiogram (TTE) revealed a highly mobile thrombus in transit, occupying a large area within the right atrium (RA) (Fig. 7.68A, Online Video 7.43). Consequently, the patient underwent ultrasound-assisted catheter-directed thrombolysis (USAT) using the Ekosonic endovascular system (EKOS, Bothell, Washington). Pulmonary angiogram was performed to enable accurate catheter insertion (Fig. 7.69A). The USAT catheters were inserted bilaterally extending up to the right and left pulmonary artery bifurcations (Fig. 7.70) and left in place to infuse tissue plasminogen activator at 1 mg/h per catheter for 12 h. Catheters were then removed and angiogram was performed again (Fig. 7.69B) and revealed improvement in pulmonary hemodynamics and perfusion of previously oligemic lobes. TTE performed 48 h

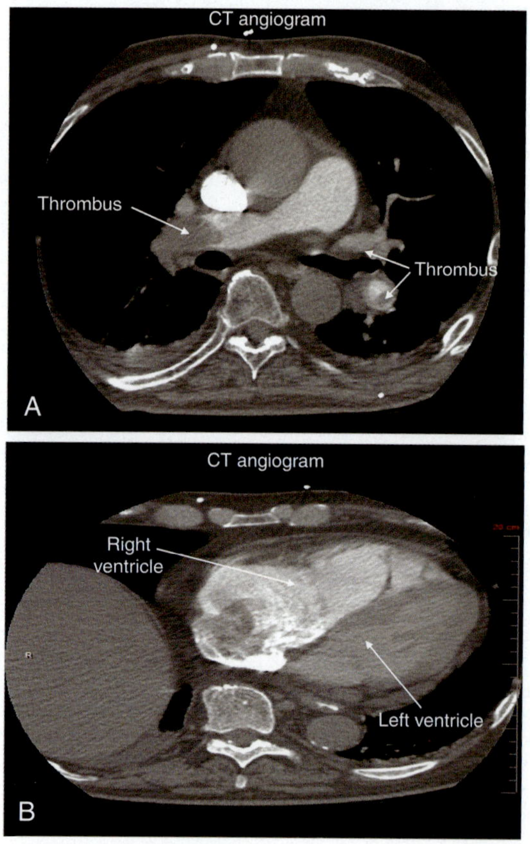

FIG. 7.67 Computed Tomography (CT) Angiogram of the Chest. (A) CT angiogram of the chest showing bilateral upper and lower lobe pulmonary emboli. (B) CT angiogram of the chest showing enlarged right ventricular size with a right ventricle to left ventricle diameter ratio ≥0.90.

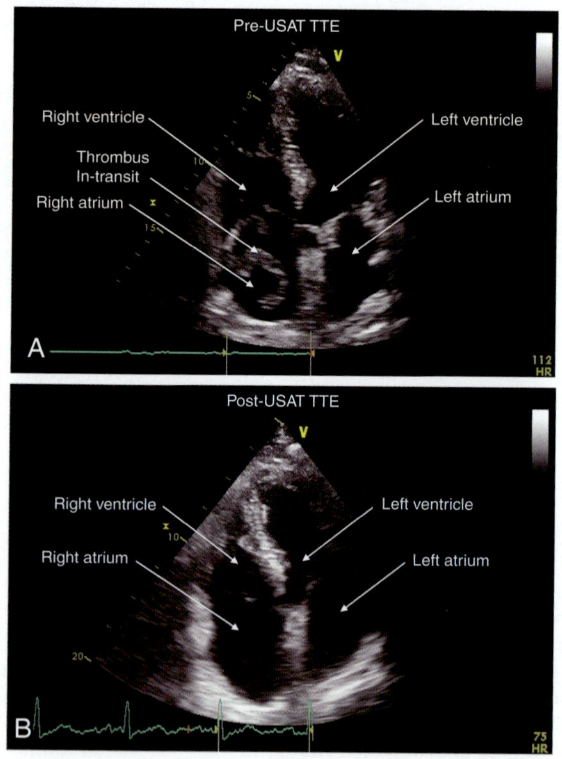

FIG. 7.68 Echocardiography Performed Before and After Ultrasound-Assisted Catheter-Directed Thrombolysis (*USAT*). (A) Pre-USAT transthoracic echocardiogram (TTE), four-chamber view, showing thrombus (identified by *arrow*) occupying a large area within the right atrium (Online Video 7.43). (B) Post-USAT TTE, four-chamber view, showing near-complete resolution of thrombus previously seen in the right atrium (Online Video 7.44).

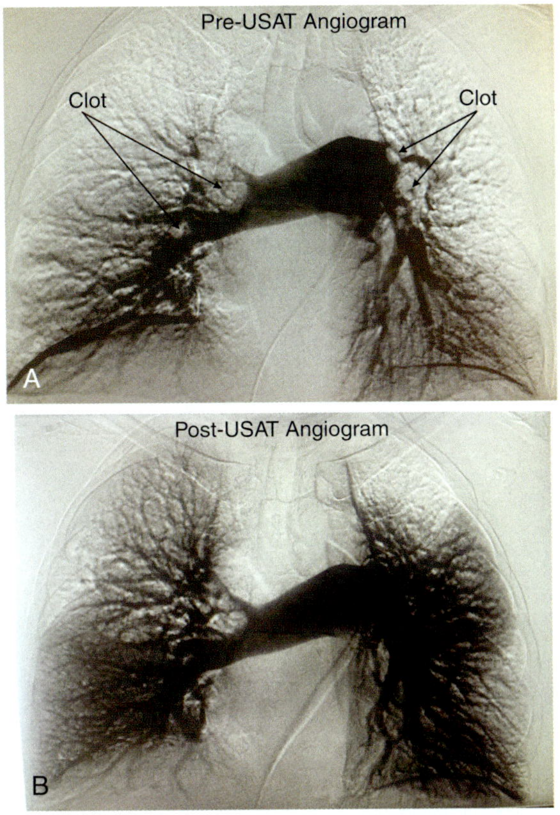

FIG. 7.69 Pulmonary Angiography Performed Before and After Ultrasound-Assisted Catheter-Directed Thrombolysis (*USAT*). (A) Pre-USAT pulmonary angiogram showing extensive pulmonary oligemia with arrows representing areas of increased clot burden. (B) Post-USAT pulmonary angiogram showing improved perfusion of bilateral lung fields.

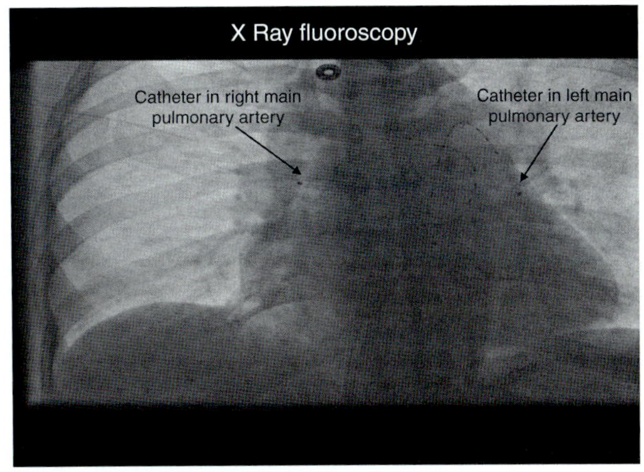

FIG. 7.70 X-Ray Fluoroscopy. Placement of the ultrasound-assisted catheter-directed thrombolysis catheters in the left and right main pulmonary arteries.

post-USAT demonstrated near-complete resolution of the RA thrombus (Fig. 7.68B, Online Video 7.44). The patient was discharged on enoxaparin to an extended-care facility. These promising results suggest that USAT could be a beneficial tool in the treatment of PE in transit.

References

1. Rose PS, Punjabi NM, Pearse DB. Treatment of right heart thromboemboli. *Chest.* 2002;121:806-814.
2. Athappan G, Sengodan P, Chacko P, Gandhi S. Comparative efficacy of different modalities for treatment of right heart thrombi in transit: a pooled analysis. *Vasc Med.* 2015;20:131-138.

Vertebral Artery Rupture Treated by Transcatheter Arterial Embolization

Zhongzhi Jia, PhD, Guomin Jiang, MD

A 27-year-old man presented with a huge hematoma in the neck that resulted from a knife wound. Vertebral artery rupture was suspected by ultrasonography. Vertebral arteriography was performed for a possible cover stent placement, and a right vertebral artery rupture was identified. A balloon was placed proximal to the right vertebral artery (Fig. 7.71A). Left vertebral arteriography showed a huge hematoma at the site of the rupture of the right vertebral artery (Fig. 7.71B), and a microcatheter was placed into the right vertebral artery via the left vertebral artery with the tip at the site of rupture (Fig. 7.71C). The distal portion of the vertebral artery was embolized by coils (Fig. 7.71D). The wound and hematoma were treated with surgical irrigation and debridement after the embolization procedure, and the patient recovered without procedure-related complications and side effects at 4-year follow-up.

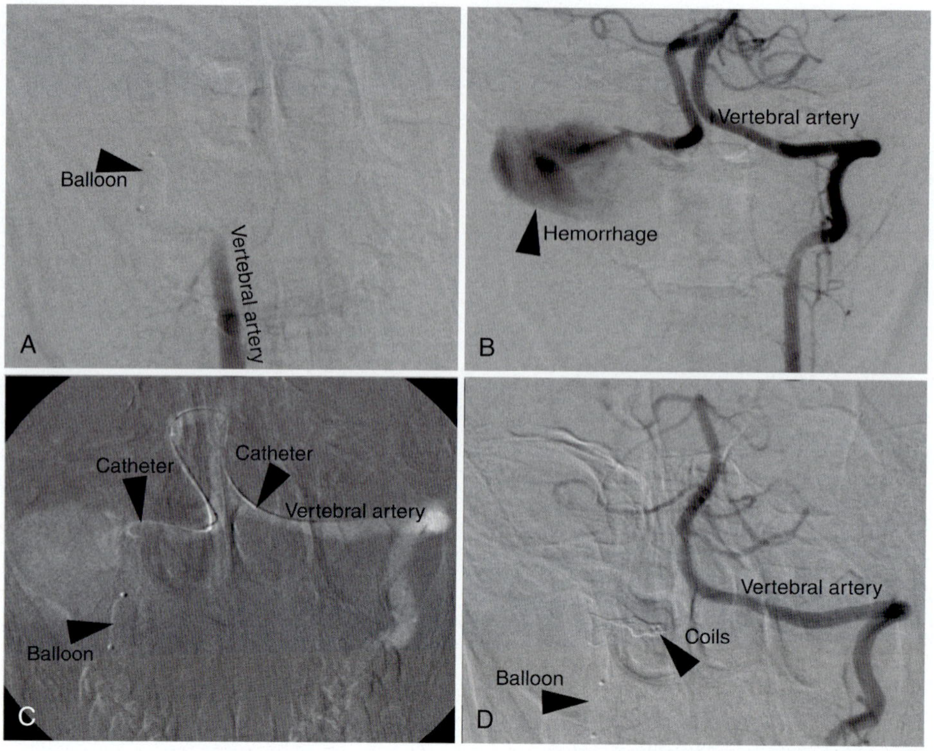

FIG. 7.71. Vertebral Arteriography and Embolization. (A) A balloon was placed proximal to the right vertebral artery to block the flow. (B) Left vertebral arteriography showed a huge hematoma at the site of the rupture of the right vertebral artery. (C) A microcatheter was placed into the right vertebral artery via the left vertebral artery with the tip at the site of rupture. (D) The distal portion of the vertebral artery was embolized by coils.

Aorta to Right Atrial Tunnel: Prenatal Diagnosis and Transcatheter Management in a Neonate

Kappanayil Mahesh, FNB, Edwin Francis, DM, Raman Krishna Kumar, DM

These images show an example of aorta to right atrial tunnel, a rare form of aorta–right atrial communication that was closed on the 4th day of life of this neonate in the catheterization laboratory. The condition was suspected on fetal echocardiogram at 31 weeks' gestation that showed the presence of a large vascular communication between the rightward aspect of the aortic root and the right atrium (Fig. 7.72), with impressive flow reversal in the ascending and descending aorta. The baby was delivered at term (birth weight, 2.7 kg) and had signs of aortic runoff and a loud continuous murmur. Postnatal echocardiogram confirmed the diagnosis of aorta to right atrial tunnel with a 3-mm opening into the right atrium. Three days after birth, the child became critically ill with congestive cardiac failure, poor systemic perfusion, and renal failure and required mechanical ventilation. The patient underwent cardiac catheterization on the next day. Angiograms in anterior-posterior view (Fig. 7.73A) and lateral view (Fig. 7.73B) showed the course and anatomy of the tunnel. The right coronary artery was seen arising separately from the right coronary sinus with normal course and branching pattern. The tunnel was successfully occluded by delivery of multiple coils into the tunnel with the assistance of a 3F bioptome, through a 5.5F long sheath passed via the femoral vein after establishment of an arteriovenous wire loop (Fig. 7.74A). An additional coil was delivered into the coil mass from the arterial route by a 4F Judkins Right catheter. Fig. 7.74B shows the final coil mass occluding the tunnel. The patient had complete clinical recovery after the procedure. Six months after the procedure she was well with no residual flows.

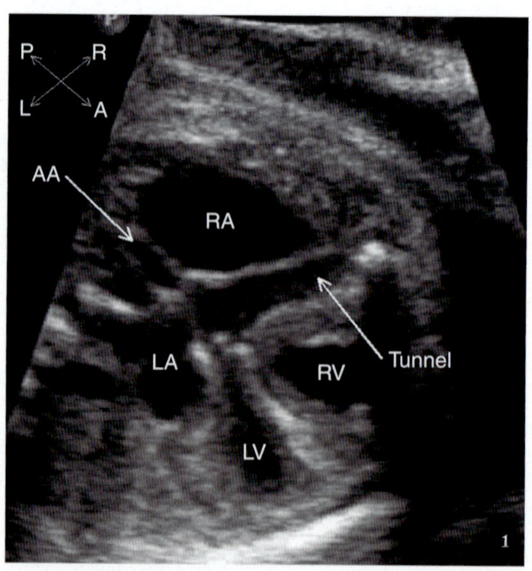

FIG. 7.72. Fetal Echocardiogram Showing a Large Vascular Communication Between the Aortic Root and the Right Atrium. *A*, anterior; *AA*, ascending aorta; *L*, left; *LA*, left atrium; *LV*, left ventricle; *R*, right; *RA*, right atrium; *RV*, right ventricle; *P*, posterior.

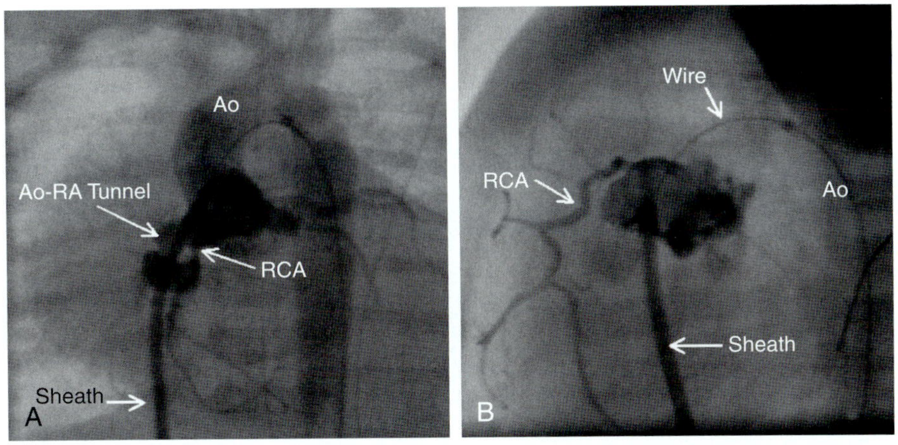

FIG. 7.73 Angiograms Showing Course and Anatomy of Tunnel. (A) Angiographic frame (posterior-anterior view) showing an arteriovenous wire loop with sheath positioned within the aorta–right atrial tunnel. The right coronary artery is seen arising separately with normal course and branching pattern. (B) Lateral view angiographic frame showing the tunnel and the separate course of the right coronary artery (*RCA*). *Ao*, aorta; *RA*, right atrium.

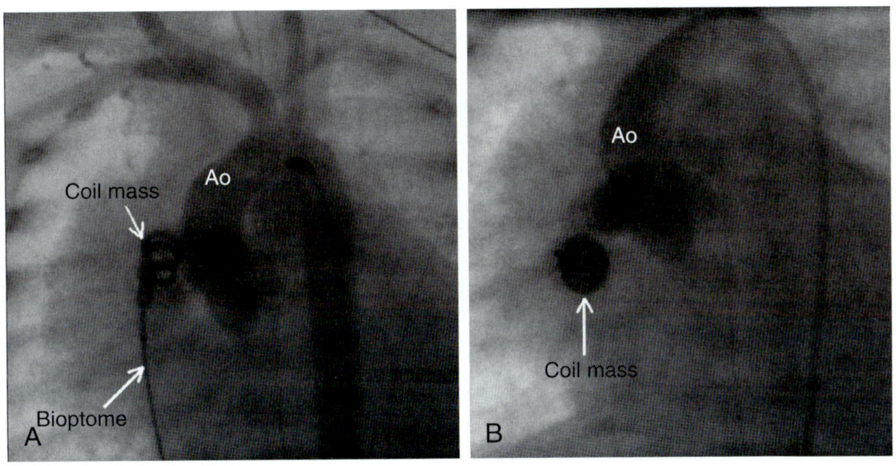

FIG. 7.74 Angiographic Frame Showing Coil Mass. (A) Angiographic frame showing the coil mass being positioned within the aorta–right atrial tunnel with a bioptome. (B) Angiographic frame showing the final position of the coil mass occluding the tunnel. *Ao*, aorta.

Closure of Ascending Aorta Pseudoaneurysm to Right Atrium Fistula

Salwa M. Gendi, MD, Damien Kenny, MD, John Hibbeln, MD, Ziyad M. Hijazi, MD, MPH

A 75-year-old man presented with worsening right-sided heart failure on the background of previous supracoronary ascending aortic replacement and bioprosthetic aortic valve replacement for bicuspid aortopathy. Transthoracic echocardiography showed continuous flow on color Doppler from an ascending aortic aneurysm fistulating into the right atrium (Fig. 7.75A). Noncontrast magnetic resonance imaging confirmed a large pseudoaneurysm of the proximal ascending aorta around the graft and fistulous connection into the right atrium (Fig. 7.75B). On intraprocedural angiography, the neck of the pseudoaneurysm was revealed at the anastomosis point of the aortic graft to the true ascending aorta (Fig. 7.76). Closure of the fistula between the pseudoaneurysm and the right atrium was achieved with a 12-mm Amplatzer Muscular Occluder (St. Jude Medical, St. Paul, Minnesota). Subsequently, the neck of the pseudoaneurysm was occluded with a 14-mm Amplatzer vascular plug II. There was no residual flow into the pseudoaneurysm or fistula seen with angiography. Postprocedural transthoracic echocardiography showed no residual flow across the pseudoaneurysm (Fig. 7.77).

ACKNOWLEDGMENT

The authors thank Dr. Q. Cao for help with images.

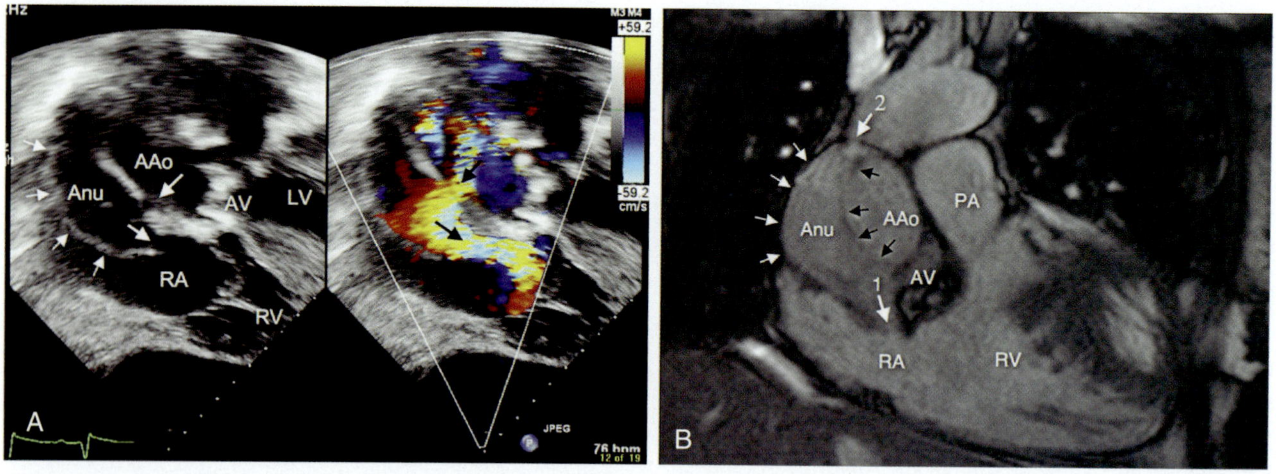

FIG. 7.75 Preprocedure Imaging of Aortic Pseudoaneurysm. (A) Transthoracic echocardiography subcostal view showing pseudoaneurysm (*Anu*) of the ascending aorta (*AAo*) (*smaller white arrows*) fistulating to the right atrium (*RA*) (*large white arrow*). Color image confirms flow from the ascending aorta to the Anu and into the RA (*black arrows*). (B) Noncontrast magnetic resonance image in the coronal plane showing the wall of the AAo (*black arrows*) and the wall of the Anu (*white arrows*). The opening of the fistula to the RA is indicated by *arrow 1*, with neck of Anu seen superiorly (*arrow 2*). *AV*, aortic valve; *LV*, left ventricle; *PA*, pulmonary artery; *RV*, right ventricle.

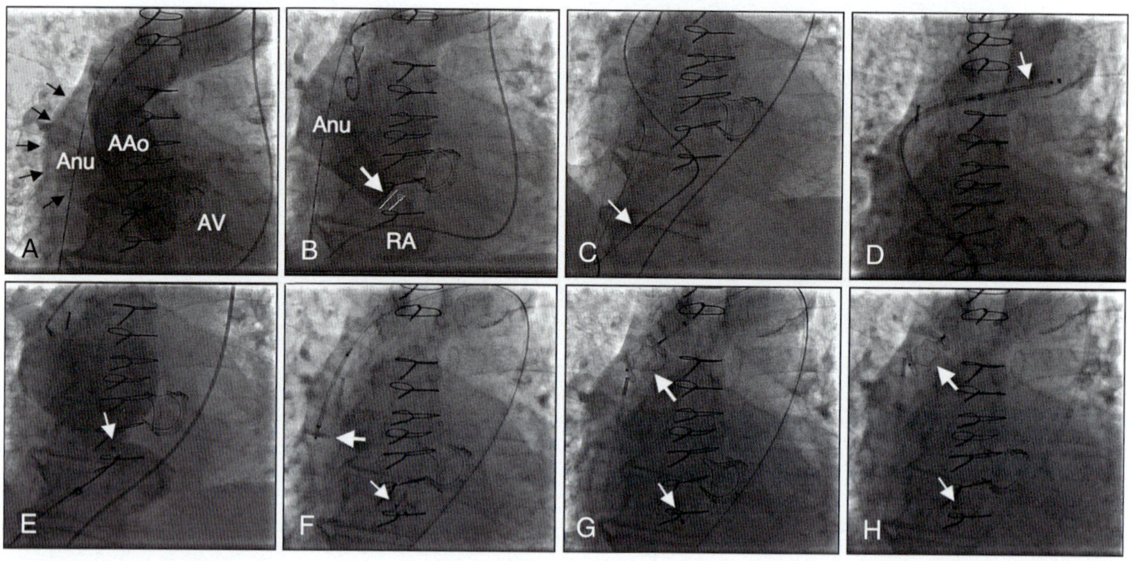

FIG. 7.76 Intraprocedural Angiography. (A) Ascending aortogram (*AAo*) indicating the pseudoaneurysm (*Anu*) (*multiple black arrows*). (B) Selective angiography within the Anu showing connection to the right atrium (*RA*) (*white arrow*). (C) Creation of an arteriovenous loop. (D) Crossing the fistula Anu with the delivery sheath. (E) After deployment of ventricular septal defect device (*white arrow*) across the neck of the fistula. (F) Deployment of the vascular plug within the Anu (*larger white arrow*). (G) Vascular plug fully deployed (*upper white arrow*). (H) Release of the vascular occluder in the neck of the Anu (*upper arrow*). *AV*, aortic valve.

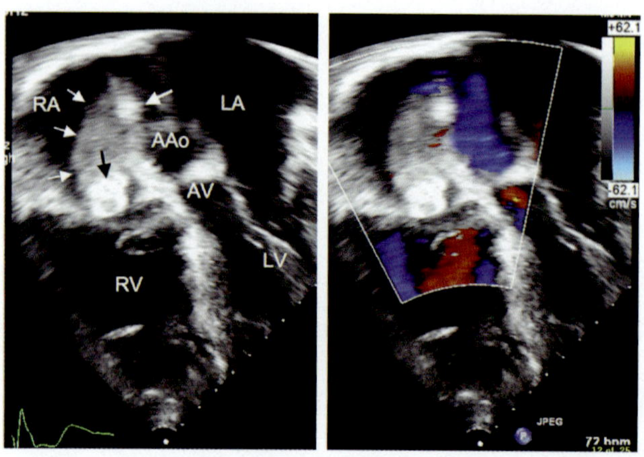

FIG. 7.77 Follow-up Transthoracic Echocardiography. Follow-up transthoracic echocardiography showing the wall of the pseudoaneurysm (*multiple white arrows*) with echogenic material within suggestive of thrombus. Ventricular septal defect device is seen across the fistula (*black arrow*) and the vascular plug superiorly (*white arrow*). No leak seen on color Doppler. *AAo*, ascending aorta; *AV*, aortic valve; *LA*, left atrium; *LV*, left ventricle; *RA*, right atrium; *RV*, right ventricle.

Percutaneous Closure of an Aortoatrial Fistula After Surgery for Infective Endocarditis

Rodrigo Estévez-Loureiro, MD, Jorge Salgado Fernández, MD, Nicolás Vázquez-González, MD, Miriam Piñeiro-Portela, MD, Ángela López-Sainz, MD, Alberto Bouzas-Mosquera, MD, Francisco Pombo, MD, Alfonso Castro-Beiras, PhD

A 44-year-old man was referred to the cardiology outpatient clinic due to dyspnea on exertion. He had undergone aortic valve replacement with a biological prosthetic valve (Carpentier-Edwards 23 mm, Edwards Lifesciences, Irvine, California) and reconstruction of the mitroaortic junction due to infective endocarditis from *Streptococcus viridians*, both events in 2004. Transthoracic echocardiogram revealed a mildly dilated left ventricle with preserved function, a biologic prosthetic valve with mild stenosis (effective area 1.3 mm^2), and an abnormal flow in the left atrium (Fig. 7.78A). A transesophageal echocardiogram confirmed a patent communication between the aortic root at the level of the noncoronary sinus and left atrium, close to the anterior mitral leaflet, with preserved prosthetic function (Fig. 7.78B, Online Video 7.45). A 64-multislice computed tomography scan demonstrated the defect and allowed the measurement of both long and short axis diameters (Fig. 7.79A–B). Angiographic evaluation showed normal coronary arteries, and a multipurpose diagnostic catheter could be placed through the defect (Fig. 7.78C), allowing the injection of contrast into the atrium (Online Video 7.46).

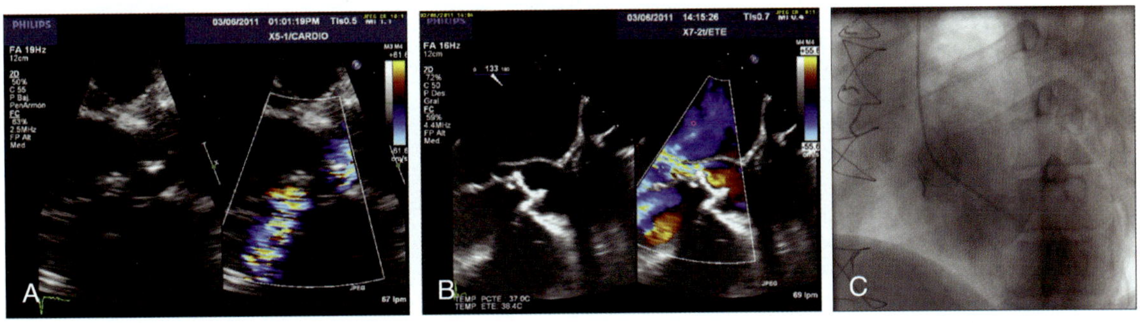

FIG. 7.78 Diagnostic Work-Up: Echocardiogram and Angiography. (A) Parasternal long axis two-dimensional transthoracic echocardiogram showing an abnormal flow in the left atrium. (B) Transesophageal echocardiogram showing a patent communication between the noncoronary sinus and the left atrium. (C) Multipurpose catheter placed through the defect and injecting contrast into left atrium. See Online Videos 7.45 and 7.46.

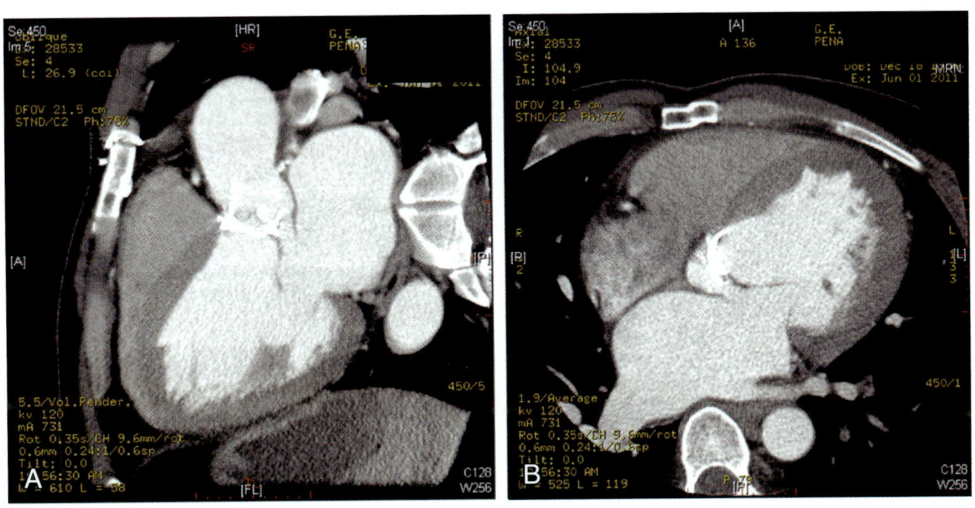

FIG. 7.79 Diagnostic Work-Up: Computed Tomography Scan. A 64-slice computed tomography scan in sagittal (A) and transverse (B) axes showing the defect close to the prosthetic valve and the anterior mitral leaflet.

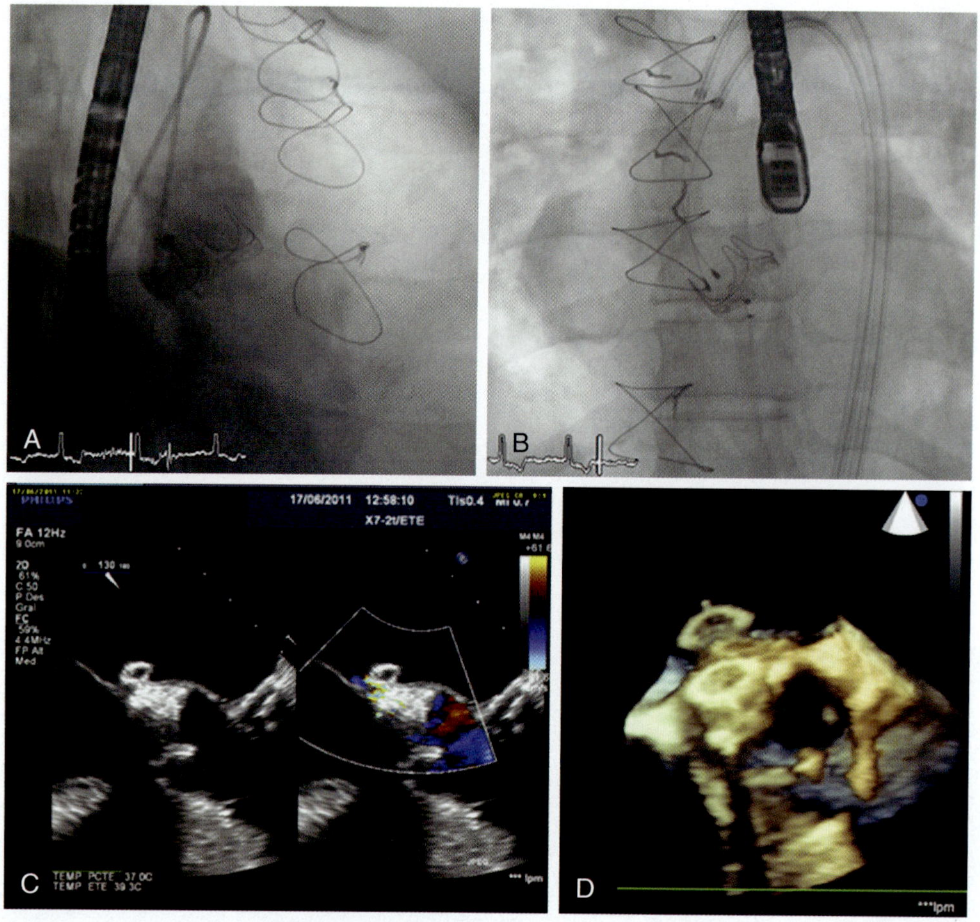

FIG. 7.80 Percutaneous Closure of the Fistula With the Vascular Plug. (A) Pigtail contrast injection showing the defect at the beginning of the closure procedure. (B) Two Amplatzer vascular plug III devices positioned through the fistula and ready to be deployed. (C) A three-dimensional real-time transesophageal echocardiogram with the closure devices placed in the fistula and with minimum shunt detected with Doppler. (D) Three-dimensional transesophageal echocardiogram reconstruction of the closure device deployed in the aortocavitary communication. See Online Video 7.47.

Using a right femoral approach, interventional cardiologists were able to cross the defect and deployed two Amplatzer vascular plug III occluders (AGA Medical Corp., Plymouth, Minnesota) (Fig. 7.80A–B). Monitorization with real-time three-dimensional transesophageal echocardiography showed a marked decrease in the shunt magnitude and that both devices did not interfere with the mitral valve or aortic prosthetic valve function (Fig. 7.80C–D, Online Video 7.47).

Fistulae between the aorta and cardiac cavities after infective endocarditis are rare. These aortocavitary communications create intracardiac shunts, which may result in clinical deterioration.[1,2] Although surgery is the treatment of choice, such a therapeutic option may cause serious complications, and the mortality could be high.[3] Percutaneous treatment represents an attractive alternative, and the improvement of recent occlusion devices has placed this technique in the frontline for the treatment of these defects.[4]

References

1. Anguera I, Miro JM, Vilacosta I, et al., for the Aorto-Cavitary Fistula in Endocarditis Working Group. Aorto-cavitary fistulous tract formation in infective endocarditis: clinical and echocardiographic features of 76 cases and risk factors for mortality. *Eur Heart J.* 2005;26:288-297.
2. Anguera I, Miro JM, San Roman JA, et al., for the Aorto-Cavitary Fistula in Endocarditis Working Group. Periannular complications in infective endocarditis involving prosthetic aortic valves. *Am J Cardiol.* 2006;98:1261-1268.
3. Ananthasubramaniam K. Clinical and echocardiographic features of aortoatrial fistulas. *Cardiovasc Ultrasound.* 2005;3:1.
4. Lu TL, Beregi JP, Rey C, Midulla M, Lions C. Percutaneous closure of an aorto-right ventricular fistula with an Amplatzer plug. *J Vasc Interv Radiol.* 2011;22:100-101.

Index

A

B

C

D

E

R

S

T